Adult-Gerontology Nurse Practitioner Certification Intensive Review

Maria T. Codina Leik, MSN, ARNP, FNP-C, AGPCNP-BC (ANP, GNP), designed and developed materials for the nurse practitioner review courses that she has presented nationally since 1997 through her company, National ARNP Services, Inc. (www.npreview.com). She is board-certified as an Adult Gerontology Primary Care Nurse Practitioner (AGPCNP-BC) with the American Nurses Credentialing Center (ANCC). She is also board-certified by the American Academy of Nurse Practitioners (AANP) as Family Nurse Practitioner (FNPC). She has been in the field of nursing for the past 23 years and has been in active practice as a nurse practitioner since 1991 in the South Florida area. Ms. Leik is also a speaker and twice-published chapter author.

Adult-Gerontology Nurse Practitioner Certification Intensive Review

Fast Facts and Practice Questions
Second Edition

Maria T. Codina Leik, MSN, ARNP, FNP-C, AGPCNP-BC (ANP, GNP)

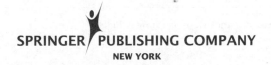

SPRINGER PUBLISHING COMPANY
NEW YORK

Springer Publishing Company, LLC
11 West 42nd Street
New York, NY 10036
www.springerpub.com

Acquisitions Editor: Margaret Zuccarini
Composition: Newgen Imaging

ISBN: 978–0-8261–3426-4
e-book ISBN: 978–0-8261–3427-1

13 14 15 / 5 4 3 2 1

The author and the publisher of this Work have made every effort to use sources believed to be reliable to provide information that is accurate and compatible with the standards generally accepted at the time of publication. Because medical science is continually advancing, our knowledge base continues to expand. Therefore, as new information becomes available, changes in procedures become necessary. We recommend that the reader always consult current research and specific institutional policies before performing any clinical procedure. The author and publisher shall not be liable for any special, consequential, or exemplary damages resulting, in whole or in part, from the readers' use of, or reliance on, the information contained in this book. The publisher has no responsibility for the persistence or accuracy of URLs for external or third-party Internet websites referred to in this publication and does not guarantee that any content on such websites is, or will remain, accurate or appropriate.

Library of Congress Cataloging-in-Publication Data
Codina Leik, Maria T.
 Adult-gerontology nurse practitioner certification intensive review : fast facts and practice questions / Maria T. Codina Leik. – 2nd ed.
  p. ; cm.
 Rev. ed. of: Adult nurse practitioner certification intensive review. c2008.
 Includes bibliographical references and index.
 ISBN 978-0-8261-3426-4 – ISBN 978-0-8261-3427-1 (e-book)
 I. Codina Leik, Maria T. Adult nurse practitioner certification intensive review. II. Title.
 [DNLM: 1. Geriatric Nursing–Examination Questions. 2. Certification–Examination Questions. 3. Nurse Practitioners–Examination Questions. WY 18.2]
 RT82.8
 610.73076–dc23

2013007390

Special discounts on bulk quantities of our books are available to corporations, professional associations, pharmaceutical companies, health care organizations, and other qualifying groups. If you are interested in a custom book, including chapters from more than one of our titles, we can provide that service as well.
For details, please contact:
Special Sales Department, Springer Publishing Company, LLC
11 West 42nd Street, 15th Floor, New York, NY 10036–8002
Phone: 877–687-7476 or 212–431-4370; Fax: 212–941-7842
E-mail: sales@springerpub.com

Printed in the United States of America by Bradford & Bigelow.

This book is dedicated to all my review course students, past and present, who have worked so hard to pass the certification exam. It is the result of hundreds of hours of work by many. Thank you all. I want to extend my gratitude to Springer Publishing Company, New York. I especially want to thank my wonderful and endlessly patient editor, Margaret Zuccarini. Without her support and dedication, I do not know if this book would have been possible. The feedback I received from my former review course and webinar students has been invaluable. My secret weapon is my wonderful husband Edward, whose love and support and infinite patience helped me keep going. I want to thank my two daughters, Christina and Maryfaye, for giving up some "mommy" time so that I could complete this book. They have been so very patient with me. The book is finally done, girls! I will always love you both, even when you are very naughty. Last, but not least, I want to extend my gratitude to my dear parents, Ricardo and Thelma Codina.

Contents

SECTION V: GERONTOLOGY REVIEW

SECTION VI: PRACTICE QUESTIONS AND ANSWERS

Preface

Welcome to the second edition of my review book. This book is designed to help you study effectively and efficiently for the family nurse practitioner certification exam from both the American Nurses Credentialing Center (ANCC) and the American Academy of Nurse Practitioners Certification Program (AANPCP).

The goal for all of my nurse practitioner certification review books is to provide you, the student and/or nurse practitioner test-taker, a tool to effectively and rapidly review for both the ANCC and the AANPCP certification exams. This book is also a good resource for current NP students. Many students credit these books with helping them pass not only their certification exam but also quizzes and tests while they are students. Students report that the review book has helped them successfully pass their school's dreaded "exit" exam.

A new section, Geriatrics, is designed to address the gerontologic-related issues of the new exams. Discussion of nonclinical topics has been greatly expanded in this new edition. The total number of nonclinical questions has also been increased so that those taking the ANCC exam are more adequately prepared. The answers to all the questions now include rationales. The question dissection section has been expanded. New diseases topics, tables, and pictures have been added.

The book's format remains the same as the popular and best-selling first edition, which was published 5 years ago by Springer Publishing. The book is styled as a "mega review" study guide because it combines six different resources in one: (a) specific certification exam information that is highly specific for both the ANCC and AANPCP exams, (b) test-taking techniques, (c) a question dissection and analysis section that breaks down questions for further study, (d) a review of primary care diseases and conditions, (e) a review of pertinent normal physical exam findings, and finally (f) a total of 645 questions with rationales to practice your new skills.

My two books, the *Adult Gerontology Nurse Practitioner Certification Intensive Review* and the *Family Nurse Practitioner Certification Intensive Review,* have become the most successful and relied-upon review books to study for both the ANCC and the AANPCP certification exams.

If you have any comments or suggestions for this book, or want me to teach a review course in your school, please contact me at npreviews@gmail.com. If you want to attend one of my webinars or live review courses, please visit my website at npreview.com. When they become available, I will post the treatment updates for the book (i.e., JNC 8) on my website at www.npreview.com.

Maria T. Codina Leik

Contributors and Reviewers

CONTRIBUTORS

Jill C. Cash, MSN, APN, FNP-BC
Nurse Practitioner

Cheryl A. Glass, RN, MSN, WHNP, BC
Clinical Research Specialist

REVIEWERS

Donna Bowles, MSN, EdE, RN, CNE
Associate Professor, Indiana University Southeast

Linda Carman Copel, PhD, RN, PMHCNS, BC, CNE, NCC, FAPA
Professor, Villanova University College of Nursing

Jill C. Cash, MSN, APN, FNP-BC
Nurse Practitioner

Lucille R. Ferrara, EdD, MBA, RN, FNP-BC
Assistant Professor and Director, Family Nurse Practitioner Program
Lienhard School of Nursing

Frank L. Giles, PhD, CRC, CCM, NCC, LMFT
President, Giles & Associates, Inc.

Cheryl A. Glass, RN, MSN, WHNP, BC
Clinical Research Specialist

Pamela L. King, PhD, FNP, PNP
MSN Program Director, Spalding University

Liza Marmo, RN-BC, MSN, CCRN, ANP-C
Director, Clinical Services, Lehigh Valley Health Network

JoAnne M. Pearce, MS, RNC, APRN-BC
Nursing Education Consultant, Idaho State University

Sue Polito, RN, MSN, ANPC, GNPC
Specialist Professor, Monmouth University

Cirese Webster, RN, CPN, FNP-BC
Nurse Practitioner, Metro Medical and Midwest Physicians
Certified Pediatric Nurse, St. Louis Children's Hospital

Exam and Health Screening Overview

I

Certification Exam Information

AMERICAN NURSES CREDENTIALING CENTER

www.nursecredentialing.org
Credentials: ANP-BC and AGPCNP-BC
Phone: 1-800-284-2378
Local and International: 301-628-5250

The American Nurses Credentialing Center (ANCC) is the independent credentialing body of the American Nurses Association (ANA). It is the largest nurse credentialing organization in the United States. The new ANCC Adult-Gerontology Primary Care Nurse Practitioner (AGPCNP) exam released on January 2013. The dates when some of the NP specialty exams will be retired are listed in Table 1.1.

The ANCC currently offers certification exams for the following nurse practitioner (NP) specialties: Family Nurse Practitioner (FNP), Pediatric NP, Adult Nurse Practitioner (ANP; until 2015), Gerontological NP (until 2015), Acute Care NP (ACNP), Family or Adult Psychiatric and Mental Health NP (PMHPNP-BC), and Diabetes Management (Advanced). The School NP exam was retired a few years ago. The application forms and *General Testing and Renewal Handbook* are available at the ANCC website.

AMERICAN ACADEMY OF NURSE PRACTITIONERS CERTIFICATION PROGRAM

www.aanpcertification.org
Credentials: NP-C, A-GNP
Phone: (512)-442-5202
Fax: (512)-442-5221
Email: certification@aanp.org

The American Academy of Nurse Practitioners Certification Program (AANPCP) is the independent credentialing body for the American Academy of Nurse Practitioners (AANP). The AANP merged with the American College of Nurse Practitioners (ACNP) in January 2013. They are releasing their new specialty exam for the Adult-Gerontological Nurse Practitioner (A-GNP) on January 2013. Their Gerontology NP exam was retired in December 28, 2012); the ANP exam will be retired in 2015.

The AANPCP is currently offering three specialty exams: the ANP (retirement date of 2015), A-GNP exam, and the FNP exam. The AANPCP released the new edition of the ANP exam and their FNP exam in 2012. The entire application packet and their *Candidate and Renewal Handbook* (containing sample questions) can be downloaded from their website.

Table 1.1 Certification Exams: Launch and Retirement Dates

Nurse Practitioner Exam	Credentials	Date Launched	Application Deadline	Retirement Date
ANCC adult-gerontology primary care NP	AGPCNP-BC	Jan. 31, 2013		
Adult NP	ANP-BC		Dec 31, 2014	Early 2015
Gerontologic NP	GNP-BC		Dec. 31, 2014	Dec. 2015
FNP	FNP-BC	New edition Aug 6, 2013		
AANPCP adult-gerontology NP	A-GNP-C	Jan 2013		
Gerontologic NP	GNP-C		Oct 12, 2012	Dec 28, 2012
Adult NP	ANP-C		Not yet known	2015

The ANCC is retiring several exams. The complete list is available on their website.

PROMETRIC COMPUTER TESTING CENTERS

www.prometric.com
Phone: 1-800-350-7076
National Registration Center: Monday to Friday (8:00 AM–8:00 EST)
Special Conditions Department (Special Accommodations): 1-800-967-1139

Both certifying organizations use Prometric to administer their exams. You can schedule your exam in real time and receive immediate confirmation. You can also reschedule or cancel an appointment online (available 24/7) or by calling their National Phone Registration Center.

There are Prometric Testing Centers located in the United States, Puerto Rico, the U.S. Virgin Islands, Guam, Canada, and the Republic of Korea. Bulk registration (five or more appointments) is also available online at their website.

International Testing for Military Personnel

Military nurses who want to take the exam outside of the United States are allowed to take their exams at one of Prometric's "global" testing centers.

Prometric Eligibility ID Number

All test candidates must first have an assigned a Prometric Eligibility ID number before they can schedule an appointment to take the exam. For both the ANCC and the AANPCP, the letter with your Prometric ID number will arrive 2 weeks after you receive their "acceptance" or the "authorization to test" letter. If it does not arrive, it is important that you call the ANCC or AANPCP as soon as possible.

If you are taking the ANCC exam, your letter will come directly from Prometric. For those taking the AANPCP exam, your letter will be from the Professional Examination Service (ProExam).

Qualifications

Must be a graduate of an approved master's, post-master's, or a doctorate degree program with a specialization in adult NP or adult-gerontology specialty NP program (plus the required clinical practice hours) from an institution of higher learning. The program must be accredited by the Commission on Collegiate Nursing Education (CCNE) or the National League for Nursing Accrediting Commission (NLNAC). In addition, the candidate must possess an active registered nurse (RN) license in any state or territory of the United States. The ANCC will, on an individual basis, accept the professional legally recognized equivalent (of NP status) from another country if the applicant meets their certification criteria.

FAST FACTS

Background Information

The ANCC and the AANPCP usually release a new edition of their exams every 2 to 3 years. Furthermore, each exam edition has several versions that are very similar to each other. The version of the exam that you are taking is assigned at random by the Prometric computer system.

What this means is that you may be taking a different version of the exam (but the same edition) than your classmate even though both of you are taking the same exam on the same date and time at the same Prometric Testing Center.

Exam Format

Both exams are computer-based tests (CBTs) designed in a multiple-choice format. The exam does not shut down automatically after you have earned enough points, as does the NCLEX-RN® exam. Each question has four answer options and each option has only one answer. You will not see multiple answers for one option such as "Both A and C are correct." There may be one case scenario question that is followed by two questions per exam.

Test Content Outline and Reference List

The Test Content Outline (TCO) is a list of the domains (major subject areas) that will be on the exam. It is important that you print out a copy of both these documents. Read each carefully and concentrate your studies on the designated topic areas.

Total Number of Questions

ANP Exams (Released on March 2010)

ANCC: There are 175 total questions (only 150 questions are graded). The exam contains 25 questions that are being evaluated for statistical data only (not graded).
AANPCP: There are 150 total questions (only 135 questions are graded). The exam contains 15 questions that are being evaluated for statistical data only (not graded).

Adult-Gerontology Nurse Practitioner Exams (Released January 2013)

ANCC: There are 200 total questions (only 175 questions are graded). The new exam contains 25 more questions than the older exam. There are 25 questions that are not graded (for statistical data).
AANPCP: There are 150 total questions (only 135 questions are graded). The new exam contains the same number of questions as previous exams. There are 15 questions that are not graded (for statistical data only).

Total Time

ANP Exams (Released March 2010)

ANCC: Total counted testing time is 3.5 hours.
AANPCP: Total counted testing time is 3 hours.

Adult-Gerontology Nurse Practitioner Exams (Released in January 2013)

ANCC: Total counted testing time of 4 hours (exam is 30 minutes longer than the previous exam).
AANPCP: Total counted testing time is 3 hours (remains the same as the previous exam).

Computer Tutorial

For both exams, each testing session starts with a 10- to 15-minute computer tutorial session. This time period is not counted as part of the testing time (it is "free" time). When the tutorial time period expires, the computer will automatically start the exam and the first question will appear on the screen. The countdown clock (upper corner of the screen) will start counting down the time. The countdown clock will not stop for "breaks," but if you need a break, inform the Prometric staff member who is monitoring the testing area. Watch the time clock closely because when the allotted testing time expires, the computer will automatically shut down the exam.

Time Allotted per Question

For both the ANCC and AANPCP certification exams, each question is allotted about 60 seconds. If you find yourself spending too much time on one question, pick an answer (best guess) and move on to the next question. Never leave any question unanswered. If you guess correctly, it will get counted; if you leave it blank, it is marked as an error (0 points).

Sample Exam Questions

I highly recommend that you try the sample exams because they are very similar to the actual exam questions. The ANCC's sample exam is web-based and contains 25 questions. It can be taken as many times as desired at no charge (and it is scored every time). The AANPCP also has free questions, which are listed on the last two pages of their 2012 candidate handbook.

Both the AANPCP and ANCC now offer additional web-based practice exams for a fee. These practice exams can be taken several times; all have expiration dates.

COMPARING THE ANCC VERSUS THE AANPCP EXAM

1) **Which board certification exam is better?**

   Both certifications are equally recognized as being from national specialty certifying bodies and are acceptable to governmental entities such as state boards of nursing, Medicare, Medicaid, and the Veterans Administration, as well as private health insurance plans. If you are a new graduate, it may be a good idea to speak to NPs as well as faculty in your area to find out whether one certification is preferred over the other in your area of practice. In Canada, it is best to check with the governing board of the province where you plan to practice.

2) What is the major difference between the two exams?

ANCC: The ANCC exam always contains more nonclinical questions compared with the AANPCP exam. The ANCC markedly increased the percentage of nonclinical questions to 50% of the total (71 questions) on both their ANP and FNP exams. The ANP exam will be phased out soon and the FNP exam will be replaced with the new edition (to be released on August 6, 2013).

AANPCP: The AANPCP exam has two major differences from the ANCC exam. The most important difference is the percentage of nonclinical questions. Students who have taken the exam through the years have consistently reported that there are few nonclinical questions on the exams. Another major difference between the two exams is the style of questioning. The questions on the AANPCP exam are usually "shorter" in length compared with the ANCC's exam questions.

3) How many nonclinical questions will be in the new Adult-Gerontology nurse practitioner exams?

The ANCC Adult-Gerontology Primary Care NP exam (AGPCNP) test content outline indicates that 25% of the questions are nonclinical, but the total percentage is much higher. I arrived at this conclusion because some of the nonclinical topics (such as culture) are included under a clinical domain. Therefore, I think that their new exam may contain up to 28% nonclinical questions (49 out of the 175 graded questions).

The AANPCP exams are considered more "clinical" by the majority of test-takers and contains few nonclinical questions (5% or less). But their new Adult-Gerontology Nurse Practitioner exam (A-GNP) may contain a few more nonclinical items compared with the older ANP exams because of the gerontological topics. The tendency over the years has been that the ANCC exams always contain more nonclinical questions compared with the AANPCP's exams.

4) Is it possible to take the exam at any time of the year?

ANCC and AANPCP: You can take both certification exams at any time of the year whenever the Prometric Testing Centers are open (they only close during major holidays). The majority of Prometric Testing Centers are also open evenings and weekends.

5) How do I apply for the ANCC or the AANPCP certification exam?

Most test-takers prefer to apply online, but first you must open an account on their website. You can also apply by mail (the AANPCP charges an extra fee for mailed applications). All the application forms can be filled out and then saved on your desktop and printed. Another option is to download the form and fill it out by hand. If you apply by mail, do not forget to photocopy the entire contents of your application package (use a large brown envelope). You can use the U.S. Postal Service to mail your package, but I would recommend that you also pay the extra fee for registered mail.

6) How early can I apply for the certification exam?

AANPCP: Both the ANCC and AANPCP will allow NP students to apply as early as the last semester of their program. In general, students usually apply a few weeks before they graduate. When you apply for the AANPCP early, you are required to submit an official copy of your current transcript (the "interim" transcript). The interim transcript is your most recent transcript that contains all of the course work that you have completed up to that date. When the official final transcript is released, either you or your school's Registrar's Office can mail it directly to the AANPCP. Early applications to the AANPCP can get approved as early as 2 to 3 weeks after graduation.

ANCC: The ANCC will not process an application until payment has cleared and the application is completed. A completed application must contain all the required documentation, including the official final transcript and the signed "ANCC Validation of Advanced Practice Nursing Education" form.

7) **What is the ANCC's "Expedited Application" process?**

For this method to work, your final transcript must be available. This new application method can drastically shorten the processing time to 5 business days (for a $200.00 nonrefundable fee). Download and print the Expedited Review Request form and fax it to the ANCC. Follow up by calling to verify that they received your faxed application. The "Validation of Advanced Practice Nursing Education" form can be signed by electronic signature (they will explain the process to you) if you use this method.

8) **If I join their respective membership organizations, will I receive a discount on my fees?**

ANCC: Yes, you will receive a member discount. If you are applying to the ANCC, you need to be a member of the ANA. If you belong to a state nursing association, you may already be a member of the ANA. Check with your state nursing association to see if you are a member. To apply for membership, apply online at the ANA's website (www.nursingworld.org) at the same time that you apply for their certification exam.

AANPCP: Yes, you will receive a member discount if you become a member of their organization, the American Academy of Nurse Practitioners (www.aanp.org). You can apply to the AANP for membership at the same time that you apply to the AANPCP (www.aanpcertification.org).

9) **What is the final transcript and the "official" transcript?**

ANCC and AANPCP: The final transcript is the one that is issued after you graduate from your NP program. It should indicate the type of degree that you earned (e.g., master's degree) along with the NP specialty that you graduated with (e.g., family or ANP).

A transcript is considered "official" only if it remains inside the sealed envelope in which it was mailed from your college Registrar's Office or if it is mailed directly from their office to the certifying agency. The mailing address to send your final transcripts are listed on each agency's website. Order at least three to four copies of your final transcripts and keep the extras unopened to keep them official. Open one copy (yours) and check it for accuracy.

10) **What is the "ANCC Validation of Advanced Practice Nursing Education" form?**

ANCC: This one-page form is a requirement for ANCC applicants only. Most NP programs have this document signed in bulk by the current director of the NP program within 1 to 2 weeks of graduation.

Note: It is probably a good idea for all NP students to get this document signed, even if they plan to take only the AANPCP exam. Since the ANCC requires this form, it will save you precious time in the future if you decide to apply for their exam. You always have the option of applying quickly for the "other" certification exam in case you fail the first. Do not forget that you will need another official final transcript (another good reason why you should have at least four copies of your transcript).

11) **Do they require a "hard copy" of the transcripts and the education validation form?**
ANCC and AANPCP: Yes, they do require a hard copy of your transcripts. The ANCC also requires a hard-copy of the original signed education validation form.

12) **How long does it take to process a completed application?**
ANCC and AANPCP: It generally takes between 2 and 8 weeks to process a completed application. Be warned that the ANCC will not process an application until they have received the official final transcript and the original copy of the signed education validation form.

13) **After receiving an acceptance or authorization letter, how much time do I have before it expires?**
ANCC: The ANCC "authorization-to-test letter" will expire within 90 days.
AANPCP: The AANPCP "acceptance letter" will expire in 120 days.

14) **When should I schedule my exam?**
Do not wait on the last minute to schedule your exam with Prometric because the testing centers in your area may no longer have the date (or the time) that you desire. It is better to schedule yourself early, especially if you want to take your exam in the morning. Morning time slots tend to get filled very quickly. Prometric allows test-takers to schedule, reschedule, or cancel an appointment on their website or by phone. If you give them less than 24 hours' notice, Prometric requires that you also call the testing center directly to inform them of your decision to cancel.
Note: Avoid scheduling yourself at the time of the day when you tend to get tired or sleepy. For most, this is usually after lunchtime. Simply picking the wrong time can cause you to fail the exam, sometimes by as little as 2 points.

15) **What should I do if the time slot or date that I want is no longer available?**
If the testing center you chose does not have the time or date you want available, then look for another testing center as soon as possible. For some, it may mean a long drive to another city, but it may well be worth the extra time and effort if your authorization-to-test letter is about to expire.

16) **What happens if I am late or miss my scheduled appointment?**
If you are late or miss your scheduled appointment, you are considered a "no show" by the Prometric Testing Center staff. Your testing time period or "window" will automatically expire on that same day. You must call the certifying agency as soon as possible if this happens for further instructions. Both the ANCC and the AANPCP will allow you to reschedule your exam (one time only) and you will be charged a rescheduling fee.

17) **What happens if my authorization-to-test letter expires and I have not taken the exam?**
First, check out the latest instructions on their website and read the FAQs (frequently asked questions) page. Call the certifying agency for further instructions. Both the ANCC and the AANPCP will allow you to reschedule your exam (one time only). You must pay a rescheduling fee. You will be issued another authorization-to-test letter. If you are taking the AANPCP test, your "new" testing window will only be 90 days (instead of 120 days). If you still do not take the exam at this time, then you must fill out a full application (like the first time) and pay the fee.

18) **If I have a disability, how can I obtain special testing accommodations?**
Request a report from your personal health care provider about your disability using their office's letterhead, typed, dated, and signed by your health care provider. The report should document and support your specific diagnosis and contain the specific recommendations for your testing accommodation. The requirements are in the ANCC General Testing and Renewal Handbook.

Table 1.2 Application Timeline

Timeline	Recommended Activities Before Graduation
About 2 to 3 months before graduation	Open an account on the ANCC and/or the AANPCP website and start the application process. Find out about the certification requirements. Download and read the General Testing Booklet, Test Content Outline, and the Reference List. Visit your State Board of Nursing website and read the licensure requirements for NPs in your state
About 4 weeks before graduation	Order three to four copies of your official transcripts

COMMON QUESTIONS ABOUT THE NURSE PRACTITIONER CERTIFICATION EXAMS

1) **Is it possible to return to a question later and change its answer?**

    ANCC and AANPCP: Yes, it is, but only if you "mark" the question. You will learn about this simple command during the computer tutorial time at the beginning of the exam. "Marking" a question allows the test-taker to return to the question at a later time (if you want to change or review your answer). On the other hand, if you indicate to the computer that your answer is "final," then you will not be allowed to change the answer. Do not worry about forgetting to "unmark" the questions if you run out of time. As long as a question has an answer, it will be graded by the computer.

2) **Is there a penalty for guessing on the exam?**

    ANCC and AANPCP: No, there is no penalty for guessing. Therefore, if you are running out of time, answer the remaining questions at random. Please do not leave any questions "blank" or without an answer since it will be marked as an error (0 points). You may earn a few extra points if you guess correctly, which can make the difference between passing and failing the exam.

3) **Will I find out immediately if I passed the exam while I am in the Prometric Center?**

    ANCC and AANPCP: Yes, you will immediately find out whether you passed or failed. When you complete the exam (or run out of time), the computer will automatically shut down the exam. Then a document with some legal "warnings" will appear on the screen. Afterward, you will see your "unofficial" score in the "Pass" or "Fail" format. Do not expect to see a "number" score at this time. The Prometric Test Center staff will give you a copy of your unofficial score (pass or fail format). Make sure that you get it before you leave the testing center because they cannot give it to you afterward. Instead, you will need to wait for your official score letter. If you took the ANCC exam and did not receive a copy of your unofficial score, the ANCC recommends that you call them as soon as possible to report the problem.

4) **When do I receive the letter with my official scores?**

    ANCC and AANPCP: For both certifying agencies, the official letter with your scores will arrive within 1 to 2 weeks after you have taken the exam. An ANCC certificate with a pin or an AANPCP certificate with a card will arrive approximately 8 weeks later.

5) **What are the passing scores?**

    ANCC: The passing score is 350 points or higher. ANCC scores range from 100 to 500 points.

    AANPCP: The passing score is 500 points or higher. AANPCP scores range from 100 to 800 points.

6) **What are the passing rates for each exam?**

The ANCC and the AANPCP has not released the official passing rates for their exams for several years. The ranges below are my estimates.

ANCC: Their passing rates vary depending on the exam edition. On some years when the exam edition is "harder" than normal, the passing rates have gone down to as low as the mid-70th percentile. On some years, the passing rates can be as high as the upper 80th percentile.

AANPCP: The passing rates for the AANPCP usually range from the mid-80th to the low-90th percentile.

7) **How are the scores listed?**

ANCC and AANPCP: The raw scores (total number of correct answers) are converted into a scaled score. Only the total scaled score is given. For example, for the ANCC exam, the passing score is 350 points or higher. For the AANPCP exam, the passing score is 500 points or higher. The individual domains are listed from the best to the weakest domain (no number scores). Devote more study time in your "weakest" areas if you do not pass the exam. If you did not take a review course, I recommend that you buy a CD of their review course. My review courses are listed in my website at www.npreview.com.

8) **Does the certifying agency inform the state board of nursing (SBON) of my certification status?**

ANCC and AANPCP: For both certifying agencies, you must sign their release of scores consent form, which is one of the documents required when you apply for the exam. Make sure that you have signed and attached the 1-page "Release of Scores" form in your application package. The AANPCP will not automatically send your scores to your state board of nursing. You can request one free verification from their website. If you need additional verification letters, both certifying agencies will charge a nominal fee. Active duty military personnel requesting verification will not be charged verification fees. Emergency verifications may be requested for an additional fee. The ANCC processing time for these type of requests is 5 business days of receipt of the order. AANPCP does not provide emergency verification. Processing time is 10 business days.

9) **What will happen if I fail the certification exam?**

You should visit the ANCC or AANPCP website as soon as you find out and read about the latest procedures to follow for retaking the exam. You need to submit the "retake" application, which can be downloaded from their website. You will be charged a "retest" fee.

10) **How soon can I retake the exam after I fail it?**

ANCC: You must wait at least 60 days after you took the exam before you can retake it. The ANCC will allow a person to take the exam up to three times within a 12-month period.

AANPCP: Although there is no wait time requirement prior to retesting, the AANPCP requires test-takers to take 15 contact hours in their area(s) with the weakest score (your "areas of weakness"). The AANCP exam can only be taken twice a year. Choose courses that address these areas; if in doubt, call the AANPCP at (512)-442–5202. Be warned that the continuing education hours that you took before taking the certification exam are not eligible. After completing this requirement, you can mail or fax your certificates of completion as proof. Call the AANPCP certification office first before faxing any documents.

11) What happens if I fail the ANCC or AANPCP exam the second time?

ANCC and AANPCP: You must resubmit a full application along with all the required documentation (like the first time) and pay the full test fee. The AANCP exam can be taken up to twice a year and the ANCC exam can be taken up to three times within a 12-month period.

CERTIFICATION RENEWAL

1) How long is my certification valid?

ANCC and AANPCP: Certification from both the ANCC and AANPCP is valid for 5 years. A few months before your certification expires, both the ANCC and the AANPCP will send you a reminder letter. "Failure of the certificant to receive their renewal notice does not relieve the Certificant of his or her professional responsibility for renewing their certification" (AANPCP, 2012).

2) What should I do if I change my legal name or move to a new address?

ANCC and AANPCP: You need to update your online account at the ANCC or at the AANPCP website if there are any changes in your contact information such as your legal name, residence address, email, or phone number.

3) How long does it take to process renewal of certification applications?

ANCC: The average review time for renewals is 8 weeks. The ANCC recommends that you start the renewal process at least 8 weeks to 1 year before your certification expiration date so that they have enough time to review your application documents. If you submit your application later than 8 weeks before expiration, it is possible that your current certification will expire before you are issued your new certificate.

AANPCP: Starting January 2013, certificants will be allowed to apply as early as 12 months before their current AANPCP certification expires. Recertification applications should be submitted no later than 8 weeks prior to the expiration date of the current certification to allow time for reviewing, processing, and issuing the new certificate before the expiration of the current certification.

4) How many contact hours of pharmacotherapeutics (or pharmacology) are required?

ANCC: Currently, there are no specific requirements for pharmacology-related courses but starting January 1, 2014, NPs are required by the ANCC to complete a minimum of 25 contact hours of pharmacology continuing education credits. In other words, for every 75 contact hours, it is required that 25 hours come from pharmacology, *AANPCP*: Currently, they do not have specific requirements relating to pharmacology. A minimum of 75 continuing education hours from your area of specialization is required. They must be completed within the 5-year certification time period. If you submit continuing education credits that were taken before you became certified (or after your certificate expired), those credits will not be accepted by the AANPCP.

5) What type of continuing education (CE) courses are not acceptable for AANPCP recertification?

The courses that will not be accepted by the AANPCP for CE credit are the following: Basic Life Support (BLS), Advanced Cardiac Life Support (ACLS), Pediatric Advanced Life Support (PALS), Neonatal Resuscitation, and Nonclinical college courses.

6) **How many clinical hours of practice are required to renew my certification every 5 years?**

   ANCC and AANPCP: Both the ANCC and the AANPCP require a minimum of 1,000 hours of clinical practice in your area of specialty. If you plan to use your clinical volunteer hours as an NP, keep a notebook to record each clinical site's address, the number of hours that you practiced, and the name of the supervising physician. It may also be a good idea to ask the supervising physician or NP to sign your recorded time.

7) **Can I still renew my certification if I do not have enough clinical "practice" hours?**

   ANCC: Currently, the only option in these cases is to retake the certification exam along with completing the required professional development requirements for your specialty.

   AANPCP: You must retake their certification examination if you do not have enough clinical practice hours or do not have the minimum requirement for continuing education hours.

8) **What happens if I forget to renew my certification and it has expired?**

   ANCC: The ANCC does not have a grace period nor does it allow "backdating" of your certification dates. On the day when your certification expires, you are prohibited from using your ANCC designation after your name. In addition, you will have a gap in your certification dates. The ANCC recommends that you check with your state licensing board to determine whether you can continue to practice as an NP. They also recommend that you check with your employer and with the agencies that are reimbursing your services.

   AANPCP: The AANPCP has a grace period, but this policy can change at any time. For the latest information, call their customer service staff at (512)-442–5202.

9) **Since the ANP and GNP certification exams will be retired, what other options do I have if my certification is expired?**

   ANCC: Unfortunately, the ANCC does not have a grace period. Call them for more information. It is important to periodically check the website for updates or changes in the renewal process, especially if your certification exam is no longer available.

   AANPCP: If your AANPCP certification has expired, you may still be within their grace period. Call the AANPCP for further instructions as soon as possible.

10) **Is there any reciprocity between the ANCC and the AANPCP?**

   No, there is not. Both the ANCC and the AANPCP have discontinued their reciprocity program.

EXAM QUESTION CLASSIFICATION

American Nurses Credentialing Center

Adult Nurse Practitioner Exam (March 2010 Edition)

Table 1.3 shows a breakdown of the domains used in the ANCC ANP exam. Starting on March 1, 2010, there was a marked increase in the percentage of questions that I consider the "nonclinical" domains (professional role and policy, research, etc.). For their ANP exam, they increased it to 47% (71 out of the 150 graded questions) come from the nonclinical domains.

Summary

1) These are the top three domains in the ANCC ANP certification exam:
   - Clinical Management (30%, or 45 questions)
   - Foundations of Advanced Nursing Practice (23%, or 35 questions)
   - Health Assessment (23%, or 35 questions)
2) Test-takers who score low in these three domains will fail the exam because together they account for 76% of the questions (114 out of 150 graded questions).
3) Clinical-related questions make up 53% of questions (80 questions out of 150).
4) The percentage of nonclinical questions is now at 47% (72 out of 150 graded questions).
   - Foundations of Advanced Nursing Practice (23%, or 35 questions)
   - Professional Role (14%, or 21 questions)
   - Health Care Policy and Delivery (11%, or 16 questions)

Adult-Gerontology Primary Care Nurse Practitioner Exam

The ANCC released the new specialty exam on January 2013. It contains a total of 200 questions, but only 175 of the questions will be graded. Table 1.4 shows the domain breakdown of the new exam.

Summary

1) The domain with the most questions is "independent practice" which has 84 questions. This domain makes up 42% of the exam's questions.
2) The nonclinical domain is "professional roles" which has 50 questions. This domain makes up 25% of the exam questions.
3) The ANCC Adult-Gerontology NP exam will cover the following age groups: adolescents (age 13–18 years), adults (age 21–64 years), and the elderly (age 65 years and older).

Table 1.3 ANCC Exam Domains: ANP Exam

ANP Exam	%	
Foundations of advanced nursing practice	23%	34 Questions
Professional role	14%	21 Questions
Health care policy and delivery	11%	16 Questions
Health assessment	23%	34 Questions
Clinical management	30%	45 Questions
TOTAL		150 Graded Questions

Adapted from the ANCC Adult Nurse Practitioner Board Certification Exam Content Outline; retrieved September 29, 2012, from http://www.nursecredentialing.org

Table 1.4 ANCC Exam Domains: AG-NP Exam

AG-NP Exam	%	
Foundations of advanced practice nursing	33%	58 Questions
Professional roles	25%	44 Questions
Independent practice	42%	73 Questions
TOTAL		175 Graded Questions

Adapted from the ANCC Adult Nurse Practitioner Board Certification Exam Content Outline; retrieved October 31, 2012, from http://www.nursecredentialing.org.

American Academy of Nurse Practitioners Certification Program

Adult Nurse Practitioner Exam

The AANPCP exam has a total of 150 questions, but only 135 of these are graded. The AANPCP releases both the domain and age breakdown of their exams.

Domains

1) The percentage of their exam questions by domain is listed below.

I	Assessment (36%)	48 Questions
II	Diagnosis (24%)	33 Questions
III	Plan (23%)	31 Questions
IV	Evaluation (4%)	6 Questions
TOTAL		135 Graded Questions

2) Percentage breakdown by age group of the AANPCP's Adult NP exam questions is listed below.

Age Groups (FNP Exam)	
Late adolescence (6%)	8 Questions
Adults (43%)	58 Questions
Elderly (39%)	53 Questions
Frail elderly (12%)	16 Questions

1) The ANP and A-GNP exams will start at the age of 16 years (late adolescence).
2) On the ANP exam, half of the questions (51%) are on the elderly (65 years and older) and 43% of the questions are on adults (21–64 years).

Summary

The majority of the questions on the ANP exam are on the elderly (69 out of 135 graded questions). The next largest group is the adult age group (age 21–64 years), which has 58 questions. The majority of their exam questions are clinically based.

Adult-Gerontology Nurse Practitioner Exam

The AANPCP released the Adult-Gerontology NP exam on January 2013. The exam has a total of 150 questions, but only 135 questions are graded.

Domains

The breakdown by domain of the type of questions on the Adult-Gerontology NP exam has not been released as yet but the four domains remain the same for all the exams. They are: assessment, diagnosis, plan, and evaluation.

Age Groups (Adult-Gerontology NP Exam)

- Late Adolescence (16–20 years)
- Adults (21–64 years)
- Elderly (65–84 years)
- Frail Elderly (85 years and older)

Summary

The Adult-Gerontology NP exam, like the ANP exam, will start with late adolescent age group. The youngest age on their exam for this specialty is 16 years. The percentage breakdown by age group has not yet been released as yet. When the information becomes available, I will post it on my website at www.npreview.com.

FAST FACTS

Testing Center Details
1) Call the testing center 1 to 2 weeks before to verify your appointment date and time.
2) Locate and drive to the testing center 1 to 2 weeks before taking the exam.
3) Arrive at least 30 minutes before your scheduled time to get checked in.
4) Acceptable forms of primary identification (photo with signature):
   - Driver's license, passport, U.S. Military ID, or identification card issued by the Department of Motor Vehicles (DMV).
   - Your secondary ID (nonphoto) includes a credit card or check cashing card.
   - Expired IDs are not acceptable. If you forget your IDs, you will not be allowed to take the exam.
5) Biometrics are used for enhanced security. Your fingerprint is scanned before testing and every time you re-enter the test area (it is erased in 24 hours to ensure privacy). The test-taking room is also monitored closely by videotape and microphones.
6) Scratch paper and pencils are given to you by the testing center staff (and collected after you are done). Ask for extra paper if you tend to write a lot of notes.
7) You can request noise-reducing headsets; consider this option if you are sensitive to noise.
8) Testing computers are predetermined. Each test taker is assigned one small cubicle with one computer. If you are having problems with seeing the computer screen, bring it to the proctor's attention as soon as possible.
9) Verify that you are given the correct examination as soon as you sit down. Check that the title and the examination code on the screen match the information the testing agency sent.
10) Do not forget your computer glasses if you need them to read text on the computer.
11) No food or drink is allowed inside the testing room. If you need to drink water, you can go to the restroom, but you must first sign out with the testing center staff.
12) Special testing accommodations are available if requested in advance.

FAST FACTS

ANCC and AANPCP Exams
1) The ANCC and AANPCP NP certification tests are designed for entry-level practice (not expert-level practice). The majority of test-takers who sit for the NP certification exams are new graduates.
2) The new ANCC Adult-Gerontology exam will contain fewer nonclinical questions (about 25% to 30%) compared with the March 2010 ANP exam, which had 50% questions about nonclinical topics (75 questions out of 150 graded questions).
3) You only need to answer about 65% of the questions correctly to pass the certification exam.

4) Keep in mind that the questions will be on primary care disorders (doctors' clinics, public health clinics, etc.). If you are guessing, avoid picking an exotic diagnosis as an answer.

5) Most of the questions on the AANPCP exam are about clinical topics.

6) New clinical information (treatment guidelines or new drugs) released within the past 6 months of the current exam will most likely not be included.

7) Expect to find a large number of culture-related questions on the ANCC exam.
   - *Example:* If a traditional Muslim woman refuses to undress and use a hospital gown, an alternative is to examine her with her clothes on (modified physical exam).

8) The other cultures that may be addressed on the ANCC exam are Hispanics, Chinese, Cambodian/Thai (Hmong tribe), and Native Americans (Navajo).
   - *Example*: A Navajo woman has an appointment for a follow-up visit, but she does not show up for the appointment. One of the most common causes for Navajo patients to skip health visits is the lack of transportation.

9) The AANPCP exams will list the normal lab results when it is pertinent to a question, but they will only be listed once. Write them down on your scratch paper. When a related question comes up later, these pertinent labs will not be listed again.

10) Follow the norms given by the AANPCP. For example, they may list their mean corpuscular volume (MCV) normal value between 82 and 102 fL (femoliters). The usual norm taught in NP schools is an MCV of 80 to 100 fL (use this norm for the ANCC's exam).

11) Unlike the AANPCP, the ANCC does not list the normal lab results. If you are taking the ANCC exam, it is important to memorize some normal laboratory results and to write them down on your scratch paper during the computer tutorial time period.

12) Learn the significance of abnormal lab results and the type of follow-up needed to further evaluate the patient.
   - *Example*: An elderly male complains of the new onset of left-sided temporal headache accompanied by scalp tenderness and indurated temporal artery. The NP suspects temporal arteritis. The screening test is the sedimentation rate, which is expected to be much higher than normal (elevated value).

   A patient with an elevated WBC (greater than $12,000/mm^3$) accompanied by neutrophilia (greater than 70%) and the presence of bands ("shift to the left") most likely has a serious bacterial infection.

13) There may be a question on epidemiologic terms.
   - *Example*: Sensitivity is defined as the ability of a test to detect a person who has the disease. Specificity is defined as the ability of a test to detect a person who is healthy (or to detect the person without the disease).

14) Learn the definition of some of research study designs.
   - *Example:* A cohort study follows a group of people over time who share some common characteristics to observe the development of disease (e.g., The Framingham Nurses' Health Study).

15) Sometimes, there will be one unexpected question relating to a dental injury.
   - *Example*: A completely avulsed permanent tooth should be reimplanted as soon as possible. It can be transported to the dentist in cold milk (not frozen milk) or in normal saline.

16) Several emergent conditions that may present in the primary care area will be on the exam.
   - *Example*: Cauda equina syndrome, anaphylaxis, angioedema, meningococcal meningitis, etc.

17) Become familiar with the names of some anatomic areas.
   - *Example*: Trauma to Kiesselbach's plexus will result in an anterior nosebleed (epistaxis).
18) There are many questions asking for an initial "action." Depending on the question, the initial action might be to interview the patient (get subjective data or the history).
19) If the question is asking for the initial lab test, it will probably be a "cheap" test such as the CBC (complete blood count) to screen for anemia.
20) Some questions may ask about the "gold standard test" or the diagnostic test for a condition.
   - *Example*: The diagnostic or gold standard test for sickle cell anemia, G6PD anemia, and alpha or beta thalassemia is the hemoglobin electrophoresis.
21) Distinguish between first-line antibiotics and second-line antibiotics.
   - *Example*: A patient who is treated with amoxicillin returns in 48 hours without improvement (complains of ear pain, bulging TMP). The next step is to discontinue the amoxicillin and start the patient on a second-line antibiotic (for otitis media) such as amoxicillin-clavulanate (Augmentin) BID × 10 to 14 days.
22) Become knowledgeable about alternative antibiotics for penicillin-allergic patients. If the patient has a gram-positive infection, the possible alternatives are macrolides or clindamycin.
23) If a patient has an infection that responds well to macrolides, but thinks that she is "allergic" to erythromycin (symptoms of nausea or GI upset), educate her that she had an adverse reaction, not a true allergic reaction (hives, angioedema).
   - *Example*: Switch the patient from erythromycin to azithromycin (usually a Z-Pack).
24) If a patient fails to respond to the initial medication, add another medication (follow the steps of the treatment guideline).
   - *Example*: A patient with COPD is prescribed ipratronium bromide (Atrovent) for dyspnea. On follow up, the patient complains that his symptoms are not relieved. The next step would be to prescribe an albuterol inhaler (Ventolin).
25) Disease states are usually presented in their full-blown "classic" textbook presentations.
   - *Example*: In a case of acute mononucleosis, the patient will most likely be a teen presenting with the classic triad of sore throat, prolonged fatigue, and enlarged cervical nodes.
26) Ethnic background may give a clue for some diseases.
   - *Example*: Alpa thalassemia is more common among Southeast Asians (such as Filipinos).
27) No asymptomatic or "borderline" cases of disease states are presented in the test.
   - *Example*: In real life, most patients with iron-deficiency anemia are asymptomatic and do not have either pica or spoon-shaped nails. In the exam, they will probably have these clinical findings plus the other findings of anemia.
28) Become familiar with lupus or systemic lupus erythematosus (SLE).
   - *Example*: A malar rash (butterfly rash) is present in most patients with lupus. These patients should be advised to avoid or to minimize sunlight exposure (photosensitivity).
29) Become familiar with polymyalgic rheumatica (PMR).
   - *Example*: First-line treatment for PMR is long-term steroids. Long-term, low-dosed steroids are commonly used to control symptoms (pain, stiffness on shoulders and hip girdle). PMR patients are also at higher risk for temporal arteritis.

30) The gold standard exam for temporal arteritis is a biopsy of the temporal artery. Refer patient to an ophthalmologist for management.

31) Learn the disorders for which maneuvers are used and what a positive report signifies.
   - *Example:* Finkelstein's test: Positive in De Quervains tenosynovitis. Anterior Drawer maneuver and Lachman maneuver: Positive if anterior cruciate ligament (ACL) of the knee is damaged. The knee may also be unstable. McMurray's sign: Positive in meniscus injuries of the knee.

32) Some conditions need to be evaluated with a radiologic test.
   - *Example*: Damaged joints: Order an x-ray first (but the MRI is the gold standard)

33) The abnormal eye findings in diabetes (diabetic retinopathy) and hypertension (hypertensive retinopathy) should be memorized. Learn to distinguish each one.
   - *Example*: Diabetic retinopathy (neovascularization and microaneurysms). Hypertensive retinopathy (AV nicking, silver and/or copper wire arterioles).

34) Become knowledgeable about physical exam "normal" and "abnormal" findings.
   - *Example*: When checking deep tendon reflexes (DTRs) in a patient with severe sciatica or diabetic peripheral neuropathy, the ankle jerk reflex (Achilles reflex) may be absent or hypoactive. Scoring: absent (0), hypoactive (1), normal (2), hyperactive (3), and clonus (4).

35) There are only a few questions on benign or physiologic variants.
   - *Example:* A benign S4 heart sound may be auscultated in some elderly patients. Torus palatinus and fishtail uvula may be seen during the oral exam in a few patients.

36) Some commonly used drugs have rare (but potentially life-threatening) adverse effects.
   - *Example*: A rare but serious adverse effect of angiotensin-converting enzyme (ACE) inhibitors is angioedema. A common side effect of ACE inhibitors is a dry cough (up to 10%).

37) Learn about the preferred and/or first-line drug to treat some diseases.
   - *Example:* ACE inhibitor (ACEI) or angiotensin-receptor blockers (ARBs) are the preferred drugs to treat hypertension in diabetics and patients with mild renal disease because of their renal-protective properties.

38) When medications are used in the answer options, they will be either listed by name (generic and brand name) or by drug class alone.
   - *Example:* Instead of using the generic/brand name of ipratropium (Atrovent), it may be listed as a drug class (an anticholinergic).

39) Most of the drugs mentioned in the exam are the well-recognized drugs.
   - *Example:*
     Penicillins: amoxicillin (broad-spectrum penicillin), penicillin VK.
     Macrolide: erythromycin, azithromycin (Z-Pack) or clarithromycin (Biaxin).
     Cephalosporins: first-generation (Keflex); second-generation (Cefaclor, Ceftin, Cefzil); third-generation (Rocephin, Suprax, Omnicef).
     Quinolones: ciprofloxacin (Cipro); ofloxacin (Floxin).
     Quinolones with gram-positive coverage: levofloxacin (Levaquin); moxifloxacin (Avelox).
     Sulfa: trimethoprim/sulfamethazole (Bactrim, Septra).
     Nitrofurantoin (Macrobid).
     Tetracyclines: tetracycline; doxycycline; minocycline (Minocin).

Nonsteroidal anti-inflammatory drug (NSAID): ibuprofen; naproxen (Aleve, Anaprox).

Cox-2 inhibitor: celecoxib (Celebrex).

Anti-tussives: dextromorphan (Robitussin), benzonate (Tessalon Perles).

Other examples are listed in both Chapters 2 and 3.

40) Category B drugs are allowed for pregnant or lactating women and may be included in the ANP exam.

 ■ *Example:* For pain relief, pick acetaminophen (Tylenol) instead of NSAIDs such as ibuprofen (Advil) or naproxen (Aleve, Anaprox). Avoid nitrofurantoin and sulfa drugs during the third trimester (increases risk of hyperbilirubinemia).

41) One or two questions on bioterrorism topics have appeared in the exam. Remember that the best method for spreading viruses or bacteria is to make them airborne or nebulized. The preferred treatment for cutaneous anthrax is ciprofloxacin 500 mg orally BID for 60 days or for 8 weeks. If the patient is allergic to ciprofloxacin, use doxycycline 100 mg BID.

42) There may be a few questions on theories and conceptual models.

 ■ *Example*: Stages of Change or "Decision" theory (Prochaska) includes concepts such as pre-contemplation, contemplation, preparation, action, and maintenance.

43) Other health theorists who have been included on the exams in the past are (not inclusive): Alfred Bandura (self-efficacy), Erickson, Freud, systems theory, family theory, Elizabeth Kübler-Ross, the Health Belief Model, and others.

44) Starting at the age of about 11 years, most people can understand abstract concepts and are better at logical thinking.

 ■ *Example*: When performing the Mini-Mental Exam, when the NP is asking about "proverbs," the nurse is assessing the patient's ability to understand abstract concepts.

45) Keep these good communication rules in mind: Ask open-ended questions, do not reassure patients, avoid angering the patient, and respect the patient's culture. There may be two to three questions relating to "abuse" (child abuse, domestic abuse, elderly abuse).

46) Follow national treatment guidelines for certain disorders. Following is a list of treatment guidelines used as references by the ANCC and the AANPCP.

National Treatment Guidelines*

Asthma: Guidelines for the Diagnosis and Management of Asthma. Expert Panel Report 3. National Asthma Education and Prevention Program (2007).

Diabetes: American Diabetes Association (ADA). Clinical Practice Recommendations (2012). ANP exam (March 2010): ADA Clinical Practice Recommendations (2009).

Ethics: Guide to the Code of Ethics for Nurses: Interpretation and Application. Silver Spring, MD: Nursesbooks.org; 2008.

Geriatrics: American Geriatric Society (AGS). Geriatric Nursing Review Syllabus: A Core Curriculum in Advanced Practice Geriatric Nursing (2011).

---

*Not an all-inclusive list.

Hyperlipidemia: National Cholesterol Education Panel (2002). Third Report of the Expert Panel on Detection, Evaluation, and Treatment of High Cholesterol in Adults.

Hypertension: Joint National Committee on Prevention, Detection, and Treatment of High Blood Pressure (JNC) 7th Report.

Sexually Transmitted Diseases (or Sexually Transmitted Infections): Sexually Transmitted Disease Treatment Guidelines (2010). Centers for Disease Control and Healthy People 2020. U.S. Department of Health and Human Services.

Health Promotion: The Guide to Clinical Preventive Services (2012): Recommendations of the U.S. Preventive Services Task Force.

FAST FACTS

Maximizing Your Score

1) The most important advice is to make sure that you get enough sleep the night before the exam. Aim for at least 7 to 8 hours of sleep. Better yet, make sure that you get enough sleep the few days before you take the exam.
2) Read each question very carefully. Avoid reading questions too rapidly. You will go into "autopilot" mode. Remind yourself to read slowly and carefully throughout the test.
3) The first few questions are usually harder to solve. This is a common test design. Do not let it shake your confidence. Guess the answer and "Mark" it so that you can return to it later.
4) Save yourself time (and mental strain) by reading the last sentence (or stem) of long questions and case scenarios *first*. Then read the question again from the beginning. The advantage of this "backward reading" technique is that you know ahead of time what the question is asking for. When you read it again "normally," it becomes easier to recognize important clues that will help you answer the question.
5) If you are having problems choosing or understanding the answer options, try to read them from the bottom up (from option D to A or from 4 to 1).
6) Just because a statement or an answer is true does not mean that it is the correct answer. If it does not answer the question, then it is the wrong answer.
7) Assume that each question has enough information to answer it correctly. Questions and answers are carefully designed. Take the facts at face value.
8) Eliminate the wrong answers. If an answer option contains all-inclusive words ("all," "none," "every," "never," "none"), then it is probably wrong.
9) Be careful with certain words such as "always," "exactly," "often," "sometimes" and "mostly."
10) Design and memorize your "scratch paper" a few weeks before you take the exam. Choose what you want on it wisely. Remember that the scratch paper that is used at Prometric Centers is smaller (one-fouth the size of standard paper).
11) Use the time left from the "free" computer tutorial time to write down the facts that you memorized for your scratch paper. If you run out of time, skip this step.

12) Some suggestions of facts to write down on the scratch paper are lab results (hemoglobin, hematocrit, MCV, platelets, WBC count, neutrophil percentage, potassium, urinalysis, etc.). Others popular choices are the murmurs, mnemonics, and cranial nerves.

13) Do not leave any of the questions unanswered because there is no penalty for guessing. Questions that are left blank are marked as errors (0 points). If you have only have 15 minutes left and you are not done, quickly answer the remaining questions at random.

14) If you spend more than 60 seconds on a question, you are wasting time. Answer it at random and then "Mark" it so that you can return to it later (after you finish the entire test).

15) Each question is allotted about 60 seconds. Most finish the exam within 2.5 hours.

16) One method of guessing is to look for a pattern. Pick the answer that does not fit the pattern. Another is to pick the answer that you are most "attracted" to. Go with your gut feeling and do not change the answer unless you are very sure of the answer.

17) Consider a quick break (if you have enough time) if you get too mentally fatigued. Go to the bathroom and get a drink of water, and splash cold water on your face. This can take less than 5 minutes. Eat some hard candy or chocolate inside the restroom.

18) The countdown clock in the computer does not stop for breaks. Do not use more than 5 minutes for your quick bathroom break.

19) If you have failed the test before, try not to memorize what you did on the previous exam you took. The answers you remember may be wrong. Pretend that you have never seen the test before so that you can start out fresh mentally.

20) Do not panic or let your anxiety take over. Learn to use a calming technique such as deep breathing to calm yourself quickly before you take the exam.

21) Consider using a test-anxiety hypnosis CD and use it every night for maximum effect.

FAST FACTS

Review Timeline

1) Start seriously reviewing for the exam at least 2 to 3 months in advance. Study time can range from 1 to 3 hours per day. Buy a digital copy of a review/textbook and download to your cell phone and review it when you have free time.

2) Prepare a study time schedule by organ system. Copy the table of contents of your primary care textbook. Place check marks next to the diseases that you want to concentrate on, then schedule the date and time for each system.

3) I highly recommend that you attend at least one review course. Another option is to buy review course CDs. I teach review courses live and by webinar. You can view my class schedule at my website at www.npreview.com.

4) Buy a new notebook. If you find that you are having a problem understanding a concept, write it down in your notebook, then research and find the answer to your question.

5) Purchase at least two different review books. You will get two different views of how to study for the exam.

6) Note the disease and topics that I have highlighted in this review book. Some organ systems have more "weight" on the exam than others. Become more familiar with these areas.

7) If you are taking the ANCC exam, I highly recommend that you devote at least 50% of your study time learning about the nonclinical topics.

8) If you learn better in a group, organize one. Decide ahead of time what organ systems or diseases to cover together so that you do not waste time.

FAST FACTS

Testing Center Details

1) Call the testing center 1 to 2 weeks before to verify your appointment date and time.

2) Locate and drive to the testing center 1 to 2 weeks before taking the exam.

3) Arrive at least 30 minutes before your scheduled time to get checked in.

4) Acceptable forms of photo identification:
   - Driver's license, passport, U.S. Military ID, or employee identification card.
   - Your secondary ID (nonphoto) includes a credit card or check cashing card.
   - Expired IDs are not acceptable. If you forget your IDs, you will not be allowed to take the exam.
   - The name that is printed on your primary ID must match the name that you used when you applied for the exam.

5) Biometrics are used for enhanced security. Your fingerprint is scanned before testing and every time you re-enter the test area (it is erased in 24 hours to ensure privacy). The test-taking room is also monitored closely by videotape and microphone.

6) Scratch paper and pencils are given to you by the testing center staff (and collected after you are done). Ask for extra paper if you tend to write a lot.

7) You can request noise-reducing headsets; consider this option if you are sensitive to noise.

8) Testing computers are predetermined. Each test taker is assigned one small cubicle with one computer. If you are having problems with seeing the computer screen, bring it to the proctor's attention as soon as possible.

9) Verify that you are given the correct examination as soon as you sit down. Check that the title of the exam and the code is for your NP specialty.

10) Do not forget your computer glasses if you need them to read text on the computer.

11) No food or drink is allowed inside the testing room. If you need to drink water, you can go to the restroom, but you must first sign out with the testing center staff.

12) Special testing accommodations are available if requested in advance.

The Night Before the Exam

1) Check that both your primary and secondary IDs and the letter with your Prometric identification number match. Make sure that all your IDs are inside your wallet/handbag.

2) Avoid eating a heavy meal or consuming alcoholic drinks the night before the exam. Avoid eating 3 to 4 hours before bedtime (prevents heartburn).

3) Get enough sleep. Aim for at least 7 to 8 hours. Getting adequate sleep is probably one of the most important things you can do to help you pass the exam.

4) If you are scheduled to take your exam in the morning, set two alarms to wake you up on time. Give yourself extra time if it is a weekday (traffic congestion).

The Day of the Exam

1) If you are very drowsy, there are several ways to "wake up" rapidly. For example, you can wash your face using cold water and drink a glass of ice cold water. You can perform 10 to 20 "jumping jacks." Drinking a caffeinated beverage or coffee can be very helpful.

2) Avoid eating a heavy breakfast or eating only simple carbs. The best meals are a combination of a protein with a complex carbohydrate (eggs, whole wheat bread, nuts, cheese, etc.). If you eat only simple carbs, you can become hypoglycemic within 1 hour.

3) Avoid drinking too much fluid and do not forget to empty your bladder before the exam.

4) If you get drowsy and "fuzzy" during the exam, you may need to "wake up" quickly. Excuse yourself and go the bathroom to drink cold water and to splash cold water on your face. If you still feel drowsy, do some jumping jacks in the bathroom.

5) Wear comfortable clothing and dress in layers.

OTHER TEST-TAKING ISSUES

Test Anxiety

It is normal to feel anxious before taking an exam. A little anxiety helps us to become alert and vigilant, but too much anxiety can wear you down both emotionally and physically.

Your internal beliefs about how well you will do in the exam are very important. If you tend to become very anxious (or you are now more anxious because you previously failed the exam), there are calming methods that may prove helpful in helping control your anxiety. Following are some suggestions to help reduce test-taking anxiety a few weeks before the exam.

1) Make sure that you have devoted enough time for your review studies. If you feel in your gut that you have not studied "enough" or that you are not ready, it will worsen anxiety.

2) Consider signing up for both the ANCC and the AANPCP exams. It can help to reduce your anxiety level because you feel like you have a "back-up" exam.

3) If you have a firm job offer, I also recommend that you sign up for both exams to decrease test-taking anxiety.

4) Consider taking one to two review courses. My review courses and webinars are listed at my website www.npreview.com.

5) Avoid negative "self-talk." When you catch yourself doing it, silently tell yourself to "Stop it. Now!"

6) Improve the nutritional content of your diet, especially about 4 weeks before the exam. Vitamins and supplements which may be helpful for the brain are omega-3 fatty acids (fish oil), B-complex vitamins, vitamins C, D, E, choline, and others.

Your Panic Button

When you find yourself feeling panicky during the exam, please try the following calming technique. Practice this exercise at home until you feel comfortable doing it.

Breathing Exercise

1) Close your eyes. Tell yourself very firmly to "Stop it" at least three times.
2) Consciously slow down your breathing and inhale deeply through your nose.
3) Exhale slowly and deeply through your mouth (count slowly from 1 to 5).
4) Complete one cycle of three inhalations and three exhalations. Repeat as needed.

Question Dissection and Analysis

CULTURE

I. Discussion

There will be several questions on the American Nurses Credentialing Center (ANCC) exam that address culture. The questions will address knowledge of cultural practices that influence health-seeking behavior. Some of the cultures that may be included in the ANCC exam are Hispanic/Latino, Muslim, Chinese, Native American (Navajo), and Southeast Asian (Vietnamese, Hmong, Filipinos, and others).

II. Example

An elderly woman immigrant from Vietnam who recently has been diagnosed with hypertension is returning for a 4-week follow-up visit. The patient is on a prescription of hydrochlorothiazide 12.5 mg daily. Her blood pressure during the visit is 150/94. The nurse practitioner queries the patient whether she is taking her medication. The patient looks down at the floor and does not directly answer the question. All of the following statements are true regarding the health behaviors of Southeast Asians except:

A) The patient may have difficulty verbalizing questions about his/her treatment.
B) The patient may ask to consult with an older family member about major health decisions.
C) If the patient is not compliant with taking medications, he/she will not directly communicate it with the health provider.
D) The patient will directly verbalize his/her disagreement in a loud voice.

III. Correct Answer: Option D

D) The patient will directly verbalize his/her disagreement in a loud voice.

IV. Question Dissection

Best Clues

1) The patient's behavior (assertive behavior, loud voice is not usually found among Vietnamese and other Southeast Asian cultures).

Notes

1) The Hmong ethnic group who immigrated to the United States came from several countries (i.e., Laos, Vietnam, Thailand). A traditional household has a male (i.e., father) who is the head of the household. The family identifies with a clan group, which is headed by an older male.
2) For major health decisions, the head of the family is always involved in the health decision. If the father is dead, then another older male relative (i.e., uncle) may be consulted.
3) Most Asians have high regard for physicians (and college education). Because of this cultural value, they may not directly disagree or question the health care provider. A prescription for medicine may be accidentally "left" in the physician's office if the person does not want to take the medicine.
4) Another large ethnic group from Southeast Asia is the Filipinos (from the Philippine Islands). Alpha thalassemia is more common in this ethnic group compared with beta thalassemia, which is more common in people of Mediterranean descent.

LAB RESULTS AND DIAGNOSTIC TESTS

I. Discussion

Laboratory tests such as hemoglobin and hematocrit, mean corpuscular volume (MCV), total white blood cell (WBC) count, percentage of neutrophils in the WBC differential, the thyroid-stimulating hormone (TSH), prostate-specific antigen (PSA), and urinalysis are commonly encountered in the exams. Learn the significance of the abnormal results and the follow-up tests that are needed to evaluate them further.

The American Academy of Nurse Practitioners Certification Program (AANPCP) exam does list the norms for some of the common laboratory tests. They will appear only when needed to answer a question (such as an anemia question). It is important that you copy the lab norm that is given (on your scratch paper) because it will be listed only once.

In contrast, the ANCC exam does not list any of the normal results in their certification exams. Therefore, if you plan to take the ANCC exam, it is important for you to memorize the normal results of these laboratory tests.

Be warned that lab results are also used as distractors; the labs listed may not be necessary to solve the exam question correctly. The normal results for these labs are also under the pertinent chapter (e.g., TSH will be under Endocrine System).

II. Example

An elderly male of Mediterranean descent has a routine complete blood count (CBC) done for an annual physical. The following are his lab test results: hemoglobin of 13.0 g/dL, a hematocrit of 39%, and an MCV of 72 fL. His PSA result is 3.2 ng/mL. The urinalysis shows no leukocytes and few epithelial cells. Which of the following laboratory tests are indicated for this patient?

A) Serum iron, serum ferritin, total iron binding capacity (TIBC), and the red cell differential width (RDW).
B) Serum B12 and folate level with a peripheral smear.

C) CBC with white cell differential and urinalysis.

D) Urine culture and sensitivity with microscopic exam of the urine (Tables 2.1 and 2.2).

III. Correct Answer: Option A

A) Serum iron, serum ferritin, TIBC, and the red cell differential width (RDW).

Table 2.1 List of Laboratory Norms

CBC	Reference Ranges
Hemoglobin	
Males	14 to 17.4 g/dL
Females	12.0 to 16 g/dL
Hematocrit	
Males	42% to 52%
Females	36% to 48%
MCV	80 to 100 fL
RDW (red cell distribution width)	>14.5%
Platelet count	<140,000/mm³ (increased risk bleeding, ITP)
Reticulocytes	0.5% to 1.5% of red cells (↑ acute bleeds), starting tx for vitamin deficiencies (iron, B12, folate), acute hemolytic episodes
Total WBC count	4,500 to 11,000/mm³ (↑ bacterial infections)
Neutrophils (or segs)	>50% (↑ bacterial infections)
Band forms (immature WBCs)	>6% (↑ severe bacterial infections) Also called "shift to the left"
Eosinophils	>3% (↑ allergies, intestinal parasites)

Adapted from the NIH Medline Plus, 2011.

Table 2.2 List of Blood Chemistry

Laboratory Test	Reference Ranges
TSH	>5.0 mU/L (hypothyroidism, also has low serum total T4 and low T-3 resin uptake)
	<0.1mU/L (hyperthyroidism, also has high serum total/ free T4, high T3 resin uptake)
PSA	>4.0 (BPH, prostate cancer)
Ferritin	<15 µg/L (iron-deficiency anemia)
ESR (sed rate)	Elevated (rheumatoid arthritis/RA, lupus, temporal arteritis, inflammation)
CRP	Elevated (inflammation, autoimmune diseases, a risk factor for heart disease)
Cardiac troponins (cTnT)	Elevated in MI, heart damage, heart failure Sensitive test for myocardial cell damage
B-type natriuretic peptide	Elevated (elevated in heart failure).
Potassium	< 3.0 or > 5.5 mEq/L (risk of cardiac arrest).

IV. Question Dissection

Best Clues

1) Low hemoglobin and hematocrit for gender (male) and age (abnormal CBC result).
2) An MCV of 72 fL is indicative of microcytic anemia (assessment).
3) The ethnic background of the patient (demographics).
4) Ignore the urinalysis and PSA tests since they are not necessary to solve the problem.

Notes

1) You must go through three steps to answer this question correctly:
   First step: A hemoglobin of less than 13.5 g/dL in males (but not in females) is indicative of anemia. An MCV of 72 fL is indicative of microcytic anemia (norm 80–100 fL).
   Second step: The MCV will direct you in the differential diagnosis (microcytic, normocytic, or macrocytic).
   Third step: The differential diagnosis for microcytic anemia is iron deficiency and alpha/beta thalassemia trait/minor for the exams.
2) In iron-deficiency anemia, the following results are found:
   - Decreased (serum ferritin and serum iron levels).
   - Elevated (TIBC/transferrin levels and the RDW).
3) In alpha or beta thalassemia trait or minor, the following results are found:
   - Normal to high (serum ferritin and serum iron levels)
   - Normal (TIBC/transferrin levels)
4) The gold standard test to diagnose any anemia involving abnormal hemoglobin (thalassemia, sickle cell, etc.) is the hemoglobin electrophoresis.
5) The red cell distribution width (RDW) is a measure of the variability in size of RBCs (or anisocytosis). An elevated RDW is indicative of iron-deficiency anemia (for the exam).
6) In clinical practice, rule out iron-deficiency anemia first (most common anemia in the world for all ages/races/gender) before ordering a hemoglobin electrophoresis.

NONCLINICAL TOPICS

I. Discussion

Nonclinical topics now make up about half of the questions on the ANCC's ANP and FNP certification exams (released March 2010). The new Adult-Gerontology Nurse Practitioner and FNP exams that are being released during 2013 will have less nonclinical content (about 30% vs. 50% in the older test). If you plan on taking the ANCC exam, it is important that you study the topics in this area well.

One common topic that is frequently included in the certification exam is the Health Insurance Portability and Accountability Act (HIPAA) of 1996. The questions are designed to determine whether you know how to apply HIPAA regulations in primary care practice. Your job is to determine whether the activity is compliant (or not) with HIPAA regulations.

II. Example

According to the HIPAA of 1996, which of the following examples demonstrates noncompliance?

A) The sign-in sheet on the front desk is covered so that other patients' names are not visible to new patients.
B) The medical assistant calls the patient who is in the waiting room using his/her first name.
C) A patient's chart that is hanging on the door of the examination room is turned backward.
D) The nurse practitioner calls the daughter of an elderly diabetic patient and leaves a detailed message on her answering machine regarding her mother's laboratory results.

III. Correct Answer: Option D

D) The nurse practitioner calls the daughter of an elderly diabetic patient and leaves a detailed message on her answering machine regarding her mother's laboratory results.

IV. Question Dissection

Best Clues

1) For Option D, the words "detailed message on her answering machine" is a good clue of HIPAA noncompliance.
2) The question does not specify whether the patient authorized that her information could be released to her daughter. Therefore, assume that no authorization was given by the patient.
3) Option B is HIPAA compliant since only the patient's first name is used.

Notes

1) Option D demonstrates two examples of HIPAA noncompliance. First, there is no mention that the patient gave consent for her daughter to have access to her medical information. Second, the NP did not follow the "minimum necessary requirement" rule when she left a detailed message on the daughter's answering machine.
2) The best action in this case is for the NP to call the elderly patient's home and to leave only her name, the name of the clinic, and phone number that the patient can call back.
3) When speaking to a patient in the waiting room area (or any public area), use only the patient's first name. If both the patient's first and last names are used, then Option C would be an example of HIPAA noncompliance.

DISEASE PREVENTION

I. Discussion

The prevention of disease is grouped into three levels (primary, secondary, and tertiary). If you are not sure whether the action or condition is primary or secondary, ask yourself this question: "Will performing this action prevent the disease or the social condition from happening?" If it does, then it is considered as primary prevention (if it does not, then it is secondary prevention). Primary prevention can be performed by individuals, or by nations (federal programs such as Women, Infants, and Children [WIC]), as well as on a global level (WHO health promotion programs).

Remember that the breast self-exam (BSE) and the genital self-exam (GSE) are both considered as secondary prevention. Tertiary prevention involves not only rehabilitation, but also includes activities that will help to prevent complications from disease treatment, such as patient education about medication side effects or the proper use of equipment such as a cane. Support groups for a disease/condition are all considered as part of a tertiary prevention activity.

Primary Prevention (Prevent Disease/Injury/Condition)

- Youth violence prevention (e.g., youth recreational center for high-risk inner-city youth, mentoring teens, teaching teens better communication skills).
- Bullying prevention (e.g., antibullying school programs).
- Personal safety promotion (e.g., seatbelts, airbags, helmets).
- Disease prevention (e.g., immunizations, using sunscreen).
- Healthy lifestyle promotion (e.g., sleep 7–8 hours/night, avoid sunlight 10 a.m. to 4 p.m., healthy diet, exercise).
- Promotion of OSHA laws (e.g., workplace safety) and EPA laws (e.g., clean water, anti-pollution laws).

Secondary Prevention (Detect Disease/Condition as Early as Possible)

- Any laboratory test to screen for a disease (e.g., CBC for anemia, TSH for thyroid disease).
- U.S. Preventive Services Task Force (USPSTF) screening recommendations (e.g., mammograms, PSA, purified protein derivative [PPD]).
- Screening for high-risk behavior (e.g., asking a patient about the number of sexual partners), screening for suicide risk (e.g., assess suicide risk, check for signs and symptoms of depression).
- Personal actions to detect cancer (e.g., BSE, GSE).

Tertiary Prevention (Limiting Further Harm and Disability)

- All types of rehabilitation (e.g., cardiac rehab, PT, OT, speech therapy, addiction/drug rehab).
- Support groups (e.g., breast cancer patients, alcoholics with Alcoholics Anonymous).
- Exercise for an obese person (if the person is healthy, then it is primary prevention).

Patient Education

- Self-management of disease (e.g., insulin self-injection, dietary education).
- Medications (e.g., drug–food interactions, side effects).
- Equipment safety (e.g., how to use wheelchairs/cane).

WOMEN'S HEALTH

I. Discussion

Expect to see several questions addressing gynecological conditions. The topics that are covered include sexually transmitted infections (STIs or STDs) treatment, oral contraceptives issues, abnormal Pap smears, menopausal conditions, and many more.

For example, there will be questions about vaginal disorders such as bacterial vaginosis (BV), Candida vaginitis, trichomoniasis, and atrophic vaginitis.

Be aware that a clinical finding can be described in detail instead of using its common name.

For example, the term "clue cell" is not used in the question below. Instead it is described in detail ("mature squamous epithelial cells with numerous bacteria noted on the cell borders").

II. Example

An 18-year-old female presents in the college health clinic complaining of a strong odor in her vagina. She reports that she had an abortion about 3 weeks ago and recently completed her prescription of antibiotics. The NP performs a vaginal speculum exam and notes a large amount of grayish to off-white discharge coating the patient's vaginal walls. It has a milk-like consistency. During microscopy, the slide reveals mature squamous epithelial cells with numerous bacteria noted on the cell borders. The vaginal pH is at 6.0. Which of the following conditions is most likely?

A) Trichomoniasis
B) Bacterial vaginosis
C) Candida vulvovaginitis
D) Hormonal changes

III. Correct Answer: Option B

B) Bacterial vaginosis

IV. Question Dissection

Best Clues

1) The vaginal pH is alkaline (pH of 6.0).
2) Rule out *Candida* because it is classified as a yeast organism (not a bacteria).
3) Rule out *Trichomonas* because it is a protozoa or unicellular flagellated organism.
4) The odor and discharge are not due to hormonal changes in an 18-year-old female.

Notes

1) Bacterial vaginosis (BV) has an alkaline pH (vagina normally has an acidic pH of 4.0). BV is the only vaginal condition with an alkaline pH for the exam.
2) BV is not considered an STD (it is caused by an imbalance of vaginal bacteria). The sex partner does not need to be treated. It is a vaginosis (not a vaginitis).
3) BV does not cause inflammation (the vulvovagina will not be red or irritated). The microscopy slide will have very few WBCs and a large number of clue cells.

(Continued)

> **Notes** (*Continued*)
> 4) The vaginal discharge in *Candida* infection is of a white color with a thick and curd-like consistency. It frequently causes redness and itching in the vulvovagina due to inflammation.
> 5) The microscopy in candidiasis will show a large number of WBCs, pseudo-hyphae, and spores ("spaghetti and meatballs").
> 6) Candida yeast is normal flora of the gastrointestinal (GI) tract and in some women's vaginas.
> 7) Trichomonas infection (or trichomoniasis) vaginal discharge is copious, bubbly, and green in color. It causes a lot of inflammation resulting in itching and redness of the vulvovagina. It is considered a sexually transmitted infection. The sex partner also needs treatment.
> 8) Microscopy is the gold standard of diagnosis for BV, candida vaginitis, and trichomoniasis for the exam.

MEDICATIONS

I. Discussion

When studying pharmacology for the exam, it is generally not important to memorize the specific drug doses. What is more important is to study a drug's "safety" issues such as the drug's contraindications, major drug/food interactions, and the well-known side effects.

You will need to be familiar with the drug's indications and the duration of treatment. Become familiar with a "first-line drug" and the alternative drug (if applicable). For example, the first-line (or preferred) drug for treating strep throat is still penicillin VK PO for 10 days. If the patient has a penicillin allergy, macrolides can be used instead.

The majority of the medicines seen on the exam are the well-known drugs that have been in use for a few years to many decades (i.e., doxycycline, penicillin, amoxicillin). Memorize the drug class and some representative drugs from that class. For example, under the quinolone drug class are the drugs such as ofloxacin (Floxin), moxifloxacin (Avelox), and levofloxacin (Levaquin). You can memorize a drug either by its generic name or by both its generic and brand name. In addition, you need to become familiar with some of the FDA Category X drugs (listed in Chapter 3).

II. Examples

Example A

Using the drug class as the answer option:

A previously healthy 30-year-old complains of an acute onset of fever and chills accompanied by a productive cough with purulent sputum and a loss of appetite. The patient denies receiving an antibiotic in the previous 3 months. The NP diagnoses community-acquired pneumonia (CAP). The Infectious Diseases Society of America (IDSA) and the American Thoracic Society (ATS) treatment guidelines recommend which of the following as the preferred first-line treatment for this patient?

A) Macrolides
B) Antitussives
C) Cephalosporins
D) Fluoroquinolones with gram-positive bacteria activity

Example B

Which of the following antibiotics is preferred treatment for healthy adults diagnosed with uncomplicated CAP?

A) Azithromycin (Zithromycin) 500 mg on day 1, then 250 mg daily for 4 days.
B) Dextromethorphan with guaifenesin (Robitussin diabetes mellitus [DM]) 1 to 2 teaspoons PO QID as needed
C) Cephalexin (Keflex) 500 mg PO QID × 10 days
D) Levofloxacin (Levaquin) 500 mg PO daily × 7 days

Example C

The following is an example of a question about a common side effect:

   Possible side effects that may be seen in a patient who is being treated with hydrochlorothiazide for hypertension are:

A) Dry cough and angioedema
B) Swollen ankles and headache
C) Hyperuricemia and hyperglycemia
D) Fatigue and depression

III. Correct Answers

Example A: Option A

A) Macrolides

Example B: Option A

A) Azithromycin (Zithromax) 500 mg on day 1, then 250 mg daily for 4 days

Example C: Option C

C) Hyperuricemia and hyperglycemia

IV. Question Dissection

Best Clues

1) Lack of comorbidity ("healthy adults") is an important clue for Examples A and B.
2) Your knowledge of the latest IDSA and the ATS treatment guidelines helps to correctly answer Examples A and B (covered in the Chapter 8: Pulmonary review).
3) For Example C, you must memorize the adverse side effects of the thiazide diuretics.

Notes

1) According to the IDSA and the ATS treatment guidelines, outpatient treatment of CAP in healthy patients (no comorbidities) are the macrolides (azithromycin, clarithromycin, or erythromycin).
2) Example A is caused by angiotensin-converting enzyme (ACE) inhibitors. Look for a sudden or new onset of a dry cough in a patient with hypertension (without signs of the common cold). Angioedema is a rare adverse effect and can be life-threatening.
3) Example B is caused by calcium channel blockers (CCBs). Look for a hypertensive patient with swollen ankles (not associated with heart failure) and headache.

(Continued)

Notes (*Continued*)

4) Example C is caused by the thiazide diuretics (hyperuricemia and hyperglycemia).

5) Example D is caused by beta-blockers. Look for a patient with hypertension who complains of increased fatigue and depression (avoid if possible in depressed patients).

U.S. CENTERS FOR DISEASE CONTROL AND PREVENTION STATISTICS

I. Discussion

It is important that you memorize these U.S. Centers for Disease Control and Prevention (CDC) statistics. The questions will be short and to the point. Determine if a question is asking about the most common cause of death (mortality) or if it is asking about the most common cause of a certain disease in a population (prevalence). For example, the most common cause of cancer death overall is lung cancer (mortality), but the most common cancer overall (prevalence) is skin cancer. The most common type of skin cancer is basal cell skin cancer.

Sometimes, a question will ask about gender-specific cause. For example, the most common cancer in females is breast cancer and the most common cancer in males is prostate cancer (prevalence). But the cancer causing the most deaths overall for both males and females is still lung cancer (mortality).

CDC Mortality Statistics
- Disease causing the most deaths overall: heart disease.
- Cancer with the highest mortality: lung cancer.
- Cancer with the highest mortality in males (lung cancer) and in females (lung cancer).
- Most common cause of death for adolescents: motor vehicle accidents.

Prevalence
- Most common cancer in females: breast cancer.
- Most common cancer in males: prostate cancer.
- Most common type of cancer overall (males/females): skin cancer.
- Most common type of skin cancer (males/females): basal cell cancer.
- Skin cancer with the highest mortality: melanoma.
- Gynecological cancer (vulva/vagina/cervix/uterus/ovary).
  - Uterine/endometrial cancer (most common gynecological cancer).
  - Ovarian cancer (second most common gynecological cancer).

II. Example

What is the most common type of gynecological cancer?
A) Uterine cancer
B) Cervical cancer
C) Breast cancer
D) Ovarian cancer

III. Answer
Correct answer is Option A.
A) Uterine cancer

IV. Question Dissection
Best Clues
1) This question is based on your recall of facts that you memorized (rote memory).
2) Rule out breast cancer because it is not considered a gynecological cancer.

Notes
1) There may be a question about the gynecologic cancers (see example). These types of cancers are located in the pelvis (labia, vagina, uterus, fallopian tubes, ovaries).
2) Breast cancer is not classified as a gynecological cancer.

BENIGN PHYSIOLOGIC VARIANTS

I. Discussion
A benign variant is a physiological abnormality that does not interfere with bodily process or function. There are very few questions on benign variants. Some examples of the benign variants that have been seen on the exams include the geographic tongue, torus palatinus, and a split or fishtail uvula (listed in Chapter 5: HEENT). Benign variants are listed under the appropriate organ system.

II. Example
A 45-year-old patient complains of a sore throat. Upon examination, the NP notices a bony growth midline at the hard palate of the mouth. The patient denies any changes or pain. It is not red, tender, or swollen. She reports a history of the same growth for many years without any change. Which of the following conditions is most likely?
A) Torus palatinus
B) Geographic tongue
C) Acute glossitis
D) Leukoplakia

III. Correct Answer: Option A
A) Torus palatinus

IV. Question Dissection
Best Clues
1) Description of a chronic bony growth located midline in the hard palate.
2) Rule out glossitis, geographic tongue, and hairy leukoplakia because they are all located on the tongue and not on the hard palate (roof of the mouth).

Notes

1) A torus palatinus is a benign growth of bone (an exostosis) located midline on the hard palate and covered with normal oral skin. It is painless and does not interfere with function.

2) A "geographic tongue" has multiple fissures and irregular smoother areas on its surface that makes it look like a topographic map. The patient may complain of soreness on the tongue after eating or drinking acidic or hot foods.

3) Leukoplakia is not a benign variant. It appears as a slow-growing white plaque that has a firm to hard surface that is slightly raised on the tongue or inside the mouth. It is considered a precancerous lesion. It is due to chronic irritation of the skin or to precancerous changes on the tongue and inside the cheeks. Its causes include poorly fitting dentures, chewing tobacco (snuff), and using other types of tobacco. Refer the patient for a biopsy because it can sometimes become malignant.

4) Oral hairy leukoplakia (OHL) of the tongue is a painless white patch (or patches) that appears corrugated. It is located on the lateral aspects of the tongue and is associated with HIV and AIDS infection. It is caused by Epstein-Barr virus (EBV) infection of the tongue. It is not considered a premalignant lesion.

U.S. PREVENTIVE SERVICES TASK FORCE SCREENING GUIDELINES

I. Discussion

USPSTF screening guidelines are graded as A, B, C, D, or I (insufficient evidence or evidence is lacking or of poor quality). The highest rating is a Grade A (routine screening is advised—high certainty that the net benefit is substantial). A rating of Grade D means that the harm outweighs the benefits (or there is no benefit) to the service and the use of the service is discouraged.

Both the ANCC and the AANPCP exam use the USPSTF screening recommendations. Regarding breast cancer screening, the USPSTF (2009) currently recommends that a screening baseline mammogram (with or without clinical breast exam) start at age 50 years, then every 2 years (biennially) until the age of 75 years. For women aged 40 to 49 years, mammograms should be based on individual factors (such as risk factors, preferences, risk vs. benefits of mammograms).

II. Example

What is the USPSTF screening recommendation for ovarian cancer?

A) Annual bimanual pelvic exam with pelvic ultrasound
B) Pelvic and intravaginal ultrasound
C) Intravaginal ultrasound with CA 125 tumor marker
D) The USPSTF does not recommend routine screening of women for ovarian cancer.

III. Correct Answer: Option D

D) The USPSTF does not recommend routine screening of women for ovarian cancer.

IV. Question Dissection

Best Clues

1) Do not "over read" the question. Assume that the question is asking about routine screening of the general population.
2) "High-tech" tests (ultrasounds, CA 125) are not used for routine screening due to the cost.
3) Although the bimanual pelvic exam is "low tech," it is being used as a distractor.

Notes

1) The USPSTF does not recommend routine screening for ovarian cancer, lung cancer, etc.
2) If there is a case scenario of an older woman who complains of vague abdominal/pelvic symptoms (stomach bloating, low back ache, constipation) and is found to have a palpable ovary during the bimanual exam, rule out ovarian cancer.
3) Always rule out ovarian cancer in a postmenopausal female who has a palpable ovary.
4) The initial workup for ovarian cancer is the intravaginal ultrasound and the CA 125.
5) The risk factors for ovarian cancer are: early menarche or late menopause, nulliparity, endometriosis, PCOS, and family history of ovarian cancer. Women with *BRCA 1* and *2* mutations are also at higher risk for both breast and ovarian cancer (Table 2.3).

Table 2.3 USPSTF Screening Guidelines

Disease	Screening Test
Breast cancer (2009)	Baseline at age 50 years. Screen every 2 years until 74 years. Stop at age 75 years or older. After age 74 years (no recommendation)
Cervical cancer (2012)	Baseline at age 21 years. Age 21 to 65 years every 3 years. Pap smear/cytology. Age of 21 or less (do not screen)
Hysterectomy (no cervix)	Do not screen (if no history of pre-cancer or cervical cancer)
Prostate cancer (2012)	Routine screening is not recommended
Testicular cancer (2011)	Routine screening is not recommended
Colon cancer (2008)	Age 50 to 75 years. Baseline age 50 years. Use *high-sensitivity* fecal occult blood test (yearly) or sigmoidoscopy (every 5 years) or colonoscopy (every 10 years)
Skin cancer counseling (2012)	Age 10 to 24 years. Educate fair-skinned persons to avoid sunlight (10 a.m.–3 p.m.), use sunblock SPF 15 or higher
Smoking cessation (2009)	Ask all adolescents and adults about tobacco use
Fall prevention in community-dwelling older adults (2012)	Age 65 years or older, moderate-intensity aerobic activity for 150 minutes or 2.5 hours per week (i.e., brisk walking).
Ovarian cancer (2012)	Do not screen. High-risk (Ashkenazi Jew, *BRCA* gene, family history of two or more first- or second-degree relative)
AAA	One-time screening (only men aged 65–75 years) who are cigarette smokers. Screening test is ultrasound of the abdomen

FOLLOWING UP ON A PRESCRIPTION MEDICINE

I. Discussion

In these cases, a patient who is taking prescription medicine is running out of their supply or does not have refills left. The test-taker must decide what type of initial follow-up is needed. Depending on the case scenario, for a patient who is fully symptomatic due to the abrupt cessation of medicine (either due to running out of refills or discontinuation of health insurance), a reasonable initial action is to continue the prescription medicine.

II. Example

A 65-year-old female smoker presents with a history of Barrett's esophagus, and gastroesophageal reflux disease (GERD). The patient reports that her gastroenterologist's prescription for esomeprazole (Nexium) 40 mg daily ran out a few days ago. She is complaining of severe heartburn and a sore throat. During the physical exam, the NP notes an erythematous posterior pharynx without tonsillar discharge and mild dental enamel loss on the rear molars. What is the best initial action for the NP to follow?

A) Refer the patient to an oncologist for a biopsy to rule out esophageal cancer.
B) Give the patient a refill of her proton pump inhibitor (PPI) prescription.
C) Recommend that the patient take an OTC ranitidine (Zantac) twice a day until she can be seen by her gastroenterologist.
D) Switch the patient's prescription to another brand of PPI because her symptoms are not getting better.

III. Correct Answer: Option B

B) Give the patient a refill of her PPI prescription and advise her to schedule an appointment with her gastroenterologist.

IV. Question Dissection

Best Clues

1) Rule out option A because the patient is already under the care of a gastroenterologist.
2) OTC ranitidine (Zantac) is not potent enough to control the symptoms of erosive esophagitis. A PPI is the preferred treatment for erosive esophagitis.
3) Do not switch the patient to another PPI brand. Her worsening symptoms are caused by rebound.
4) The best initial action in this case is to refill the PPI prescription because the patient is fully symptomatic (erosive esophagitis) until she can see her gastroenterologist.

Notes

1) The patient's severe symptoms are caused by the sudden discontinuation of the high-dose PPI (rebound-type of reaction).
2) Barrett's esophagus is the "precancerous" lesion of esophageal cancer. It is best managed by gastroenterologists (not oncologists).
3) Patients diagnosed with Barrett's esophagus typically have endoscopic examinations with biopsy by a gastroenterologist annually (or every 6 months for high-grade lesions).

4) Patients with Barrett's esophagus are treated with high-dose PPIs for a "lifetime."

5) The first-line treatment of mild, uncomplicated GERD is lifestyle changes (avoid eating 3 to 4 hours before bedtime, dietary changes, weight loss if overweight, etc.).

6) If a patient is at high risk for esophageal cancer (aged 50 years or older, smoker, chronic GERD for decades), consider referral to a gastroenterologist for an upper endoscopy.

TANNER STAGES

I. Discussion

Expect to see at least two questions regarding Tanner stages in girls and boys. Because Tanner Stage I is prepuberty and Tanner Stage V is the adult pattern for both boys and girls, the only stages to memorize for the exams is from Tanner Stage II to Tanner Stage IV.

For girls, memorize the pattern of breast development and for boys, the genital development (testes and penis). It is not as important to memorize pubic hair development for both.

Tanner Stages
Girls:
Stage I: Prepubertal pattern.
Stage II: Breast bud and areola starts to develop.
Stage III: Breast continues to grow with nipples/areola (one mound/no separation).
Stage IV: Nipples and areola become elevated from the breast (a secondary mound).
Stage V: Adult pattern.

Boys:
Stage I: Prepubertal pattern.
Stage II: Testes with scrotum starts to enlarge (scrotal skin starts to get darker/more ruggae).
Stage III: Penis grows longer (length) and testes/scrotum continues to become larger.
Stage IV: Penis become wider and continues growing in length (testes are larger with darker scrotal skin and more ruggae).
Stage V: Adult pattern.

II. Example

A 14-year-old boy is brought in by his mother for a physical exam. Both are concerned about his breast enlargement. The teen denies breast tenderness. On physical exam, the NP palpates soft breast tissue that is not tender. No dominant mass is noted. The skin is smooth and there is no nipple discharge with massage. The teen has a BMI of 29. Which of the following statements is correct?

A) The patient has physiologic gynecomastia and should return for a follow-up exam.

B) Order an ultrasound of both breasts to further assess the patient's breast tissue development.

C) Reassure the mother that the patient's breast development is within normal limits.

D) Educate the mother that her son has pseudo-gynecomastia.

III. Correct Answer: Option D

D) Educate the mother that her son has pseudo-gynecomastia.

IV. Question Dissection

Best Clues

1) The boy is very overweight (BMI 29) and is almost obese.
2) The clinical breast exam does not show palpable breast tissue. Instead, the breast palpation reveals soft fatty tissue.
3) It is wrong to "reassure" a patient or a family member in the exam (poor therapeutic communication technique).

Notes

1) Physiologic gynecomastia physical exam findings will show disc-like breast tissue that is mobile under each nipple/areola, the breast may be tender, and the breast can be asymmetrical (one breast larger than the other).
2) A BMI of 25 to 29.9 is considered overweight. Obesity is a BMI of 30 or higher.
3) Overweight to obese males are at highest risk for pseudo-gynecomastia.

QUESTIONS ABOUT FOOD

I. Discussion

There are basically three kinds of food-related questions on the exam. You may be asked to pick the foods that have high levels of certain minerals, such as potassium, calcium, or magnesium. Other questions will address food interactions (tetracycline and dairy), drug interactions (MAOI and high tyramine-content foods such as fermented foods), or foods that should be avoided for a particular disease (avoid wheat products in case of celiac disease).

Certain foods are recommended for certain diseases (e.g., salmon/omega-3 for heart disease) because of their favorable effect. In contrast, certain foods are contraindicated for some conditions because of adverse or dangerous effects.

II. Example

Which of the following foods are known to have high potassium content?

A) Low-fat yogurt, soft cheeses, and collard greens.
B) Aged cheese, red wine, and chocolate.
C) Potatoes, apricots, and Brussels sprouts.
D) Black beans, red meat, and citrus juice.

III. Correct Answer: Option C

C) Potatoes, apricots, and Brussels sprouts.

IV. Question Dissection

Best Clues

1) First, look at the answer option pairs for inconsistencies in the list of foods.
2) Rule out Option A because it is inconsistent and these foods do not contain high levels of potassium: low-fat yogurt and soft cheeses (calcium) with collard greens (vitamin K).
3) Rule out Option B because these foods have high tyramine content, not potassium.
4) Rule out Option D because it is inconsistent. Although citrus juices are high in potassium, both black beans and red meat are not (iron).
5) If Options A, B, and D are incorrect, then the only one left is Option C (potatoes, apricots, and Brussels sprouts. A large number of fruits and vegetables are rich in potassium and vitamins).

Notes

1) Foods with high tyramine content can cause dangerous food–drug interactions with MAOI inhibitors (Marplan, Nardil, and Parnate).
2) Foods and supplements containing stimulants such as caffeine and ephedra are best avoided by patients with hypertension, arrhythmias, high risk for MI, thyroid disease, etc.
3) If one of the food choices in an answer option is incorrect, rule out this answer option because all of the foods on the list have to be correlated.

Examples of Food Groups

1) Gluten (avoid with celiac disease/celiac sprue): Wheat (including spelt and kamut), rye, barley, oats (breads, cereals, pasta, cookies, cakes).
   - Gluten-free (safe carbohydrates): Corn, rice, potatoes, quinoa, tapioca, soybeans.
2) Plant sterols and sterols (reduces cholesterol, low-density lipoprotein [LDL], triglycerides): Benecol spread, wheat germ, sesame oil, corn oil, peanuts.
3) Monounsaturated fats/fatty acids (decreases risk of heart disease):
   - Olive oil, canola oil, some nuts (almonds, walnuts), sunflower oil/seeds.
   - The Mediterranean diet is high in monounsaturated fats.
4) Saturated fats or trans fats (increases risk of heart disease): lard, beef fat (fatty steak), deep-fried fast foods.
5) Omega-3 or fish oils (decrease risk of heart disease): fatty cold-water marine fish (salmon), fish oils, flaxseed oil, and krill oil.
6) Magnesium (decreases BP, dilates blood vessels): some nuts (almonds, peanuts, cashews), some beans, whole wheat. Also found in laxatives, antacids, milk of magnesia.
7) Potassium (helps decreases BP): most fruits (especially apricot, banana, orange, prune juice), some vegetables.
8) Folate (decreases homocysteine levels and fetal neural tube defects): breakfast cereals fortified with folate, green leafy vegetables (i.e., spinach), liver.
9) Iron (treats iron-deficiency anemia): beef, liver, black beans, black-eyed peas.
10) Vitamin K (control intake if on anticoagulants): green leafy vegetables, (kale, collard greens, spinach), broccoli, cabbage.
11) High sodium content (increases water retention, can increase BP): cold cuts, pickles, preserved foods, canned foods, hot dogs, chips.
12) Calcium (helps with osteopenia and osteoporosis, helps decrease BP): low-fat dairy, low-fat milk, low-fat yogurt, cheeses.

Common Disorders Associated With Certain Foods

1) Celiac disease
   - Lifetime avoidance of gluten-containing cereals such as wheat, rye, barley, and oats.
   - Gluten-free: rice, corn, potatoes, peanuts, soy, beans, meat, dairy, all fruits/vegetables.
2) Hypertension
   - Maintain an adequate intake of calcium, magnesium, and potassium.
   - Calcium: low-fat dairy, low-fat yogurt, cheeses.
   - Magnesium: wheat bread, nuts (almonds, peanuts, cashews), some beans.
   - Potassium: most fruits (apricot, banana, oranges, cantaloupes, raisins), green vegetables.
   - Avoid high-sodium foods: cold cuts, pickles, preserved foods, canned foods, preservatives.
3) Migraine headaches and MAOIs (Marplan, Nardil, and Parnate)
   - High-tyramine foods: aged cheeses/meats, red wine, fava beans, draft beer, fermented foods.
4) Anticoagulation therapy (i.e., warfarin sodium or Coumadin)
   - Avoid or limit high intake of vitamin K foods such as green leafy vegetables (kale/collard greens, spinach, cabbage), broccoli. Vitamin K decreases the effectiveness of warfarin sodium. Avoid excessive intake of vitamin K-rich foods.

CASE MANAGEMENT

I. Discussion

Medical case managers are experienced RNs who work for hospitals, health care plans, and health insurance companies. Their job is essentially to coordinate the outpatient health care of patients with high-cost chronic conditions. The goal of case management is to decrease disease exacerbations and decrease the risk of hospitalization.

II. Example

Asthma

A good outcome for children with asthma is their ability to attend school full-time and to play normally every day.

A poor case management outcome is if the child misses school and/or is unable to play due to poor control of asthma symptoms.

> **Notes**
> 1) With asthma, a good case outcome is for the child (or adult) to return to normal function. For children, it means the child is attending school and can play daily. If the child is not able to attend school full time (frequent absences), it is a poor case management outcome.
> 2) The risk factors for asthma fatality includes a history of emergency department (ED) of short-acting beta agonist use (i.e., albuterol), nocturnal awakenings, increased dyspnea and wheezing, respiratory viral infection, etc.
> 3) Diseases that are picked for case management are usually chronic conditions such as asthma, congestive heart failure (CHF), HIV infection, chronic psychiatric conditions, and so on. A good outcome will show good symptom control, no exacerbations or hospitalizations.

ALL QUESTIONS HAVE ENOUGH INFORMATION

I. Discussion Only

Assume that all the questions on the exams contain enough information to answer them correctly. Do not read too much into a question or assume that it is missing some vital information. As far as the ANCC and AANPCP are concerned, all questions contain enough information to allow you to solve them correctly. Unless it is indicated, consider a patient is in good health unless a disease or other health condition is mentioned in the test question.

EMERGENT CASES

I. Discussion

The ability to recognize and initially manage emergent conditions that may present in the primary care arena is a skill that is expected of all NPs. It is important to memorize not only the presenting signs and symptoms of a given condition, but also its initial management in primary care.

Learn how these conditions present so that you can recognize them in the exam. The following is a list of emergent conditions that will be on the exam. (They are discussed in detail under each "Danger Signals" section under the appropriate organ system under the Systems Review section in the next section.).

Danger Signals

Cardiovascular System
- Acute myocardial infarction (MI)
- Congestive heart failure (CHF)
- Deep vein thrombosis (DVT)
- Abdominal aortic aneurysm (AAA)

Skin and Integumentory System
- Angioedema/Anaphylaxis
- Stevens–Johnson syndrome
- Meningococcemia
- Rocky Mountain spotted fever (RMSF)
- Lyme disease

Gastrointestinal System
- Acute abdomen (surgical abdomen)
- Acute appendicitis
- Acute pancreatitis

Men's Health
- Testicular torsion
- Priapism

Psychosocial Mental Health
- Depression with suicidal plan
- Acute mania with psychosis
- Severe anorexia

Nervous System
- Cerebrovascular accident (CVA)
- Temporal arteritis headache
- Subarachnoid bleeding "headache"

Head, Eyes, Ears, Nose, and Throat
- Sudden vision loss or rapid worsening of vision
- Herpes keratitis
- Temporal arteritis
- Acute angle-closure glaucoma

Pulmonary System
- Anaphylaxis
- Severe asthmatic exacerbation (impending respiratory failure)
- Pulmonary emboli

Renal System
- Acute pyelonephritis

Women's Health
- Dominant breast mass that is attached to surrounding tissue
- Ruptured tubal ectopic pregnancy

II. Example

An asthmatic male complains of a sudden onset of itching and coughing after taking two aspirin tablets for a headache in the waiting room. The patient's lips and the eyelids are becoming swollen. The patient complains of feeling hot. Bright red wheals are noted on his chest and arms and legs. Which of the following is the best initial intervention to follow?

A) Call 911.

B) Check the patient's blood pressure, pulse, and temperature.

C) Give an injection of aqueous epinephrine 1:1000 (1 mg/mL) 0.5 mg IM (intramuscular) into the vastus lateralis muscle immediately.

D) Initiate a prescription of a potent topical steroid and a Medrol Dose Pack.

III. Correct Answer: Option C

C) Give an injection of aqueous epinephrine 1:1000 dilution (1 mg/mL) 0.5 mg IM into the vastus lateralis muscle immediately.

IV. Question Dissection

Best Clues
1) The quick onset of symptoms such as angioedema after taking aspirin.
2) The classic signs and symptoms of anaphylaxis are described in this case.
3) Severe anaphylactic episodes occur almost immediately or within 1 hour after exposure.

Notes

1) Treatment of anaphylaxis (in primary care):
   - If only one clinician is present: Give an injection of epinephrine 1:1000 dilution 0.3 to 0.5 mg IM STAT, and then call 911. May repeat dose within 5 minutes in case of poor response.
2) ED treatment medications: epinephrine IM, 100% oxygen by face mask, an antihistamine (H1 blocker) such as diphenhydramine (Benadryl), an H2 antagonist such as ranitidine; a bronchodilator such as albuterol (short-acting beta-2 agonist); and systemic glucocorticosteroids such as prednisone.
3) Patients with an atopic history (asthma, eczema, allergic rhinitis) with nasal polyps are at higher risk for aspirin and NSAID allergies.
4) Anaphylaxis is classified as a Type I IgE-dependent reaction.
5) Biphasic anaphylaxis occurs in up to 23% of cases (symptoms recur within 8–10 hours after initial episode). This is the reason why these patients are prescribed a Medrol Dose Pack and a long-acting antihistamine after being discharged from the ED.
6) The most common triggers for anaphylaxis in children are foods. Medications and insect stings are the most common triggers in adults.

PRIORITIZING OTHER EMERGENT CASES

I. Discussion

During life-threatening situations, managing the airway, breathing, and circulation (the ABCs) is always the top priority. If the question does not describe conditions requiring the ABCs, then the next level of priority is the acute or sudden change in the mental status and the level of consciousness (LOC). One of the most important clues in such problems is the acute timing of onset of symptoms or the sudden change of the LOC from the patient's "baseline." The mnemonic device to use if the ABCs do not apply is AMPICILLIN.

A	Acute
M	Mental status changes
P	Pain
I	Infection
CILLIN	No meaning. Makes mnemonic easier to remember

II. Example

A 16-year-old male presents to a community clinic accompanied by his grandmother, who reports that the patient fell off his bike this morning. The patient now complains of a headache with mild nausea. The patient's grandmother reports that he did not wear a helmet. The health history is uneventful. Which of the following statements is indicative of an emergent condition?

A) The patient complains of multiple painful abrasions that are bleeding on his arms and legs.

B) The patient complains of a headache that is relieved by acetaminophen (Tylenol).

C) The patient makes eye contact occasionally and answers with brief statements.

D) The patient is having difficulty with following normal conversation and answering questions.

III. Correct Answer: Option D

D) The patient is having difficulty with following normal conversation and answering questions.

IV. Question Dissection

Best Clues

1) History of recent trauma that is followed by a headache with nausea.
2) The patient did not wear a bicycle helmet.

Notes

1) Any recent changes in LOC, even one as subtle as difficulty with normal conversation, should ring a bell in your head and remind you of the AMPICILLIN mnemonic.
2) Notice the words "normal conversation." Do not overread the question and ask yourself what they mean by "normal conversation." Take it at face value.
3) Changes in LOC on the test are usually subtle changes. Signs to watch for: has difficulty answering questions, has slurred speech, seems confused, does not understand instructions/conversation, is sleepy/lethargic, and so forth.
4) Even though the patient is bleeding, note that he has "abrasions," which are superficial.
5) The behavior under Option C is considered "normal" for an adolescent male (or female).

GERIATRICS

I. Discussion

The ANCC does not give any information about the number of questions by age group, but the AANPCP does. Elderly patients are broken down into two age categories on the AANPCP exam. Between the ages of 65 and 84 years are the "young gerontologicals." From the age of 85 years and older are the "frail elderly."

The AANPCP's FNP exam has a total of 23 questions (15%) on gerontological topics. The AANPCP ANP exam has a total of 62 questions (42%).

II. Example

A 92-year-old woman has recently been diagnosed with community-acquired bacterial pneumonia. During the follow-up visit, the son reports that the patient seems to be getting better. Which of the following statements about the patient is *not* indicative of a serious condition?

A) The patient is sleeping less in the daytime and is more alert when awakened (positive/positive).

B) The patient complains of double vision and is sleeping more (negative/negative).
C) The patient is eating less and she has lost 10% of her previous body weight (negative/negative).
D) The patient has become more agitated and confused at night (negative/negative).

III. Correct Answer: Option A

A) The patient is sleeping less in the daytime and is more alert when awakened (positive/positive).

IV. Question Dissection

Best Clues

1) The patient's LOC is "alert when awakened."
2) Both halves of the complex sentence under option A are positive findings.
3) Rule out Options B, C, and D because they are all negative findings.

Notes

1) The answers are all written as complex sentence and have two "parts." Under Options B, C, and D, both parts of the sentence indicate serious clinical findings. Both parts are "negative/negative."
2) Elderly patients who lose weight are at higher risk of complications and death. An unintentional weight loss of 10% is considered pathologic in any age group.
3) An elderly patient who becomes agitated and confused at night is probably experiencing "sundowning." Sundowning is seen in patients who have dementia. In addition, elderly patients are also at higher risk for delirium (temporary mental state, not a disease).
4) Some elderly patients with bacterial infections (such as a UTI) can become acutely confused. Elderly patients with UTIs may not exhibit fever or the other classic symptoms of a UTI.

CHOOSING THE BEST INITIAL INTERVENTION

I. Discussion

Numerous questions on the exam will ask test takers about the best initial intervention to perform in a given case scenario. The question may ask you to pick out the best initial evaluation, treatment, or statement to say to a patient.

One of the reasons why some test takers answer these questions incorrectly is because they skip a step in the "SOAPE" process (Subjective, Objective, Assessment, Planning, and Evaluation). The first step of the patient evaluation is to find "subjective" information such as asking about the patient's symptoms and other historical/demographic information. The next step is to find "objective" information. This means performing a physical examination or other tests. It is best to start out "low-tech," such as performing a physical exam or a low-tech maneuver.

For example, in a case of peripheral vascular disease (PVD), it makes sense to check the pulse and blood pressure first on the lower and upper extremities before ordering an expensive test such as an ultrasound Doppler flow study. The following are examples of actions that can be done using the "SOAPE" mnemonic as a guide.

S: Look for Subjective Evidence (S)

1) Interview the patient and/or family member about the history of the present illness.
2) Ask about the presentation of the illness (timing, signs and symptoms, etc.).
3) Ask if the patient is on any medication, the past medical history, diet, etc.
4) Be alert for the historical findings because they provide important clues that help point to the correct diagnosis (or differential diagnosis).

O: Look for Objective Evidence (O)

1) Perform a physical exam (general or targeted to the present complaints).
2) If applicable, perform a physical maneuver (Tinels, Kernigs, Drawer, etc.).
3) Order laboratory/other tests to "rule in" (or "rule out") the differential diagnosis.
4) If the laboratory test result is abnormal, you may be asked about the next step (such as a follow-up lab test that is more sensitive or specific).

A: Diagnosis or Assessment (A)

1) What is the most likely diagnosis based on the history, disease presentation, and physical exam findings?
2) If applicable, figure out if the lab or other testing results point to a more specific diagnosis (or rule out a diagnosis).
3) Decide if the condition is emergent or not (if applicable).

P: Treatment Plan (P)

1) Initiate or prescribe medications and symptomatic treatment (if applicable).
2) Patient education.
3) Follow-up visit to assess response to treatment, etc.

E: Evaluate Response to the Treatment/Intervention or Evaluate the Situation (E)

1) Poor or no response to treatment (or worsens). An exception is a strep pharyngitis patient who is not responding to amoxicillin after 3 days. Switch to second-line antibiotics such as Augmentin or second- to third-generation cephalosporin.
2) If emergent, refer to ED/call 911.

II. Example

A 21-year-old woman with a history of mild intermittent asthma and allergic rhinitis complains of a cough that has been waking her up very early in the morning. She reports that she is wheezing more than usual. Her last office visit was 8 months ago. Which of the following is the best initial course of action?

A) Initiate a prescription of a short-acting beta-2 agonist QID PRN.
B) Refer the patient to an allergist for a scratch test.
C) Discuss her symptoms and other factors associated with the asthmatic exacerbation.
D) Perform a thorough physical examination and obtain blood work.

III. Correct Answer: Option C

C) Discuss her symptoms and other factors associated with asthmatic exacerbation.

IV. Question Dissection

Best Clues

1) The patient's asthma appears to be getting worse (asthmatic exacerbation).
2) There is a lack of information because of poor follow-up (none for 8 months).

3) There is a need to find out about precipitating factors, medication compliance, comorbid conditions, what is precipitating her asthma, and so on.

Notes

The correct order of actions to follow in this case scenario is the following:

1) Interview the patient to find out more about her symptoms, etc. (subjective).
2) Perform a thorough physical examination (objective).
3) Administer a nebulizer treatment. Check peak expiratory flow (PEF) before and after treatment to assess for effectiveness.
4) Initiate a prescription of a short-acting beta-2 agonist and steroid inhaler BID. Dose depends on severity of asthma (planning).
5) Refer the patient to an allergist for a scratch test if you suspect the patient has allergic asthma (evaluation).
6) Patients with asthmatic exacerbations whose PEF is less than 50% of predicted value after being given nebulized albuterol/saline treatments should not be discharged. Consider calling 911.
7) The differential diagnosis for an early morning cough includes postnasal drip, allergic rhinitis, sinusitis, GERD, and so forth.

ASSESSMENT QUESTIONS

I. Discussion

The ANCC's name for this area in their FNP exam is "Clinical Assessment." This domain contains 30 questions (20%) out of the total of 150 graded questions in their exam.

On their ANP exam, it is called "Health Assessment." This domain contains 34 questions (23%) out of the total 150 graded questions in their exam. Therefore, test takers who are weak in this area are more likely to fail the certification exam (the ANCC or the AANPCP) because it makes up a large percentage of the questions.

PICK OUT THE MOST SPECIFIC SIGN/SYMPTOM

I. Discussion

Always pick out the most specific answer to a question when it is asking about the signs and/or symptoms of a disease. Learn the unique or the most specific signs/symptoms associated with the disease. The following is a good example of this concept.

II. Example

Which of the following is most likely to be found in patients with a long-standing case of iron-deficiency anemia?

A) Pica
B) Fatigue
C) Pallor
D) Irritability

III. Correct Answer: Option A

A) Pica

IV. Question Dissection

Best Clues

1) The diagnosis (iron-deficiency anemia).
2) Knowledge that pica is also associated with iron-deficiency anemia.

> **Notes**
>
> 1) If you are guessing, use common sense. Fatigue and irritability are found in many conditions.
> 2) Pallor is also seen in many disorders such as shock, illness, and anemia.
> 3) By the process of elimination, you are left with option A, the correct choice.
> 4) Another specific clinical finding in iron-deficiency anemia is spoon-shaped nails (or koilonychia). Do not confuse this finding with pitted nails (psoriasis).

DERMATOLOGY QUESTIONS

I. Discussion

Many of the questions from this area will test your skill diagnosing skin diseases. The rash or skin lesion is described in detail. Some of the questions will ask about how to treat the skin condition. One of the problems that students have with these questions is their unfamiliarity with the dermatologic terms used to describe the skin condition. A list and description of the primary and secondary skin lesions is available in the Skin and Integumentary section.

- Maculopapular: a skin rash that has both color (macular) and texture (small papules or raised skin lesions—the color ranges from red [erythematous] to bright pink)
- Maculopapular rash in a lace-like pattern (fifth disease)
- Maculopapular rashes with papules, vesicles, and crusts (varicella)
- Maculopapular rashes that are oval-shaped with a herald patch (pityriasis rosea)
- Vesicular rashes on an erythematous base (herpes simplex, genital herpes)

II. Example

A male nursing assistant who works in a nursing home is complaining of multiple pruritic rashes that have been disturbing his sleep at night for the past few weeks. He reports that several members of his family are starting to complain of pruritic rashes. On physical examination, the NP notices multiple small papules, some vesicles, and maculopapular excoriated rashes on the sides and the webs of the fingers, on the waist, and on the penis. Which of the following is the most likely diagnosis?

A) Scarlatina
B) Impetigo
C) Erythema migrans
D) Scabies

III. Correct Answer: Option D

D) Scabies

IV. Question Dissection

Best Clues

1) The history (pruritic rashes disturb sleep at night, several family members with same symptoms, and works in a higher-risk area such as nursing homes)
2) Classic location of the rashes (finger webs, waist, penis)

Notes

1) Assume that a patient has scabies if excoriated pruritic rashes are located in the finger webs and the penis until proven otherwise. Higher-risk groups are health care givers or any person working with large populations such as schools, nursing homes, group homes, or prisons.
2) The usual recommendation is that all family members and close contacts be treated at the same time as the patient (spread by skin-to-skin contact). Wash used clothes/sheets in hot water, then dry or iron in high heat.
3) The rash of scarlatina has a sandpaper-like texture and is accompanied by a sore throat, strawberry tongue, and skin desquamation (peeling) of the palms and soles. It is not pruritic.
4) Impetigo rashes initially appear as papules that develop into bullae that rupture easily, becoming superficial, bright red "weeping" rashes with honey-colored exudate that becomes crusted as it dries. The rashes are very pruritic and are located on areas that are easily traumatized, such as the face, arms, or legs. Insect bites, acne lesions, and varicella lesions can also become secondarily infected, resulting in impetigo.
5) Cutaneous larva migrans (creeping eruption) rashes are shaped like red raised wavy lines (serpinginous or snakelike) that are alone or few. They are red and very pruritic, and become excoriated from scratching (appears maculopapular).
6) The areas of the body that are commonly exposed directly to contaminated soil and sand, such as the soles of the feet, extremities, or the buttocks, are the most common locations for larva migrans.
7) Systemic treatment with either ivermectin once a day (for 1 to 2 days) or albendazole (for 3 days) is the preferred therapy for larva migrans.

CHOOSING THE CORRECT DRUG

I. Discussion

Test takers are expected to know not only the drug's generic and/or brand name, but also its drug class. If you are only familiar with the drug's brand name or generic form, you will still be able to recognize the drug on the test because both names will be listed.

In addition, the drug's action, indication(s), common side effects, drug interactions, and contraindications are important to learn. Drugs may only be listed as a drug class.

II. Example

A 14-year-old female student complains of pain and fullness in her left ear that is getting steadily worse. She has a history of allergic rhinitis and is allergic to dust mites. On physical exam, the left tympanic membrane is red with cloudy fluid inside. The landmarks are displaced in the same ear. The student denies frequent ear infections, and the last antibiotic she took was 8 months ago for a urinary tract infection. She is allergic to sulfa and tells the NP that she will not take any erythromycin because it makes her very nauseated. Which of the following is the best choice of treatment for this patient?

A) Amoxicillin 500 mg PO three times a day for 10 days
B) Pseudoephedrine (Sudafed) 20 mg PO as needed every 4 to 6 hours
C) Fluticasone (Flonase) nasal inhaler 1 to 2 sprays each nostril every 12 hours
D) Biaxin (clarithromycin) 500 mg PO two times a day for 10 days

V. Correct Answer: Option A

A) Amoxicillin 500 mg PO three times a day for 10 days

VI. Question Dissection

Best Clues

1) Red tympanic membrane with cloudy fluid inside and displaced landmarks.
2) Last antibiotic taken was 8 months ago and ear infections were infrequent (lack of risk factors for beta-lactamase resistant bacteria).

Notes

1) This question is more complicated compared with the first example. Although the question is regarding the correct drug treatment, it also lists the signs/symptoms of the disease. In order to answer this question correctly, you must first arrive at the correct diagnosis, which is AOM.
2) Amoxicillin is the preferred first-line antibiotic for both AOM and acute sinusitis in both children and adults (for patients with no risk factors for resistant organisms).
3) The ideal patient is someone who has not been on any antibiotics in the past 3 months and/or does not live in an area with high rates of beta-lactam resistant bacteria.
4) If the patient is a treatment failure, or was on an antibiotic in the previous 3 months, then a second-line antibiotic such as Augmentin BID or cefdinir (Omnicef) BID should be given.
5) If penicillin-allergic, an alternative is azithromycin (Z-Pack) and clarithromycin (Biaxin) BID.
6) Pseudoephedrine (Sudafed) is for symptoms only. Do not use for infants, young children, or patients with hypertension.
7) Nasal steroid spray BID is a good adjunct treatment for this patient because of allergic rhinitis, which causes the eustachian tube to swell and get blocked.

DIAGRAMS

I. Discussion

Currently, neither chest x-ray (CXR) films nor electrocardiogram (EKG) strips have been seen on the NP certification exams. The only diagram seen on the test at the moment is one of a chest with the four cardiac auscultory areas (aortic, pulmonic, tricuspid, and mitral) marked. The diagram is used for questions on either cardiac murmurs or the heart sounds.

II. Example

Which of the following is the best location to auscultate for the S3 heart sound?
A) Aortic area
B) Pulmonic area
C) Tricuspid area
D) Mitral area

III. Correct Answer: Option B

B) Pulmonic area

IV. Question Dissection

Best Clues
1) Memorization of the S3 heart sound facts.

> **Notes**
> 1) The best place to listen for the S3 heart sound is the pulmonic area (the pulmonic area is near the ventricles).
> 2) The S3 heart sound is pathognomic for heart failure.

"GOLD STANDARD" TESTS

I. Discussion

Learn to distinguish between a screening test and a diagnostic test (the "gold standard"). Diagnostic tests are highly specific and/or very sensitive. Depending on the disease process, the preferred diagnostic test might be a biopsy (e.g., melanoma), blood culture (e.g., septicemia), or an MRI scan (e.g., meniscus cartilage damage).

In contrast, screening tests are generally less sensitive and/or specific, but are more available and cost effective. Some examples of screening tests are the CBC (anemia), blood pressure (hypertension), Mantoux test (tuberculosis), or a urinalysis (UTI). The ideal screening test is one that can detect a disease at an early enough stage so that it can help to decrease the mortality. A good example of a disease with no approved screening test is ovarian cancer. Although the CEA 125 and intravaginal ultrasound are widely available, these two tests are not sensitive enough to pick up ovarian cancer during the early stages of the disease when it is potentially curable.

II. Example

A middle-aged nurse is having his PPD or Mantoux test result checked. A reddened area of 10.5 mm is present. It is smooth and soft and does not appear to be indurated. During the interview, the patient denies fever, cough, and weight loss. Which of the following is a true statement?

A) The PPD result is negative.
B) The PPD result is borderline.
C) The PPD should be repeated in 2 weeks.
D) A chest x-ray and sputum culture are indicated.

III. Correct Answer: Option A

A) The PPD result is negative.

IV. Question Dissection

Best Clues

1) Knowledge that skin induration, not the red color, is the best indicator of a positive reaction.
2) Lack of signs or symptoms of TB.

Notes

1) When some test takers see the 10.5 mm size and the red color, they assume automatically that it is a positive result.
2) The PPD result is negative because of the description of the soft and smooth skin (it is not indurated). Erythema alone is not an important criterion. The PPD result must be indurated and the correct size to be valid.
3) For pulmonary TB, a sputum culture is the gold standard. Treatment is started with at least three antitubercular drugs because of high rates of resistance. When the sputum culture and sensitivity result are available, the antitubercular antibiotic treatment can be narrowed down, changed, or another drug can be added.
4) TB is a reportable disease. Noncompliant patients who refuse treatment can be quarantined to protect the public.
5) A baseline LFT level and follow-up testing are recommended for patients on isoniazid (INH).

ARE TWO NAMES BETTER THAN ONE?

I. Discussion

Some diseases and conditions are known by two different names that are used interchangeably in both the clinical area and the literature. Sometimes the alternate name is the one being used in the exam questions. This can fool the test taker who is familiar with the disease but only recognizes it under its other name.

II. Examples

1) Degenerative joint disease (DJD) or osteoarthritis
2) Atopic dermatitis or eczema
3) Senile arcus or arcus senilis

4) AOM or purulent otitis media
5) Serous otitis media or otitis media with effusion (OME) or middle ear effusion (MEE)
6) Group A beta streptococcus or strep pyogenes
7) Tinea corporis or ringworm
8) Enterobiasis or pinworms
9) Vitamin B12 or cobalamin or cyanocobalamin (chemical name)
10) Vitamin B1 or thiamine
11) Scarlet fever or scarlatina
12) Otitis externa or swimmer's ear
13) Condyloma acuminata or genital warts
14) Tic douloureux or trigeminal neuralgia
15) Tinea cruris or jock itch
16) Thalassemia minor or thalassemia trait (either alpha or beta)
17) Giant cell arteritis or temporal arteritis
18) Psoas sign or ilipsoas muscle sign
19) Tinea capitis or ringworm of the scalp
20) Light reflex or the Hirschsprung test
21) Sentinel nodes or Virchow's nodes
22) PPD or the Mantoux test or TB skin test (TST)
23) Erythema migrans or early Lyme disease
24) Sinusitis or rhinosinusitis

SUICIDE RISK AND DEPRESSION

I. Discussion

All depressed patients should be screened for suicidal and/or homicidal ideation. This is true in the clinical arena as well as on the exam. Avoid picking statements that do not directly address the patient's suicidal and homicidal plans. Risk factors for suicide and depression are discussed in Chapter 15.

Incorrect answers are statements that are judgmental, reassuring to the patient, vague, disrespectful, or do not address the issue of suicide (or homicide) in a direct manner.

II. Example

A nurse practitioner working in a school health clinic is evaluating a new student who has been referred to him by a teacher. David is a 16-year-old male with a history of attention deficit disorder (ADD). He complains that his parents are always fighting and he thinks that they are getting divorced. During the interview, he is staring at the floor and avoiding eye contact. He reports that he is having problems falling asleep at night and has stopped seeing friends, including his girlfriend. Which of the following statements is the best choice to ask this teen?

A) "Do you want me to call your parents after we talk?"
B) "Do you have any plans of killing yourself or hurting other people?"
C) "Do you have any close male or female friends?"
D) "Do you want to wait to tell me about your plans until you feel better?"

III. Correct Answer: Option B

B) "Do you have any plans of killing yourself or hurting other people?"

IV. Question Dissection

Best Clues

1) Classic behavioral cues (avoidance of eye contact, insomnia, social isolation)
2) Parents fighting and getting divorced

Notes

1) Option B is the most specific approach in the evaluation for suicide in this case.
2) Although option C ("Do you have any close male or female friends?") is a common question asked of depressed patients, it is incorrect because it does not give specific information about specific plans of suicide or of homicide.
3) Always avoid picking answer choices in which an intervention is delayed. The statement "Do you want to wait to tell me about your plans until you feel better?" is a good example. This advice is applicable to all areas of the test.
4) Teenagers are separating from their parents emotionally and value their privacy highly. When interviewing a teen, do it privately (without parents) and also with the parent(s) present.

OTHER PSYCHIATRIC DISORDERS

I. Discussion

Other psychiatric disorders such as obsessive compulsive disorder (OCD), bipolar disorder, minor depression, anxiety, panic disorder, alcohol addiction, attention deficit hyperactivity disorder (ADHD), and ADD may be included in the exams. Not all of these disorders are usually seen together in one exam. The most common psychiatric conditions on the exam are major depression, alcohol abuse, and suicide risk. The question may be as straightforward as querying about the correct drug treatment for the condition, as illustrated in this example.

II. Example

Which of the following drug classes is indicated as first-line treatment of both major depression and OCD?

A) Selective serotonin reuptake inhibitors (SSRIs)
B) Tricyclic antidepressants (TCAs)
C) Mood stabilizers
D) Benzodiazepines

III. Correct Answer: Option A

A) SSRIs

IV. Question Dissection

Best Clues

1) Rule out benzodiazepines, which are used to treat anxiety or insomnia (process of elimination).

2) Mood stabilizers such as lithium salts are used to treat bipolar disorder (process of elimination).

3) The stem is asking for the "first-line treatment" for depression, which is the SSRIs.

Notes

1) TCAs are considered second-line treatment for depression.

2) TCAs are also used as prophylactic treatment of migraine headaches, chronic pain, and neuropathic pain (i.e., tingling, burning) such as post-herpetic neuralgia. *Example of TCA:* amitriptyline (Elavil), nortriptyline (Pamelor).

3) Do not give suicidal patients a prescription for TCAs because of the high risk of hoarding the drug and overdosing. Overdose of TCAs can be fatal (cardiac and CNS toxicity).

4) SSRIs are also first-line treatment for OCD, generalized anxiety disorder (GAD), panic disorder, social anxiety disorder (extreme shyness), and premenstrual mood disorder (fluoxetine or Prozac). *Examples of SSRIs:* citalopram (Celexa), escitalopram (Lexapro), fluoxetine (Prozac), sertraline (Zoloft), paroxetine (Paxil).

5) Anticonvulsants such as carbamazepine (Tegretol) are also used for chronic pain and trigeminal neuralgia.

ABUSIVE SITUATIONS

I. Discussion

Health care workers are required by law to report suspected and actual child abuse to the proper authorities. Abuse-related topics may include domestic violence, physical abuse, child abuse, child neglect, elderly abuse, elderly neglect, and sexual abuse.

II. Example

A 16-year-old teenager with a history of ADHD is brought in to the ED by his mother. She does not want her son to be alone in the room. The NP doing the intake notes several burns on the teen's trunk. Some of the burns appear infected. The NP documents the burns as mostly round in shape and about 0.5 cm (centimeter) in size. Which of the following questions is most appropriate to ask the child's mother?

A) "Your son's back looks terrible. What happened to him?"
B) "Does your son have more friends outside of school?"
C) "Did you burn his back with a cigarette?"
D) "Can you please tell me what happened to your son?"

III. Correct Answer: Option D

D) "Can you please tell me what happened to your son?"

IV. Question Dissection

Best Clues
1) Option D is the only open-ended question in the group.
2) In addition, it is not a judgmental statement.

Notes

1) In general, open-ended questions are usually the correct answer in cases where an NP is trying to elicit the history in an interview.
2) "Your son's back looks terrible. What happened to him?" and "Did you burn his back with a cigarette?"
   - Both are considered judgmental questions and are always the wrong choice.
3) These types of questions are more likely to make people defensive and/or hostile and cause them to end the conversation.
4) "Does your son have more friends outside of school?"
   - This question does not address the immediate issue of the burn marks on the boy's back.
5) Communication tips:
   Questions on Abuse:
   - If a history is being taken, pick the open-ended question first. Interview both the patient and possible "abuser" together, and then interview the patient separately.

   Questions on Depression:
   - Pick the statement that is the most specific to find out if the patient is suicidal or homicidal.
   - Any answer considered judgmental or confrontational is wrong.
   - Do not pick answers that "reassure" patients about their issues, because this discourages them from verbalizing more about it.
   - In addition, do not ignore cultural beliefs. Integrate them into the treatment plan if they are not harmful to the health of the patient.

THE "CAGE" MNEMONIC

I. Discussion

The CAGE is a screening tool used to screen patients for possible alcohol abuse. Scoring two out of four questions is highly suggestive of alcohol abuse. In the exam, you are expected to use higher-level cognitive skills and apply the concepts of CAGE. Examples of this concept are the questions that ask you to pick the patient who is most likely (or least likely) to abuse alcohol.

CAGE Screening Tool (A Score of Two or More Positive Answers Is Suggestive of Alcoholism)

C: Do you feel the need to cut down?
A: Are you annoyed when your friends/spouse comment about your drinking?
G: Do you feel guilty about your drinking?
E: Do you need to drink early in the morning? (Eye-opener)

II. Example

Which of the following individuals is least likely to have an alcohol abuse problem?

A) A housewife who gets annoyed if her best friend talks to her about her drinking habit.
B) A carpenter who drinks one can of beer nightly when playing cards with friends.

C) A nurse who feels shaky when she wakes up, which is relieved by drinking wine.

D) A college student who tells his friend that he drinks only on weekends but feels that he should be drinking less.

III. Correct Answer: Option B

B) A carpenter who drinks one can of beer nightly when playing cards with friends.

IV. Question Dissection

Best Clues

1) Lack of risk factor (one drink of beer at night is considered normal consumption for males).

2) There is no description of any negative effects on the carpenter's daily functioning, social environment, or mental state.

Notes

Any person who feels compelled to drink (or use drugs) no matter what the consequences are to their health, finances, career, friends, and family is addicted to the substance.

1) "A housewife who gets annoyed if her best friend talks to her about her drinking habit." This is the "A" in CAGE ("Annoyed"), a good example of an alcohol abuser getting annoyed when someone close remarks about her drinking problem.

2) "A nurse who feels shaky when she wakes up, which is relieved by drinking wine." This is the "E" in CAGE ("Eye-opener"). The patient is having withdrawal symptoms and must drink in order to feel better.

3) "A college student who tells his friend that he drinks only on weekends but feels that he should be drinking less." This fits the "C" in CAGE ("Cut down"). This student is aware that he is drinking too much.

"FACTOID" QUESTIONS

I. Discussion

Questions that simply ask for facts are what I call "factoid" questions. Some of my review course students in the past have remarked about these types of questions that "you either know the answer or you don't." Unfortunately, this statement is applicable in these types of questions. The correct answer is either based on your memorization of the facts (rote memory) or from a lucky guess. No reasoning or higher-level thinking is required.

II. Example

Which of the following drugs is considered the first-line treatment for an uncomplicated case of Stage I hypertension according to the Joint National Commission on the Evaluation, Management, and Treatment of High Blood Pressure (JNC 7)?

A) ACE inhibitors

B) Thiazide diuretics

C) Calcium channel blockers

D) Beta blockers

III. Correct Answer: Option B

B)   Thiazide diuretics

IV. Question Dissection

Best Clues

1)   There are no clues in the question. It is based on memorization of facts.

> **Notes**
> 1)   Thiazide diuretics are considered the first-line treatment for uncomplicated Stage I hypertension (JNC 7). New guidelines (JNC 8) will be released in the fall/winter of 2013.
> 2)   These drugs are also preferred for hypertensive patients with osteopenia or osteoporosis.
> 3)   The mechanism of action of thiazide on the bone is that it decreases calcium excretion by the kidneys and it stimulates osteoclast activity that helps with bone formation.
> 4)   ACE inhibitors are first-line drugs for hypertensive patients with DM and patients with mild to moderate renal disease.
> 5)   Hypertensive patients with migraines or diabetics who do not have chronic lung disease are good candidates for beta-blocker therapy.
> 6)   Beta blockers are contraindicated in asthmatics or patients with chronic lung diseases such as asthma, chronic obstructive pulmonary disease (COPD), emphysema, or chronic bronchitis.

PHYSICAL ASSESSMENT FINDINGS

I. Discussion

Questions about physical exam findings are plentiful. Learn the classic presentation of disease and emergent conditions. The knowledge of normal findings, as well as some variants, is important for the exam. In addition, if the question style used is negatively worded, careful reading is essential.

II. Example

An older woman complains of a new onset of severe pain in her right ear after taking swimming classes for 2 weeks. On physical exam, the right ear canal is red and swollen. Purulent green exudate is seen inside. All of the following are true statements except:

A)   Pulling on the tragus is painful.
B)   The tympanic membrane is translucent with intact landmarks.
C)   The external ear canal is swollen and painful.
D)   Pain on palpation of the mastoid area.

III. Correct Answer: Option D

D)   Pain on palpation over the mastoid area.

IV. Question Dissection

Best Clues

1)   Positive risk factor (history of swimming)
2)   Classic signs (reddened and swollen ear canal with green exudate)

Notes
1) Acute otitis externa is a superficial infection of the skin in the ear canal. It is more common during warm and humid conditions such as swimming and summertime.
2) The most common bacterial pathogen is *Pseudomonas* (bright green pus).
3) Otitis externa does not involve the middle ear or the tympanic membrane.
4) Acute mastoiditis is a possible complication of AOM.

NEGATIVE POLARITY QUESTIONS

I. Discussion

The current item-writing guidelines discourage the use of negative polarity question design. The use of all-inclusive words such as "all," "always," and "never" or "except" is also avoided. Questions now are usually written in a positive format. Answer options such as "all of the above" or "none of the above" are now rarely used.

An example of a negatively worded question is "All of the following are false statements about colonic diverticula except." An example of the same question written with a positive stem is "Which of the following is the correct statement about colonic diverticula?"

II. Example

"Which of the following is a correct statement about colonic diverticula?"
A) Diverticula are more common in young adults.
B) Diverticula formation happens over a period of months.
C) Mild cases of diverticulitis can be managed outside the hospital.
D) Dietary fiber supplementation is not recommended.

III. Correct Answer: Option C

C) Mild cases of diverticulitis can be managed outside the hospital.

IV. Question Dissection

Best Clues
1) The words "mild cases" of diverticulitis is the most important clue.
2) Know the difference between "diverticula" and "diverticulitis."

Notes
1) Diverticula are diagnosed by colonoscopy. Diverticula are asymptomatic, small, polyp-like pouches on the wall of the colon.
2) They are more common in Western society due to low intake of dietary fiber.
3) Diverticula and diverticulitis are rarely seen below the age of 50 years.
4) Mild cases of acute diverticulitis in stable patients are managed in the outpatient setting with antibiotics such as ciprofloxacin 500 mg PO BID plus metronidazole PO TID × 10 to 14 days.
5) Recommend fiber supplementation such as psyllium (Metamucil) and soluble fibers such as guar gum fiber, inulin, and apple pectin.
6) Diverticulitis infections can become life-threatening.

TWO-PART QUESTIONS

I. Discussion

Fortunately, there are usually only one to two questions of this type per exam. These questions are problematic because the two questions are dependent on each other.

To solve both correctly, the test taker must answer the first portion by figuring out the diagnosis in order to solve the second question correctly.

II. Example

Part One

An adolescent male reports the new onset of symptoms 1 week after returning from a hiking trip in North Carolina. He presents with complaints of high fever, severe headache, muscle aches, and nausea. The symptoms are accompanied by a generalized red rash that is not pruritic. The rash initially appeared on both ankles and wrists and then spread toward the patient's trunk. The rash involves both the palms and the soles. Which of the following conditions is most likely?

A) Meningococcemia
B) Rocky Mountain spotted fever (RMSF)
C) Idiopathic thrombocytopenic purpura (ITP)
D) Lyme disease

Part Two

Which of the following is the best treatment plan to follow?

A) Refer the patient to the hospital ED.
B) Refer the patient to an infectious disease specialist.
C) Initiate a prescription of oral glucocorticoids.
D) Collect a blood specimen for culture and sensitivity.

III. Correct Answers

Part One: Option B

B) Rocky Mountain spotted fever (RMSF)

Part Two: Option A

A) Refer the patient to the hospital ED.

IV. Question Dissection

Best Clues
Part One

1) Location and activity (south central U.S., outdoor activity)
2) Classic rash (red rash on both wrists and ankles that spreads centrally with involvement of the palms and the soles)
3) Systemic symptoms (high fever, headache, myalgia, nausea)

Part Two

1) Knowledge of the emergent nature of RMSF (can cause death if not treated within the first 8 days of symptoms).

Notes

1) Early treatment is important and empiric treatment should be started early if RMSF is suspected. Refer the patient to the closest ED as soon as possible.
2) It may be difficult to distinguish RMSF from meningococcemia before the blood culture results and the CSF culture results are available.
3) RMSF:
   - Dog/wood tick bite; spirochete called *Rickettsia rickettsia*.
   - Treat with doxycycline 100 mg PO/IV for a minimum of 7 days.
4) Early Lyme disease (erythema migrans rash stage):
   - Ixodes (deer) tick bite; spirochete called *Borrelia burgdorferi*.
   - Treat with doxycycline × 21 days.
   - Majority of the cases are in the Mid-Atlantic and New England states (i.e., CT, MA, NY, NJ, PA).
5) ITP severity ranges from mild to severe (platelet count less than 30,000/μL). Platelets are broken down by the spleen, causing thrombocytopenia. Look for easy bruising, petechiae, purpura, epistaxis, and gingival bleeding (combined with low platelet count).
6) Initial treatment for ITP is glucocorticoids (i.e., prednisone) based on platelet response.

NORMAL PHYSICAL EXAM FINDINGS

I. Discussion

A good review of normal physical exam findings and some benign variants is necessary. Pertinent physical exam findings are discussed at the beginning of each organ system review.

A good resource to use in your review is the advanced physical assessment textbook that was used in your program. Keep in mind that sometimes questions about normal physical findings are written as if they were a pathological process. This is important when you encounter these types of questions.

II. Example

A 13-year-old girl complains of an irregular menstrual cycle. She started menarche 6 months ago. Her last menstrual period was 2 months ago. She denies being sexually active. Her urine pregnancy test is negative. Which of the following would you advise the child's mother?

A) Consult with a pediatric endocrinologist to rule out problems with the hypothalamus, pituitary, and adrenal (HPA) axis.
B) Advise the mother that irregular menstrual cycles are common during the first year after menarche.
C) Advise the mother that her child is starting menarche early and has precocious puberty.
D) Ask the medical assistant to get labs drawn for TSH, follicle stimulating hormone (FSH), and estradiol levels.

III. Correct Answer: Option B

B) Advise the mother that irregular menstrual cycles are common during the first year after menarche.

IV. Question Dissection

Best Clues
1) Patient recently started menarche 6 months ago (knowledge of pubertal changes).
2) The teen is not sexually active (rule out pertinent negative, such as the negative pregnancy test).

Notes
1) This question describes normal growth and development in adolescents.
2) When girls start menarche, their periods may be very irregular for several months up to 2 years.

ADOLESCENCE

I. Discussion

During this period of life, numerous changes are occurring, both physically and emotionally. Adolescents are thinking in more abstract ways and are psychologically separating from their parents. The opinions of peers are more important than those of the parents. Privacy is a big issue in this age group and should be respected.

II. Example

Which of the following is the second highest cause of mortality among adolescents and young adults in this country?
A) Suicide
B) Smoking
C) Homicide
D) Illicit drug use

III. Correct Answer: Option C

C) Homicide

IV. Question Dissection
Best Clues
1) Rote memory (homicide is now the second highest cause of mortality among adolescents).

Notes
1) The number one cause of mortality in this age group is motor vehicle accidents.
2) The second most common cause of mortality from age 15 to 24 years in the United States is homicide (CDC, 2013).

3) Screening for depression in all adolescents is recommended. Signs of a depressed teen include falling grades, acting out, avoiding socializing, moodiness, and so forth.
4) Smoking is ruled out because its health effects take decades (i.e., COPD).
5) Most deaths from congenital heart disease are during infancy. Mortality from illicit drug use is more common among adults.

LEGAL RIGHTS OF MINORS

I. Discussion

Certain legal issues that are not seen in adult patients exist in this age group. These are the issues of confidentiality and right to consent without parental involvement.

II. Example

All of the following can be considered emancipated minors except:
A) A 15-year-old who is married
B) A 16-year-old who is married and has one child
C) A 17-year-old who is on active duty with the U.S. Army
D) A 16-year-old who has his own job.

III. Correct Answer: Option D

D) A 16-year-old who has his own job.

IV. Question Dissection

Best Clues
1) No clues. Knowledge of adolescent legal issues is needed to answer this question.

Notes

1) *Minor:* a person who is under the age of 18 years. The "age of majority" or the age of 18 years is when an adolescent is considered as a legal adult in the United States. Some exceptions exist (in some states, the age of majority is 19 years).
2) *Emancipated minors:* a person under the age of 18 years who has the full legal rights of an adult such as signing legal contracts and consents.
3) Minors who are parents are not considered emancipated unless they are legally married. Minors who are single parents may give consent for the care of their children, but not for their own medical care.
4) Criteria for an emancipated minor (United States):
   - Any minor who is legally married
   - Any minor who is enlisted on active duty in the U.S. military
   - A minor who has obtained emancipation through the court or a "Declaration of Emancipation"

DIFFERENTIAL DIAGNOSIS

I. Discussion

Differential diagnoses are the conditions whose presentations share many similarities. For example, the differential diagnoses to consider for chronic cough (a cough lasting more than 8 weeks) are: asthma, GERD, ACE inhibitors, chronic bronchitis, and lung infections such as TB (and many more). In this type of question, the differential diagnoses are the distractors.

II. Example

A 57-year-old male walks into an urgent care center. The patient complains of an episode of chest pain in his upper sternum that is relieved after he stops the offending activity. He has had several episodes of the chest pain before. A fasting total lipid profile is ordered. The result reveals total cholesterol of 180 mg/dL, an LDL of 120 mg/dL, and a high-density lipoprotein (HDL) of 25 mg/dL. Which of the following is most likely?

A) Acute esophagitis
B) MI
C) GERD
D) Angina

III. Correct Answer: Option D

C) Angina

IV. Question Dissection

Best Clues

1) Classic presentation (chest pain that is precipitated by exertion and is relieved by rest)
2) History (several episodes of the same chest pain)
3) Positive risk factors (low HDL, elevated lipid levels, age, and gender)

> ### Notes
>
> All four answer options are some common conditions that can mimic angina (differential diagnoses). Rule out the pertinent negatives.
>
> 1) Pain is relieved by rest (angina). If pain not relieved by rest, then rule out angina.
> 2) Presence of risk factors for heart disease and chest pain (angina, MI).
> 3) Physical activity aggravates condition (angina, MI).
> 4) Lack of history of aggravating factors such as intake of certain meds such as NSAIDs, aspirin, bisphosphonates, or alcohol (rule out esophagitis).
> 5) Chest pain is not related to meals (rule out GERD).

CLASSIC PRESENTATION

I. Discussion

Since certification exams are administered all over the country, the questions are written to conform to the classic "textbook presentation." This allows the test to be valid and statistically sound. All of the questions on the exam are referenced by at least two to three reliable sources. For both exams, a large number of clinical questions are referenced by popular medical and nursing textbooks.

The disease process is described at its height, although in real-life practice, the signs and/or symptoms are dependent upon the stage of the illness. For example, for the majority of disease processes, usually the prodromal period or the early phase is asymptomatic or mildly symptomatic, while during the height of the illness, the full signs and symptoms are usually present.

II. Example

While performing a routine physical exam on an older White male with a history of cigarette smoking, the NP palpates a pulsatile mass in the patient's midabdominal area. A bruit is auscultated over the soft mass. Which of the following is the recommended imaging method?

A) CT scan
B) Abdominal ultrasound
C) Radiography of the chest
D) Plain film of the abdomen

III. Correct Answer: Option B

B) Abdominal ultrasound

IV. Question Dissection

Best Clues

1) Pulsatile mass located in the middle of the abdomen that is associated with a bruit
2) Patient demographics

Notes

1) This question describes the classic case of an abdominal aortic aneurysm (AAA).
2) Risk factors for AAA are male gender, elderly, smoker, hypertension, White race, and family history.
3) Signs and symptoms of AAA rupture are abrupt onset of severe abdominal pain with low back pain and abdominal distension with signs and symptoms of shock.
4) The initial imaging diagnostic test to order is the abdominal ultrasound.

ETHNIC BACKGROUND

I. Discussion

Ethnic background is an important clue for certain genetic disorders. For example, Tay-Sachs, a rare and fatal genetic disorder, is most common among Eastern European (Ashkenazi) Jews.

A warning about ethnic background: It can also be used as a distractor. In the majority of medical conditions, the patient's ethnic background does not affect the treatment plan or the patient's response to treatment. The next question is an example of this concept.

II. Example

Which of the following laboratory tests is a sensitive indicator of renal function in people of African descent?

A) Serum blood urea nitrogen (BUN)
B) Serum creatinine concentration
C) Estimated glomerular filtration rate (GFR)
D) Serum BUN-to-creatinine ratio

The question in this example can also be phrased as:

Which of the following laboratory tests is a sensitive indicator of renal function in people of Hispanic descent? Or Asian descent?

III. Correct Answer: Option C

C) Estimated GFR

IV. Question Dissection

Best Clues

1) Knowledge that the estimated GFR is a better test of renal function compared with the serum creatinine concentration.

Notes

1) A GFR value of 60 or less is a sign of kidney damage (refer to a nephrologist).
2) The GFR is an "estimated" value (it is not measured directly) and is computed by using the serum creatinine value in the Cockcroft–Gault (or the MDRD Study) equations.
3) The serum creatinine is affected by age (less sensitive in elderly), gender (higher in males), ethnicity (higher with African background), and other factors.
4) The BUN is a waste product of the protein from foods that you have eaten. If you eat more protein before the test, it will increase (or decrease with low protein intake).
5) Dehydration will elevate the BUN value.

3

Pharmacology Review

During your review, memorize both the drug class and the representative drug(s) for that particular class. The reason is that sometimes drugs are listed by class only. Memorizing drug doses is generally not emphasized to the same extent as the NCLEX-RN® examination. Higher-level thinking skills, such as knowledge of drug indications and drug safety issues, are considered more important in the NP examinations.

Learn about clinically important drug "safety" issues, such as drug–drug interactions, disease–drug interactions, and the adverse reactions that are seen in the primary care area. For example, one of the most common drug interactions in the primary care area is between warfarin sodium (Coumadin) and Bactrim (trimethoprim-sulfamethoxazole). Sulfa drugs will interact with warfarin (increases the blood level), which results in an elevation of the INR and the risk of bleeding.

The most common question about drugs (prescription and over-the-counter [OTC]) is related to disease management. These questions will involve the correct drug(s) used to treat a condition.

The drugs that are included in the examinations are usually the "older" drugs that have been in use for several years to several decades (e.g., amoxicillin). Drugs that have been recently released (past 6 to 12 months or less) will not be included on the examinations. Lately, there have been a few questions about pharmacokinetics (e.g., first-pass metabolism, excretion).

This section is not meant to be a comprehensive review of pharmacology. The goal is to help you understand certain basic pharmacologic concepts, drug interactions, disease–drug interactions, types of laboratory tests needed for certain medications, and various other issues.

ORAL DRUGS: FIRST-PASS HEPATIC METABOLISM (OR FIRST-PASS EFFECT)

All oral drugs must go through "first-pass metabolism" before they can be used by the body. When a drug is swallowed, it is absorbed through the gastrointestinal (GI) tract where it enters the portal circulation. After the drug enters the liver, it is metabolized (biotransformation) and then released into the systemic circulation.

"First-pass metabolism" lowers the amount of active drug available to the body. If a drug has a high first-pass effect, most of it becomes "inactivated" and cannot be used by the body.

Drugs that have extensive first-pass metabolism cannot be given by the oral route. A good example is insulin, which, if given by the oral route, is completely broken down in the GI tract (by enzymes). To bypass first-pass metabolism, insulin must be given by injection.

DRUG METABOLISM (BIOTRANSFORMATION)

The most active organ is the liver (cytochrome P450 enzyme system). The other organ systems are the kidneys, the GI tract (breakdown by gut bacteria), and the lungs (CO_2).

DRUG EXCRETION

Almost all drugs/chemicals are broken down by the liver and excreted from the body in the bile, urine, feces, respiratory gas (CO_2), and as sweat (sweat glands). It is unusual to have a drug that is totally (100%) broken down by only one organ (e.g., kidneys only). Most drugs are excreted by both the liver and the kidneys. For example, oral furosemide is excreted mainly through the kidneys (50%) and some through feces.

PHARMACOLOGY TERMS

- Half-life (t½): the amount of time in which drug concentration decreases by 50%.
- Area under the curve (AUC): the average amount of a drug in the blood after a dose is given. It is a measure of the availability (bioavailability) of a drug after it is administered.
- Minimum inhibitory concentration (MIC): the lowest concentration of an antibiotic that will inhibit the growth of organisms (after overnight incubation).
- Maximum concentration: the highest concentration of a drug after a dose.
- Trough (minimum concentration): the lowest concentration of a drug after a dose.

POTENT INHIBITORS OF THE CYTOCHROME P450 (CYP450) SYSTEM

The following are some "problematic" drugs. These drugs are responsible for a large number of drug–drug interactions. Drugs that act as inhibitors slow down drug clearance (increase drug concentration). When this happens, the patient is at high risk for a drug overdose and adverse effects. When a test question is asking about a drug interaction, think of these drugs.

- Macrolides (erythromycin, clarithromycin, pediazole)
- Antifungals (ketoconazole, fluconazole)
- Cisapride (Propulsid). This drug has been pulled from the U.S. market.
- Cimetidine (Tagament)
- Citaprolam (Celexa)

NARROW THERAPEUTIC INDEX DRUGS*

- Warfarin sodium (Coumadin): monitor INR.
- Digoxin (Lanoxin): monitor digoxin level, EKG, electrolytes (potassium, magnesium, calcium).
- Theophylline: monitor blood levels.
- Carbamezapine (Tegretol) and phenytoin (Dilantin): monitor blood levels.
- Levothyroxine: monitor TSH.
- Lithium: monitor blood levels, TSH (risk of hypothyroidism).

---

* List is not all-inclusive.

Table 3.1 Safety Issues With Some Prescription Drugs*

Drug Class and Generic and Trade Names	Exam Tips
Thiazolidinediones (TZDs)	Black Box Warning: cause or exacerbate CHF in some patients. Do not use if NYHA Class III or IV heart failure
Pioglitazone (Actos)	Stop if: c/o dyspnea, weight gain, cough (heart failure)
Atypical antipsychotics Risperidone (Risperdal) Olanzapine (Zyprexa) Quietipine (Seroquel)	High risk of weight gain, metabolic syndrome, and type 2 diabetes. Monitor weight every 3 months. Black Box Warning: higher mortality in elderly patients. Monitor: TSH, lipids, weight/body mass index (BMI)
Bisphosphonates Alendronate (Fosamax) Risedronate (Actonel)	Jaw pain (jaw necrosis). Chest pain, difficulty swallowing, burning mid-back (perforation). Take alone upon awakening with 8 oz glass water (NOT juice) before breakfast. Do not lie down × 30 minutes afterward. Do not mix with other drugs). Take first thing in the morning before breakfast
Statins Atorvastatin (Lipitor) Lovastatin (Mevacor) Rosuvastatin (Crestor) Simvastatin (Zocor)	Do not mix with grapefruit juice Drug-induced hepatitis or rhabdomyolysis higher if mixed with azole antifungals High-dose Zocor (80 mg) has highest risk of rhabdomyolysis (muscle pain/tenderness) CK (creatine kinase) level goes up.
Lincosamides Clindamycin (Cleocin)	Higher risk of *Clostridium difficile*-associated diarrhea (CDAD) Metronidazole (Flagyl) PO TID × 10–14 days Probiotics daily—BID × few weeks

* List is not all-inclusive.

DRUGS USED TO TREAT HEART DISEASE

Cardiac Glycosides: Digoxin (Lanoxin)

- Treats atrial fibrillation.
  - Digoxin has a narrow therapeutic range (0.5–2.0 ng/mL). Not a first-line drug for heart rate control in atrial fibrillation.
- Signs and symptoms of digoxin overdose:
  - Initial symptoms are gastrointestinal (anorexia, nausea/vomiting, abdominal pain). Others are arrhythmias, confusion, and visual changes (yellowish green tinged-color vision, scotomas).
  - Severe toxicity is treated with digoxin-binding antibodies (Digibind).
- What laboratory test should be ordered if digoxin toxicity is suspected?
  - Order a digoxin level, electrolytes (potassium, magnesium, calcium), creatinine, and serial EKGs.
- Potassium values (adult to elderly):
  Critical: Less than 2.5 or greater than 6.5 mEq/L.
  Normal: 3.5 to 5.0 mEq/L.

Anticoagulants: Warfarin Sodium (Coumadin)

- Decreases emboli/thrombi formation (atrial fibrillation, stroke, pulmonary emboli).
- For atrial fibrillation, the target INR is from 2.0 to 3.0.

- A patient has an INR of 8.0. Physical examination is negative for petechiae, bleeding gums, bruising, or dark stools. What is the best treatment plan for this patient?
  - INR between 5.0 and 9.0 (without bleeding): Hold the warfarin for 1 to 2 doses. Recheck INR every 2 to 3 days until it is stable (INR between 2.0 and 3.0). Another option is to hold the warfarin and add a small dose of oral vitamin K. Limit and/or avoid high vitamin K foods (green leafy vegetables, broccoli, brussels sprouts, cabbage). After the INR becomes stable, recheck it monthly.*

📋 CLINICAL TIPS

- INR values below 2.0 increase stroke risk sixfold.
- There is a higher risk of hemorrhage with high INRs in the elderly (age greater than 70 years).
- Mayonnaise, canola oil, and soybean oil also have high levels of vitamin K.

DIURETICS

Thiazide Diuretics

- Uncomplicated hypertension (first line), heart failure (first line), edema.
- Hypertension accompanied by osteoporosis.
- Hydrochlorothiazide (HCTZ) 12.5 to 25 mg PO daily.
- Chlorthalidone 12.5 to 25 mg PO daily.
- Indapamide (Lozol) PO daily.

Adverse Effects

- Hyperglycemia (careful with diabetics).
- Elevates triglycerides and LDL (careful if preexisting hypertriglyceremia).
- Elevates uric acid (can precipitate a gout attack).
- Hypokalemia (muscle weakness, arrythymia).

Pharma Notes

- Patients with both hypertension and osteoporosis have an extra benefit from thiazides.
- Thiazide diuretics decrease calcium excretion by the kidneys and stimulate osteoclast formation.
- Patients with serious sulfa allergies should avoid thiazide diuretics. Potassium-sparing diuretics such as triamterene and amiloride (Midamor) are the alternative options for these patients.
- Chlorthalidone is longer acting and more potent than HCTZ.

Potassium-Sparing Diuretics

- Hypertension, alternative diuretic for patients with severe sulfa allergy.
- Triamterene (Dyrenium).
- Amiloride (Midamor).

---

* UpToDate.com. Correcting excess anticoagulation after warfarin (May 2012).

- Combination: triamterene and HCTZ (Dyazide), amiloride and HCTZ (Moduretic).
- Black Box Warning: Hyperkalemias, which can be fatal. Higher risk with renal impairment, diabetes, elderly, severely ill.
- Monitor serum potassium frequently (baseline, during, dose changes, illness).

Pharma Notes
- Do not give potassium supplement. Avoid using salt substitutes that contain potassium.
- Be careful with combinations of ACEI/angiotensin-receptor blockers (ARBs); increases risk of hyperkalemia.
- Avoid with severe renal disease (increases risk of hyperkalemia).

Loop Diuretics
- Edema from heart failure, cirrhosis, renal disease, hypertension.
- Loop diuretics are excreted via the loop of Henle of the kidneys and are more potent than HCTZ.
- Furosemide (Lasix) PO BID.
- Bumetanide (Bumex).
- More potent than thiazides, but with shorter duration of action (BID).
- Black Box Warning: excessive amounts of furosemide may lead to profound diuresis. Medical supervision required, individualized dose schedule.

Adverse Effect
- Electrolytes (hypokalemia, hyponatremia/low sodium, low levels of chlorine).
- Hypovolemia and hypotension (dizziness, lightheadedness).
- Pancreatitis, jaundice, rash.
- Ototoxicity (worsens aminoglycoside ototoxicity effect if combined).

Aldosterone Antagonists
- Hirsuitism, hypertension, severe heart failure
- Spironolactone (Aldactone)

Pharma Notes
- Adverse effects are galactorrhea and hyperkalemia. Spironolactone is rarely used to treat hypertension in primary care due to adverse effects and higher risk of certain cancers.
- Black Box Warning: increases risk of both benign and malignant tumors.

DRUGS USED TO TREAT HYPERTENSION
Beta-Blockers (Beta Antagonists)
- Hypertension, post-myocardial infarction (first line), angina, arrhythmias, migraine prophylaxis.
- Adjunct treatment: hyperthyroidism/thyrotoxicosis (decreases heart rate, anxiety).

- Migraine prophylaxis.
  - Non-cardioselective (blocks beta-1 and beta-2).
- Propanolol immediate release (Inderal) or extended release (Inderal LA).
- Timolol oral (Blocadren) or timolol ophthalmic drops (glaucoma).
- Cardioselective (blocks beta-1 only).
  - Atenolol (Tenormin) daily.
  - Metoprolol immediate release (Lopressor) or extended release (Toprol XL).

Adverse Effects

- Bronchospasm
- Bradycardia
- Depression, fatigue (careful with elderly)
- Erectile dysfunction (ED)
- Blunts hypoglycemic response (warn diabetic patients)
- Contraindications:
  - Asthma (causes bronchoconstriction)
  - COPD (causes bronchoconstriction)
  - Chronic bronchitis (causes bronchoconstriction).
  - Emphysema (causes bronchoconstriction).
  - Bradycardia and AV-block (second- to third-degree block; Table 3.2).

Table 3.2 Drug Contraindications*

Drug Class and Generic and Trade Names	Contraindications
ACE Inhibitors	Avoid potassium supplements
Lisinopril (Zestril)	Careful with potassium-sparing diuretics
Captoril (Capoten)	ACE inhibitor cough—new onset of dry cough (not accompanied by URI symptoms)
ARBs	First-line choice for diabetics
Valsartan (Diovan)	First-line choice for mild to moderate renal disease
Losartan (Cozaar)	
Potassium-sparing diuretics	Higher risk of hyperkalemia if combined with ACEI or ARBs and with severe renal disease
Triamterene (Dyrenium)	Diuretics may worsen urinary incontinence
Triamterene + HCTZ (Dyazide)	
Amiloride (Midamor)	
Beta Blockers Propranolol (Inderal), atenolol (Tenormin), metoprolol (Lopressor), pindolol (Visken)	Contraindicated if patient has chronic lung diseases (asthma, COPD, emphysema, chronic bronchitis) Do not discontinue beta-blockers abruptly due to severe rebound (hypertensive crisis)
Sildenafil (Viagra)	Do not mix with nitrates (nitroglycerine, isosorbide dinitrate) and some alpha-blockers. Erection greater than 4 hours—refer to ED
Tadalafil (Cialis)	Do not give within 3 to 6 months of an MI, stroke

* List is not all-inclusive.

ACE INHIBITORS (ACEIs) AND ARBs

- Hypertension, diabetes (renal), chronic kidney disease (CKD), others.
- Category C (first trimester) and Category D (second to third trimesters).
- ACE inhibition blocks conversion of angiotensin I to angiotensin II (potent vasoconstrictor).
- ARBs block angiotensin II (less aldosterone). ACEI suffix of "pril." ARB suffix of "sartan."
- Black Box Warning: ACEI can cause death/injury to the developing fetus during the second and third trimesters. Discontinue ACEIs and ARBs immediately if pregnant.

ACEIs

- Lisinopril (Zestril, Prinivil)
- Combination: lisinopril and HCTZ (Zestoretic)
- Benazepril (Lotensin)
- Captopril (Capoten)
- Enalapril (Vasotec)

ARBs

- Losartan (Cozaar)
- Irbesartan (Avapro)
- Contraindication: ACEI-/ARB-associated angioedema, hereditary angioedema

Adverse Effects

- Angioedema and anaphylactoid reactions
- ACEI cough
- Hyperkalemia

Pharma Notes

- ACEI cough occurs within the first few months of treatment. It is a dry and hacking cough (without other symptoms of URI). Stop ACEI and switch to an ARB.
- First-line drug for hypertension in diabetics (diabetic nephropathy).
- First-line drug for patients with (proteinuric) CKD.
- Avoid using salt substitutes that contain potassium.
- Captopril associated with agranulocytosis, neutropenia, leukopenia (rare). Monitor CBC.
- Both ACEIs and ARBs are excreted in breast milk (breastfeeding mothers should avoid them).

📋 CLINICAL TIP

Be careful prescribing ACEIs/ARBs to sexually active, reproductive-aged females who are not consistently using birth control (Category C and Category D during the second and third trimester).

CALCIUM CHANNEL BLOCKERS

- Hypertension, Raynauds phenomenon (first line)
- Amlodipine (Norvasc)
- Diltiazem (Cardizem)
- Nifedipine (Procardia)
- Verapamil (Calan): Do not mix with erythromycin and clarithromycin (drug interaction)
- Contraindications
  - AV-block (second- to third-degree block)
  - Bradycardia
  - Congestive heart failure (CHF)

Pharma Notes

- Educate patients to avoid grapefruit juice (toxicity results as it will increase drug level).
- Possible drug interactions: intraconazole, macrolides (except azithromycin).

Adverse Effects
- Headache (vasodilation)
- Peripheral edema (not due to fluid overload)
- Bradycardia
- Heart failure and heart block
- Hypotension, QT prolongation
- Constipation is the most commonly reported side effect

ALPHA-BLOCKERS

- Hypertension with coexisting BPH.
- Terazosin (Hytrin) 1 mg PO at bedtime (lowest dose).

Pharma Notes

- Not a first-line choice except for males with both hypertension and BPH.
- Potent vasodilator. Common side effects are dizziness and hypotension. Give at bedtime at very low dose and slowly titrate up. Careful with frail elderly (risk of syncope and falls).

ANTIBIOTICS

Antibiotic Case Scenarios

Case 1

Penicillin-Allergic Patient With Strep Throat (A Gram-Positive Bacterial Infection)
An 18-year-old female has a positive throat C&S for *Strep pyogenes* (Group A beta strepto-cocci). The patient reports a history of an allergic reaction to penicillin with "swollen lips" accompanied by urticaria. Which of the following is the most appropriate treatment?

A) Clarithromycin (Biaxin) 250 mg PO BID × 10 days
B) Gargle with salt water 3 times a day
C) Cephalexin (Keflex) 250 mg PO QID × 10 days
D) Doxycycline 100 mg PO BID × 10 days

Question Dissection

The correct answer is Option A.

Best Clues

- Positive C&S for strep.
- Report of a penicillin allergy.
- Rule out the following options because:
  - Option B (gargling with salt water is for symptoms and will not eradicate strep).
  - Option C (penicillin-allergic patients may also be allergic to cephalosporins).
  - Option D (doxycycline not effective for gram-positive infections).

Pharma Notes

- Become familiar with alternative antibiotics for penicillin-allergic patients. A good alternative antibiotic for PCN-allergic patients with gram-positive bacterial infections are macrolides such as azithromycin × 5 days (Z-Pack) or clarithromycin (Biaxin) PO BID.
- Clindamycin (Cleocin) is also an alternative, but it is associated with slightly higher risk for *C. difficile* colitis.

Case 2

Patient With Both Mononucleosis and Strep Throat Infection

A 16-year-old high school athlete is returning for follow-up for a severe sore throat. The test result reveals a positive throat culture for Group A beta hemolytic strep and a positive Monospot test (heterophile antibody test). What is the best *initial* clinical management of this patient?

A) Initiate a prescription of amoxicillin 500 mg PO TID × 10 days.
B) Initiate a prescription of penicillin VK 250 mg PO QID × 10 days.
C) Order an Epstein-Barr virus (EBV) titer to determine whether the patient has an acute or a reactivated mononucleosis infection.
D) Write a prescription for an abdominal ultrasound to determine the size of the patient's liver and spleen.

Question Dissection

Correct answer is Option B.

Best Clues

- Positive test results (Monospot and strep).
- Rule out:
  - Option A (avoid using amoxicillin due to high risk of a "drug rash" that is not due to an allergy).

– Option C (not for initial management; strep infection must be treated first before ordering labs).
– Option D (not for initial management; only for cases where the PE reveals an enlarged liver and/or spleen).

Pharma Notes

In the case of rash in mononucleosis patients, it is very hard to determine whether the rash is due to a true allergy or whether the patient has a benign nonallergic drug rash. About 70% to 90% of patients with mono taking amoxicillin may break out with a "nonallergic" generalized maculopapular rash (mechanism is not well understood). If a patient has both mono and strep throat, avoid using amoxicillin or ampicillin. Instead, use penicillin (if not allergic) or a macrolide to treat the patient.

📋 CLINICAL TIP

Up to 10% of patients may report being allergic to penicillin. A very small percentage (0.17%–8.4%) will also react to a cephalosporin.

Case 3

Young Adult With History of GI Symptoms After Taking Erythromycin

A 25-year-old healthy adult is diagnosed with atypical pneumonia by the NP. The patient reports a history of nausea, upset stomach, and vomiting with erythromycin. The patient is complaining of a sore throat. The vital signs are temperature of 99°F, pulse of 80/minute, and respiratory rate of 12 breaths/minute. What is the most appropriate treatment plan for this patient?

A) Initiate a prescription of azithromycin (Z-Pack) PO × 5 days.
B) Initiate a prescription of trimethoprim-sulfamethazole (Bactrim) 1 tab PO BID × 10 days.
C) Order a chest x-ray with the anterior–posterior and lateral views.
D) Order a sputum for culture and sensitivity.

Question Dissection

Correct answer is Option A.

Best Clues

Because the patient has a definite diagnosis of atypical pneumonia, ordering additional tests will not change the treatment outcome (rule out Options C and D). Bactrim is not effective against *Mycoplasma* or *Chlamydia* bacterial infections (rule out Option B), but it is an excellent drug for certain gram-negative infections. For community-acquired pneumonia, ordering a sputum for C&S is not recommended (rule out Option D).

Pharma Notes

GI upset (N/V, abdominal pain) are common side effects of erythromycin—it is not an allergic reaction (such as angioedema, hives, anaphylaxis). If a patient who needs a macrolide is not allergic, azithromycin (Z-Pack) is a good choice. It usually does not cause GI side effects, has fewer drug interactions, and a broader spectrum of activity. If the patient is allergic to macrolides, an alternative is doxycycline PO BID or the new generation quinolones (Levaquin, Avelox).

CLINICAL PEARL

Consider macrolide-resistant *Strep pneumoniae* if the patient was on a macrolide the previous 3 months.

Case 4

Answer Options Listed by Drug Class

A 65-year-old male presents with a history of a chronic cough that is productive of large amounts of off-white to light-yellow colored sputum. The patient reports a history of cigarette smoking. The chest x-ray reveals hyperinflation with flattened diaphragms and several small bullae. Which of the following drug classes is the initial treatment of choice for this condition?

A) Short-acting B2 agonists.
B) Anticholinergics.
C) Pneumococcal polysaccharide vaccine (Pneumovax).
D) Oxygen by nasal cannula.

Question Dissection

The correct answer is Option B.

Best Clues

Arriving at the correct answer is based on your knowledge of the step-wise approach to COPD treatment. Notice that the stem of the question is asking for the "initial treatment" (rule out options A, C, and D).

Pharma Notes

The initial treatment of choice for chronic bronchitis/COPD is ipratropium bromide or Atrovent (an anticholinergic). If the question is asking you for the next step (if symptoms are not better with Atrovent), then add a short-acting beta-2 agonist (albuterol) or both drugs combined (Combivent). Pneumovax is recommended for all with COPD—it is considered a primary prevention measure.

Antibiotics

Antibiotic drugs are either bacteriostatic or bactericidal. Bactericidal antibiotics kill bacteria. Bacteriostatic antibiotics limit bacterial growth and replication (limits the infection). The result is a lower bacterial count, which helps the immune system clear the infection.

TETRACYCLINES (CATEGORY D)

Tetracyclines may cause permanent discoloration of teeth (yellow-brown to gray) and skeletal defects if taken during the last half of pregnancy, in infancy, or by children less than 8 years of age.

Generally, tetracycline is used to treat acne starting at age 13 to 14 years. By this age, all of the permanent teeth have erupted (except wisdom teeth).

- Doxycycline PO BID (first-line chlamydial and atypical bacterial infections).
- Minocycline (has more side effects and adverse reactions).
- Tetracycline (first-line moderate to severe acne, rosacea).

Adverse Reactions

- Photosensitivity reaction (severe sunburns) from minimal sunlight exposure. Avoid or minimize sunlight exposure; use sunblock, wide-brim hats, and sunglasses.
- Esophageal ulcerations (rare). Swallow tablet completely using a full glass of water.
- Contraindications: Avoid use in pregnancy, infancy, and in children aged 8 years or younger.

Pharma Notes

1) Do not use oral tetracycline for mild acne (comedones). Use only topicals.
2) For mild acne not responding to OTCs, trial prescription topicals (Benzamycin, Retin-A).
3) Consider adding tetracycline if a patient with moderate acne is not responding to topical prescriptions (Benzamyzin, Retin-A) after 2 to 3 months.
4) Tetracycline binds to some minerals (calcium, dairy products, iron, magnesium, zinc). It's best to take it on an empty stomach. Take 1 hour before or 2 hours after a meal.
5) Tetracyclines may decrease effectiveness of oral contraceptive pills.
6) Doxycycline is first line for chlamydial infections (i.e., cervicitis, PID, atypical pneumonia) and other atypical bacteria like ureaplasma or mycoplasma (i.e., nongonococcal urethritis).

CLINICAL NOTES

- A common side effect of minocycline (Minocin) is vertigo and dizziness (vestibular dysfunction).
- Advise patients to throw away expired tetracycline pills (they degenerate and may cause nephropathy or Fanconi syndrome; Table 3.3).

MACROLIDES (CATEGORY B)

Compared with other antibiotic drug classes, macrolides (and quinolones) are associated with more drug interactions. Both erythromycin and clarithromycin (Biaxin) are potent CYP 34A inhibitors, but not azithromycin (which has fewer drug interactions). All macrolides are Category B except clarithromycin and telithromycin (both are Category C; avoid using in pregnancy).

- Erythromycin PO QID.
- Azithromycin (Z-Pack).
- Clarithromycin PO BID.

Table 3.3 Macrolides and Tetracyclines

Generic Name Trade	Drug Interactions
Macrolides	
Erythromycin QID	Many major drug interactions. Careful with myasthenia gravis.
Azithromycin (Z-Pack)	Anticoagulants: warfarin (Coumadin)
Clarithromycin BID	QT prolongation/bradyarrhythmias: verapamil (Calan), amlodipine (Norvasc), diltiazem (Cardizem), amiodarone, others
	Benzodiazepines: Triazolam (Halcion), midazolam (Versed)
	Asthma: Salmeterol (Serevent), theophylline
	Others: anticonvulsants (carbamezapine, phenytoin), ergotamine, statins, carbamexapine (Tegretol), statins (rhabdomyolysis), and others
Ketolide	
Telithromycin (Ketek) once a day	*Black Box Warning*: Myasthenia gravis patients—do not use on these patients
	Same drug interactions as macrolides
Tetracyclines	
Tetracycline QID	Photosensitivity reactions (use hat, sunblock)
Doxycycline BID	Binds with iron, calcium, magnesium, zinc
Minocycline (Minocin) BID	Antacids, sucralfate, and bile-acid sequestrants markedly decrease absorption. Oral contraceptives (may decrease effectiveness). Can cause pseudotumor cerebril.

Adverse Effects

- GI distress (especially erythromycin).
- Ototoxicity, cholestatic jaundice.
- QTc prolongation (risk of torsades de pointes).

Telithromycin (Ketek)

Classified as a ketolide (a type of macrolide). Indicated for treatment of mild to moderate CAP for adults (do not use if less than 18 years old). Of all the macrolides, Ketek has the narrowest indication.

- Black Box Warning: Contraindicated in patients with myasthenia gravis.
  - Cases of liver failure have been reported.
- Contraindications: History of jaundice/hepatitis from previous macrolide use.

Pharma Notes

1) Erythromycin's GI side effects are common (nausea, vomiting, abdominal pain, diarrhea).
2) If a condition must be treated with a macrolide (i.e., atypical bacteria) and the patient cannot tolerate erythromycin or Biaxin, switch the patient to azithromycin (Z-Pack).
3) Many drug interactions (anticoagulants, digoxin, theophylline, astimizole, carbamazepine, cisapride, triazolam, terfenadine).

CLINICAL PEARLS

1) Advise patients to use only one pharmacy so that all the drugs they take are on one database. It makes it easier for the pharmacy to check for drug interactions (your back-up system).
2) May prolong INR and increase risk of bleeding if warfarin is mixed with erythromycin or clarithromycin.
3) Macrolides (and quinolones) will prolong QT intervals (risk of torsade de pointes—variant type of VT).

CEPHALOSPORINS (CATEGORY B)

- Cephalosporins and penicillins belong to the beta-lactam family of antibiotics.
- Beta-lactams are bactericidal and work by interfering with the cell wall synthesis of actively growing bacteria.

First-Generation Cephalosporins

- Activity against gram-positive bacteria. Used to treat infections caused mainly by gram-positive bacteria (cellulitis, mastitis).

Second-Generation Cephalosporins

- Considered as "broad-spectrum" antibiotics. Used to treat infections caused by both gram-positive and gram-negative bacteria (i.e., sinusitis, otitis media).

Third-Generation Cephalosporins

- Less activity against gram-positive infections compared to the first-generation cephalosporins.
- Better coverage for gram-negative bacteria (i.e., *Neisseria gonorrheae* infections) and against enteric bacteria.

Pharma Notes
1) Rocephin (ceftriaxone) IM is first-line treatment for gonorrheal infections.
2) MRSA skin infections (boils, abscesses)—do not use cephalosporins. First line is either trimethoprim-sulfa (Bactrim DS) BID or clindamycin TID. Treat for at least 5 to 10 days.
3) Patients who have a true allergy to penicillin (history of anaphylaxis, angioedema) are more likely to have an allergic reaction to cephalosporins (especially first-generation).
4) Anaphylaxis and angioedema are type 1 IgE-mediated reactions (Table 3.4).

PENICILLINS (CATEGORY B)

There is a chance of cross-reactivity, especially with first-generation cephalosporins.

Amoxicillin and ampicillin are extended-spectrum penicillins. They are effective against gram-positive bacteria as well some gram-negative bacteria (*Haemophilus influenzae, Escherichia coli, Proteus mirabilis*).

- Penicillin V PO QID
- Amoxicillin PO BID to TID
- Amoxicillin plus clavulanic acid (Augmentin) PO BID

- Benzathine penicillin G IM
- Dicloxacillin PO QID

Adverse Reactions

- Diarrhea
- *Clostridium difficile*-associated diarrhea (CDAD)
- Vaginitis (usually candida)

Pharma Notes

1) Avoid using amoxicillin for patients with mononucleosis (causes a generalized rash not related to allergy). Use penicillin VK instead (if not allergic).
2) Dicloxacillin is for penicillinase-producing staph skin infections (mastitis and impetigo).
3) Patients who have a true allergy to penicillin (history of anaphylaxis, angioedema) are more likely to have an allergic reaction to cephalosporins (especially, first generation).
4) Anaphylaxis and angioedema are type 1 IgE-mediated reactions.
5) Some women will complain of candida vaginitis with amoxicillin. Recommend probiotic capsules or eating yogurt daily.

Table 3.4 Cephalosporins and Penicillins*

Generic Name (Trade Name)	Indications
Cephalosporins	
First generation	
Cephalexin (Keflex) PO QID	Pregnancy: UTI (if sensitive) pregnancy
	Skin: Cellulitis (not caused by MRSA), impetigo
Second generation	
Cefuroxime axetil (Ceftin) PO BID	ENT: Sinusitis, otitis media
Cefprozil (Cefzil) PO BID	Respiratory: CAP, exacerbation chronic bronchitis
Cefaclor (Ceclor) PO BID	Others: AOM, sinusitis, skin infections
Third generation	
Ceftriaxone (Rocephin) IM	STDs: Gonorrhea cervicitis, urethritis, PID
Cefixime (Suprax) daily to BID	ENT: AOM in children, acute sinusitis, otitis media
Cefdinir (Omnicef) daily to BID	GU: Pyelonephritis, CAP
Penicillins	
Penicillin V PO QID	Strep throat (first line)
Amoxicillin BID to TID	Otitis media (first line)
Amoxicillin plus clavulanic acid (Augmentin PO BID)	Otitis media/sinusitis (first to second line)
Benzathine penicillin G IM	Syphillis (first line)
Dicloxacillin PO QID	Cellulitis (not caused by MRSA), impetigo, erysipelas

* Not an all-inclusive list.

FLUOROQUINOLONES (QUINOLONES)

Effective against gram-negative bacteria and some atypical bacteria (*Chlamydia, Mycoplasma, Legionella*). Newer-generation quinolones (levofloxacin, moxifloxacin, gatifloxacin) are also active against gram-positive bacteria. Levofloxacin and moxifloxacin are also known as the "respiratory quinolones" due to their excellent activity against strep pneumonia.

- Norfloxacin (Noroxin) BID.
- Ciprofloxacin (Cipro) BID.
- Ofloxacin (Floxin) BID.
- Broad-spectrum quinolones.
- Levofloxacin (Levaquin) daily.
- Moxifloxacin (Avelox) daily.
- Gemifloxacin (Factive) daily.
- *Black Box Warning*: Increased risk of Achilles tendon rupture. Avoid strenuous activity while on the drug. Stop drug if develops tendon pain/swelling.

Drug Interactions

Avoid concomitant use of quinolones with other QT-prolonging drugs (amiodarone, macrolides, TCAs, antipsychotics, others) or with electrolyte imbalance (hypomagnesemia, hypokalemia) since these will elevate the risk of sudden death from arrhythmias (torsades de pointes).

Coadministration of antacids (aluminum/magnesium/calcium) or sucralfate drastically reduces effectiveness of quinolones due to binding (inactivation).

Contraindications:

- Children (less than 18 years of age).
- Myasthenia gravis.
- Pregnant women, breastfeeding.

Adverse Effects

- CNS (dizziness, headache, insomnia, mood changes).
- QT prolongation and others.

Pharma Notes

1) Achilles tendon rupture is a serious complication of quinolone therapy.
2) Do not use quinolones on children (less than 18 years) due to adverse effects on growing cartilage.
3) If a patient on quinolone reports a new onset of difficulty in walking, order an ultrasound to rule out Achilles tendon rupture and discontinue the medicine.
4) Bioterrorism-related inhalation of anthrax is treated with ciprofloxacin 500 mg BID × 60 days.
5) Cutaneous anthrax is treated with ciprofloxacin 500 mg BID × 7–10 days.
6) Traveler's diarrhea is treated with Cipro 500 mg BID × 3 days.
7) Ciprofloxacin has the best activity against *Pseudomonas aeruoginosa* (gram-negative) and is the first-line drug for treating pseudomonal pneumonia.
8) Per the CDC (2009), stop using quinolones to treat gonorrheal infections.

CLINICAL PEARL

Quinolones have three to four times the risk of tendon rupture (especially the Achilles tendon). Patients with the highest risk for tendon rupture are those on steroids and older patients (older than 60 years; Table 3.5).

SULFONAMIDES (CATEGORY C)

- Active against gram-negative bacteria (*E. coli*, *Klebsiella*, *H. influenzae*).
  - Bacteriostatic.
- Trimethoprim-sulfamethoxazole (TMP-SMX) Bactrim DS BID.
- Other sulfa-type drugs:
  - Diuretics (furosemide, HCTZ).
  - Sulfonylureas (glyburide, glipizide, etc.).
  - COX-2 inhibitor (celecoxib or Celebrex).
  - Dapsone (for HIV).
- Contraindications:
  - G6PD anemia (a genetic hemolytic anemia) causes hemolysis.
  - Newborns and infants less than 2 months of age.
  - Pregnancy in late third trimester (increased risk of hyperbilirubinemia/kernicterus).
  - Hypersensitivity to sulfa drugs.
- Drug interactions:
  - Warfarin (increases INR).

Adverse Effects

Skin rash, Stevens–Johnson syndrome, and others.

> ### Pharma Notes
> 1) Patients with a UTI who are on warfarin (Coumadin) should not be given TMP-SMX (increased risk of bleeding). Monitor INR closely.
> 2) Pregnant woman (or suspected pregnancy) with a UTI can be treated with amoxicillin or cephalosporins.

Table 3.5 Quinolones*

Generic Name (Trade Name)	Indications
Ciprofloxacin (Cipro) BID	Anthrax infection and prophylaxis (Cipro)
Ofloxacin (Floxin) BID	Traveler's diarrhea (Cipro)
	UTIs, pyelonephritis, epididymitis, prostatitis
	Black Box Warning: Risk of tendinitis and Achilles tendinopathy/rupture
Broad-spectrum quinolones	Levofloxacin has increased risk of hypoglycemia
Levofloxacin (Levaquin) daily	CAP, acute exacerbation of chronic bronchitis, pyelonephritis, epididymitis, prostatitis
Moxifloxacin (Avelox) daily Gemifloxacin (Factive) daily	Osteomyelitis, sinusitis, AOM
Topical formulations Floxin Otic (gtts)	OM with perforated TM, otitis externa
Ocuflox ophthalmic (gtts)	Bacterial conjunctivitis

* List is not all-inclusive.

CLINICAL PEARLS

1) HIV patients are at high risk (25%–50%) for sulfa-related Stevens–Johnson syndrome.
2) The typical G6PD patient in the United States is a Black male (10%) who presents with hemolysis/jaundice secondary to being treated with a sulfa drug. Look for a low H&H and jaundice.
3) Sulfonamide antibiotics are the second most frequent cause of allergic drug reactions (penicillins and cephalosporins are the first; Table 3.6).

OVER-THE-COUNTER (OTC) DRUGS AND HERBS

Topical Nasal Decongestants

Oxymetazoline Nasal Spray (Afrin), Phenylephrine (Neo-Synephrine).

- Short-term use of topical nasal decongestants (BID PRN × 3 days) is considered safe treatment for nasal congestion (common cold, allergic rhinitis).
- Rhinitis medicamentosa is due to chronic use (greater than 3 days) of nasal decongestants.

Antihistamines

Diphenhydramine (Benadryl), Loratadine (Claritin), Cetrizine (Zyrtec)

- Avoid using diphenhydramine (Benadryl) with the elderly.
- For elderly patients, use loratadine (Claritin) since it has a lower incidence of sedation.
- Zyrtec is more potent and long acting. It is very effective for acute and chronic urticaria.

Cold, Cough, and/or Sinus Medicines

Decongestants: Pseudoephedrine (Sudafed), Phenylephrine
Antitussives: Dextromethorphan (Robitussin, Delsym), benzonatate (Tessalon).
Mucolytics: Guaifenesin.

- Decongestants contraindicated with hypertension, CAD (angina, MI).
- Avoid mixing decongestants with other stimulants (caffeine, Ritalin) since they can elevate blood pressure and cause palpitations, arrythymias, tremors, and anxiety.
- Dextromethorphan is contraindicated within 14 days of a MAOI and seligiline (Eldepryl).

NSAIDs

- Ibuprofen (Advil, Motrin), naproxen sodium (Aleve).

Table 3.6 Sulfonamides

Generic Name	Indications
Trimethoprim-sulfamethoxazole (TMP-SMX) Bactrim DS BID	Prophylaxis/ treatment of PCP (HIV-patients)
	MRSA cellulitis
	UTIs, pyelonephritis
Topical sulfas Silver sulfadiazine (Silvadene)	Burns

Prescription NSAIDs

- Naproxen (Naprosyn, Anaprox), diclofenac (Voltaren) oral and topical gel
- Indomethacin (Indocin), ketoprofen (Orudis), ketorolac (Toradol)
- COX-2 inhibitors: Celecoxib (Celebrex)

NSAID Warnings

- NSAIDs should be avoided in heart failure, severe heart disease, GI bleeding, severe renal disease.
- Ketorolac (Toradol) IM, IV, or tablets is for short-term use only (up to 5 days).
- *Contraindications*: Ketorolac should not be used before surgery, with concurrent ASA, pediatric patients, active or recent GI bleed, stroke, labor/delivery, and others.
- For long-term use, document informed consent such as the higher risk of serious MI, stroke, emboli, GI bleeds, acute renal failure.
- COX-2 inhibitors (celecoxib) have lower risk of GI bleeding compared with the other NSAIDs. They are not a first-line NSAID except for patients at high risk for GI bleeding.
- Increased risk of bleeding if NSAIDs are combined with: warfarin, steroids, aspirin, alcohol. For long-term use, consider prescribing concurrent PPIs, H2-receptor antagonists, or misoprostol (Cytotec). Cytotec is a synthetic prostaglandin.
- Avoid long-term use of NSAIDs if patient is on aspirin prophylaxis (interferes with aspirin's cardioprotective effect).
- NSAIDs may worsen hypertension in patients who were previously well controlled.

Salicylates

- Aspirin (Bayer), magnesium salicylate (Doan's Pills).
- *Topical:* Methyl salicylate and menthol (BenGay gel/cream).
- *Nonacetylated salicylates:* Salsalate (Disalcid), namebutone (Relafen).

✍ EXAM TIPS

1) Aspirin irreversibly suppresses platelet function for up to 7 days (due to irreversible acetylation).
2) Discontinue ASA if patient complains of tinnitus (possible aspirin toxicity).
3) For chronic use, the recommended dose is 81 mg/day (some exceptions exist).
4) Aspirin given post-MI or after a stroke/TIA is considered tertiary prevention.
5) Avoid using in children with viral infections who are less than 16 years of age (Reye's syndrome).

Acetaminophen (Tylenol)

Maximum dose up to 4 g/day (or 1,000 mg QID or 650 mg every 4 hours).

- *Avoid if:* chronic hepatitis B/C/D, dehydration, liver disease, cirrhosis, heavy drinker (alcoholic).
- Considered first-line drug for pain from osteoarthritis.
- The antidote for acetaminophen overdose is acetylcysteine.

IMMUNE SYSTEM

Glucocorticoids (Steroids)

- Rheumatoid arthritis and other autoimmune disorders.
- Polymyalgia rheumatica (dramatic relief of symptoms).

- Asthma or acute asthmatic exacerbations.
- Temporal arteritis (high doses × several weeks to months) and uveitis.
- Skin (eczema, psoriasis, contact dermatitis).

Oral Steroids

- Prednisone 40 to 60 mg/day (high-dosed) for 3–4 days. Can be used for short-term treatment (i.e., asthma exacerbation). There is no need to taper if patient is not on chronic steroids.
- Methylprednisolone (Medrol Dose Pack) × 7 days. Does not need to be weaned.

Topical Steroids

- Classification: (Class 1 (superpotent) to Class 7 (least potent)
  - Superpotent (Class 1) —clobetasol (Temovate)
  - Potent—halocinonide (Halog)
  - Moderate—triamcinolone (Kenalog)
  - Least potent (Class 7)—hydrocortisone

Pharma Notes
Topical Steroids

- Use *low potency* steroid for children, and on the face, intertriginous areas, and the genitals.
  - *Example:* Use hydrocortisone 1% cream (OTC) to treat rashes on the face. May need to use ophthalmic-grade ointments for rashes around the eyes/eyelids.
- Use *moderate to high potency* steroids for thicker skin (scalp, soles of feet, palms of the hands) or for plaques (psoriasis). Taper topical steroids (or will rebound).
- What is "occlusion"?
  Thick resistant psoriatic plaques are sometimes treated by using occlusion (increases absorption). The topical steroid is applied to the plaque and is covered with plastic wrap. Ultrapotent steroids (Temovate, etc.) should not be occluded for more than 2 weeks (risk of hypothalamic-pituitary-axis [HPA] suppression).

Acutely inflamed joints (knees/hips/shoulders/elbows) can be treated with intra-articular triamcinolone (Kenalog) injections up to 3 times per year. Septic joint—do not inject steroids.

Side Effects of Glucocorticoids/Steroids (Chronic Use)

- HPA suppression.
- Cushing's disease (dorsal hump, rounded face, etc.).
- Osteoporosis (advise weight-bearing exercises, vitamin D, calcium 1,200 mg/day, bisphosphonates).
- Immunosuppression (increased risk of infection).
- Skin changes from long-term topical therapy (skin atrophy, striae, telangiectasia, acne).

CLINICAL PEARL

A severe case of poison ivy or poison oak rash may require 14 to 21 days of an oral steroid to clear.

OTHER DRUGS AND SAFETY ISSUES

Drugs That Require Eye Examination

The following drugs require careful monitoring of vision due to adverse effects. Check that the patient has baseline examination with regular eye exams done by an ophthalmologist.
- Digoxin (yellow to green vision, blurred vision, halos if blood level too high).
- Ethambutal and linezolid (optic neuropathy).
- Corticosteroids (cataracts, glaucoma, optic neuritis).
- Fluoroquinolones (retinal detachment).
- Viagra, Cialis, Levitra (cataracts, blurred vision, ischemic optic neuropathy, others).
- Accutane (cataracts, decreased night vision, others).
- Topamax (acute angle-closure glaucoma, increased ICP, mydriasis).
- Plaquenil (neuropathy and permanent loss of vision).

Cisapride (Propulsid):
- Available only by limited-access protocol in the United States.
- *Block Box Warning*: Serious cardiac arrhythmias (ventricular fibrillation/tachycardia, torsades de pointes, prolongation of QT interval). Check: 12-lead EKG at baseline. Check serum electrolytes and creatinine.
- Numerous drug contraindications (macrolides, antifunglas, TCAs, etc.).

Theophylline drug interactions:
- Theophylline level (adults): 5–15 mcg/mL.
- Drug interactions (cimetidine, alprazolam, macrolides, fluvoxamine, others).
- Avoid combining with other stimulants (theophylline, pseudoephedrine, caffeine, Ritalin).
- Disorders worsened by stimulants: hypertension, arrhythmias, stroke, seizures.
- BPH: causes urinary retention, worsening of symptoms.
- Suspect toxicity if: persistent vomiting.

Tapering (weaning) drugs:
- Certain drugs that are used long term need to be tapered. Abrupt discontinuation will cause the treated condition to flare up (exacerbation), rebound, and/or have adverse effects:
  - Beta-blockers (rebound hypertension or hypertensive crisis).
  - Benzodiazepines (severe anxiety, insomnia, seizures, tremors).
  - Oral steroids.
  - Anticonvulsants (seizures).
  - Paroxetine or Paxil.
  - Antiarrythmics (refer to cardiologists).
  - Antipsychotics and many others.

ILLEGAL DRUG OVERDOSE

All of these drugs will cause euphoria, sociability, talkativeness, more energy, need for less sleep or no sleep, anorexia, others. The most common cause of death (cocaine,

Ecstasy, amphetamines) is cardiac-related (hypertension, MI, sudden death, arrhythymias, seizures resulting in respiratory arrest, stroke, others).

Cocaine

- Euphoria, sociability, more energy, decreased appetite, insomnia.
- Pupils appear constricted and are very small in size. Nasal cartilage ulcers/nosebleeds.

Ecstasy (MDMA)

- A powerful stimulant. Colors look brighter. Vivid dreams and hallucinations.
- Enlarged pupils. May cause dehydration (due to low sodium) if poor fluid intake.

Methamphetamines ("Crystal Meth")

- Chronic use results in severe dental carries with loss of front teeth on the upper jaw and drastic weight loss. Pupils appear constricted.

U.S. FDA DRUG ENFORCEMENT AGENCY (DEA)

Controlled Substances Act

- *Schedule I drugs* (heroin, Ecstasy/MDMA, PCP, etc.).
  - Illegal to prescribe. No currently accepted medical use. High abuse potential.
- *Schedule II drugs* (Demerol, Dilaudid, OxyContin, cocaine, amphetamines, etc.).
  - Only the original prescription with the physician's signature (not stamped) is acceptable.
  - The total number of pills must be indicated. No refills are allowed.
- *Schedule III drugs* (Tylenol with codeine, Vicodin, anabolic steroids, testosterone, etc.).
- *Schedule IV drugs* (benzodiazepines, Ambien, Lunesta, Soma, etc.).
- *Schedule V drugs* (cough medicines with less than 200 mg of codeine, Lomotil, Lyrica).
- *Schedule IV, V*: can be mailed to the patient. Some states allow NPs to prescribe lower-level controlled substances.
- For all controlled substances: Must have the prescriber's and the supervising physician's name/DEA number with the clinic address on the pad. Cannot be pre-dated or post-dated. Some states do not require a supervising physician's signature.

List of FDA Category X Drugs

- Finasteride (Proscar, Propecia): Reproductive-aged or pregnant women should not handle crushed/broken finasteride tablets
- Isotretinoin (Accutane)
- Warfarin sodium (Coumadin)
- Misoprostol (Cytotec)
- Androgenic hormones: Birth control pills, HRT, testosterone
- Live virus vaccines (measles, mumps, rubella, varicella, rotavirus, FluMist)
- Thalidomide, DES, methimazole, and so on

FDA Category Classifications

- *Category A:* Adequate well-controlled human studies show no risk to the fetus in all trimesters of pregnancy (especially first trimester of pregnancy).
- *Category B:* Adequate well-controlled animal studies show no risk to the fetus and there are no adequate human studies in pregnant women.

- *Category C:* Animal studies show adverse effect on the fetus and there are no adequate well-controlled studies in humans, but the potential benefits may outweigh the risks.
- *Category D:* There is evidence of harm to the human fetus based on data from investigational studies and/or marketing experience, but potential benefits may still warrant use of the drug despite its risks.
- *Category X:* Studies in animals or humans demonstrate fetal abnormalities (teratogenicity). The risks from using the drug outweigh its benefits.

Pharma Notes

In general, FDA category X drugs are those that interfere with or block hormones (finasteride, misoprostol, Lupron), contain estrogen (birth control pills, HRT), are live virus vaccines, interfere with cell growth (methotrexate, chemo, radiation), or are derivatives of vitamin A (e.g., Accutane, high-dosed Vitamin A supplements).

✍ EXAM TIPS

1) Memorize the FDA category and dose of finasteride (Proscar 5 mg PO once a day).
2) Accutane is a potent teratogen. Reproductive-aged females must use 2 reliable forms of birth control and must have a negative pregnancy test 1 month before, during, and 1 month after Accutane.
3) High-dose vitamin A is teratogenic in animal studies—avoid "mega-doses" of vitamins in pregnancy.
4) Avoid mixing warfarin with sulfa drugs—can increase INR and bleeding risk.

PRESCRIPTION PADS

The NP's prescription pads should contain the following information:
- NP's name/designation/license number
- Supervising physician's name (some states do not require a supervising physician)/designation/license number
- Clinic address (if multiple sites, the sites where the NP works should be listed on the pad)

Writing a Prescription

- Date and name of the patient. The name of the drug, dose, frequency, and the quantity. If a refill, indicate how many times. Avoid using initials/shortcuts (i.e., daily instead of QD).
- If a controlled substance, the quantity of the drug is written in both number and written word form:
  - *Example:*
    Lunesta tablets 3 mg by mouth at bedtime as needed.
    Dispense: #20 (twenty). Refills: 1 (one).

    Bactrim DS 1 (one) tablet by mouth twice a day for 10 (ten) days.
    Dispense: #20 (twenty). Refills: 0 (none).

The "Five Rights"

- There are "Five Rights" that help to prevent or decrease the chances of a medical error:
  1) Right patient
  2) Right drug
  3) Right dose
  4) Right time
  5) Right route
- What is "e-prescribing"? The process of sending and receiving prescriptions by electronic means. Clinicians write the prescription in their offices on the computer or by personal digital assistant (PDA) using e-prescribing software. Preferred method for drug prescriptions by Medicare.

COMPLEMENTARY AND ALTERNATIVE MEDICINE

Conventional medicine (or allopathic medicine) is also known as modern medicine or "Western" medicine. Alternative medicine is the treatments and substances that are not part of standard medicine.

- *Examples*: Herbal supplements, probiotics, chiropractic, homeopathy, meditation, yoga, massage therapy.

Complementary and alternative medicine (CAM) is the term used when Western medicine is combined with alternative medicine or "medical products and practices that are not part of standard care" (NIH, 2010). CAM is using both Western medicine with alternative medicines (herbs) or with another healing system such as homeopathy, ayurveda (from India), or traditional Chinese medicine (or TCM).

Herbal Supplements

- Glucosamine (with/without chondroitin): osteoarthritis.
- Natural progesterone cream (from wild yam root extract): PMS symptoms (hot flashes)
- Isoflavones (from soy beans): Estrogen-like effects
- Saw palmetto: Urinary symptoms of BPH
- Kava kava, valerian root: Anxiety and insomnia
- St. John's wort: For mild depression. Do not use with SSRIs, MAOIs, sumatriptan, HIV protease inhibitors (indinavir), others.

Homeopathy

Founder: physician Samuel Hahnemann (1755–1843). This healing system is based on the "Law of Similars" or "Let likes be cured by likes."

- What is the *Homeopathic Pharmacopoeia of the United States* (HPUS)? The HPUS is a list of approved homeopathic substances used in this country.
- How are homeopathic substances made? Extremely small amounts of a substance are diluted (ultradilution). For example, the herb *Arnica montana*, which is used to prevent or treat bruises, can be diluted by 30X (e.g., *Arnica montana* 30X dilution).

Ayurveda

An ancient healing system that is based on Hindu beliefs of the people from India.

Systems Review

II

Health Screening and Health Promotion Review

UNITED STATES HEALTH STATISTICS

Mortality Statistics*

Leading cause of death (all ages/genders):
- Heart disease (or diseases of the heart)
- Cancer (or malignant neoplasms)
- Chronic lung diseases (or chronic lower respiratory diseases)

Cancer Mortality

Leading cause of cancer deaths:
- Lung cancer

Leading cause of cancer deaths in men:
- Lung cancer

Leading cause of cancer deaths in women:
- Lung cancer

Leading Causes of Death in Adolescents

Death rate for teen males is higher than for females.
- Accidents/injuries (48%). The most common cause is car accidents.
- Homicide (13%).
- Suicide (11%). Watch teens for signs of depression, excess stress, and suicidal behavior. Open communication between the adolescent and the parents/caretakers (or persons they trust) is extremely important in preventing teenage suicide.
- Unintentional injuries (accidents) are the leading cause of death in the United States for persons aged 1 to 19 years.

Life Expectancy

Average life expectancy is 78.5 years.

---

* CDC *Morbidity and Mortality Report Weekly* (MMWR), April 16, 2012.

CANCER STATISTICS

Prevalence

Most common cancer:
- Skin cancer.

Most common type of skin cancer:
- Basal cell cancer (but melanoma causes 75% of deaths from skin cancers)

Most common cancer by gender (prevalence):

Males
- Prostate cancer

Females
- Breast cancer

SCREENING TESTS

Sensitivity

- These screening tests detect individuals who have the disease.
- Highly sensitive tests have higher risk of "false positives."
- For example, the HIV ELISA has a 99% sensitivity for HIV antibodies, but it is too sensitive and can be "false positive" (especially in low-risks populations).
- The next step is the Western Blot test, which is very specific for HIV (the confirmatory test).

Specificity

- These screening tests detect individuals who do not have the disease.
- For example, a positive HIV ELISA result is always "confirmed" with the Western Blot test, which is very specific for HIV antibodies.
- The Western Blot is the "confirmatory test" for HIV. It is better at ruling out a person who does not have the disease.

HEALTH PROMOTION/DISEASE AND DEATH PREVENTION

Primary Prevention (Prevention of Disease/Injury)

- Individual actions (healthy individuals): Eat a nutritious diet, exercise, use seatbelts, helmets.
- Gun safety: Safety locks for guns, keep guns out of reach of children/teens.
- National programs: Immunizations, OSHA job safety laws, EPA environmental laws.
- Other: Building a youth center in an urban high-crime area, Habitat for Humanity (shelter).

Secondary Prevention (Early Detection of a Disease to Minimize Bodily Damage)

- Screening tests (Pap smears, mammograms, CBC for anemia, etc.).
- Screening for depression (interviewing a patient about feelings of sadness, hopelessness).
- Screening for sexually transmitted infections (STIs; sexual history, partners, signs and symptoms).
- Screening for alcohol abuse (interview a patient using the CAGE questionnaire).

Tertiary Prevention (Rehabilitation, Support Groups, Education on Equipment)

- Support groups: Alcoholics Anonymous (AA), breast cancer support groups, HIV support groups.
- Education for patients with preexisting disease (i.e., diabetes, hypertension): Avoidance of drug interactions, proper use of wheelchair or medical equipment, and so on.
- Rehabilitation: Cardiac rehab, physical therapy (PT), occupational therapy (OT).
- Exercise programs for obese children and adults.

U.S. PREVENTIVE SERVICES TASK FORCE

Breast Cancer (2009)

- Baseline mammogram: Start at age 50 years then every 2 years (biennially) until the age of 74 years.
- Age 75 years or older: Insufficient evidence for routine mammogram.

Notes

Age 40 to 49 years (individualize based on risk factors, biennial schedule if done).

The American Cancer Society recommends starting routine screening at age 40 years.

Source: U.S. Preventive Services Task Force (USPSTF) Recommendation Statement (Dec. 2009 addendum).

Cervical Cancer

- Baseline Pap smear/liquid cytology: Start at age 21 years then every 3 years until age 65 years.
- Age greater than 65 years: No routine screening (if history of prior screening and no risk factor for cervical cancer).
- Hysterectomy with removal of the cervix: Against routine screening (if no past history of high-grade precancer or cancer of the cervix).

Notes

Age 21 years or younger: Against routine screening (cervical cancer rare before age 21 years).

Note: These recommendations do not apply to women who are immunocompromised (i.e., HIV infection), had in-utero exposure to diethylstilbestrol (DES), or have a diagnosis of high-grade precancerous cervical lesion or cervical cancer.

Source: Screening Recommendations for Cervical Cancer (March 2012).

Colorectal Cancer

- Baseline: Start at age 50 years until the age of 75 (older age is the most common risk factor).
- Age 76 to 85 years: Against routine screening but "there may be considerations." Individualize.
- Older than age 85 years: Against screening for colorectal cancer.

> ### Notes
>
> These three methods are all acceptable. The screening intervals of each method differ:
>
> - High-sensitivity fecal occult blood test (FOBT) × 3 consecutive stool samples annually.
> - Flexible sigmoidoscopy every 5 years.
> - Colonoscopy every 10 years.
>
> ---
>
> *Source:* Screening for Colon Cancer (October 2008).

Lipid Disorders

- Total lipid profile after a 9-hour (minimum) fast.

Males

- *Age 35 years or older:* Screen for lipid disorder.
- *Age 20 to 35 years:* Screen if at increased risk of heart disease.

Females

- *Age 45 years or older:* Screen for lipid disorder.
- *Age 20 to 45 years:* Screen if at increased risk of heart disease (i.e., hypertensive, strong family history of MI, or stroke).

Prostate Cancer*

- The USPSTF does not recommend prostate-specific antigen (PSA) screening for prostate cancer. The new recommendation "applies to men in the general U.S. population, regardless of age."
- Exception: Males diagnosed or undergoing treatment for prostate cancer (PSA test for surveillance).

Skin Cancer Counseling

- Recommended for children, adolescents, and young adults (ages 10 to 24 years) with fair skin.
- Education includes avoidance of sunlight from 10 a.m. to 4 p.m., use of SPF 15 or higher sunblock, protective clothing, wide-brim hats.

Other

Routine screening is not recommended by the USPSTF for the following conditions:

- Lung cancer
- Ovarian cancer

---

* Screening for Prostate Cancer (May 2012).

Table 4.1 USPSTF Health Screening Recommendations

	Baseline	Notes
Breast cancer	Start at age 50 years	Mammogram every 2 years (biennial) until age 74 years
	Age 75 years or older*	Stop routine screening. Individualize*
	Breast self-exam (BSE)	Against teaching BSE (Grade D rec.)
Cervical cancer	Start at age 21 years	Every 3 years (Pap smear) until age 65 years. Against routine screening if younger than 21 years
	Age 65 year (or older) Hysterectomy with removal of cervix (benign disease)	Stop routine screening if history of adequate screening (and not high risk for cervical cancer) Can stop routine Pap smear screening
Colon/colorectal cancer	Start at age 50 years	High-sensitivity FOBT (every year), or sigmoidoscopy (every 5 years), or colonoscopy (every 10 years)
	Age 76 to 85 years	Individualize*
	Age older than 85 years	Stop routine screening
Depression	Adolescents (12–18 years)	Start screening for depression. Look for signs/symptoms. Beck Depression Inventory Geriatric Depression Scale
Obesity	Start at age 6 years; adolescents to adults	Offer or refer for intensive behavioral interventions
Sexually transmitted infections (STIs)	Start at the onset of sexual activity	High-intensity behavioral counseling
Lung cancer	Against routine screening	Insufficient evidence for routine screening
Skin cancer	Insufficient evidence	
Ovarian/testicular cancer	Against routine screening	
Pancreatic cancer	Against routine screening	

* Decision to screen is based on risk factors, life expectancy (greater than 10 years), risk versus benefits.

- Oral cancer
- Prostate cancer
- Testicular cancer (adolescents or adult males; Table 4.1)

RISK FACTORS

Breast Cancer

- Older age: Greater than 50 years (most common risk factor).
- Previous history of breast cancer.
- Two or more first-degree relatives with breast cancer.
- Early menarche, late menopause, nulliparity (longer exposure to estrogen).
- Obesity (adipose tissue can synthesize small amounts of estrogen).

Cervical Cancer

- Multiple sex partners (defined as greater than four lifetime partners).
- Younger age onset of sex (immature cervix easier to infect).
- Immunosuppression and smoking.

Colorectal Cancer

- History of familial polyposis (multiple polyps on colon).
- First-degree relative with colon cancer.
- Crohn's disease (ulcerative colitis).

Prostate Cancer

- USPSTF against routine PSA-based screening regardless of age.
- Exceptions are men diagnosed or undergoing treatment for prostate cancer.

Sexually Transmitted Infections or STDs

- Multiple sexual partners.
- Earlier age onset of sex.
- New partners (defined as less than 3 months).
- History of STD.
- Homelessness.

VACCINES AND IMMUNIZATIONS

Hepatitis B Vaccine

Total of three doses. If series not completed, catch up until three-dose series is completed. The CDC does not recommend a restart of the hepatitis B series.

FAST FACT

If a patient had only one dose of hepatitis B vaccine, what is recommended?
Do not restart the hepatitis B series again. If only one dose, give the second dose. Catch up until the three-dose series is completed.

Influenza Vaccine

November: Start giving flu vaccines (fall to winter seasons).

Formulations
- Live attenuated inactivated virus influenza vaccine (LAIV form).
- Given by nose spray (intranasal). Contains live virus. For healthy persons aged 2 to 49 years.

LAIV Safety Issues
- Do not give aspirin to children within the 4 weeks following vaccination.
- Some antivirals (amantadine, rimantadine, zanamivir, or osletamivir) should be avoided 48 hours before and 14 days after vaccination because they interfere with antibody production.

LAIV Contraindictions
- Pregnancy, chronic diseases (i.e., asthma, COPD, renal failure, diabetes, immunosuppression).
- Contraindicated in children on aspirin therapy (age 2 to 17 years).

Flu Vaccines (Injection Forms)
- Trivalent inactivated influenza vaccine (TIV form): give by intramuscular (IM) injection.
- Fluzone intradermal formulation: Give by intradermal route.

Safety Issues

Avoid if severe egg allergy, gentamicin or gelatin allergy, or in children or adolescents receiving concomitant aspirin or aspirin-containing therapy.

FAST FACTS

1) *What is the youngest age at which flu vaccine (injection) can be given?*
   At the age of 6 months. The liver flu vaccine (FluMist) can be given at age 2 to 49 years.
2) *What types of medications are avoided after receiving the LAIV flu vaccine (intranasal form)?*
   Some antivirals (amantadine, rimantadine, zanamivir, or osletamivir) should be avoided 48 hours before and 14 days after vaccination because they interfere with antibody production.

Tetanus Vaccine

- Give every 10 years for lifetime.
- Boosters: For "dirty"/contaminated wounds, give a booster if the last dose was more than 5 years prior.
- Age 7 years and older: Use only tetanus and diphtheria (Td) and tetanus, diphtheria, and acellular pertussis (Tdap) forms of the vaccine.
- Td: Given by IM route. Start using this form at the age of 7 years.
- Tdap: Given by IM route.

Safety Issue

Avoid if egg allergy or history of Guillain–Barré syndrome.

FAST FACTS

1) *When can the Tdap be used as a booster in adolescents and adults?*
   The Tdap can be substituted for a single dose of Td (once in a lifetime).
2) *What is done if a patient has a tetanus-prone wound and vaccination status is unknown?*
   Administer immediate dose of Td vaccine and the tetanus immunoglobulin (TIG) injection.
3) *Which wounds are considered as highest risk for tetanus infection?*
   Puncture wounds, wounds with devitalized tissue, soil-contaminated wounds, crush injuries, others.

Pneumococcal Vaccine

- Pneumococcal vaccine polyvalent (Pneumovax-23): Given by IM route.
- Age 65 years or older and persons at high risk: Give one dose for a lifetime.
- Highest risk (of fatal pneumococcal infection):
  - Chronic diseases (alcoholism, diabetes, CSF leaks, asthma, chronic hepatitis).
  - Anatomic or functional asplenia (including sickle cell disease).
  - Immunocompromised or on medications causing immunocompromised state.
  - Generalized malignancy or cancers of the blood (leukemia, lymphoma, multiple myeloma).
  - Renal diseases (i.e., chronic renal failure, nephrotic syndrome).
  - History of organ or bone marrow transplant.

FAST FACTS

1) *What vaccine is recommended for persons who are 65 years of age?*
   - Give one dose of Pneumovax (lifetime). No booster is needed.
2) *If a person is vaccinated before the age of 65, what is recommended?*
   - Give a booster dose of Pneumovax 5 years after the initial dose.
   - Zoster vaccine (Zostavax) is a live attenuated virus vaccine (LAIV).
   - Age 60 years: give one-time dose SC.
   - Do not use vaccine if no history of chickenpox or shingles (seronegative). The patient will become ill with chickenpox. However, if a person had shingles before, the vaccine can still be administered. Certain antivirals (acyclovir, famciclovir, valacyclovir) can decrease immunologic response if taken 24 hours before or 14 days after vaccination. May cause exacerbation of asthma and polymyalgia rheumatica (PMR).
   - *Contraindications:*
     - Pregnancy and breastfeeding.
     - Leukemia, lymphomas, or other malignancies of the bone/bone marrow.
     - Immunocompromise (high-dosed steroids greater than 2 weeks, anti-TNF meds such as etanercept).

FAST FACTS

What age group should receive the vaccine?
- Give a one-time dose at the age of 60 years or older (even if patient already had shingles).
- The youngest age that Zostavax can be given is 50 years of age.
- *Varicella vaccine*:
  - Varicella live attenuated virus (Varivax): Given by SC route. Need two doses (4 to 8 weeks apart).
  - Exposure to chickenpox: Give within 5 days after incident for postexposure prophylaxis.
  - Acceptable evidence for varicella infection.
  - Written documentation of two doses of varicella vaccine (at least 28 days apart).
  - Written diagnosis of chickenpox or shingles based on health care provider diagnosis.
  - Positive laboratory varicella titer.
  - Born in the United States before 1980.

Safety Issues

Avoid giving to pregnant patients; patients with immunosuppression or on drugs that affect the immune system (steroids, biologics such as Humira, Enbrel); patients having radiation treatment or with any type of cancer.

Health Care Personnel Vaccination Recommendations

These recommendations also apply to students who are in training.

Td or Tdap

Give one-time dose of Tdap for all health care personnel who have not received the Tdap when due for a tetanus booster. Continue giving Td boosters every 10 years for a lifetime.

MMR

Proof of immunity necessary (born before 1957, laboratory confirmation such as positive titers). If not vaccinated for MMR, need two doses (at least 4 weeks apart).

Varicella

Proof of immunity necessary (positive varicella titer, documentation of two doses of varicella vaccine or diagnosis of varicella by physician/health care provider).

Table 4.2 CDC Immunization Recommendations for Adults and Teens (2012)*

Vaccine	Schedule	Notes
Hepatitis B	Total of three doses	If incomplete series, do not restart. If had one dose, give the second dose during the visit. If had two doses, give the third dose
Tetanus/diphtheria (Td) Tetanus/diphtheria/ acellular pertussis (Tdap)	Every 10 years for lifetime Dirty wounds, give tetanus booster if last dose more than 5 years	Substitute one-time dose of Tdap for Td booster for persons younger than age 65 years (once in a lifetime)
Flu (influenza) Trivalent inactivated vaccine (TIV) Live attenuated influenza vaccine (LAIV) intranasal**	Give once a year in the fall or winter Universal recommendation	Give in fall/winter starting in November Give flu to everyone 6 months or older Do not give FluMist to pregnant women. Use injection form For healthy persons (not pregnant) from the age of 2 years to 49 years
Varicella**	Give two doses at least 4 weeks apart	Healthy teenagers to adults with no history of chickenpox; health care workers
Shingles/zoster	Single dose at age 60 years	Give single dose at age 60 years or older (regardless if reports history of shingles)
Meningococcal conjugate vaccine quadrivalent (MCV4)	Depends: For adults, give one to two doses (at least 2 months apart)	First-year college students through age 21 years who will be living in residence halls (give one dose)
Pneumococcal polysaccharide vaccine (PPSV)	One dose age 65 years	Age 65 years, give one dose (lifetime) If vaccinated before age of 65 years, give a booster in 5 years

* Not all-inclusive.

** Live virus vaccines contraindications apply.

Hepatitis B

Hepatitis B titers should be checked within 60 days of the third dose. If incomplete hepatitis B series (fewer than three doses), complete the series (do not restart) and check the titer as recommended.

Influenza

All health care personnel should have an annual flu shot during the fall/winter.

Other Types of Vaccines

Bacille-Calmette-Guerin

Bacille-Calmette-Guerin (BCG) is a vaccine against tuberculosis (TB) infection. BCG is made from live attenuated (or weakened) tuberculosis mycobacterium. BCG vaccine is used in some countries (i.e., Asia, Africa) where TB disease is common.

■ *What is the follow-up if a person with a history of BCG immunization has a positive PPD?*

Evaluate the person for signs and symptoms of TB. Rule out latent infection. Order a chest x-ray and check for signs and symptoms of TB such as a "chronic" cough, weight loss, and night sweats. Do not assume the reaction is from the BCG vaccine since the effect of the vaccine declines over time.

5

Head, Eyes, Ears, Nose, and Throat Review

⚠ DANGER SIGNALS

EYES

Herpes Keratitis

Acute onset of severe eye pain, photophobia, and blurred vision in one eye. Diagnosed by using fluorescein dye. A black lamp in a darkened room is used to search for fernlike lines in the corneal surface. In contrast, corneal abrasions appear more linear.

Infection permanently damages corneal epithelium, which may result in corneal blindness.

Acute Angle-Closure Glaucoma

Elderly patient with acute onset of severe eye pain accompanied by headache, nausea/vomiting, halos around lights, and decreased vision. Examination reveals a mid-dilated pupil(s) that is oval shaped. The cornea appears cloudy. Fundoscopic examination reveals cupping of optic nerve. Ophthalmologic emergency. If the rise in intraocular pressure (IOP) is slower, patient may be asymptomatic.

Acute Vision Loss

May complain of sudden onset of floaters or black dots in visual field, scotoma (retinal detachment), blurred vision, photophobia, eye pain, or severe discomfort (uveitis, glaucoma).

EARS/NOSE/SINUS

Cholesteatoma

"Cauliflowerlike" growth accompanied by foul-smelling ear discharge. Hearing loss on affected ear. On examination, no tympanic membrane or ossicles are visible because of destruction by the tumor. History of chronic otitis media infections. The mass is not cancerous, but it can erode into the bones of the face and damage the facial nerve (CN 7). Treated with antibiotics and surgical debridement. Refer to head, eyes, ears, nose, and throat (HEENT) specialist.

Battle Sign

Acute onset of a bruise behind the ear over the mastoid area after a recent history of trauma. Indicates a fracture of the basilar skull. Search for a clear golden serous discharge from the ear or nose (see below). Refer to emergency department (ED) for skull x-rays and antibiotics.

Clear Golden Fluid Discharge From the Nose/Ear

Indicative of a basilar skull fracture. Cerebrospinal fluid (CSF) slowly leaks through the fracture. Testing the fluid with a urine dipstick will show that it is positive for glucose, whereas plain mucus or mucupurulent drainage will be negative. Refer to ED.

Cavernous Sinus Thrombosis

A rare but life-threatening complication with a high mortality rate. Patients with a history of a sinus or facial infection will manifest with a severe headache accompanied by a high fever. Rapid decline in level of consciousness terminating in coma and death. Refer to ED.

PHARYNX

Peritonsillar Abscess

Severe sore throat and difficulty swallowing, odonophagia, trismus, and a "hot potato" voice. One-sided swelling of the peritonsillar area and soft palate. Affected area is markedly swollen and appears as a bulging red mass with the uvula displaced from the mass. Accompanied by malaise, fever, and chills. Refer to ED for incision and drainage (I&D).

Diphtheria

Sore throat, fever, and markedly swollen neck ("bull neck"). Low-grade fever, hoarseness, and dysphagia. The posterior pharynx, tonsils, uvula, and soft palate are coated with a gray- to yellow-colored pseudomembrane that is hard to displace. Very contagious. Refer to ED.

☑ NORMAL FINDINGS

EYES

- *Fundi:* The veins are larger than arteries.
- *Cones:* For color perception, 20/20 vision, sharp vision.
- *Rods:* For detecting light and shadow, depth perception, night vision.
- *Macula (and fovea):* The macula is the area responsible for central vision. The fovea (which contains large numbers of cones) is set in the middle. This is the area of the eye that determines 20/20 vision.
- *Cobblestoning:* Inner conjunctiva with mildly elevated lymphoid tissue resembling "cobblestones." May be seen in atopic patients, allergic rhinitis, allergic conjunctivitis.
- *Presbyopia:* Age-related visual change due to a decreased ability of the eye to accommodate and stiffening of the lenses. Usually starts at the age of 40 years. There is difficulty focusing, which results in markedly decreased ability to read print at close range.

EARS

- *Tympanic membrane (TM):* Translucent off-white to gray color with the "cone of light" intact.
- *Tympanogram:* Most objective measure for presence of fluid inside middle ear (results in a straight line vs. a peaked shape).

- *External portion of the ear:* Has large amount of cartilage. Refer injuries to plastic surgeon.
- *Cartilage:* Does not regenerate; refer injuries to plastic surgeon.

NOSE

- Only the inferior nasal turbinates are usually visible. The medial and superior turbinates are not visible without special instruments.
- Bluish, pale, and/or boggy nasal turbinates seen in allergic rhinitis.
- Lower third of the nose is cartilage. Cartilage tissue does not regenerate; if damaged, refer to plastic surgeon.

MOUTH/TONGUE

- *Leukoplakia:* Appear on the surface and under the tongue. May be cancerous. Patients with a history of chewing tobacco are at high risk of oral cancer.
- *Apthous stomatitis (canker sores):* Painful and look like shallow ulcers of soft tissue (Figure 5.1).
- *Avulsed tooth:* Store in cool milk (no ice) and see dentist ASAP for reimplantation.

TONSILS

Butterfly-shaped glands with small porelike openings that may secrete white- to yellow-colored exudate. Purulent exudate may be seen with tonsillitis.

POSTERIOR PHARYNX

- Look for postnasal drip (acute sinusitis, allergic rhinitis).
- Posterior pharyngeal lymph nodes that are mildly enlarged and distributed evenly on the back of the throat (allergies, allergic rhinitis).
- Hard palate: Look for any openings (cleft palate), ulcers, redness.

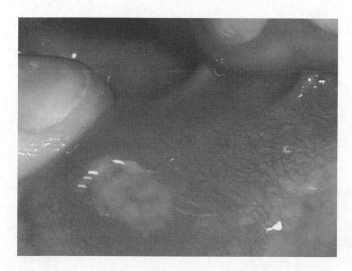

FIGURE 5.1 Apthous stomatitis (canker sore).

BENIGN VARIANTS

Geographic Tongue

- Cause unknown. Map-like appearance on tongue surface. Patches may move from day to day. May complain of soreness with acidic foods, spicy foods.

Torus Palatinus

- Painless bony protuberance midline on the hard palate (roof of the mouth). May be asymmetrical. Skin should be normal. Does not interfere with normal function.

Fishtail or Split Uvula

- Uvula is split into two sections ranging from partial to complete. May be a sign of an occult cleft palate (rare).

Nystagmus

- A few beats of nystagmus on prolonged extreme lateral gaze that resolve when the eye moves back toward midline is normal. Vertical nystagmus is always abnormal.

ABNORMAL FINDINGS

Papilledema

- Optic disc swollen with blurred edges due to increased intracranial pressure (ICP) secondary to bleeding, brain tumor, abscess, pseudotumor cerebri.

Hypertensive Retinopathy

- Copper and silver wire arterioles.

Diabetic Retinopathy

- Microaneurysms caused by neovascularization (new arteries in the retina fragile).

Cataracts

- Opacity of the corneas. Chronic steroid use can cause cataracts.

Allergic Rhinitis

- Blue-tinged or pale and swollen (boggy) nasal turbinates.

Koplik's Spots

- Small-sized red papules with blue-white centers inside the cheeks by the lower molars.

Pathognomic for Measles

Hairy Leukoplakia

Elongated papilla on the lateral aspects of the tongue that are pathognomic for HIV infection. Caused by Epstein–Barr virus (EBV) infection.

Leukoplakia of the Oral Mucosa/Tongue

■ A bright white plaque caused by chronic irritation such as chewing tobacco or snuff (rule out oral cancer) or on the inner cheeks (buccal mucosa).

Vocabulary

■ *Buccal mucosa:* Mucosal lining inside the mouth.
■ *Palpebral conjunctiva:* Mucosal lining inside eyelids.
■ *Bulbar conjunctiva:* Mucosal lining covering the eyes.
■ *Soft palate:* Refers to the area where uvula, tonsils, anterior of throat are located.
■ *Hard palate:* The "roof" of the mouth.
■ *Hyperopia:* "Farsightedness."
■ *Nystagmus:* Abnormal (rule out strabismus). A few beats of horizontal nystagmus on extreme lateral gaze that disappears when the eyes return to midline is normal.

EVALUATION AND TESTING

VISION

Distance Vision

The Snellen chart measures central distance vision. If the person is illiterate, use the Tumbling E chart. Patient must stand 20 feet away from the chart. If the patient wears glasses, test the vision with the glasses with both eyes (OU), the right eye (OD), and the left eye (OS).

■ *Abnormal:* Two-line difference between each eye; less than four letters out of six correct.

Near Vision

■ Ask patient to read small print.

Peripheral Vision

■ The "visual fields of confrontation" exam.
■ Look for blind spots (scotoma) and peripheral visual field defects.

Color Blindness

■ Use the Ishihara chart.

Visual Test Results

■ Definition of a Snellen test result 20/60.
  – *Top number (or numerator):* The distance in feet at which the patient stands from the Snellen or picture eye chart (always 20 feet and never changes).
  – *Bottom number (or denominator):* The number of feet that the patient can see compared to a person with normal vision (20/20 or less). Number changes, dependent on patient's vision. In this example, the patient can see at 20 feet what a person with normal vision can see at 60 feet.
■ *Legal blindness:* Defined as a best corrected vision of 20/200 or less or a visual field less than 20° (tunnel vision).

HEARING TESTS

Weber Test

■ Place the tuning fork midline on the forehead (Figure 5.2).
■ *Normal finding:* No lateralization. If lateralization (hears the sound in only one ear), abnormal finding.

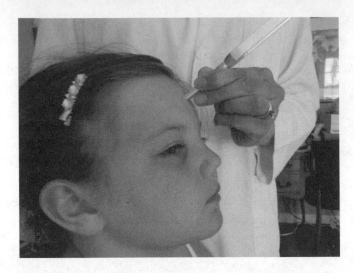

FIGURE 5.2 Weber test.

Rinne Test

- Place tuning fork first on mastoid process, then at front of the ear. Time each area.
- *Normal finding:* Air conduction lasts longer than bone conduction (i.e., can hear longer in front of ear than on mastoid).

☰ DISEASE REVIEW

EYES

Herpes Keratitis and Corneal Abrasion

Damage to corneal epithelium due to herpes virus infection secondary to shingles. Corneal abrasion will report sudden onset of symptoms with foreign body sensation.

Classic Case
Herpes Keratitis

Complains of acute onset of eye pain, photophobia, and blurred vision of the affected eye. Look for a herpetic rash on the side of the temple and on the tip of the nose (rule out shingles of the trigeminal nerve or CN 5).

Corneal Abrasion

Complains of acute onset of severe eye pain and keeps affected eye shut. Reports feeling of a foreign body sensation with increased tearing of affected eye. May be caused by contact lens.

Contact lens abrasions at very high risk of bacterial infection (treated differently—refer ASAP).

Objective

Use fluorescein dye strips with a black lamp in darkened room. Herpes keratitis appears as fernlike lines. In contrast, corneal abrasions usually appear more linear.

Treatment Plan

- Refer herpes keratitis patient to ED or ophthalmologist STAT (Zovirax or Valtrex BID).
- Avoid steroid ophthalmic drops for herpes keratitis.
- If corneal abrasion, rule out penetrating trauma, vision loss, soil/dirt. Check vision.

- Flush eye with normal saline to remove foreign body. If unable to remove, refer.
- If corneal abrasion, use topical ophthalmic antibiotic (erythromycin or Polytrim applied to affected eye × 3 to 5 days). Do not patch eye. Follow up in 24 hours. If not improved, refer.
- Consider eye pain prescription (hydrocodone with acetaminophen; prescribe enough for 48 hours of use).

Hordeolum (Stye)

A painful acute bacterial infection of a hair follicle on the eyelid.

Classic Case

Complains of an itchy eyelid and an acute onset of a pustule on either upper or lower eyelid that eventually becomes painful.

Treatment Plan

- Antibiotic drops or ointment (i.e., sulfa drops, erythromycin gtts, etc.).
- Warm packs BID to TID until pustule drains.

Chalazion

A chronic inflammation of the meibomian gland (specialized sweat gland) of the eyelids.

Classic Case

Complains of a gradual onset of a small superficial nodule that is discrete and movable on the upper eyelid that feels like a bead. Painless. Can slowly enlarge over time. Benign.

Treatment Plan

- If nodule enlarges or does not resolve in a few weeks, biopsy to rule out squamous cell cancer. If large and affects vision, surgical removal is an option.

Pinguecula

A yellow triangular thickening of the bulbar conjunctiva (skin covering eyeball). Located on the inner and outer margins of the cornea. Caused by ultraviolet (UV) light damage to collagen.

Pterygium

A yellow triangular (wedge-shaped) thickening of the conjunctiva that extends to the cornea on the nasal or temporal cornea. Due to UV-damaged collagen from chronic sun exposure. Usually asymptomatic. Can be red/inflamed at times.

Treatment Plan (Both Pinguecula and Pterygium)

- If inflamed, use weak steroid eye drops only during exacerbations.
- Recommend use of good-quality sunglasses.
- Remove surgically if encroaches cornea and affects vision.

Subconjunctival Hemorrhage

Blood that is trapped underneath the conjunctiva and sclera secondary to broken arterioles. Can be caused by coughing, sneezing, heavy lifting, vomiting, or can occur spontaneously. Resolves within 1 to 3 weeks (blood reabsorbed) like a bruise with color changes from red, to green, to yellow. Increased risk if on aspirin, anticoagulants, and has hypertension.

Classic Case

Complains of sudden onset of bright red blood in one eye after an incident of severe coughing, sneezing, or straining. May also be due to trauma such as a fall. Denies visual loss and pain.

Treatment Plan

■ Watchful waiting and reassurance of patient. Follow up until resolution.

Primary Open-Angle Glaucoma

Gradual onset of increased intraocular pressure (IOP) greater than 22 mm Hg due to blockage of the drainage of aqueous humor inside the eye. The retina (CN 2) undergoes ischemic changes and, if untreated, becomes permanently damaged. Most common type of glaucoma (60%–70%).

Classic Case

Most commonly seen in elderly patients, especially those of African background or diabetics. Usually asymptomatic. Gradual changes in peripheral vision (lost first) and then central vision. If fundoscopic exam shows cupping, IOP is too high. Refer to ophthalmologist.

Treatment Plan

■ Check IOP. Normal range IOP: 10 to 22 mm Hg.
■ Refer patient to ophthalmologist for follow-up.

Medications

■ *Betimol (timolol):* Beta-blocker eyedrops that lower IOP.
■ *Side effects and contraindications:* Same as oral form. Include bronchospasm, fatigue, depression, heart failure, bradycardia.
■ *Contraindicated:* Asthma, emphysema, chronic obstructive pulmonary disease (COPD), second- to third-degree heart block, heart failure.

Complication

■ Blindness due to ischemic damage to retina (CN 2).

Primary Angle Closure Glaucoma

Sudden blockage of aqueous humor causes marked increase of the IOP, causing ischemia and permanent damage to the optic nerve (CN 2).

Classic Case

An older patient complains of acute onset of a severe frontal headache or severe eye pain with blurred vision and tearing. Seeing halos around lights. May be accompanied by severe nausea and vomiting.

Objective

Eyes: Fixed and mid-dilated cloudy pupil that looks more oval than round-shaped. Conjunctival injection with increased lacrimation.

Treatment Plan

Refer to ED.

Anterior Uveitis (Iritis)

Higher risk with autoimmune disorders (RA, lupus, ankylosing spondylitis), sarcoidosis, syphilis, others. Complains of red sore eyes. Appears like red eye but with increased tearing.

No purulent discharge (as in bacterial conjunctivitis). Refer to ophthalmologist for management.

Age-Related Macular Degeneration

Age-related macular degeneration (AMD) can either be atrophic (dry form) or exudative (wet form). The dry form of AMD is more common (85%–90%) and is "less severe" compared to the wet form. The wet form of AMD is responsible for 80% of vision loss (choroidal neovascularization). Caused by gradual damage to the pigment of the macula (area of central vision) that results in severe visual loss to blindness. Leading cause of blindness in the elderly. More common in smokers.

Classic Case

Elderly smoker complains of gradual or sudden and painless central vision loss. During the early phase of visual loss, may not notice central vision loss (asymptomatic) until a large area is involved. Reports that straight lines (doors, windows) appear distorted. Peripheral vision is usually preserved.

Treatment Plan

Refer to ophthalmologist. Patient is given a copy of the Amsler Grid (focus eye on center dot and view grid 12 inches from eyes) (Figure 5.3). Patient checks visual field loss daily to weekly (center of grid is distorted, blind spot or scotoma, or wavy lines).

"AREDS" formula ocular vitamins: High-dose antioxidants and zinc. Patients should consult their ophthalmologist before taking ocular vitamins.

Sjogren's Syndrome

Chronic autoimmune disorder characterized by decreased function of the lacrimal and salivary glands. It can occur alone or with another autoimmune disorder (i.e., with rheumatoid arthritis).

Classic Case

The classic symptoms are daily symptoms of dry eyes and dry mouth for several months (greater than 3 months). Complains of chronic "dry eyes" and that both eyes have sandy or gritty sensation (keratoconjunctivitis sicca). Ocular symptoms are associated with chronic dry mouth. Oral examination shows swollen and inflamed salivary glands.

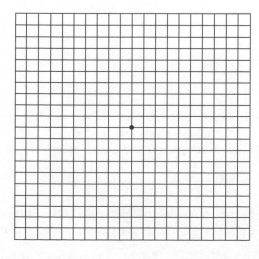

FIGURE 5.3 Amsler grid.

Treatment Plan

- OTC tear substitute eye gtts TID. Refer to ophthalmologist (keratoconjunctivitis sicca).
- *Labs:* CBC, sedimentation rate and/or C-reactive protein, autoimmune disease panel.
- Refer to rheumatologist for management.

Blepharitis

A chronic condition of the base of the eyelashes caused by inflammation. Complains of itching or irritation in the eyelash area (upper/lower or both), eye redness, sometimes crusting.

Treatment Plan

Johnson's Baby Shampoo with warm water: Gently scrub eyelid margins until resolves. Consider topical antibiotic solution (erythromycin eye gtts) to eyelids 2× to 3×/day.

NOSE

Allergic Rhinitis

Inflammatory changes of the nasal mucosa due to allergy. Atopic family history. May have seasonal or daily symptoms.

Classic Case

Complains of chronic nasal congestion with clear mucus discharge or postnasal drip. Accompanied by nasal itch and, at times, frequent sneezing. Coughing worsens when supine due to postnasal drip. May be allergic to dust mites, mold, pollen, others.

Objective

Nose has blue-tinged or pale boggy nasal turbinates. Mucus clear. Posterior pharynx reveals thick mucus, with colors ranging from clear, white, yellow, or green (rule out sinusitis).

Treatment Plan

- Nasal steroid sprays daily (i.e., fluticasone/Flonase) BID.
- Decongestants (i.e., pseudoephedrine or Sudafed) PRN. Do not give to infants/young children.
- Zyrtec 10 mg daily or PRN or combined antihistamine with decongestants.
- Dust mite allergies: Avoid using ceiling fans, no stuffed animals or pets in bed, use a HEPA filter, and the like.

Complications

- Acute sinusitis.
- Acute otitis media.

Rhinitis Medicamentosa

- Prolonged use of topical nasal decongestants (greater than 3 days) causes rebound effects that result in severe and chronic nasal congestion.
- Patients present with daily severe nasal congestion and clear, watery, mucus nasal discharge.

Epistaxis (Nosebleeds)

Trauma and/or laceration to nasal passages results in bleeding. Posterior nasal bleeds can result in severe hemorrhage. Anterior nasal bleeds are milder. Aspirin use, cocaine abuse, severe hypertension, and anticoagulants (i.e., warfarin sodium or Coumadin) place patients at higher risk.

Classic Case

Complains of acute onset of nasal bleeding secondary to trauma. Bright red blood may drip externally through the nasal passages and/or the posterior pharynx. Profuse bleeding can result in vomiting of blood.

Treatment Plan

Tilt head slightly forward and apply pressure over nasal bridge for several minutes. Use nasal decongestants (i.e., Afrin) to shrink tissue. Nasal packing. Antibiotic prophylaxis for staph and strep as needed.

Complications

- Posterior nasal bleeds may hemorrhage (refer to ED).

THROAT

Strep Throat

An acute infection of the pharynx caused by beta streptococcus (gram positive) Group A bacteria. Rare sequelae are scarlet fever and rheumatic fever.

Classic Case

All ages are affected, but most common in children. Acute onset of pharyngitis, pain on swallowing, and mildly enlarged submandibular nodes. Not associated with rhinitis, watery eyes, or congestion (coryza) as seen in the common cold. Anterior cervical nodes mildly enlarged. Adult may report having a small child attending preschool.

Objective

- Pharynx dark pink to bright red. Adults usually afebrile (or mild fever).
- May have tonsillar exudate that is yellow to green color. May have pettechiae on the hard palate (roof of the mouth). Anterior cervical lymph nodes mildly enlarged.

Treatment Plan

- Throat culture and sensitivity (C&S) or Rapid Strep testing.
  - First line: Penicillin QID × 10 days.
  - Ibuprofen (Advil) or acetaminophen (Tylenol) for throat pain and fever.
  - Symptomatic treatment: Salt water gargles, throat lozenges. Drink more fluids.
  - Repeat culture if high risk: History of mitral valve prolapse (MVP) or heart valve surgery.
- PCN allergy.
  - Z-Pack (azithromycin) × 5 days.
  - Levaquin (levofloxacin) × 10 days (contraindicated if age less than 18).

Complications

- *Scarlet fever:* Sandpaper-textured pink rash, acute pharyngitis findings.
- *Rheumatic fever:* Inflammatory reaction to strep infection that may affect the heart and the valves, joints, and the brain.
- *Peritonsillar abscess:* Displaced uvula, red bulging mass on one side of anterior pharyngeal space, dysphagia, fever. Refer to ED STAT.

EARS

Acute Otitis Media (Purulent or Suppurative Otitis Media)

An acute infection of the middle ear cavity with bacterial pathogens due to mucus that becomes trapped in the middle ear secondary to temporary eustachian tube dysfunction. The infection is usually unilateral, but may at times involve both ears. Most have middle ear effusion (MEE).

Organisms

- *Streptococcus pneumoniae* (gram positive). High rates of beta-lactam resistant strains.
- *Haemophilus influenzae* (gram negative).
- *Moraxella catarrhalis* (gram negative).

Classic Case

Complains of ear pain (otalgia), popping noises, muffled hearing. Recent history of a cold or flare-up of allergic rhinitis. Adult infections usually develop much more slowly than in children. Afebrile or low-grade fever.

Bullous Myringitis

A type of acute otitis media infection, but causes more pain. Presence of blisters (bulla) on a reddened and bulging tympanic membrane. Conductive hearing loss. Caused by different types of pathogens (mycoplasma, viral, bacteria). Treat the same as bacterial AOM.

Objective

- Weber exam will show lateralization in the affected ear (conductive hearing loss).
  - Tympanic membrane (TM): Bulging or retraction with displaced light reflex (displaced landmarks). May look opaque.
  - Erythematous TM (may be due to coughing or crying in children).
  - Decreased mobility with flat-line tracing on tympanogram (most objective finding).
  - If TM is ruptured, purulent discharge from affected ear (and relief of ear pain).
- Acute sinusitis (acute rhinosinusitis).
- The maxillary and frontal sinuses are most commonly affected. Reports a history of a "bad cold" or flare-up of allergic rhinitis.

Organisms

- *Streptococcus pneumoniae* (gram positive). Beta-lactam resistant strains common.
- *Haemophilus influenzae* (gram negative).
- *Moraxella catarrhalis* (gram negative).

Classic Case

Complains of unilateral facial pressure that worsens when bending down, along with pain in the upper molar teeth (maxillary sinusitis) or frontal headache (frontal sinusitis). Coughing is made worse when supine (post-nasal drip cough). Self-treatment with over-the-counter cold and sinus remedies provides no relief of symptoms.

Objective

- Posterior pharynx: Purulent dark yellow- to green-colored postnasal drip.
- Infected sinus: Tender to palpation.
- If with allergy flare-up, may have boggy swollen nasal turbinates.
- Transillumination: Positive ("glow" of light on infected sinus is duller compared with normal sinus).

- Follow-up: Within 48 to 72 hours, symptoms will start to improve. If not getting better, check ears again for bulging and erythema. Switch to second-line drug (Augmentin, Ceftin).
- Treatment plan (both AOM and acute sinusitis).
- Duration of treatment: 10 to 14 days.

Treatment Plan

First-Line

- Amoxicillin is the gold standard for any age group.
  - First line: Amoxicillin 500 mg to 875 mg BID to TID × 10 to 14 days.
- OR consider starting with second-line antibiotic (Augmentin, Ceftin, Cefzil) if severe disease (severe ear pain, fever).
- Most patients will respond within 48 to 72 hours. If no improvement noted (TM same with symptoms), then switch to second-line drug (Augmentin, Ceftin, Cefzil).
- Use adjunct for symptoms such as a decongestant (pseudoephedrine or phenylephrine), saline nasal spray (Ocean spray), or mucolytic (guaifenesin), analgesic for ear pain. If allergic rhinitis, consider steroid nasal spray (Flonase, Vancenase).
- Educate about auto-insufflation (pinch nose and blow hard). Popping noises may be heard.
- The use of systemic steroids is not recommended.

Note

The FDA withdrew a large number of OTC cold medications in March 2011.

Second-Line

Second-line antibiotic treatment criteria: History of antibiotic use in the past 3 months, no response to amoxicillin, or severe case of AOM (high fever, severe ear pain).

Time duration is from 10 to 14 days.

- Amoxicillin/clavulanate (Augmentin) PO BID.
- Or third-generation cephalosporins.
  - Cefdinir (Omnicef) PO BID.
  - Cefpodoxime (Vantin) PO BID.
  - Ceftriaxone (Rocephin) 3 g IM × 1 dose.
- OR Cefuroxime (Ceftin) PO BID—second-generation cephalosporin.

Penicillin-Allergic Patients

- Azithromycin (Z-Pack) × 5 days or clarithromycin (Biaxin) PO BID.
- Trimethoprim sulfamethazole (Bactrim DS) PO BID.
- Levofloxacin (Levaquin) or moxifloxacin (Avelox) if 18 years or older. Increases risk for tendinitis/Achilles tendon rupture.

Pain

- Naproxen sodium (Anaprox DS) PO BID or ibuprofen (Advil) PO QID as needed.
- Acetaminophen (Tylenol) every 4 to 6 hours PRN.

Drainage

- Oral decongestants such as pseudoephedrine (Sudafed) or pseudoephedrine combined with guaifenesin (Mucinex D).
- Topical decongestants (i.e., Afrin); use only for 3 days maximum or will cause rebound.

- Saline nasal spray (Ocean spray).
- Steroid nasal spray (Flonase, Vancenase).
- Mucolytic (guaifenesin) and increase fluid to thin mucus.

Complications

- *Cholesteatoma:* Cauliflowerlike growth accompanied by foul-smelling ear discharge. No tympanic membrane or ossicles are visible (destroyed). History of chronic otitis media infections. Mass is not cancerous, but it can erode into the bones of the face and cause damage to the facial nerve (CN 7).
- *Mastoiditis:* Red and swollen mastoid that is tender to palpation. Treat with antibiotics. Refer.
- *Preorbital or orbital cellulitis* (more common in children).
  - Edema and redness periorbital area and diplopia.
  - Abnormal EOM (extraorbital muscles) testing of affected orbit.
  - Pain, fever, toxicity. Refer to ED.
- *Meningitis:* Acute onset of high fever, stiff neck, severe headache, photophobia, toxic. Positive Brudzinski or Kernig's sign. Refer to ED STAT.
- *Cavernous sinus thrombosis:*
  - Life-threatening medical emergency with high mortality; refer to ED.
  - Complains of acute headache, abnormal neurological exam, confused, febrile, toxic.

Otitis Media With Effusion

May follow acute otitis media. Can also be caused by chronic allergic rhinitis. Complains of ear pressure, popping noises, and muffled hearing in affected ear. Serous fluid inside middle ear is sterile.

Objective

- Tympanic membrane may bulge or retract. Tympanogram abnormal (flat line or no peak).
- TM should not be red.
- Fluid level with bubbles.

Treatment Plan

- Oral decongestants (pseudoephedrine or phenylalanine).
- Steroid nasal spray BID to TID × few weeks or saline nasal spray (Ocean spray) PRN.
- Allergic rhinitis, steroid nasal sprays with long-acting oral antihistamine (Zyrtec).

Otitis Externa (Swimmer's Ear)

Bacterial infection of the skin of the external ear canal (rarely fungal). More common during warm and humid weather (i.e., summer).

Organisms

- *Pseudomonas aeruginosa* (gram negative).
- *Staphylococcus aureus* (gram positive).

Classic Case

Complains of external ear pain, swelling, and green purulent discharge. History of recent activities that involve swimming or wetting ears.

Objective

Ear pain with manipulation of the external ear or tragus. Purulent green discharge. Erythematous and swollen ear canal that is very tender.

Treatment Plan

Cortisporin Otic suspension QID × 7 days. Keep water out of ear during treatment. If patient has recurrent episodes, prophylaxis is Otic Domedoro (boric) or alcohol and vinegar (Vosol).

Complications

- Malignant otitis media:
  - Seen in diabetics/immunocompromised; aggressive spread of infection to surrounding soft tissue/bone. A cellulitis infection.
  - Hospitalize for high-dose antibiotics and surgical debridement.

Infectious Mononucleosis

Infection by the Epstein-Barr virus (herpes virus family). Peak ages of acute infection are between ages 15 and 24 years. After acute infection, EBV virus lies latent in oropharyngeal tissue. Can become reactivated and cause symptoms. Virus is shed mainly through saliva. *Classic triad:* fatigue, acute pharyngitis, lymphadenopathy.

Classic Case

Teenage patient presents with new onset of sore throat, enlarged posterior cervical nodes, and fatigue. Fatigue may last weeks to months. May have abdominal pain due to hepatomegaly and/or splenomegaly. History of intimate kissing.

Objective

- *CBC:* Atypical lymphocytes and lymphocytosis (greater than 50%). Repeat CBC until resolves.
- *Heterophile antibody test (Monospot):* Positive.
- *Nodes:* Large cervical nodes that may be tender to palpation.
- *Pharynx:* Erythematous.
- *Tonsils:* Inflamed, sometimes with cryptic exudate (off-white color).
- *Hepatomegaly and splenomegaly:* Avoid vigorous palpation of the abdomen until resolves.
- *Skin:* Occasionally a generalized red maculopapular rash is present.

Treatment Plan

- Order abdominal ultrasound if splenomegaly/hepatomegaly is present, especially if patient is an athlete, a physically active adult, or an athletic coach.
- Educate athlete to avoid contact sports and heavy lifting until hepatomegaly and/or splenomegaly resolves (repeat abdominal ultrasound in 4 to 6 weeks).
- Symptomatic treatment.
- Avoid using amoxicillin if patient has strep throat (drug rash from 70% to 90%).

Complications

- Splenomegaly/splenic rupture (rare) but serious complications of mononucleosis.
- Airway obstruction (hospitalized and given high-dose steroids to decrease swelling).
- Neurologic (Guillain–Barré, aseptic meningitis, optic neuritis, others).
- Blood dyscrasias (atypical lymphocytes). Repeat CBC until lymphocytes normalized.

Cheilosis

Skin fissures and maceration at the corners of the mouth. Multiple etiologies such as over-salivation, iron-deficiency anemia, secondary bacterial infection, vitamin deficiencies.

Treatment Plan

- Apply triple antibiotic ointment BID to TID until healed.
- Remove or treat underlying cause.

✍ EXAM TIPS

- Treatment for otitis externa is Cortisporin Otic drops.
- Otitis externa's common bacterial pathogen is *Pseudomonas.*
- Ruptured spleen is a catastrophic event. Avoid contact sports (i.e., 4 weeks) until ultrasound documents resolution.
- Betimol (timolol) has the same contraindications as oral beta blockers.
- Cholesteatoma, periorbital sinusitis complication.
- Do not use amoxicillin if used in the past 3 months. Advance to second-line antibiotics such as Augmentin or Ceftin.
- Penicillin-allergic patients, use macrolides, sulfas (avoid cephalosporins, especially if had Class I reaction or anaphylaxis from penicillins).
- Learn to recognize a description of eye findings such as pinguecula, pterygium, chalazion.
- Rinne test result of BC greater than AC with conductive hearing loss (i.e., cerumenosis, AOM).
- Weber test result is lateralization to the "bad" or affected ear with conductive hearing loss.
- Weber or Rinne are testing the acoustic or CN 8.
- Lateralization on the Weber exam is an abnormal finding.
- Normal finding in Rinne test is air conduction that lasts longer than bone conduction (AC greater than BC).
- Remember what 20/40 vision means: patient can see at 20 feet what a person with normal vision can see at 40 feet.
- Carbamide peroxide (similar to hydrogen peroxide) is one of the most common OTC treatments for cerumenosis.

Skin and Integumentary System Review

⚠ DANGER SIGNALS

Rocky Mountain Spotted Fever

The classic rash looks like small red spots (petechiae) and starts to erupt on both the hands and feet (including the palms and soles), rapidly progressing toward the trunk until it becomes generalized. The rashes appear on the third day after the abrupt onset of high fever (103 to 105 degrees) accompanied by a severe headache, myalgia, conjunctival injection (red eyes), nausea/vomiting, and arthralgia. Rocky Mountain spotted fever (RMSF) can be fatal, with a mortality rate ranging from 3% to 9%. In the United States, the highest incidence is in southeastern/south central areas of the country. Most cases of RMSF occur during the spring and early summer season.

Actinic Keratosis

Older to elderly fair-skinned adults complain of numerous dry, round, and red-colored lesions with a rough texture that do not heal. Lesions are slow growing. Most common locations are sun-exposed areas such as the cheeks, nose, face, neck, arms, and back. The risk is highest for those with light-colored skin, hair, and/or eyes. In some cases, a precancerous lesion of squamous cell carcinoma is a possibility. Patients with early childhood history of severe sunburns are at higher risk for squamous cell, basal cell carcinoma, and melanoma.

Meningococcemia

Symptoms include sudden onset of sore throat, cough, fever, headache, stiff neck, photophobia, and changes in LOC (drowsiness, lethargy to coma). The appearance could be toxic. In some cases, there is abrupt onset of petechial to hemorrhagic rashes (pink to purple colored) in the axillae, flanks, wrist, and ankles (50% to 80% of cases). Rapid progression in fulminant cases results in death within 48 hours. The risk is higher for college students residing in dormitories (the CDC recommends vaccination for this higher-risk group). It is spread by aerosol droplets. Rifampin prophylaxis is recommended for close contacts.

Erythema Migrans (Early Lyme Disease)

The classic lesion is an expanding red rash with central clearing that resembles a target. The "bulls-eye" rash usually appears within 7 to 14 days after a deer tick bite (range between 3 to 30 days). The rash feels hot to the touch and has a rough texture. Common locations are the belt line, axillary area, behind the knees, and in the groin area. It is accompanied by flu-like symptoms. The lesion spontaneously resolves within a few weeks. It is most common in the northeastern regions of the United States. Use of DEET-containing repellent on clothes and skin can repel deer ticks.

Shingles Infection of the Trigeminal Nerve (Herpes Zoster Ophthalmicus)

A sight-threatening condition caused by reactivation of the herpes zoster virus that is located on the ophthalmic branch of the trigeminal nerve (CN 5). Patient reports sudden eruption of multiple vesicular lesions (ruptures into shallow ulcers with crusts) that are located on one side on the scalp, forehead, and the sides and the tip of the nose. If herpetic rash is seen on the tip of the nose, assume it is shingles until proven otherwise. The eyelid on the same side is swollen and red. The patient complains of photophobia, eye pain, and blurred vision. This is more common in elderly patients. Refer to an ophthalmologist or the ED as soon as possible.

Melanoma

Dark-colored moles with uneven texture, variegated colors, and irregular borders with a diameter of 6 mm or larger are observed. They may be pruritic. If melanoma is in the nailbeds (fungal melanoma), it may be very aggressive. Lesions can be located anywhere on the body including the retina. Risk factors include family history of melanoma (10% of cases), extensive/intense sunlight exposure, blistering sunburn in childhood, tanning beds, high nevus count/atypical nevus, and light skin/eyes.

Basal Cell Carcinoma (BCC)

Superficial form (30%) of BCC looks like a pearly or waxy skin lesion with an atrophic or ulcerated center that does not heal. The color could be white, light pink, brown, or flesh colored. It may bleed easily with mild trauma. This is more common in fair-skinned individuals with long-term daily sun exposure. An important risk factor is severe sunburns as a child.

Acral Lentiginous Melanoma

This is the most common type of melanoma in African Americans and Asians, and is a subtype of melanoma (<5%). These dark brown to black lesions are located on the nailbeds (subungual), palmar, and plantar surfaces, and rarely the mucous membranes. Subungual melanomas look like longitudinal brown to black bands on the nailbed.

Subungual Hematoma

Direct trauma to the nailbed results in pain and bleeding that is trapped between the nailbed and the finger/toenail. If the hematoma involves >25% of the area of the nail, there is a high risk of permanent ischemic damage to the nail matrix if the blood is not drained. One method of draining (trephination) a subungual hematoma is to straighten one end of a steel paperclip or to use an 18-gauge needle and heat it with a flame until it is very hot. The hot end is pushed down gently until a 3 to 4 mm hole is burned on the nail. The nail is pressed down gently until most or all of the blood is drained or suctioned with a smaller needle. Blood may continue draining for 24 to 36 hours.

Stevens–Johnson Syndrome (Erythema Multiforme Major)

The classic lesions appear target-like (or "bulls-eye"). Multiple lesions start erupting abruptly and can range from hives, blisters (bullae), petechiae, purpura, and hemorrhagic lesions that are painful. Extensive mucosal surface involvement (eyes, nose, mouth, esophagus, and bronchial tree) is observed. There could be a prodrome of fever with flu-like symptoms before rashes appear. Stevens–Johnson syndrome (SJS) is a severe and rare hypersensitivity reaction caused by medicines, infections, and malignancies. The drug classes associated with SJS are the penicillins, sulfas, barbiturates, and phenytoin (Dilantin). Mortality rate is 25% to 35%. HIV-infected patients have a 40-fold increased risk of SJS due to trimethoprim/sulfamethoxazole compared with the general population.

NORMAL FINDINGS

Anatomy of the Skin

Three layers: epidermis, dermis, and subcutaneous layer.
- *Epidermis:* No blood vessels; gets nourishment from the dermis. Consists of two layers:
  - Top layer consists of keratinized cells (dead squamous epithelial cells)
  - Bottom layer is where melanocytes reside and vitamin D synthesis occurs
- *Dermis:* Blood vessels, sebaceous glands, and hair follicles.
- *Subcutaneous layer:* Fat, sweat glands, and hair follicles.

Vitamin D Synthesis

People with darker skin require longer periods of sun exposure to produce vitamin D. A deficiency in pregnancy results in infantile rickets (brittle bones, skeletal abnormalities).

Screening for Melanoma

The "A, B, C, D, E" of melanoma:
  A (asymmetry)
  B (border irregular)
  C (color varies in the same region)
  D (diameter >6 mm)
  E (enlargement or change in size)
  Other symptoms to watch for include intermittent bleeding with mild trauma and itching.

Skin Cancer Stats

Skin cancer is the most common cancer in the United States. Basal cell skin carcinoma is the most common type of skin cancer.

Skin Lesion Review

- *Bulla:* Elevated superficial blister filled with serous fluid and >1 cm in size
  Example: Impetigo, second-degree burn with blisters, SJS lesions
- *Vesicle:* Elevated superficial skin lesion <1 cm in diameter and filled with serous fluid
  Example: Herpetic lesions

- *Pustule:* Elevated superficial skin lesion <1 cm in diameter filled with purulent fluid
  Example: Acne pustules
- *Macule:* Flat nonpalpable lesion <1 cm diameter
  Example: Freckles, lentigenes, small cherry angiomas
- *Papule:* Palpable solid lesion up to 0.5 cm
  Example: Nevi (moles), acne
- *Plaque:* Flattened elevated lesions with variable shape that is >1 cm in diameter
  Example: Psoriatic lesions

SKIN CLINICAL FINDINGS

Seborrheic Keratoses

Soft and round wart-like fleshy growths in the trunk that are located mostly on the back. Lesions on the same person can range in color from light tan to black. It is asymptomatic.

Xanthelasma (Figure 6.1)

Raised and yellow-colored soft plaques that are located under the brow or upper and/or lower lids of the eyes on the nasal side. It may be a sign of hyperlipidemia if present in persons younger than 40 years of age.

Melasma (Mask of Pregnancy)

Brown- to tan-colored stains located on the upper cheeks and forehead in some women who have been or are pregnant or on oral contraceptive pills (estrogen). It is more common in darker-skinned women. Stains are usually permanent but can lighten over time.

Vitiligo

Hypopigmented patches of skin with irregular shapes. It is progressive and can involve large areas. It can be located anywhere on the body and is more visible on darker skin.

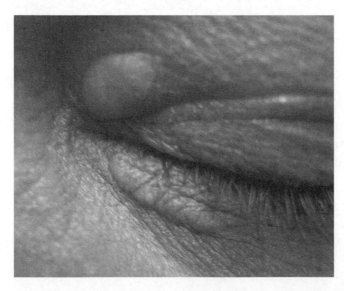

FIGURE 6.1 Xanthelasma.

Cherry Angioma

Benign small and smooth round papules that are a bright cherry-red color. The sizes range from 1 to 4 mm. Lesions are due to a nest of malformed arterioles. It is asymptomatic.

Lipoma

Soft fatty cystic tumors located in the subcutaneous layer of the skin. These could be of round or oval shape. These tumors can be large and are located mostly on the neck, trunk, legs, and arms. They are painless unless they become too large or are irritated or ruptured.

Nevi (Moles)

Round macules to papules (junctional nevi) in colors ranging from light tan to dark brown. Their borders may be distinct or slightly irregular.

Xerosis

Inherited skin disorder that results in extremely dry skin and may involve mucosal surfaces such as the mouth (xerostomia) or the conjunctiva of the eye (xerophthalmia).

Acanthosis Nigricans

Diffuse velvety thickening of the skin that is usually located behind the neck and on the axilla. It is associated with diabetes, metabolic syndrome, obesity, and cancer of the gastrointestinal (GI) tract.

TOPICAL STEROIDS

- Avoid steroids in case of suspected fungal etiology because it will worsen the infection.
- Infants, children, and adults with thin facial skin:
  – Do not use fluorinated topical steroids. Use 0.5% to 1% hydrocortisone.
- Topical steroids: HPA (hypothalamus–pituitary–adrenal) axis suppression may occur with excessive or prolonged use. It can cause striae, skin atrophy, telangiectasia, acne, and hypopigmentation.

⋮≣ DISEASE REVIEW

Psoriasis

An inherited skin disorder in which squamous epithelial cells undergo rapid mitotic division and abnormal maturation. The rapid turnover of skin produces the classic psoriatic plaque.

Special Findings
- *Koebner phenomenon:* New psoriatic plaques form over areas of skin trauma.
- *Auspitz sign:* Pinpoint areas of bleeding remain in the skin when a plaque is removed.

Classic Case
The patients complains of pruritic erythematous plaques covered with fine silvery-white scales along with pitted fingernails and toenails. The plaques are distributed in the scalp, elbows, knees, sacrum, and the intergluteal folds. Partially resolving plaques

are pink colored with minimal scaling. Patients with psoriatic arthritis will complain of painful red, warm, and swollen joints (migratory arthritis) in addition to the skin plaques.

Medications
Topical steroids, topical retinoids (tazorotene), tar preparations (psoralen drug class).

Black Box Warning (Topical Tacrolimus)
- Rare cases of malignancy (including skin and lymphoma). Use sunblock. Avoid if patient is immunocompromised.
  - *Severe disease:* Antimetabolites (i.e., methotrexate), biologics/antitumor necrosis factor (TNF) agents
  - *Black Box Warning* (biologics/anti-TNF agents)
- Humira, Enbrel, and Remicade are associated with higher risk of serious/fatal infections, malignancy, TB, fungal infections, sepsis, etc. (baseline PPD, CBC with differential).
- Goeckerman regimen (UVB light and tar-derived topicals) may induce remission in severe cases.

Complications
- *Guttate psoriasis (drop-shaped lesions)*: Severe form of psoriasis resulting from a beta-hemolytic streptococcus Group A infection (usually due to strep throat).

Actinic Keratoses

Precancerous precursors to squamous cell carcinoma.

Classic Case
Older to elderly adult complains of numerous dry round and red-colored lesions with a rough texture that do not heal; lesions slow growing; most common locations are sun-exposed areas such as the cheeks, nose, face, neck, arms, and back; highest risk if light-colored skin, hair, and/or eyes; a precancerous lesion of squamous cell carcinoma. Early childhood history of frequent sunburns places person at higher risk.

Medications
If there are only a small number of lesions, they can be treated with cryotherapy. With larger numbers, fluorouracil cream 5% (5-FU cream), a topical antineoplastic agent, is used over several weeks.

Tinea Versicolor

A superficial skin infection caused by yeasts *Pityrosporum orbiculare* or *Pityrosporum ovale*.

Classic Case
Complains of multiple hypopigmented round macules on the chest, shoulders, and/or back that "appear" after skin becomes tan from sun exposure; asymptomatic.

Labs
Potassium hydroxide (KOH) slide: hyphae and spores ("spaghetti and meatballs").

Medications
Topical selenium sulfide or ketoconazole (Nizoral) shampoo or cream BID × 2 weeks. Oral antifungals have also been used.

Atopic Dermatitis (Eczema)

A chronic inherited skin disorder marked by extremely pruritic rashes that are located on the hands, flexural folds, and neck (older child to adult). The rashes are exacerbated by stress and environmental factors (i.e., winter). The disorder is associated with atopic disorders such as asthma, allergic rhinitis, and multiple allergies (family history).

Classic Case

Infants up to age 2 years have a larger area of rash distribution compared to teens and adults. The rashes are typically found on the cheeks, entire trunk, knees, and elbows.

Older children and adults have rashes on the hands, neck, and antecubital and popliteal space (flexural folds). The classic rash starts as multiple small vesicles that rupture, leaving painful, bright red, weepy lesions. The lesions become lichenified from chronic itching and can persist for months. Fissures form that can be secondarily infected with bacteria.

Medications

- Topical steroids are first-line treatment.
  - *Mild:* Hydrocortisone 1% to 2.5%.
  - *Medium:* Triamcinolone.
- Medium to high potency (Halog) use × 10 days and taper to weaker steroids, then stop.
- Systemic oral antihistamines for pruritis (Benadryl, hydroxyzine).
- Skin lubricants (Eucerin, Keri Lotion, baby oil). Avoid drying skin/xerosis since it will exacerbate eczema (i.e., no hot baths, harsh soaps, chemicals, wool clothing).
- Hydrating baths (avoid hot water/soaps) followed immediately by application of skin lubricants (Eucerin, Keri Lotion, Crisco). Do not wait until skin is dry before applying.

Contact Dermatitis

An inflammatory skin reaction due to contact with an irritating external substance; can be a single lesion or generalized rash (i.e., sea-bather's itch). Common offenders are: poison ivy (rhus dermatitis) and nickel. Onset can occur within minutes to several hours after skin contact.

Classic Case

Acute onset of one to multiple bright red and pruritic lesions that evolve into bullous or vesicular lesions; easily ruptures, leaving bright red moist areas that are painful. When rash dries, it becomes crusted; very pruritic and gets lichenified from chronic itching. The shape may follow a pattern (i.e., a ring around a finger) or have asymmetric distribution.

Medications

- Stop exposure to substance. Calamine lotion; topical steroids; oatmeal baths (Aveeno).
- Severe rash: Oral prednisone for 12 to 14 days (wean). Avoid reexposure.

Superficial Candidiasis

Superficial skin infection from the yeast *Candida albicans*. Environmental factors promoting overgrowth are: increased warmth and humidity, friction, and decreased immunity;

can infect skin (candidal intertrigo), mucous membranes (thrush, vaginitis), and systemically. Intertrigo/intertriginous areas of the body (or apposed areas of skin that rub together) can be infected by either fungal and/or bacterial organisms.

Classic Case

External: An obese adult complains of bright red and shiny lesions that itch or burn, located on the intertriginous areas (under the breast in females, axillae, abdomen, groin, the web spaces between the toes). The rash may have satellite lesions (small red rashes around the main rash).

Oral-Thrush: Complains of a severe sore throat with white adherent plaques with a red base that are hard to dislodge on the pharynx. Thrush in "healthy adults" who are not on antibiotics may signal an immunodeficient condition.

Treatment Plan

- Nystatin powder and/or cream in skin folds (intertriginous areas) BID. OTC topical antifungals are miconazole, clotrimazole. Prescription needed for terconazole, ciclopirox.
- Keep skin dry and aerated.
- Nystatin (Mycostatin) oral suspension for oral thrush (swish and swallow) QID.
- "Magic Mouthwash" (viscous lidocaine, diphenhydramine, Maalox) is compounded by pharmacists and is for severe sore throat (thrush, canker sores, mouth ulcers).

> **Note**
>
> HIV esophageal *Candida* infections should be treated with systemic antifungals (fluconazole).

Acute Cellulitis

An acute skin infection of the deep dermis and underlying tissue, usually caused by gram-positive bacteria. There are two forms of cellulitis (purulent and nonpurulent). Points of entry are skin breaks, insect bites or abrasions, and surgical wounds. Community-acquired type of MRSA strain also called "USA 300."

- *Purulent form of cellulitis: Staphyloccus aureas* (gram-positive). Community-acquired MRSA now common. Most cases are located on the lower leg (85%).
- *Nonpurulent form of cellulitis:* Usually due to streptococci (but may also be staph).
- *Dog and cat bites: Pasteurella multicoda* (gram-negative).
- *Erysipelas:* Group B streptococcus.
- *Puncture wounds (foot):* Contaminated with soft-foam liner material or puncture wounds through sneakers. Rule out *Pseudomonas aeruginosa*.
- *Vibrio vulnificus*: Saltwater contamination, higher risk if liver disease or immunocompromised.

Classic Case (Staphylococcal Cellulitis)

Most common location is the legs/feet. Acute onset of diffused pink- to red-colored skin on the "traumatized" site with poorly demarcated margin that grows larger. The lesion feels hot and does not have a distinct border (as seen in erysipelas). There may be abscesses or draining of purulent green discharge. Deeper infection of the skin is manifested by red streaks radiating from infected area under the skin (lymphagitis) and regional lymphadenopathy. Patients may have systemic symptoms. Tinea pedis increases risk of lower-extremity cellulitis.

Clenched Fist Injuries (Fist Fights)

High risk of infection to joints (i.e., knuckles), fascia, nerves, and the bones. Refer to ED for treatment. There may be a foreign body embedded, such as a tooth (x-ray needed) and/or a fracture.

- Necrotizing fasciitis: usually Group A strep or polymycrobial.
- Reddish to purple color lesion that increases rapidly in size. Infected area appears indurated ("woody" induration) with complaints of severe pain on affected site.

Boils (Furuncles)

A furuncle/boil is an infected hair follicle that fills with pus (abscessed). It looks like a round red bump that is hot and tender to touch. When it is fluctuant, it can rupture and drain purulent green-colored discharge. Apply antibiotic ointment BID and cover with dressing until healed.

CARBUNCLES (COALESCED BOILS)

Carbuncles are several boils that coalesce to form a large boil or abscess. Sometimes, they may form several "heads." They are usually treated with systemic antibiotics.

Labs

- Culture and sensitivity (C&S) advancing edge of lesion (if fluid or pus, vesicles, drainage)
- Lower-extremity cellulitis, also fungal culture for tinea pedis (swab interdigital spaces)
- CBC (complete blood count) if fever or toxic or suspect necrotizing fasciitis (refer to ED)

Treatment Plan

- *Non-MRSA nonpurulent cellulitis:* Dicloxacillin PO (orally) QID × 10 days (preferred due to high rate of beta-lactam resistance). Cephalexin QID or clindamycin TID × 10 days.
- *Penicillin allergic:* Erythromycins (macrolides), second-generation cephalosporins, clindamycin.
- *Suspect MRSA:* Bactrim DS one tablet BID × 10 days, Doxycycline PO BID × 10 days or clindamycin 3 to 4×/day for 10 days.
- *Td booster:* If last dose was more than 5 years ago.
- *Recurrent cellulitis:* Consider decolonozation. Muciprocin BID on nares × 5 to 10 days.
- Elevate affected limb.

Follow Up

Follow up with the patient within 48 hours. Refer cellulitis cases if:

- Systemic symptoms develop (i.e., fever, toxic) or worsen.
- The cellulitis is not responding to treatment within 48 hours.
- Cellulitis is spreading quickly or is a small lesion with gangrenous center associated with large amount of pain (necrotizing fasciitis).
- Patient is a diabetic, immunocompromised, or taking anti-TNF (rheumatoid arthritis).

Complications
- Osteomyelitis; septic arthritis; sepsis.
- Tendon and fascial extension.
- Rarely, death (*V. vulnificus* infections have high fatality rates).

Erysipelas

A subtype of cellulitis involving the upper dermis and superficial lymphatics that is usually caused by Group A *Streptococcus*.

Classic Case

Sudden onset of one large hot and indurated red skin lesion that has clear demarcated margins. It is usually located on the lower legs (the shins) or the cheeks. It is accompanied by fever and chills. Hospitalization may be needed for severe cases, infants, the elderly, and the immunocompromised.

Bites: Human and Animal

Human Bites

The "dirtiest" bite of all. Watch for closed-fist injuries of the hands (may involve joint capsule and tendon damage). *Eikenella corrodens* and numerous bacteria may be involved.

Dog and Cat Bites

P. multicoda (gram-negative). Cat bites have a higher risk of infection than dog bites. If infection is severe, redness, swelling, intense pain, and systemic symptoms may develop within 12 to 24 hours.

Treatment Plan (Both Human and Animal Bites)

- Amoxicillin/clavulanate (Augmentin) PO × 10 days (penicillin allergy, use clindamycin plus fluoroquinolone).
- All bites and infected wounds need wound cultures with sensitivity testing (C&S).
- Do not suture wounds at high risk for infection: puncture wounds, wounds >12 hours old (24 hours on face), cat bites, bites wounds on compromised hosts.
- Cartilage injuries (cartilage does not regenerate); refer to plastic surgeon.
- Tetanus prophylaxis (if last booster >5 years, needs booster).
- Follow up with patient within 24 to 48 hours after treatment.

Referral of Wounds

- Closed-fist injuries or crush injuries
- Cartilage damage or wounds with cosmetic effects; refer to plastic surgeons
- Compromised hosts: adult diabetics, absent/dysfunction of the spleen, immunocompromised

Rabies

- Bats, raccoons, skunks, foxes, coyotes (domestic animals can also have rabies).
- Rabies immune globulin plus rabies vaccine may be required. Call local health department for advice. Consider if wild animal acts tame, copious saliva, unprovoked attack, or animal looks ill.
- *Option:* Quarantine a domestic animal for 10 days (look for signs/symptoms of rabies).

Hidradenitis Suppurativa (Figure 6.2)

A bacterial infection of the sebaceous glands of the axilla (or groin) by *Staphylococcus aureus* (gram positive) that frequently becomes chronic. It is marked by flare-ups and resolution. Usually both axillae are involved. Chronic episodic infection eventually leaves sinus tracts and heavy scarring.

Classic Case

Patient complains of an acute onset of painful, large, dark-red nodules and papules under one or both axillae that become abscessed. Ruptured lesions drain purulent green-colored discharge. Pain resolves when the abscess drains and heals. History of recurrent episodes on the same areas in the axilla results in sinus tracts and multiple scars.

Labs

C&S of purulent discharge.

Treatment Plan

- Amoxicillin/clavulanate (Augmentin) PO BID or dicloxacillin TID × 10 days.
- Mupirocin ointment to lower third of nares and under fingernails BID × 2 weeks.
- Use antibacterial soap (e.g., Dial), especially on axilla and groin areas.
- Avoid underarm deodorants during acute phase.

Impetigo

Acute superficial skin infection caused by gram-positive bacteria such as strep pyogenes (beta strep) or *S. aureus*. It is very contagious and pruritic, and is more common in warm and humid weather. Two types: bullous and nonbullous forms.

Classic Case

It is more common in children and teens. There may be acute onset of itchy pink to red lesions that become bullous, then crusty and maculopapular. The bullae are thin-roofed and easily ruptured.

After rupture, lesions are covered with honey-colored crusts (dried serous fluid).

Labs

C&S of crusts/wound.

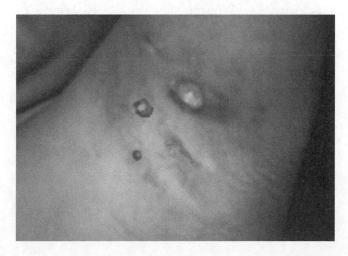

FIGURE 6.2 Hidradenitis suppurativa (mild).

Treatment Plan

- Cephalexin (Keflex) QID, dicloxacillin QID × 10 days.
- *PCN allergic:* Azithromycin 250 mg × 5 days (macrolides), clindamycin × 10 days.
- If very few lesions with no bulla, may use topical 2% mupirocin ointment (Bacitracin) × 10 days.
- Frequent hand-washing, shower/bathe daily to remove crusts.

Meningococcemia

A serious life-threatening infection caused by *Neisseria meningitides* (gram-negative diplococci) that are spread by respiratory droplets. Bacterial meningitis is a medical emergency.

- Do not delay treatment if high index of suspicion—refer to emergency department STAT.
- College students living in dormitories are at higher risk. If treated early, mortality is less than 5%. The bodily damage is due to the endotoxin's effects on the endothelium of blood vessels.

Classic Case

- Described earlier under "Danger Signals."

Prophylaxis

- *Close contacts:* Rifampin PO every 12 hours × 2 days.
- Meningococcal vaccination recommended for all college students living in dormitories.

Labs

- Lumbar punctures: culture cerebrospinal fluid (CSF).
- Blood cultures, throat cultures, etc.
- CT or MRI of the brain.

Treatment Plan

- Ceftriaxone (Rocephin) 2 g IV every 12 hours plus vancomycin IV every 8–12 hours
- Hospital; isolation precautions; supportive treatment

Complications

- Tissue infarction and necrosis (i.e., gangrene of the toes, foot, fingers, etc.) causing amputation
- Death

Early Lyme Disease

Erythema migrans is a skin lesion caused by the bite of an *Ixodes* tick infected with *Borrelia burgdorferi*. If untreated, infection becomes systemic and affects multiple organ systems.

Classic Case

- Described earlier under "Danger Signals."

Labs

- Serum antibody titers IgM (early) and IgG (late)

Treatment Plan
- Early Lyme only: Doxycycline BID (twice daily) or tetracycline × 14 days (amoxicillin if pregnant).

Complications
- Neurological system problems such as Guillain–Barré syndrome
- Migratory arthritis, chronic fatigue, and so forth

Rocky Mountain Spotted Fever

Caused by the bite of a dog tick or wood tick that is infected with the parasite *Rickettsia rickettsii*. If high index of suspicion, do not delay treatment (do not wait for lab results). Treatment most effective if started within first 5 days of symptoms. Doxycycline is the first-line treatment for all age groups (CDC, 2011). Most cases occur in the spring and early summer.

Classic Case
Described earlier under "Danger Signals."

Labs
- Diagnostic: antibody titers to *R. rickettsii* (by indirect fluorescent antibodies)
- Biopsy of skin lesion (3 mm punch biopsy). CBC, LFTs, CSF, others

Medications
Doxycycline BID or tetracycline QID (4 times daily) × 21 days. Refer STAT.

Complications
- Death. Neurological sequelae (hearing loss, paraparesis, neuropathy, others).

Varicella-Zoster Virus Infections

Chickenpox (varicella) and herpes zoster (shingles) are both caused by the same virus. The primary infection is called chickenpox (varicella) and the reactivation of the infection is known as shingles (herpes zoster). After primary infection (chickenpox), the virus becomes latent within a dermatome (sensory ganglia) and is kept under control by an intact immune system.
- *Chickenpox:* Contagious from 1 to 2 days before the onset of the rash and until all of the lesions have crusted over (chickenpox and shingles). Duration of illness is 1 or 2 weeks.
- *Shingles:* Contagious with the onset of the rashes until all the lesions have crusted over.

Classic Case
Chickenpox/Varicella
Prodrome of fever, pharyngitis, and malaise that is followed within 24 hours by the eruption of pruritic vesicular lesions in different stages of development over a period of 4 days. The rashes start on the head/face and quickly spread to the trunk and extremities. It takes 1 to 2 weeks for the crusts to fall off and the skin to heal.

Shingles
Elderly patient reports of the sudden onset of groups of small vesicles on a red base that becomes crusted. Crusted lesions follow a dermatomal pattern on one side of the body.

Patient complains of pain, which can be quite severe. Some with prodrome may have severe pain/burning sensation at the site before the breakout. Shingles can last from 2 to 4 weeks. Immunocompromised and elderly patients are at higher risk for post-herpetic neuralgia (PHN). Early treatment reduces risk. Treat within 48 to 72 hours after onset of breakout if patient is above age 50 years or immunocompromised.

Labs

Gold standard: Viral culture, polymerase chain reaction (PCR) for ZDV.

Medications

Acyclovir (Zovirax) 5 × per day or valacyclovir (Valtrex) BID × 10 days for initial break-outs and 7 days for flare-ups. Most effective when started within 48 to 72 hours of when rash appears.

Complications

- *PHN:* More common in elderly and immunocompromised patients. Treat PHN with tricyclic antidepressants (i.e., low-dose amitriptyline), anticonvulsants (i.e., Depakote), or gabapentin TID. Lidocaine 5% patch (Lidoderm) to intact skin.
- *Herpes zoster ophthalmicus (CN 5):* Can result in corneal blindness. Refer immediately to ophthalmologist or ED (described under "Danger Signals").
- *Others:* Ramsay Hunt syndrome (herpes zoster oticus or CN 8), refer to neurologist.

Vaccines

- *Varicella vaccine (1995):* A person can still become infected with VZV but will have very mild disease with fewer lesions (compared with the unvaccinated). Advise reproductive-aged women not to get pregnant within the next 3 months.
- *Shingles/zoster vaccine (2006):* One dose is recommended for persons aged 60 years or older.
- *Contraindications:* AIDS, chronic high-dosed steroids, radiation, chemo, immuno-compromised.

📋 CLINICAL TIPS

- Only a person who has had chickenpox (rarely the chickenpox vaccine) can get shingles.
- About one in five people with shingles will suffer from PHN.

Herpetic Whitlow

A viral skin infection of the finger(s) that is caused by herpes simplex (type 1 or type 2) virus infection, from direct contact with either a cold sore or genital herpes lesion.

Classic Case

Patient complains of the acute onset of extremely painful red bumps and small blisters on the sides of the finger or the cuticle area or on the terminal phalanx of one or more fingers; may have recurrent outbreaks. Ask patient about coexisting symptoms of oral herpes or genital herpes.

Management
Usually symptomatic treatment.
- *Self-limited infection:* Analgesics or nonsteroidal anti-inflammatory drugs (NSAIDs) for pain PRN.
- *Severe infections:* Treat with acyclovir (Zovirax).

Patient Education
- Avoid sharing personal items, gloves, towels.
- Cover skin lesion completely with large Band-Aid/bandage until the lesions heal.

Paronychia (Figure 6.3)
An acute local bacterial skin infection of the proximal or lateral nail folds (cuticle) that resolves after the abscess drains. Causative bacteria are *S. aureus*, streptococci, or pseudomonas (gram negative). Chronic cases are associated with coexisting onychomycosis (fungal infection of nails).

Classic Case
Complains of acute onset of a painful and red swollen area around the nail on a finger that eventually becomes abscessed. The most common locations are index finger and thumb. Reports a history of picking on a hangnail, biting off hangnail, or of trimming of the cuticle during a manicure.

Management
- Soak affected finger in warm water for 20 minutes 3 times a day.
- Apply topical antibiotic such as triple antibiotic or mupirocin to affected finger after soaking.
- *Abscess:* Incision and drainage (use #11 scalpel) or use the beveled edge of a large-gauge needle to gently separate the cuticle margin from the nail bed to drain the abscess.

Pityriasis Rosea
Cause unknown. Self-limiting illness (4 to 8 weeks) and asymptomatic.

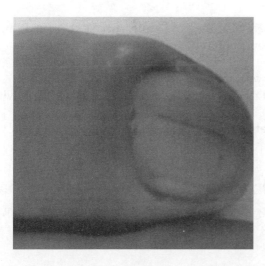

FIGURE 6.3 Paronychia.

Classic Case

Complains of oval lesions with fine scales that follow skin lines (cleavage lines) of the trunk or a "Christmas tree" pattern. Salmon-pink color in Whites. May be pruritic.

- *"Herald patch"*: First lesion to appear and largest in size; appears 2 weeks before full breakout.

Medications

- No medications. Advise patient that lesions will take about 4 weeks to resolve.
- If high risk of STDs, check rapid plasma reagent (RPR) to rule out secondary syphilis.

Scabies

An infestation of the skin by the *Sarcoptes scabiei* mite. The female mite burrows under the skin to lay her eggs; transmitted by close contact. May be asymptomatic the first 2 to 6 weeks. Even after treatment, the pruritis may persists for 2 to 4 weeks (sensitivity reaction to mites and their feces).

- *Norwegian scabies:* Lesions covered with fine scales (looks like white plaques) and crusts; involves the nails (dystrophic nails), scalp, body; absent to mild pruritis; very contagious.

Classic Case

Complains of pruritic rashes located in the interdigital webs of the hands, axillae, breasts, buttock folds, waist, scrotum, and penis. Severe itching that is worse at nighttime and interferes with sleep. Other family members may also have the same symptoms.

Objective

The rash appears as serpinginous (snakelike) or linear burrows. Lesions can be papular, vesicular, or crusted. Higher incidence in crowded conditions (i.e., nursing homes, etc.) and among the homeless.

Labs

Scrape burrow or scales with glass slide, use coverslip (wet mount). Look for mites or eggs.

Medications

- Permethrin 5% (Elimite); apply cream to entire body (head to soles); wash off at 8 to 14 hours.
- Treat everyone in the same household at the same time. Any clothes/bedding used 3 days before and during treatment should be washed and dried using the hot settings.
- Pruritis usually improves in 48 hours, but can last up to 2 to 4 weeks (even if mites are dead). Do not retreat (do wet mount to check for live mites). Treat itch with Benadryl and topical steroids.
- *Long-term care facility:* Treat all patients, staff, family members, and frequent visitors for scabies.

Tinea Infections (Dermatophytoses)

An infection of superficial keratinized tissue (skin, hair, nails) by tinea yeast organisms. Tinea yeasts organisms are classified as dermatophytes.

Labs for Tinea Infections
Gold Standard: Fungal Culture of Scales/Hair/Nails/Skin Lesions
KOH slide microscopy (low to medium power) reveals pseudohyphae and spores.

Medications
- OTC topicals such as azoles and allylamines
  - *OTC azoles:* Clotrimazole (Lotrimin) BID, miconazole (Monistat) BID
  - *Prescription topical azole:* Terconazole (Terazol) cream BID
  - *OTC allylamines:* Terbinafine (Lamisil AT) or naftifine cream (Naftin) once a day to BID

Tinea Capitis (Ringworm of the Scalp)

Black dot tinea capitis (BDTC) is the most common type in the United States. African American children are at higher risk. Spread by close contact, fomites (shared hats, combs).

Classic Case
School-aged child with asymptomatic scaly patch that gradually enlarges. The hairs inside the patch breaks off easily by the roots (looks like black dots) causing patchy alopecia.
Black dot sign: broken hair shafts leave dot-like pattern on scalp.

Medications
- Baseline LFTs and repeat 2 weeks after initiating systemic antifungal treatment. Monitor.
- *Gold standard:* Griseofulvin (microsize/ultramicrosize) daily to BID × 6 to 12 weeks.
- Avoid hepatotoxic substances (alcohol, statins, acetaminophen).

Table 6.1 Common Skin Rashes

Disease	Description
Impetigo	"Honey-colored" crusts. Fragile bullae. Pruritic.
Measles	Koplik's spots are small white round spots on a red base on the buccal mucosa by the rear molars.
Scabies	Very pruritic, especially at night. Serpenginous rash on interdigital webs, waist, axilla, penis.
Scarlet fever	"Sandpaper" rash with sore throat (strep throat).
Tinea versicolor	Hypopigmented round to oval macular rashes. Most lesions on upper shoulders/back. Not pruritic.
Pityriasis rosea	"Christmas tree" pattern rash (rash on cleavage lines). "Herald patch" largest lesion, appears initially.
Molluscum contagiosum	Smooth papules 5-mm size that are dome-shaped with central umbilication with a white "plug."
Erythema migrans	Red target-like lesions that grow in size. Some central clearing. Early stage of Lyme disease.
*Meningococcemia	Purple-colored to dark red painful skin lesions all over body. Acute onset high fever. Headache. LOC changes. Rifampin prophylaxis for close contacts.
*Rocky Mountain spotted fever (*Rickettsia rickettsii* from tick bite)	Red spot-like rashes that first break out on the hand/palm/wrist and on the feet/sole/ankles. Acute onset high fever. Severe headache. Myalgias.

* These are life threatening and are CDC Reportable Diseases.

Complications

- Kerion: Inflammatory and indurated lesions that permanently damage hair follicles causing patchy alopecia.

Tinea Pedis (Athlete's Foot)

Two types: Scaly and dry form or moist type (strong odor). Dry type with fine scales only.

Moist lesions between toe webs, which are white-colored with strong unpleasant odor.

Tinea Corporis or Tinea Circinata (Ringworm of the Body)

Ring-like pruritic rashes with a collarette of fine scales that slowly enlarge with some central clearing. Large numbers or severe cases can also be treated with oral antifungals.

Tinea Cruris ("Jock Itch")

Perineal and groin area has pruritic red rashes with fine scales; may be mistaken for candidal infection (bright red rashes with satellite lesions) or intertrigo (bright red diffused rash due to bacterial infection).

Tinea Manuum (Hands)

Pruritic round rashes with fine scales on the hands. Usually infected from chronic scratching of foot that is also infected with tinea (athlete's foot).

Tinea Barbae (Beard Area)

Beard area affected. Scaling with pruritic red rashes.

Onychomycosis (Nails)

Nail becomes yellowed, thickened, and opaque with debris. Nail may separate from nailbed (onycholysis). Great toe is the most common location. Treated with systemic antifungals, except for mild cases. If mild, trial of topical treatment (Penlac "nailpolish").

Labs

Fungal cultures of nails and nail debris.

Medications

- Pulse therapy with systemic antifungals. Baseline LFTs. Monitor periodically.
- Oral fluconazole 150 mg to 300 mg weekly or terbinafine (Lamisil) weekly × several weeks.
- *Mild cases:* Penlac nail lacquer × several weeks. Works best in mild cases of the fingernails.

Acne Vulgaris (Common Acne)

Inflammation and infection of the sebaceous glands. Multifactorial causes such as high androgen levels, bacterial infection (*Propionibacterium acnes*), and genetic influences. Found mostly on the face, shoulders, chest, and back. Highest incidence during puberty and adolescence.

Mild Acne (Topicals Only)

Open comedones (blackheads), closed comedones, small papules, small pustules.

- *Prescription meds:* Isotretinoin (Retin-A), benzoyl peroxide with erythromycin (Benzamycin) cream, clindamycin topical (Cleocin).

- *Start at lowest dose:* Retinoic acid (Retin-A) 0.25% cream every other day at bedtime × 2 to 3 weeks, then daily application at bedtime. Photosensitivity reaction possible (use sunscreen).

Moderate Acne (Topicals Plus Antibiotic)
Same as indicated for mild acne plus large numbers of papules and pustules.

Treatment Plan
- Use prescription topicals (i.e., Benzamycin) plus oral tetracycline (Category D), or minocycline (Minocin), or doxycline.
- Tetracyclines can be given for acne starting at about age 13. Growth of permanent teeth is finished except wisdom teeth (or third molars), which erupt between the ages of 17 to 25 years.
- *Tetracyclines* (Category D): Permanent discoloration of growing tooth enamel. Tetracyclines decrease effectiveness of oral contraceptives (use additional method). Not given during pregnancy or to children under age 13.
- *Others:* Certain oral contraceptives (Desogen, Yaz) are indicated for acne.

Severe Cystic Acne

All of the preceding findings plus painful indurated nodules and cysts over face, shoulders, and chest.

Medications

Isotretinoin (Accutane) is a category X drug (extremely teratogenic). Need to sign special consent forms. Females must enroll in approved pregnancy prevention program (iPLEDGE). Use two forms of reliable contraception. Prescribe 1-month supply only. Monthly pregnancy testing and show results to pharmacist before refills. Pregnancy test 1 month after discontinued. Discontinue if the following are present:
- Severe depression, visual disturbance, hearing loss, tinnitus, GI pain, rectal bleeding, uncontrolled hypertriglyceremia, pancreatitis, hepatitis

Rosacea (Acne Rosacea)

Chronic and relapsing skin inflammatory disorder that is common. There is no cure for rosacea. Management is aimed at symptom control and avoidance of triggers that cause exacerbations.

Classic Case
Light-skinned adult to older patient with Celtic background (i.e., Irish, Scottish, English) complains of chronic and small acne-like papules and pustules around the nose, mouth, and chin. Patient blushes easily. Patient usually is blond or red haired and has blue eyes. Some have ocular symptoms such as red eyes, "dry eyes," or chronic blepharitis (ocular rosacea).

Medications
- Metronidazole (Metrogel) topical gel
- Azelaic acid (Azelex) topical gel
- Low-dose oral tetracycline or minocycline given over several weeks

Complications
- *Rhinophyma:* Hyperplasia of tissue at the tip of the nose from chronic severe disease
- *Ocular rosacea:* Blepharitis, conjunctival injection, lid margin telangiectasia

Burns (Thermal Burns)

Superficial Thickness (First Degree)

- Erythema only (no blisters). Painful (i.e., sunburns, mild scalds).
- Cleanse with mild soap and water (or saline): Cold packs for 24 to 48 hours.
- Topical OTC anesthetics such as benzocaine if desired.

Partial Thickness (Second Degree)

- Red-colored skin with superficial blisters (bullae). Painful (i.e., hot water/oil scalds, fire).
- Use water with mild soap or normal saline to clean broken skin (not hydrogen peroxide or full-strength Betadine). Do not rupture blisters. Treat with silver sulfadiazine cream (Silvadene) and apply dressings.

Full Thickness (Third Degree)

- *Initial assessment:* Rule out airway and breathing compromise. Smoke inhalation injury is a medical emergency. Painless. Entire skin layer, subcutaneous area, and soft tissue fascia may be destroyed.
- *Refer:* Facial burns, electrical burns, third-degree burns, cartilaginous areas such as the nose and ears (cartilage will not regenerate). Burns on greater than 10% of body.

Total Percentage of Body Surface Area (TBSA)

Rule of Nines (Adult):

- Body surface: 9% (each arm, head)
- Body surface: 18% (each leg, anterior trunk, or posterior trunk)
- *Example*: A middle-aged woman is cooking and suffers hot oil burns. The NP notes that the patient has bright red skin on the right arm and the right leg. The skin on the patient's chest and abdomen is bright red with several bullae on the surface. What is this patient's diagnosis?
  Answer: Superficial thickness burns on the right arm (9%) and right leg (18%) with partial thickness burns on the chest and abdomen (anterior trunk 18%). The TBSA is 45%.

BIOTERRORISM

Anthrax

Caused by *Bacillus anthracis* (gram-positive rods). There are three types of anthrax (cutaneous, GI, and pulmonary). Pulmonary anthrax (inhalational anthrax) is caused by inhaling aerosolized spores through working with animal/wool/hides/hair, or through bioterrorism. Fulminant inhalational anthrax causes death within days. Symptoms are flu-like and associated with cough, chest pain with cough, hemoptysis, dyspnea, hypoxia, and shock.

- Postexposure prophylaxis (exposure to bioterrorism event): Ciprofloxacin 500 mg PO BID × 60 days (alternate is doxycycline PO)
- Ideal pathogen for bioterrorism
- Pathogens have high mortality rates, are easily spread, and are airborne (i.e., aerosolized route).
- Highest-risk pathogens: anthrax bacilli and smallpox virus.

Ricin Toxin (From Castor Beans)

Inhalation causes cough, pulmonary edema, and respiratory distress within 8 hours. Oral intake of ricin can cause vomiting, bloody diarrhea, multi-organ failure in 6 hours. No known antidote.

Smallpox (Variola Virus)

Infects respiratory and oropharyngeal mucosal surfaces. "Eliminated" in 1977. Incubation period of 2 weeks. Flu-like signs/symptoms. Numerous large nodules appear mostly in the center of the face and on the arms and legs. Treatment is symptomatic. Mortality rate is 20% to 50%.

Smallpox Vaccine

If vaccine is given within 3 to 4 days postexposure, can lessen severity of illness. Vaccinia immune globulin (for pregnant, immunosuppressed, etc.) is available from special clinics.

✍ EXAM TIPS

- Differentiate between contact dermatitis and atopic dermatitis. The best clue is the unilateral location and the shape of the lesions in contact dermatitis.
- Rashes that are very pruritic at night and located on the interdigital webs and/or penis are scabies until proven otherwise. Treat entire family. Wash linens/clothes in hot water.
- Preferred antibiotic is Augmentin for human, dog, and cat bites.
- Do not confuse actinic keratosis (precursor to squamous cell cancer) with seborrheic keratoses (benign).
- Diagnose hidradenitis suppurativa, psoriasis, RMSF, meningococcemia, erythema migrans (Lyme disease), contact dermatitis, rosacea.
- Instead of silvery scales, may see "covered with fine scales" with psoriasis.
- Psoralens (tar-derived topicals) used to treat psoriasis, antimetabolite (methotrexate).
- How to treat mild and moderate acne. Mild acne is treated only with topicals.
- Accutane in females: Use two forms of reliable birth control.
- "Herald patch" or a "Christmas tree" pattern is found in pityriasis rosea.
- PHN (post-herpetic neuralgia) prophylaxis: Tricyclic antidepressants (TCA), amitriptyline (Elavil).
- A clue in a case scenario on cellulitis may involve a patient walking barefoot.
- Recognize erysipelas versus other types of cellulitis.
- Treatment for rosacea is topical metronidazole gel.
- Recognize herpetic whitlow.

📋 CLINICAL TIPS

- About 80% of cat bites become infected.
- Use ophthalmic grade/sterile cream/ointments for rashes near the eyes.
- On thin skin such as the facial and intertriginous areas (skin folds), use low-potency topical steroids (i.e., hydrocortisone 1%). On thicker skin such as the scalp, back, or soles, may use higher potency steroids.
- If beta streptococcus Group B infection in cellulitis, also at risk for developing postglomerular nephritis as seen in strep throat. Treat for 10 days.
- Not all dog bites have to be treated with antibiotics (if they are not on the extremities).

7

Cardiovascular System Review

Acute Myocardial Infarction (MI)

Middle-aged or older male complains of midsternal chest pain that feels like heavy pressure on the chest. The pain is associated with numbness and/or tingling in the left jaw and the left arm. The patient is diaphoretic with cool, clammy skin. Women with MIs are more likely to present with nonspecific symptoms such as dyspnea, fatigue, back pain, and nausea.

Dissecting Abdominal Aortic Aneurysm (AAA)

Elderly white male complains of pulsating-type sensation in abdomen and/or low back pain. With impending rupture, sudden onset of severe chest and low back pain that steadily becomes sharp and excruciating. Patients with hypertension (HTN) and smokers are at higher risk.

Congestive Heart Failure (CHF)

Elderly patient complains of an acute (or gradual) onset of dyspnea, fatigue, dry cough, and swollen feet and ankles. The patient has a sudden (or gradual) increase in weight. Lung exam will reveal crackles on both the lung bases (bibasilar crackles) along with an S3 heart sound. History of preexisting coronary artery disease (CAD), prior MI, or previous episode of CHF is possible. Usually is taking diuretics, digoxin (Lanoxin), and antihypertensive medications.

Bacterial Endocarditis

Patient presents with fever, chills, and malaise that is associated with a new murmur and the abrupt onset of CHF. Associated skin findings are found mostly on the fingers/hands and toes/feet. These are subungual hemorrhages (splinter hemorrhages on the nailbed), petechiae on the palate, painful violet-colored nodes on the fingers or feet (Osler nodes), and tender red spots on the palms/soles (Janeway lesions).

☑ NORMAL FINDINGS

Anatomy

Position of the Heart

Most of the left ventricular mass is located behind the right ventricle. The right ventricle sits anteriorly toward the chest. It is the chamber of the heart that lies closest to the sternum. A large part of the atria is located posteriorly facing the back. The lower border of the left ventricle is where the apical impulse is generated.

■ *Apical impulse:* Located at the 5th intercostal space (ICS) by the midclavicular line on the left side of the chest.

Displacement of the Point of Maximal Impulse (PMI)

■ *Severe left ventricular hypertrophy (LVH) and cardiomyopathy:* The PMI is displaced laterally on the chest, is larger (more than 3 cm) in size, and is more prominent.
■ *Pregnancy, third trimester:* As the uterus grows larger, it pushes up against the diaphragm and causes the heart to shift to the left of the chest anteriorly. The result is a displaced PMI that is located slightly upward on the left side of the chest.

Deoxygenated Blood

■ Enters the heart through the superior vena cava and inferior vena cava.
■ Right atrium → tricuspid valve → right ventricle → pulmonic valve → pulmonary artery → the lungs → alveoli (red blood cells [RBCs]) pick up oxygen and release carbon dioxide.

Oxygenated Blood

■ Exits the lungs through the pulmonary veins and enters the heart.
■ Left atrium → mitral valve → left ventricle → aortic valve → aorta → general circulation.

Systole and Diastole

The mnemonic to use is "Motivated Apples." These two words give you several clues. They will remind you of the names of the valves (which produce the sound) and the type of valve.

MOTIVATED	APPLES
M (mitral valve)	A (aortic valve)
T (tricuspid valve)	P (pulmonic valve)
AV (atrioventricular valves)	S (semilunar valves)

Heart Sounds

S1 (Systole)

■ The "lub" sound (of "lub-dub")
■ Closure of the mitral and tricuspid valves
■ Atrioventricular (AV) valves (three leaflets)

S2 (Diastole)

■ The "dub" sound (of "lub-dub")
■ Closure of the aortic and pulmonic valves
■ Semilunar valves (two leaflets)

S3 Heart Sound

- Pathognomic for CHF (CHF or heart failure).
- Occurs during early diastole (also called a "ventricular gallop" or an "S3 gallop").
- Sounds like "Kentucky."
- Always considered abnormal if it occurs after the age of 35.

This may be a normal variant in some children or young adults if there are no signs or symptoms of heart or valvular disease.

S4 Heart Sound

Caused by increased resistance due to a stiff left ventricle; usually indicates LVH; considered a normal finding in some elderly (slight thickening of left ventricle).

- S4 occurs during late diastole (also called an "atrial gallop" or "atrial kick").
- Sounds like "Tennessee."
- Best heard at the apex or apical area (mitral area) using the bell of the stethoscope.

Summation Gallop

- All heart sounds are present (from S1 to S4) and sound like a galloping horse.
- A pathologic finding.

Stethoscope Skills

Bell of Stethoscope

- Low tones such as the extra heart sounds (S3 or S4)
- Mitral stenosis

Diaphragm of the Stethoscope

- Mid- to high-pitched tones such as lung sounds
- Mitral regurgitation
- Aortic stenosis

Benign Variants

Benign Split S2

Best heard over the pulmonic area (or second ICS left side of sternum); due to splitting of the aortic and pulmonic components; a normal finding if it appears during inspiration and disappears at expiration.

Benign S4 in the Elderly

Some healthy elderly patients have an S4 (late diastole) heart sound; also known as the "atrial kick" (the atria have to squeeze harder to overcome resistance of a stiff left ventricle). If there are no signs or symptoms of heart/valvular disease, it is considered a normal variant.

SOLVING QUESTIONS: HEART MURMURS

To solve a murmur question correctly, only two pieces of information are needed.

- Look for the timing of the murmur (systole or diastole).
- Look for the location of the murmur (aortic or mitral area).

All the murmurs seen on the exams will fit into the following two mnemonics:

Timing

Systolic Murmurs

- Use the MR. AS mnemonic.

Diastolic Murmurs
- Use the MS. AR mnemonic.

Location
Auscultatory Areas
There are only two important sites to remember for the exam. It is necessary to memorize the locations of the auscultatory areas in order to correctly identify a heart murmur.

Mitral Area (Also Known as the Apex or the Apical Area of the Heart)
- Fifth left ICS is about 8 to 9 cm from the midsternal line and slightly medial to the midclavicular line.
- PMI or the apical pulse is located in this area.

Aortic Area
- Second ICS to the right side of the upper border of the sternum.
- The location of the aortic area can also be described as the "second ICS by the right side of the sternum at the base of the heart."

Heart Murmurs: Mnemonics
MR. ASH (Use for All Systolic Murmurs)
These murmurs are also described as occurring during S1, or as holosystolic, pansystolic, early systolic, late systolic, or midsystolic murmurs. Compared with diastolic murmurs, these murmurs are louder and can radiate to the neck or axillae.

MR (Mitral Regurgitation)
A pansystolic (or holosystolic) murmur:
- Heard best at the apex of the heart or the apical area
- Radiates to axilla
- Loud blowing and high-pitched murmur (use the diaphragm of the stethoscope)

AS (Aortic Stenosis)
A midsystolic ejection murmur:
- Best heard at the second ICS at the right side of the sternum
- Radiates to the neck
- A harsh and noisy murmur (use diaphragm of stethoscope)

Patients with aortic stenosis should avoid physical overexertion, as there is increased risk of sudden death.

Monitored by serial cardiac sonograms with Doppler flow studies. Surgical valve replacement if worsens.

MS. ART (Use for All Diastolic Murmurs)
Diastole is also known as the S2 heart sound, early diastole, late diastole, or mid-diastole.

Diastolic murmurs are always indicative of heart disease (unlike systolic murmurs).

MS (Mitral Stenosis)
A low-pitched diastolic rumbling murmur:
- Heard best at the apex of the heart or the apical area
- Also called an "opening snap" (use bell of the stethoscope)

AR (Aortic Regurgitation)
A high-pitched diastolic murmur:
- Best heard at the second ICS at the right side of the sternum
- High-pitched blowing murmur (use diaphragm of the stethoscope)

Heart Murmurs: Grading System
- *Grade I:* Very soft murmur. Heard only under optimal conditions.
- *Grade II:* Mild to moderately loud murmur.
- *Grade III:* Loud murmur that is easily heard once the stethoscope is placed on the chest.
- *Grade IV:* A louder murmur. First time that a thrill is present. A thrill is like a "palpable murmur."
- *Grade V:* Very loud murmur heard with edge of stethoscope off chest. Thrill is more obvious.
- *Grade VI:* The murmur is so loud that it can be heard even with the stethoscope off the chest. The thrill is easily palpated.

⋮⋮ ABNORMAL FINDINGS

Pathologic Murmurs
- All diastolic murmurs are abnormal.
- All benign murmurs occur during systole (S2).
- Benign murmurs do not have a thrill; only very loud murmurs will produce a thrill.

✍ EXAM TIPS

- There are usually 2 or 3 questions regarding murmurs on the exam.
- Learn to use the mnemonics "MR. ASH" and "MS. ART."
- Memorize the locations of the mitral area as well as the aortic area.
- Regarding mitral murmurs, the word *mitral* will not be used because it is an obvious clue.
- All murmurs with "mitral" in their names are only described as located:
  - on the apex of the heart or the apical area *or*
  - on the 5th ICS on the left side of the sternum medial to the midclavicular line.
- On the exam, only the systolic murmurs radiate (to the axilla in mitral regurgitation and to the neck with aortic stenosis).
- S3 is a sign for CHF; S4 is a sign of LVH.
- A split S2 is best heard at the pulmonic area.
- Memorize the mnemonic "Motivated Apple" to help you remember the names of the valves that are responsible for producing S1 and S2.
- Grading murmurs: First time thrill is palpated is at Grade IV.
- If you forget on which side of the sternum the aortic or pulmonic area lies (left or right?):
  - The "r" in aortic is for the "right side."
  - The "l" in pulmonic is for the "left side."
- Rule out AAA in an older male who has a pulsatile abdominal mass that is more than 3 cm in width. The next step is to order an abdominal ultrasound and CT.

☰ DISEASE REVIEW

Cardiac Arrhythmias

Atrial Fibrillation (AF)

AF is the most common cardiac arrhythmia in the United States—a major cause of stroke; classified as a supraventricular tachyarrhythmia. AF may be asymptomatic. If patient is hemodynamically unstable (chest pain, hypotension, heart failure), call 911. Risk of stroke/death is higher in the case of elderly patients.

Risk Factors

- HTN, CAD, caffeine, nicotine, hyperthyroidism, alcohol intake ("holiday heart"), heart failure, LVH, and others.
- Paroxysmal AF (intermittent or self-terminating): Episodes terminate with 7 days or less (usually in less than 24 hours). It is usually asymptomatic.

Management

Treatment depends on patient type and risk factors for stroke (use CHADS2 scores).

- CHADS2 Scoring System (score of 2 or more requires anticoagulation)
- C (CHF), H (HTN), A (age >75 years), D (diabetes), S2 (stroke/TIA).

Classic Case

Patients complain of the sudden onset of heart palpitations accompanied by feelings of weakness, dizziness, and dyspnea. They may complain of chest pain and feeling like passing out (pre-syncope to syncope). Rapid and irregular pulse may be more than 110 beats per minute with hypotension.

Treatment Plan

- Diagnostic test is the 12-lead ECG (does not show discrete P waves).
- *New onset:* ECG, TSH, and electrolytes (calcium, potassium, magnesium, sodium).
- Consider 24-hr Holter monitor if paroxysmal AF. Digoxin level (if on digoxin).
- Order echocardiogram (rule out valvular pathology, which increases risk of stroke).
- *Lifestyle:* Avoid stimulants (caffeine, nicotine, decongestants) and alcohol (some patients).

Medications

- Patients are referred to cardiologists for medical management. An option is cardioversion.
- *Rate control:* Calcium-channel blockers, beta-blockers, or digoxin.
- Antiarrhythmics such as amiodarone (Cordarone). Amiodarone has Black Box Warning of pulmonary and liver damage. Simvastatin with amiodarone can cause rhabdomyolysis.
- Warfarin (Coumadin) for anticoagulation. Baseline international normalized ratio (INR) and CBC (check platelets).
- If suspect a bleeding episode—check the INR with the prothrombin time (PT) and the partial thromboplastin time (PTT).
- Coumadin drug interactions are given in Chapter 3: Pharmacology.

Complications

- Death from thromboembolic event (i.e., stroke, pulmonary embolism), CHF, angina, etc.

Anticoagulation Guidelines (Table 7.1)
Atrial Fibrillation
- INR: 2.0 to 3.0

Synthetic/Prosthetic Valves
- INR: 2.5 to 3.5

Patient Education: Dietary Sources of Vitamin K
- Advise patients to be consistent with their day-to-day consumption of vitamin K foods.
- Give patient a list of foods with high levels of vitamin K ("greens" such as kale, collard, mustard, turnip, spinach, iceberg or Romaine lettuce, Brussels sprouts).
- Only one serving per day is recommended for very high vitamin K foods ("greens" and spinach).

Paroxysmal Atrial Tachycardia (PAT)

Also known as paroxysmal supraventricular tachycardia (PSVT). EKG shows tachycardia with peaked QRS complex with P waves present.
- *Causes:* Digitalis toxicity, alcohol, hyperthyroidism, caffeine intake, alcohol, illegal drug use, etc.

Classic Case
Patient complains of the abrupt onset of palpitations, rapid pulse, lightheadedness, shortness of breath, and anxiety. Rapid heart rate can range from 150 to 250 beats per minute.

Management
Holding one's breath and straining hard, carotid massage, or splashing ice cold water on the face (for some) can interrupt and stop this arrhythmia (Valsalva maneuvers).

Pulsus Paradoxus

Also known as a paradoxical pulse. The paradox is that the apical pulse can still be heard even though the radial pulse is no longer palpable. It is measured by using the blood pressure (BP) cuff and a stethoscope.

Certain pulmonary and cardiac conditions that compress the chambers of the heart (impair diastolic filling) can cause an exaggerated decrease of the systolic pressure of more than 10 mm Hg.

Table 7.1 Elevated INR

INR	Presence of Bleeding	Action
3.0 to 5.0	None	Skip one dose. Decrease maintenance dose. If only minimally prolonged, no need to decrease dose. Check INR in 1 to 2 days until normal.
5.0 to 9.0	None	Omit a dose and give small dose of oral vitamin K* OR omit next 1 to 2 doses of warfarin. Daily INR monitoring until normal. Decrease the Coumadin maintenance dose.

*Causes INR to decrease within 24 to 48 hours.

Source: Adapted from Guidelines for the Management of Patients with Atrial Fibrillation, 2011. Online copy of article from "Circulation." American College of Cardiology/American Heart Association. Accessed 11/23/2011.

Pulmonary Cause
- Asthma, emphysema (increased positive pressure)

Cardiac Cause
- Tamponade, pericarditis, cardiac effusion (decreases movement of left ventricle)

✍ EXAM TIPS

- No EKG strips are included in the exam. Instead, the symptoms of the arrhythmia or its appearance on the EKG strip will be described.
- Atrial fibrillation and PAT are usually in the exams.
- PAT and AF have many causes, such as alcohol intoxication, hyperthyroidism, stimulants such as theophylline, decongestants, cocaine, and heart disease.
- Learn the proper procedure to check for pulsus parodoxus.

📋 CLINICAL TIPS

- Major bleeding episodes can occur even with a normal INR. Order an INR with the PT and the PTT if you suspect bleeding.
- It may take from 2 to 3 days after changing the warfarin dose to see a change in the INR.
- Up to 15% of patients on Coumadin per year will have a bleeding episode.
- Coumadin is an FDA Category X drug.

Hypertension (HTN)

Majority of patients have essential HTN (>90%). It is usually asymptomatic. HTN is defined as an elevation of the systolic BP and/or diastolic BP measurements on at least two separate office visits. Higher risk for those with cardiovascular (CV) diseases and strokes (CVA). The new JNC 8 guidelines will be released in the fall or winter of 2013. When released, I will post on my website at www.npreview.com.

Correct BP Measurement

- Avoid smoking or caffeine intake 30 minutes before measurement.
- Patient should be seated on a chair with back and arm supported.
- Begin BP measurement after 5 minutes of rest (mercury sphygmomanometer preferred over digital machines).
- Two or more readings separated by 2 minutes should be averaged per visit.
- Higher number determines BP stage (BP 140/100 is stage II instead of stage I).

Routine BP Screening (Table 7.2)

- JNC 7 recommends routine BP measurement at least once every 2 years for adults with normal BP (BP <120/80 mm Hg).
- Annual BP screening is recommended if patient has a systolic BP of 120 to 139 mm Hg and a diastolic BP of 80 to 89 mm Hg.

BP
Peripheral Vascular Resistance (PVR) × Cardiac Output (CO)
- Any change in the PVR or CO results in a change in BP (increase/decrease)

Examples:
Na+ (Sodium):
- Water retention increases vascular volume (increased CO)

Table 7.2 Hypertension Diagnosis and Management: JNC 7 Treatment Guidelines

Stage	Systole/Diastole	Treatment Recommendations
Normal	<120 mm Hg <80 mm Hg	Healthy lifestyle. Exercise
Prehypertension	120 to 139 mm Hg 80 to 89 mm Hg	Lifestyle changes. Lose weight. Exercise
Stage I	140 to 159 mm Hg 90 to 99 mm Hg	Thiazide diuretics preferred for most cases If indicated or compelling condition: ACE inhibitors, ARBs, beta-blockers, CCB, or combination drug
Stage II	>160 mm Hg >100 mm Hg	Two-drug combination for most patients. Thiazide diuretic plus ACEI, ARB, beta-blocker, CCB, or a combination drug

Note: ACEI, angiotensin-converting enzyme inhibitor; ARB, angiotensin receptor blocker; CCB, calcium-channel blocker.

Source: Adapted from Joint National Committee on Prevention, Detection, Evaluation, and Treatment of High Blood Pressure (JNC 7); 2003.

Angiotensin I to Angiotensin II:
- Increased vasoconstriction (increased PVR)
- Younger patients have higher renin levels compared with the elderly

Sympathetic System Stimulation:
- Epinephrine secretion causes tachycardia and vasoconstriction (increased PVR)

Vasodilation (Alpha-Blockers, Beta-Blockers, Calcium-Channel Blockers):
- Decreased resistance (decreased PVR)

Severe Hemorrhage:
- Less blood volume (decreased CO)

Labs
- *Kidneys:* Creatinine, urinalysis
- *Endocrine:* Thyroid profile, fasting blood glucose
- *Electrolyte:* Potassium (K^+), sodium (Na^+), calcium (Ca^{2+})
- *Heart:* Cholesterol, HDL, LDL, triglycerides (complete lipid panel)
- *Anemia:* CBC.
- Baseline EKG and chest x-ray (to rule out cardiomegaly)
- Target organs

Rule Out Target Organ Damage
Look for the following clinical findings:

Microvascular Damage
Eyes
- Silver and/or copper wire arterioles
- AV junction nicking
- Flame-shaped hemorrhages, papilledema

Kidneys

- Microalbuminuria and proteinuria
- Elevated serum creatinine and abnormal GFR (rule out renal failure)
- Peripheral or generalized edema
- Macrovascular damage

Heart

- S3 (CHF)
- S4 (LVH)
- Carotid bruits (narrowing due to plaque, increased risk of CAD)
- CAD and acute MI
- Decreased or absent peripheral pulses (PAD or PVD)

Brain

- Transient ischemic attacks (TIAs) with ischemic brain damage
- Hemorrhagic strokes (CVA)

Secondary HTN

The causes of secondary HTN can be classified into three major groups:

- *Renal* (renal artery stenosis, polycystic kidneys, chronic kidney disease)
- *Endocrine* (hyperthyroidism, hyperaldosteronism, pheochromocytoma)
- *Other causes* (obstructive sleep apnea, coarctation of the aorta)

Renal artery stenosis is more common in younger adults. Middle-aged adults are more likely to have endocrine-related disorders. Chronic kidney disease is more common in elderly patients.

Rule out secondary cause and maintain a high index of suspicion if the following:

- Age younger than 30 years
- Severe HTN or acute rise in BP (previously stable patient)
- Resistant HTN despite treatment with at least three antihypertensive agents
- Malignant HTN (severe HTN with end-organ damages such as retinal hemorrhages, papilledema, acute renal failure, and severe headache.)

Clinical Findings: Secondary Hypertension

Kidneys

- Bruit epigastric or flank area (renal artery stenosis)
- Enlarged kidneys with cystic renal masses (polycystic kidney)
- Increased creatinine and decreased GFR (renal insufficiency to renal failure)

Endocrine

Primary Hyperaldosteronism

- HTN with hypokalemia
- Normal to elevated sodium levels

Hyperthyroidism

- Weight loss, tachycardia, fine tremor, moist skin, anxiety
- New onset of atrial fibrillation

Pheochromocytoma

- Excessive secretion of catecholamines (causes severe HTN, arrhythmias)
- Labile increase in BP accompanied by palpitations
- Sudden onset of anxiety, sweating, severe headache

Other Causes

Coarctation of the Aorta

- BP of the arms is higher than BP of the legs
- Delayed or diminished femoral pulses (check both radial and femoral pulse at the same time)

Sleep Apnea

- Sleep partner will report severe snoring with apneic episodes during sleep
- Marked hypoxic episodes during sleep increases BP

Hypertension Treatment Guidelines (JNC 7; Table 7.3)*

Stage I (Systolic 140–159 or Diastolic 90–99 mm Hg)

- Thiazide-type diuretics preferred for most patients

Stage 2 (Systolic >160 or Diastolic >100 mm Hg)

- Two-drug therapy for most patients
- Thiazide-type diuretic and another drug class antihypertensive agent.

Diabetics and CAD

- Goal BP is lower (BP <130/80 mm Hg)

Compelling Indications

Diabetes Mellitus (DM) and Chronic Kidney Disease (With Proteinuria)

Unless contraindicated, use angiotensin-converting enzyme reuptake inhibitors (ACEI) or angiotensive receptor blockers (ARBs). They reduce the risk of progression of renal damage (microalbuminuria, macroalbuminuria, reduction in GFR).

Table 7.3 Compelling Indications

Name of Disease	Initial Drug	Add Other Drug Classes
Diabetes mellitus type 2	ACE inhibitors or ARBs	Thiazide diuretics, BB, CCB
Chronic kidney disease	ACE inhibitors or ARBs	Diuretic (if needed)
Coronary artery disease	ACE inhibitors or ARBs	BB, long-acting CCB
Isolated systolic hypertension elderly	Thiazide diuretics	Long-acting CCB
		ACE inhibitor or ARBs
Post-MI	Beta-blockers	ACE inhibitor, aldosterone antagonist
		Beta-blockers, ACEI, or ARB, aldosterone antagonist, etc.
Heart failure or CHF	Thiazide diuretics	

Not an all-inclusive list.

ACEI, angiotensin-converting enzyme inhibitor; ARB, angiotensin receptor blocker; BB, beta-blockers; CCB, calcium-channel blockers.

Source: Adapted from Joint National Committee on Prevention, Detection, Evaluation, and Treatment of High Blood Pressure (JNC 7), 2003.

---

* Joint National Committee for the Assessment, Evaluation and Treatment of High Blood Pressure in Adults, 7th Report (JNC 7 2003). JNC 8 treatment guidelines will be released sometime in 2013. Check www.npreview.com for updates.

Heart Failure (or CHF)
- Thiazide diuretic, beta-blocker, ACEI or ARBs, aldosterone antagonist

Post-MI
- Beta-blockers, ACE inhibitors, aldosterone antagonists

Isolated Systolic HTN in the Elderly*
- Caused by loss of recoil in the arteries (atherosclerosis), which increases PVR.
- Pulse pressure (systolic BP – diastolic BP) increases in this disorder.
- New target for patients aged 80 years or older: systolic BP of 140 mm Hg to 145 mm Hg.
- For frail patients with severe orthostatic hypotension (falls, syncope), it is now acceptable to have a systolic BP of up to 150 mm Hg.

Treatment Plan
- Thiazide diuretics (use first).
- Add a long-acting dihydropyridine calcium-channel blocker (CCB) (amlodipine/ Norvasc, nifedipine/Procardia XL) and/or an ACE inhibitor or ARB.

Orthostatic Hypotension
Elderly are at higher risk for orthostatic hypotension due to a less active autonomic nervous system and slower metabolism of drugs by the liver (prolongs half-life of drugs).

To Check for Orthostatic Hypotension
- Important to check BP in BOTH sitting and standing positions. When the patient stands, wait for 1 to 3 minutes to measure the standing BP.
- Ask patient if dizzy or lightheaded with changes in position.

Lifestyle Recommendations
This is the first-line therapy for HTN, hyperlipidemia, and diabetes:
- Lose weight if overweight (BMI 25 to 29.9) or obese (BMI 30 or higher).
- Normal weight is a BMI of 18.5 to 24.9.
- Stop smoking.
- Reduce stress level.
- Reduce dietary sodium:
  - Less than 2.4 g per day
- Maintain adequate intake of potassium, calcium, and magnesium.
- Limit alcohol intake:
  - 1 ounce (30 mL) or less per day for men
  - 0.5 ounce or less per day for women
- Eat fatty cold-water fish (salmon, anchovy): 3 times a week
- Exercise moderately: 30 to 45 minutes most days of the week

DASH Diet (Dietary Approaches to Stop HTN)
Goal: Eat foods rich in potassium, magnesium, and calcium. Reduce sodium intake. Reduce red meat and processed foods. Eat more whole grains. Eat more fish and poultry.
- *Grains:* 7–8 daily servings
- *Fruits and vegetables:* 4–5 daily servings

---

* Adapted from the ACCF/AHA 2011 Expert Consensus Document on Hypertension in the Elderly. *J Am Coll Cardiol* 2011;20:2037–114.

- *Nuts, seeds, and dry beans:* 4–5 servings per week
- *Fats, oils, or fat-free dairy products:* 2–3 daily servings
- *Meat, poultry, and fish:* 2 or less daily servings
- *Sweets:* Try to limit to less than 5 servings per week
- Avoid high sodium foods:
  - Cold cuts, ready-made foods, any pickled foods (cucumbers, eggs, pork parts)

Dietary Sources of Recommended Minerals

- Calcium (low-fat dairy)
- Potassium (most fruits and vegetables)
- Magnesium (dried beans, whole grains, nuts)
- Omega 3 oils
  - Salmon, anchovies (sardines), flaxseed oil

Medications

Loop Diuretics
Action: Inhibit the sodium-potassium-chloride pump of the kidney in the loop of Henle.

Side Effects
- Electrolyte imbalance
- Hypokalemia (potentiates digoxin toxicity, increases risk of arrhythmias)
- Hyponatremia (hold diuretic, restrict water intake, replace K+ loss)
- Hypomagnesemia

Contraindications
- Sensitivity to loop diuretics

Examples
- Furosemide (Lasix) PO BID
- Bumetanide (Bumex) PO BID

Aldosterone Receptor Antagonist Diuretics
- *Action:* Antagonizes the action of aldosterone. Increases elimination of water in the kidneys and conserves potassium. Drug class also known as "mineralocorticoid receptor antagonists."
- *Indications:* HTN, heart failure, hirsuitism, precocious puberty.
- Avoid combining with potassium-sparing diuretics, ACE inhibitors, or potassium supplements.

Side Effects
- Gynecomastia
- Hyperkalemia
- GI (vomiting, diarrhea, stomach cramps), postmenopausal bleeding, erectile dysfunction

Contraindications
- Hyperkalemia (serum potassium greater than 5.5 mEq/L)
- Renal insufficiency (serum creatinine greater than 2.0 mg/dL in men or greater than 1.8 mg/dL for women)
- DM type 2 with microalbuminuria

Examples
- Spironolactone (Aldactone) daily
- Eplerenone (Inspra) daily

Beta-Blockers
- Avoid abrupt discontinuation after chronic use. Wean slowly. May precipitate severe rebound HTN
- *Action:* Decreases vasomotor activity, CO, inhibits renin and norepinephrine release
- Blocks beta receptors on the heart and the peripheral vasculature. Two types of beta-blocker receptors in the body: B1 (cardiac effects) and B2 (lungs and peripheral vasculature)

Contraindications
- Asthma, chronic obstructive pulmonary disease (COPD), chronic bronchitis, emphysema (chronic lung disease)
- Second- and third-degree heart block (okay to use with first-degree block)
- Sinus bradycardia

Other Uses
- *Acute MI:* Reduces mortality during acute MI and post-MI
- *Migraine headache:* For prophylaxis only (not for acute attacks)
- *Glaucoma:* Reduces intraocular pressure (Betimol Ophthalmic drops for open-angle glaucoma)
- *Resting tachycardia* (target heart rate <100 beats per minute)
- *Angina pectoris:* Treats symptoms
- *Post-MI:* Decreases mortality
- *Hyperthyroidism and pheochromocytoma:* To control symptoms until primary disease treated
- *Beta-blockers:* Ends with "-olol":
  - Metoprolol (Lopressor) 100 mg QD to BID
  - Atenolol (Ternormin) 50 mg daily
  - Propranolol (long-acting Inderal) 40 mg BID
- Do not use propranolol (plain Inderal) to treat HTN (shorter half-life)

Calcium Channel Blockers
Action: Blocks voltage-gated calcium channels in cardiac smooth muscle and the blood vessels. Results in systemic vasodilation. The nondihydropyridines depress the muscles of the heart (inotropic effect). The dihydropyridines slow down heart rate (chronotropic effect).

Side Effects
- Headaches (due to vasodilation)
- Ankle edema (caused by vasodilation and considered benign)
- Heart block or bradycardia (depresses cardiac muscle and AV node)
- Reflex tachycardia (seen with dihydropyridines like nifedipine)

Contraindications
- Second- and third-degree heart block (okay to use with first-degree block)
- Bradycardia
- CHF

Examples

Dihydropyridine CCB ("-pine" ending):
- Nifedipine (Procardia XL) daily
- Amlodipine (Norvasc) daily

Nondihydropyridine CCB:
- Verapamil (Calan SR) daily to BID
- Diltiazem (Cardizem CD) daily

ACE Inhibitors and Angiotensin Receptor Blockers (ARBs)
- Blocks conversion of angiotensin I to II (more potent vasoconstrictor)
- DM: drug of choice (protects kidneys) for diabetics

Pregnancy Category C (First Trimester) and Category D (Second and Third Trimesters)
- Fetal kidney malformations and fetal hypotension

Side Effects
- Dry hacking cough (up to 10% with ACEs; less with ARBs)
- Hyperkalemia, angioedema (rare but may be life-threatening)

Contraindications
- Moderate to severe kidney disease

Renal Artery Stenosis
- Precipitates acute renal failure if given ACE or ARB
- Hyperkalemia (this is also a side effect for ACE and ARBs, will have additive effect)

Examples

ARBs: Losartan (Cozaar)

Alpha-1 Blocker/Agonist

Also known as alpha-adrenergic blockers. Suffix of "zosin." A potent vasodilator. Common side effects are dizziness and hypotension. Give at bedtime at very low dose and slowly titrate up.

Side Effects
- "First dose orthostatic hypotension" is common (warn patient)
- Dizziness, postural hypotension (common side effect)
- Severe hypotension and reflex tachycardia
- Give at bedtime. Start at very low doses and titrate up slowly until good BP control. Advise patient to get out of bed slowly to prevent postural hypotension. Not a first-line choice for HTN except for males with both HTN and BPH. Alpha-blockers relax smooth muscle found on the bladder neck and the prostate gland and relieves obstructive voiding symptoms such as weak urinary stream, urgency, and nocturia

Examples
- Terazosin (Hytrin): Used for both HTN and BPH (starting dose 1 mg po at bedtime).
- Tamsulosin (Flomax): Used for BPH only.

Diuretics

All diuretics will decrease blood volume, venous pressure, and preload (cardiac filling).

Thiazide Diuretics

- *Action:* Changes the way that the kidney handles sodium, which increases urine output.
- Has a favorable effect with osteopenia/osteoporosis (slows down demineralization). All thiazides contain sulfa compounds. Avoid if patient has a sulfa allergy.

Side Effects

- Hyperglycemia (be careful with diabetics)
- Hyperuricemia (can precipitate a gout attack)
- Hypertriglyceremia and hypercholesteremia (check lipid profile)
- Hypokalemia (potentiates digoxin toxicity, increases risk of arrhythmias)
- Hyponatremia (hold diuretic, restrict water intake, replace K+ loss)

Contraindications

- Sensitivity to sulfa drugs and thiazides

Examples

- Hydrochlorothiazide 12.5–25 mg PO daily
- Chlorothalidone (Hygroton) PO daily
- Indapamide (Lozol) PO daily

✍ EXAM TIPS

- Follow JNC 7 guidelines for both ANCC and AANPCP exams until JNC 8* is released.
- *Eye findings:* Learn to distinguish the findings in hypertensive retinopathy (copper and silver wire arterioles, AV nicking) from those in diabetic retinopathy (neovascularization, microaneurysms, hard exudates, cotton wool spots).
- Know how to treat isolated systolic HTN in the elderly.
- To assess orthostatic hypotension, measure both the sitting AND standing BP.
- Know the side effects of thiazide diuretics such as hyperglycemia, hyperuricemia, hypertriglyceremia.
- Spironolactone side effect of gynecomastia.
- Memorize the numbers for a normal BP and for Stage I and II HTN.
- *ACE inhibitors:* The drug of choice for diabetics, causes a dry cough (10%).
- Careful when combining ACE inhibitors with potassium-sparing diuretics (i.e., triamterene, spironolactone) because of increased risk for hyperkalemia.
- Bilateral renal artery stenosis: ACE inhibitors will precipitate acute renal failure.
- Alpha-blockers are not first-line drugs for HTN except if patient has preexisting BPH.
- Women with HTN and osteopenia/osteoporosis should receive thiazides. Thiazides help bone loss by slowing down calcium loss (from the bone) and stimulating osteoclasts.

📋 CLINICAL TIPS

- High cholesterol is not considered a risk factor for heart disease over the age of 75.
- *Over age 75:* Screening depends on life expectancy and functional status.
- Start niacin at low dose and gradually titrate up to avoid unpleasant side effects of flushing and headache. Advise to take with food.

---

* JNC 8 is scheduled to be released in fall or winter of 2013. I will post the new JNC 8 treatment guidelines at my website www.npreview.com.

Acute CHF

Numerous causes and precipitating factors such as an acute MI, CAD, HTN, fluid retention, valvular abnormalities, arrhythmias, and so on. Ejection fraction (EF) less than 40%.

Left Ventricular Failure (Diminished Ventricular Systolic Emptying)
- Crackles, bibasilar rales (rales on lower lobes of the lungs), cough, dyspnea, decreased breath sounds, dullness to percussion
- Paroxysmal nocturnal dyspnea, orthopnea, nocturnal nonproductive cough, and wheezing (cardiac asthma).

Right Ventricular Failure
- Jugular venous distenstion (JVD), normal JVD is 4 cm or less.
- Enlarged spleen, enlarged liver causes anorexia, nausea, and abdominal pain.
- Lower extremity edema with cool skin.

Other PE Findings
- Presence of S3 gallop, which can be accompanied by anasarca (severe generalized edema due to effusion of fluid into the extracellular space).

Labs
- Chest x-ray result will show increased heart size, interstitial and alveolar edema, Kerley B lines, and other signs of pulmonary edema.
- ECG, CPK, troponin, beta-type natriuretic peptide.
- Echocardiogram with Doppler flow study.

Treatment Plan
- Furosemide (Lasix) 20 mg or higher dose (up to 320 mg) orally for diuresis.
- Reduce preload and afterload with sublingual nitroglycerin.
- If patient's condition is stable, initiate a prescription of ACE inhibitors or ARBs, diuretic, beta blockers, nitroglycerin, digoxin, and so on.
- Use New York Heart Association (NYHA) system to classify patient's degree of cardiac disability (Table 7.4).
- Refer to cardiologist. If in distress, refer to ED.

Summary
Here is an easy way to remember whether a sign or symptom is from the left or right side of the heart:
- Both *left* and *lung* start with the letter L. Therefore, any question asking you to identify a sign/symptom is made easier. Left is for *lung* and right is the GI tract (by default).

Deep Vein Thrombosis (DVT)

Thrombi develop inside the deep venous system of the legs or pelvis secondary to stasis, trauma to vessel walls, inflammation, or increased coagulation. Pulmonary embolus (PE) is considered another manifestation of this thromboembolic disorder.
- Etiology of DVT (divided into three categories)
  - *Stasis:* Prolonged travel/inactivity (more than 3 hours), bed rest, CHF.
  - *Inherited coagulation disorders:* Factor C deficiency, Leiden, and so forth.
  - *Increased coagulation due to external factors:* OC use, pregnancy, bone fractures especially of the long bones, trauma, recent surgery, malignancy.

Table 7.4 New York Heart Association Functional Capacity Ratings

Classification	Degree of Disability
Class I	No limitations on physical activity
Class II	Ordinary physical activity results in fatigue, exertional dyspnea
Class III	Marked limitation in physical activity
Class VI	Symptoms are present at rest, with or without physical activity

Source: November 14, 2011, meeting of the American Heart Association (Orlando, FL); http://www.medscape.com/viewarticle/753591?src=ptalk

Classic Case

A patient with risk factors for DVT complains of gradual onset of swelling on a lower extremity after a history of travel (more than 3 hours) or prolonged sitting. The patient complains of a painful and swollen lower extremity that is red and warm. If patient has PE, it may be accompanied by abrupt onset of chest pain, dyspnea, dizziness, or syncope.

Treatment Plan

- *Homan's sign:* Lower leg pain on dorsiflexion of the foot
- CBC, platelets, clotting time (PT/PTT, INR), chest x-ray, EKG

Contrast Venography (Gold Standard)

- B-mode ultrasound with Doppler flow study, MRI.
- Hospital admission, heparin IV then warfarin PO (Coumadin) for 3 to 6 months (first episode) or longer.
- For recurrent DVT or elderly, antithrombotic treatment may last a lifetime.

Complications

- Pulmonary emboli
- Stroke and other embolic episodes

✍ EXAM TIPS

- A case of DVT will have a positive Homan's sign (in the exam). In real-life practice, most cases of DVT are asymptomatic.
- Memorize INR of 2.0 to 3.0.
- Learn how to manage elevated INR (see Table 7.1).
- Memorize presentation of a patient with NYHA Class II heart disease.

Superficial Thrombophlebitis

Inflammation of a superficial vein due to local trauma. Higher risk if indwelling catheters, intravenous drugs (i.e., potassium), secondary bacterial infection (*Staphylococcus aureus*).

Classic Case

Adult patient complains of an acute onset of an indurated vein (localized redness, swelling, and tenderness). Usually located on the extremities. The patient is afebrile with normal vital signs.

Objective

- Indurated cordlike vein that is warm and tender to touch with a surrounding area of erythema.
- There should be no swelling or edema of the entire limb (think of DVT).

Treatment Plan

- NSAIDs such as ibuprofen or naproxen sodium (Anaprox DS) BID.
- Warm compresses. Elevate limb. If septic cause, admit to hospital.

Peripheral Vascular Disease (PVD) or Peripheral Arterial Disease (PAD)

Gradual (decades) narrowing and/or occlusion of medium to large arteries in the lower extremities. Blood flow to the extremities gradually decreases over time resulting in permanent ischemic damage (gangrene of the toes/foot). Higher risk with HTN, smoking, diabetes, and hyperlipidemia.

Classic Case

Older patient who has a history of smoking and hyperlipidemia complains of worsening pain on ambulation (intermittent claudication) that is instantly relieved by rest. Over time, the symptoms worsen until the patient's walking distance is greatly limited. Atrophic skin changes. Some have gangrene on one or more toes.

Objective

- *Skin:* Atrophic changes (shiny and hyperpigmented ankles that are hairless and cool to touch
- *CV:* Decreased to absent dorsal pedal pulse (may include popliteal and posterior tibial pulse), increased capillary refill time (less than 2 seconds), and bruits over partially blocked arteries

Treatment Plan

- Initial method (low tech): Ankle and brachial BP before and after exercise.
- Order a Doppler ultrasound flow study. Angiography is the gold standard for diagnosis.
- Smoking cessation (smoking causes vasoconstriction) and daily ambulation exercises.
- Pentoxifylline (Trental) if indicated. Percutaneous angioplasty or surgery for severe cases.

Complications

- Gangrene of foot and/or lower limb with amputation
- Increased risk of CAD
- Increased risk of carotid plaquing (check for carotid bruits)

Raynaud's Phenomenon

Reversible vasospasm of the peripheral arterioles on the fingers and toes. Cause is unknown. Associated with an increased risk of autoimmune disorders (i.e., thyroid disorder, pernicious anemia, rheumatoid arthritis). Most patients are females (60% to 90%) with a gender ratio of 8:1. Patients with no underlying disease have "primary" Raynaud's disease. Up to 95% of patients with scleroderma have "secondary" Raynaud's disease.

Classic Case

A middle-aged woman complains of chronic and recurrent episodes of color changes on her fingertips in a symmetric pattern (both hands and both feet). The colors range from white (pallor) and blue (cyanosis) to red (reperfusion). Complains of numbness and tingling. Attacks last for several hours. Hands and feet become numb with very cold temperatures. Ischemic changes may be present after a severe episode such as shallow ulcers (that eventually heal) on some of the fingertips.

- *Evaluate:* Distal pulses, ischemic signs (ischemic ulcers at the fingers/toes)

Treatment Plan

- Avoid touching cold objects, cold weather. Avoid stimulants (i.e., caffeine).
- Smoking cessation is important. Nifedipine (Adalat) or amlodipine (Norvasc).
- Do not use any vasoconstricting drugs (i.e., Imitrex, ergots, pseudoephedrine/decongestants, amphetamines). Avoid nonselective beta blockers.

Complications

- Small ulcers in the fingertips and toes.

✍ EXAM TIPS

- *Raynaud's phenomenon:* Think of the colors of the American flag as a reminder of this disorder.
- Medicines for Raynaud's phenomenon include calcium-channel blockers (nifedipine, amlodipine).

Bacterial Endocarditis

Presentation ranges from full-blown disease to subacute endocarditis. Bacterial pathogens are gram positives (i.e., *Viridans streptococcus*, *Staphylococcus aureus*, etc.). Also known as infective endocarditis.

Classic Case

Middle-aged male presents with fever, chills, and malaise that are associated with subungual hemorrhages (splinter hemorrhages on nailbed) and tender violet-colored nodules on the fingers and/or on the toes (Osler's nodes). Palms and soles may have tender red spots on the skin (Janeway lesions). Some may have a heart murmur.

Treatment Plan

- Refer to cardiologist or ED for hospitalization and IV antibiotics.
- Blood cultures × 3 (first 24 hours).
- CBC (elevated WBCs) and sedimentation rate greater than 20 mm per hour (elevated).

Complications

- Valvular destruction, myocardial abscess, emboli, etc.

Endocarditis Prophylaxis (Table 7.5)

- Antibiotic prophylaxis is *no* longer recommended for:
  - Mitral valve prolapse
  - GU or GI incisions/invasive procedures (exception is if there is an existing infection present such as a UTI before a cystoscopy).
- Standard regimen: Give 1 hour before procedure:
  - Amoxicillin 2 g PO × 1 dose (adults)
  - Amoxicillin 50 mg/kg 1 hour before procedure × 1 dose (children)

Table 7.5 Endocarditis Prophylaxis

High Risk Condition	Invasive Procedures
Previous history of bacterial endocarditis	Dental procedures that traumatize oral mucosa, gingiva, or the periapical area of the teeth.
Prosthetic valves	Invasive procedures on the respiratory tract (especially if tissue is infected).
Certain types of congenital heart disease	
Cardiac transplant with valvulopathy	

Source: Adapted from American Heart Association Guidelines: Prevention of infective endocarditis, (revised 2007 Jan).

Penicillin Allergy

- Clindamycin 600 mg or clarithromycin (Biaxin) 500 mg or cephalexin (Keflex) 2 g

Mitral Valve Prolapse (MVP)

The classic finding is an S2 "click" followed by a systolic murmur. Some patients with MVP are at higher risk of thromboemboli, TIAs, atrial fibrillation, and ruptured chordae tendineae. Diagnosed by cardiac echocardiogram with Doppler flow study.

Classic Case

Adult tall and thin female patient complains of fatigue, palpitations, and lightheadedness (orthostatic hypotension) that is aggravated by heavy exertion. May be asymptomatic. Associated with pectus excavatum, hypermobility of the joints, arm span greater than height (rule out Marfan's syndrome).

Treatment Plan

- Asymptomatic MVP does not need treatment.
- MVP with palpitations is treated with beta-blockers, avoidance of caffeine, alcohol, and cigarettes. Holter monitoring is useful in detecting significant arrhythmias.

Hyperlipidemia

These recommendations come from the ATP III guideline (2004). The final version of the ATP IV guidelines will be released sometime in late 2013. Although some of the preliminary recommendations have become available, it may be changed in the final version of the ATP IV. When the final version of the guideline is released, I will post it on my website at www.npreview.com.

Screening Guidelines

- Complete lipid profile (fasting) every 5 years starting at age 20.
- Over age 40 years, screen every 2 to 3 years.
- Preexisting hyperlipidemia: Screen annually or more frequently.

Total Cholesterol

- *Normal:* Less than 200 mg/dL
- *Borderline:* Between 200 and 239 mg/dL
- *High:* Greater than 240 mg/ dL

HDL (High-Density Lipoprotein)
- Greater than 40 mg/dL
- If less than 40 mg/dL, associated with increased risk of CAD even if normal LDL or cholesterol

LDL (Low-Density Lipoprotein)
- *Optimal:* Less than 100 mg/dL
- *LDL:* Less than 130 mg/dL for low-risk patients with fewer than two risk factors
- *Very high:* Greater than 190 mg/dL

Triglycerides
- *Normal:* Less than 150 mg/dL
- High risk of acute pancreatitis: greater than 500 mg/dL
- If triglycerides greater than 500 mg/dL:
  - Treat triglycerides first. Give niacin or prescribe fibrate or Niaspan. When triglycerides are under control, switch target to lowering LDL.
- Recommend a very low-fat diet (less than 15% calories from fat). Lose weight and increase physical activity.

Coronary Risk Equivalent
Patients without known coronary heart disease (CHD), but are at increased risk of MI (10-year risk of developing CHD exceeds 20%). These patients are treated the same as if they had preexisting heart disease. Conditions considered as coronary risk equivalents are: carotid artery disease, PVD, AAA, chronic kidney disease, diabetes, cigarette smoking, and others.

Risk Factors: Heart Disease
- HTN
- Family history of premature heart disease (women with MI before age 65 years or men with MI before age 55 years)
- DM (considered a CHD risk equivalent even if patient has no history of preexisting heart disease)
- Dyslipidemia
- Low HDL cholesterol: less than 40 mg/dL
- Age (men older than 45 or women older than 55)
- Cigarette smoking
- Obesity (BMI ≥ 30 kg/m^2)
- Microalbuminuria
- Carotid artery disease
- PVD

Treatment Plan: Hyperlipidemia
- First-line treatment is lifestyle changes (weight loss, exercise most days of the week, better diet low in saturated fat, smoking cessation).
- Reduction in dietary salt intake and education about the DASH diet (low salt, low saturated fat < 30%).
- Encourage use of soluble fiber in diet (i.e., inulin, guar gum, fruit, vegetables) to enhance lowering of LDL (lowers LDL by blocking absorption in GI tract up to 10%).
- Increase intake of beneficial stanols and sterols (Benecol or Smart Balance margarine).
- If no changes in lipids after a trial of 6 months of lifestyle changes, consider antilipidemic drugs if more than two risk factors.

Treatment Plan

- Target goal is to lower LDL first (except if high triglyceride levels).
- High triglycerides put patient at high risk for acute pancreatitis.
- Low HDL alone (even if normal LDL and cholesterol) is a risk factor for heart disease.
- Target goal for HDL is greater than 40 mg/dL.

Lipid-Lowering Medications

- HMG CoA reductase inhibitors (statins)
- Pravastatin (Pravachol), lovastatin (Mevacor), simvastatin (Zocor), atorvastatin (Lipitor)
- Best agents for decreasing LDL. Statins will also elevate HDL.
- Maximum dosage of simvastatin has been reduced to 40 mg/day (2011).
- Simvastatin/statin drug interactions (high risk of rhabdomyolysis):
  - Grapefruit juice
  - Other fibrates (except fenofibrate)
  - Antifungals (intraconazole, ketoconazole)
  - Macrolides (erythromycin, clarithromycin, telithromycin)
  - Amiodarone (Cardorone), some CCBs (diltiazem, amlodipine, verapamil)
- Combination regimens (especially in high doses) of statins, fibrates, niacin, and/or ezetimibe will increase the risk of rhabdomyolysis and drug-induced hepatitis.

Nicotinic Acid and Fibrates

- *Nicotinic acid:* Niacin (over the counter) daily to TID, Niaspan (slow-release niacin) daily.
- *Fibrates:* Gemfibrozil (Lopid), fenofibrate (Tricor). Do not use with severe renal disease.
- *Action:* Reduces production of triglycerides by the liver and increases production of HDL.
- Very good agents for lowering triglycerides and elevating HDL level. Less effective on LDL lowering compared with the statins.
- *Side effects of niacin:* Flushing, itching, tingling, hepatotoxicity; GI effects.
- *Side effects of fibrates:* Dyspepsia, gallstones, myopathy.

Patient Education

- *High triglycerides:* Reduce intake of simple carbohydrates, "junk foods," and fried foods.
- *Low HDL:* Increase level and frequency of aerobic-type exercise and a trial of OTC niacin.
- If no effect or more than two risk factors (for heart disease), consider prescribing fibrates or prescription niacin (Niaspan).

Bile Acid Sequestrants

- Cholestyramine (Questran Light), colestipol (Colestid), colesevelam (WelChol)
  - *Action:* Work locally in the small intestine. Interfere with fat absorption, including fat-soluble vitamins (Vitamins A, D, E, and K).
- Alternative drug for patients who cannot tolerate statins, fibrates, and niacin.
- Used alone, it is not as effective as statins in lowering LDL. No hepatotoxicity.
  - Side effects mainly from the GI tract. Advise patient to take MVI tabs daily.
  - *Side effects:* Bloating, flatulence, abdominal pain. Start at low doses and titrate up slowly.

Other Lipid-Lowering Drugs

■ Ezetimibe (Zetia) and combination of simvastatin and ezetimibe (Vytorin).
  – Can be taken alone or combined with a statin. Can also cause rhabdomyolysis (rare).
  – *Side effects:* Diarrhea, joint pains, tiredness.

Lab Tests

■ Combination regimen (especially in high doses) of statins, fibrates, niacin, ezetimibe, and drugs that affect the CYP450 system increases risk of rhabdomyolysis and drug-induced hepatitis.
■ *Labs:* Baseline LFTs and periodically. More frequent monitoring needed for higher doses (recheck lipids in 3 months, then 6 months during first year of therapy).

Rhabdomyolysis

Acute breakdown of skeletal muscle will cause acute renal failure. Triad of muscle pain, weakness, and dark urine. Look for muscle pain and aches that persist (not associated with muscular exertion). Higher doses or combination therapy have higher risk.

■ *Labs:* Order CK (creatine kinase): markedly elevated (i.e., 10,000 to 25,000).
■ *Urine:* Reddish-brown color (myoglobinuria) and proteinuria in up to 45% LFTs (will be elevated). Other labs are urinalysis, BUN, creatinine, potassium/electrolytes, EKG, others.

Acute Drug-Induced Hepatitis

Anorexia, nausea, dark-colored urine, jaundice, fatigue, flu-like symptoms.

■ *Labs:* Elevated alanine transaminase (ALT) (SGPT) and alanine aminotransferase (AST) (SGOT).

Patient Education

■ Minimize alcohol intake or other hepatotoxic substances while on statins.
■ Avoid prescribing to alcoholics.
■ Advise patient to report symptoms of hepatitis or rhabdomyolysis. If present, tell patient to stop the drug and to call or go to ED.

✍ EXAM TIPS

You must memorize some values. These are (list not all-inclusive):
■ Advise all patients with hypertension (or prehypertension) to lower dietary salt intake.
■ Borderline cholesterol, high cholesterol, HDL, LDL goal for CHD or DM.
■ Low HDL (less than 40 mg/dL) is a risk factor of CHD even though total cholesterol, triglyceride, and LDL are normal.
■ To lower triglycerides, advise patient to reduce intake of simple carbohydrates, junk foods, and fried foods.
■ To increase HDL, increase aerobic-type exercises and take niacin.
■ Become familiar with dietary sources of magnesium, potassium, and calcium.
■ Niacin and fibrates are best at lowering triglycerides.
■ If patient has markedly high triglycerides (500 or higher), lower triglyceride first (niacin or Tricor) before treating the high cholesterol and LDL levels. High triglycerides increase risk of acute pancreatitis.

CLINICAL TIPS

Muscle pain (mild to severe) from rhabdomyolysis is usually located on the calves, thighs, lower back, and/or shoulders. Urine will be darker than normal (reddish-brown color). Rule out rhabdomyolysis if patient on a statin complains of muscular pain with dark-colored urine.

Obesity

All obese and overweight patients should have their BMI and abdominal obesity calculated (Table 7.6). Evaluate for metabolic syndrome and diabetes type 2. In the United States, the mean prevalence of obesity is about 32%.

Abdominal Obesity

The "apple-shaped" body type is considered more dangerous for health compared with the "pear-shaped" body type.

Waist Circumference

- *Males:* Greater than 40 inches or 102 cm.
- *Females:* Greater than 35 inches or 88 cm.

Waist-to-Hip Ratio

- Waist-to-hip ratio: 1.0 or higher (males)
- Waist-to-hip ratio: 0.8 or higher (females)

Metabolic Syndrome

A metabolic disorder with a cluster of symptoms. These patients are at higher risk for type 2 diabetes and CV disease.

Criteria for Metabolic Syndrome (ATP III)

At least three characteristics must be present to diagnose metabolic syndrome (ATP III):
- Abdominal obesity (greater than 40 inches in men and greater than 35 inches in women)
- HTN
- Hyperlipidemia

Hypertension

- Fasting plasma glucose (greater than 100 mg/dL)
- Elevated triglycerides (greater than 150 mg/dL)
- Decreased HDL (less than 40 mg/dL)

Table 7.6 Body Mass Index

Classification	BMI
Underweight	<18.5
Normal weight	18.5 to 24.9
Overweight	25 to 29.9
Obese	30 to 39.9
Grossly obese	>40.0

Labs
- Fasting (from 9 to 12 hours) lipid profile (especially triglycerides and HDL).
- Fasting blood glucose

Fatty Liver (Steatosis)

Also known as nonalcoholic fatty liver disease (NAFLD). Caused by triglyceride fat deposits in the hepatocytes of the liver. An asymptomatic and reversible condition.
- *Risk factors:* Obesity, diabetes, metabolic syndrome, HTN, certain drugs, and so on.

Classic

Usually asymptomatic. Annual PE labs will show slight elevation of ALT and AST. Hepatitis A, B, and C profile is negative OR obese female complains of fatigue and malaise with vague right upper quadrant pain. Associated with obesity, metabolic syndrome, DM, and hyperlipidemia.

Labs
- Liver function tests. ALT and AST may be slightly elevated.
- Order hepatitis A, B, and C profile.
- Refer to GI specialist for management and a liver biopsy (*gold standard*).

Treatment Plan
- Lose weight. Exercise and watch diet.
- Discontinue alcohol intake permanently.
- Avoid hepatotoxic drugs (i.e., acetaminophen, isoniazid, statins).
- Recommend vaccination for hepatitis A and B. Recommend flu vaccine.

How Is the BMI Calculated?
The BMI is a measure of the ratio of weight to height. Muscular patients can have falsely elevated BMIs (higher muscle mass).

Formula for BMI calculation: Weight (kilograms)/Height (meters)^2

Patient Education
- All obese and overweight patients should be advised to lose weight (especially diabetics).
- Lifestyle changes are part of the first-line treatment (diet, nutrition, exercise, portion control). Daily aerobic exercise (walking, swimming, biking, etc.) for 30 to 45 minutes is recommended.
  - Weight Watchers—some patients like the support and education (tertiary prevention).

📋 CLINICAL TIPS

- Metabolic syndrome criteria (abdominal obesity, HTN, hyperlipidemia or elevated triglycerides and low HDL, elevated fasting glucose greater than 100 mg/dL) caused by hyperinsulinemia and peripheral insulin resistance.
- Fatty liver is associated with metabolic syndrome and/or obesity. Look for slight elevation of ALT and AST (not related to alcohol or medications) and negative hepatitis A, B, and C.

- If patient has high triglyceride levels, recommend avoiding or reducing intake of simple carbohydrates, "junk foods," and fried foods.
- For patients with low HDL, recommend increasing aerobic-type exercise and a trial of OTC niacin. If no effect, or greater than two risk factors (for heart disease), consider prescribing fibrates or prescription niacin (Niaspan).
- Memorize waist circumference numbers and ratios for both genders.
- Recognize fatty liver disease (mild elevation of ALT and AST not associated with alcohol, medications, drugs, or viral hepatitis in an overweight to obese patient).
- Remember BMI calculation factors (weight divided by height).
- Do not confuse BMI formula with the PEF (peak expiratory flow). PEF is calculated using the height, age, gender (mnemonic is "HAG").
- First-line treatment for overweight/obese patient is lifestyle modification (diet, nutrition, exercise).
- A person with a BMI of 27 is overweight (initiate lifestyle education).

8

Pulmonary System Review

⚠ DANGER SIGNALS

Pulmonary Emboli (PE)

An older adult complains of sudden onset of dyspnea and coughing. Cough may be productive of pink-tinged frothy sputum. Other symptoms are tachycardia, pallor, and feelings of impending doom. Any condition that increases risk of blood clots will increase risk of PE. These patients have a history of atrial fibrillation, estrogens, surgery, pregnancy, long bone fractures, and prolonged inactivity.

Impending Respiratory Failure (Asthmatic Patient)

An asthmatic patient presents with tachypnea (greater than 25/min), tachycardia or bradycardia, cyanosis, and anxiety. The patient appears exhausted, fatigued, and diaphoretic and uses accessory muscles to help with breathing. Physical exam reveals cyanosis and "quiet" lungs with no wheezing or breath sounds audible.

Treatment Plan

Adrenaline injection STAT. Call 911. Oxygen at 4 to 5 L/minute, albuterol nebulizer treatments, parenteral steroids and antihistamines (diphenhydramine and cimetidine).

After treatment, a good sign is if breath sounds and wheezing are present (a sign that bronchi are becoming more open). Usually discharge with oral steroids for several days (i.e., Medrol Dose Pack).

☑ NORMAL FINDINGS

- *Lower lobes:* Vesicular breath sounds (soft and low)
- *Upper lobes:* Bronchial breath sounds (louder)

Egophonys

- *Normal:* Will hear "eee" clearly instead of "bah."
- *Abnormal:* Will hear "bah" sound.
- *Normal:* The "eee" sound is louder over the large bronchi because larger airways are better at transmitting sounds. The lower lobes have a softer sounding "eee."

Tactile Fremitus

- Instruct patient to say "99" or "one, two, three." Use finger pads to palpate lungs and feel for vibrations.
- *Normal:* Stronger vibrations palpable on the upper lobes and softer vibrations on lower lobes.
- *Abnormal:* The findings are reversed; may palpate stronger vibrations on one lower lobe (i.e., consolidation). Asymmetrical findings are always abnormal.

Whispered Pectoriloquy

- Instruct patient to whisper "99" or "one, two, three." Compare both lungs. If there is lung consolidation, the whispered words are easily heard on the lower lobes of the lungs.
- *Normal:* Voice louder and easy to understand in the upper lobes. Voice sounds are muffled on the lower lobes.
- *Abnormal:* Clear voice sounds in the lower lobes or muffled sounds on the upper lobes.

Percussion

- Use middle or index finger as the pleximeter finger on one hand. The finger on the other hand is the hammer.
- *Normal:* Resonance.
- *Tympany or hyperresonance:* Chronic obstructive pulmonary disease (COPD), emphysema (overinflation). If empty, the stomach area may be tympanic.
- *Dull tone:* Bacterial pneumonia with lobar consolidation, pleural effusion (fluid or tumor). A solid organ such as the liver sounds dull.

Pulmonary Function Tests

Measures Severity of Obstructive or Restrictive Pulmonary Dysfunction

- Obstructive dysfunction (reduction in airflow rates).
  - Asthma, COPD (chronic bronchitis and emphysema), bronchiectasis, others.
- Restrictive dysfunction (reduction of lung volume due to decreased lung compliance).
  - Pulmonary fibrosis, pleural disease, diaphragm obstruction, others.

::= DISEASE REVIEW

Chronic Obstructive Pulmonary Disease (COPD)

COPD is a term that includes both emphysema and chronic bronchitis. Some patients may also have an asthma component (with emphysema). Most patients have a mixture; one or the other may predominate. The disease is characterized by the loss of elastic recoil of the lungs and alveolar damage that takes decades. The most common risk factor is chronic cigarette smoking and older age. COPD is the fourth leading cause of death in the United States.

Chronic Bronchitis

Defined as coughing with excessive mucus production for at least 3 or more months for a minimum of 2 or more consecutive years.

Emphysema

Permanent alveolar damage and loss of elastic recoil results in chronic hyperinflation of the lungs. Expiratory respiratory phase is markedly prolonged.

Risk Factors

- Chronic smoking (etiology in up to 90% of cases of COPD), older age (greater than 40).
- Occupational exposure (coal dust, grain dust).
- Alpha-1 trypsin deficiency (rare condition). Patients have severe lung damage at earlier ages. Alpha-1 trypsin protects lungs from oxidative and environmental damage.

Classic Case

Elderly male with a history of many years of cigarette smoking complains of getting short of breath upon physical exertion that worsens over time; accompanied by a chronic frequent cough that is productive of large amounts of white to light yellow sputum (chronic bronchitis) or progressive dyspnea with minimal cough, barrel chest, and weight loss (emphysema).

Objective

- *Emphysema component:* Increased anterior–posterior diameter, decreased breath and heart sounds, use of accessory muscles, pursed-lip breathing, and weight loss.
- *Percussion:* Hyperresonance.
- *Tactile fremitus and egophony:* Decreased.
- *Chest x-ray:* Flattened diaphragms with hyperinflation. Sometimes bullae present.
- *Chronic bronchitis component:* Productive cough, wheezing, and coarse crackles.

Treatment Plan

- New treatment guidelines are listed in Table 8.1.

Safety Issues

- *Short-acting sympathomimetics (albuterol or Xopenex):* Excessive use may be dangerous if patient has concurrent hypertension, heart disease, hyperthyroidism, convulsions, or diabetes.
- *Anticholinergics (Atrovent, Spiriva):* Avoid if patient has narrow-angle glaucoma, BPH, or bladder neck obstruction.

General Treatment of COPD

- Smoking cessation is very important!
- Annual flu vaccination. Give pneumococcal vaccine.
- Pulmonary hygiene (postural drainage, etc.). Pulmonary rehab may help some patients.
- Treat lung infections aggressively.

Referral

- Severe exacerbations/disease, less than age 40, rapid progression, weight loss, surgical consult.
- Suspect secondary bacterial infection (higher risk for *Haemophilus influenzae* pneumonia).
- Look for acute onset of fever, purulent sputum, increased wheezing, and dyspnea.
- *Treatment:* Bactrim DS, doxycyline, or Ceftin BID for 10 days. For severe infection, Augmentin or respiratory quinolones (Avelox, Levaquin) for 3 to 7 days. Medrol Dose Pack PRN.

Table 8.1 Treatment of COPD: New Guidelines (2011)

Recommendations	Medications
First-line treatment	
Inhaled anticholinergics AND/OR	Ipratropium (Atrovent) QID or tiotropium (Spiriva) daily
Long-acting B2 agonists	Salmeterol in powder form (Serevent Diskus) Formoterol (Foradil Certihaler)
Combination drugs	Ipratropium and albuterol (Combivent)
Second-line treatment	
*Inhaled corticosteroids	For mild to moderate disease
*Systemic/oral corticosteroids	Budesonide (Pulmicort), flunisolide (AeroBid), fluticasone and salmeterol (Advair)
Severe COPD	Oral prednisone (tapering depends on length of therapy) or pulse dosing (Medrol Dose Pack).
Inhaled corticosteroid, long-acting B2 agonist	Fluticasone and salmeterol (Advair)
Sympathomimetics	Theophylline up to 400 mg daily Therapeutic range is between 8 and 13 µg/mL (monitor)
Home oxygen therapy Mucolytics	Oxygen at 2 to 3 liters by nasal cannula Guaifenesin. Increase fluid intake

COPD, chronic obstructive pulmonary disease

*Stop if no benefit in 6 to 8 weeks. Start earlier if asthmatic component.

Source: Adapted from the Joint Clinical Practice Guideline on Diagnosis and Management of Stable Chronic Obstructive Disease (2011).

🖎 EXAM TIPS

- First-line treatment for COPD (2011 guidelines) is an inhaled anticholinergic (Atrovent) AND/OR a long-acting B2 agonist (salmeterol, formoterol).
- Ipratropium (Atrovent) is an anticholinergic.
- Salmeterol and formoterol are long-acting B2 agonists.
- Do not use long-acting B2 agonists (salmeterol, formotorol) for rescue treatment.
- The only drug class for rescue treatment is the short-acting B2 agonist (SABA), such as albuterol and Xopenex.
- The only treatment known to prolong life in COPD patients is supplemental oxygen therapy.

📋 CLINICAL TIPS

- Long-term use of oral corticosteroids (> 24 weeks) increases the risk of pneumonia.
- When you are treating a COPD patient, pick an antibiotic that has coverage against *H. influenzae* (gram-negative).

COMMON LUNG INFECTIONS (TABLE 8.2)

Community-Acquired Bacterial Pneumonia (CAP)

Bacterial lung infection results in inflammatory changes and damage to the lungs. The bacterium causing the most deaths in outpatients is *Pneumococcus pneumoniae* (gram-positive).

Table 8.2 Common Lung Infections

Disease	Signs and Symptoms
Acute bacterial pneumonia (community-acquired or CAP) No.1 *Streptococcus pneumoniae* (gram-postive)	Acute onset. High fever and chills. Productive cough and large amount of green to rust-colored sputum. Pleuritic chest pain w/cough Crackles; decreased breath sounds, dull CBC: leukocytosis; elevated neutrophils. Band forms may be seen CXR: lobar infiltrates
Atypical pneumonia No.1 *Mycoplasma pneumoniae*	Gradual onset. Low-grade fever. Headache, Sore throat. Cough. Wheezing. Sometimes, rash CXR: interstitial to patchy infiltrates
Viral pneumonia Influenza, RSV	Fever. Cough. Pleurisy. Shortness of breath. Scanty sputum production. Myalgias Breath sounds: decreased breath sounds, rales
Acute bronchitis	Paroxysms of dry and severe cough that interrupts sleep. Cough dry to productive. Light-colored sputum. Can last up to 4 to 6 weeks. No antibiotics. Treat symptoms

CXR, chest x-ray; RSV, respiratory syncytial virus.

Organisms
- *No. 1 Streptococcus pneumoniae* or *pneumococcus* (gram-positive)
- *No. 2 Haemophilus influenzae*: More common in smokers, COPD (gram-negative)
- *Moraxella catarrhalis* (gram-negative), *Staphylococcus aureus* (gram-positive), others
- *Cystic fibrosis:* No. 1 bacteria is *Pseudomas aeruginosa* (gram-negative)

Classic Case
Older adults presents with sudden onset of a high fever (greater than 100.4°F) with chills that is accompanied by a productive cough with purulent sputum (rust-colored sputum seen with streptococcal pneumonia). The patient complains of pleuritic chest pain with coughing and dyspnea.

Geriatrics: Elderly may have atypical symptoms.

Objective
- *Auscultation:* Rhonchi, crackles, and wheezing.
- *Percussion:* Dullness over affected lobe.
- *Tactile fremitus and egophony:* Increased.
- Abnormal whispered pectoriloquy (whispered words louder).

Labs
- Chest x-ray (CXR) is the "gold standard" for diagnosing CAP (not sputum culture). Repeat within 6 weeks to document clearing.
- CXR result shows lobar consolidation in classic bacterial pneumonia.
- Post-treatment CXR to ensure clearing of infection.
- CBC: leukocytosis (greater than 10.5) with a possible "shift to the left" (increased band forms).
- Routine diagnostic tests (sputum C&S) to identify etiologic diagnosis are an option for outpatients with CAP.

Treatment Plan
American Thoracic Society Guidelines for Outpatient CAP*:
No comorbidity (previously healthy and no risk factors for drug-resistant *S. pneumoniae* infection):

- Macrolides are preferred.
  - Clarithromycin (Biaxin) BID × 10 days.
  - Azithromycin (Z-Pack) daily × 5 days.
  - Erythromycin QID × 10 days.
- Tetracyclines.
  - Doxycycline 100 mg BID × 10 days.

With comorbidity (i.e., alcoholism, CHF, chronic heart, lung, liver or kidney disease, antibiotics previous 3 months, diabetes, splenectomy/asplenia, others):

- Respiratory fluoroquinolone as ONE drug therapy.
  - Levaquin 750 mg daily × 5 days.
  - Gatifloxacin (Tequin) 400 mg or moxifloxacin (Avelox) 400 mg once a day × 10 days.
- Beta-lactam PLUS a macrolide.
  - *Preferred:* High dose of amoxicillin (e.g., 1–3 g TID) OR amoxicillin clavulanate (Augmentin) BID × 10 to 14 days PLUS a macrolide.
  - *Alternatives:* Ceftriaxone, cefuroxime axetil (Ceftin) BID × 10 to 14 days, doxycycline PLUS a macrolide.
- *Poor prognosis* (refer for hospitalization):
  - Elderly: Age 60 years or older, acute mental status changes, CHF.
  - Multiple lobar involvement.
  - Acute mental status change.
  - Alcoholics (aspiration pneumonia).
  - Patient meets the "CURB-65" criterion for hospital admission. "CURB-65" is a tool to assess if a patient needs hospitalization: *c*onfusion, blood *u*rea nitrogen greater than 19.6, *r*espiration greater than 30 breaths/minute, systolic *b*lood pressure (BP) less than 90 mmHg, diastolic BP less than 60 mmHg, age equal to or greater than 65 years.

Prevention

- Influenza vaccine for all persons older than 50 years, contact with persons who are at higher risk for death from pneumonia, health care workers, others.
- Pneumococcal polysaccharide vaccine (Pneumovax) if age greater than 65 years or with high-risk condition.

Pneumococcal Vaccine (Adults)
Polyvalent pneumococcal vaccine (Pneumovax 23, Pnu-Immune 23)

Healthy Patients

- Single dose usually sufficient at age 65 years (lifetime).
- 60% to 70% effective.

Underlying Disease

- 50% effective.

---

* Adapted from the Infectious Diseases Society of America/American Thoracic Society consensus guidelines on the management of community-acquired pneumonia in adults. Mandell LA, Wunderink RB, Anzueto A, et al. *Clinic Infectious Disease,* 2007.

Severely Immunocompromised
- Only 10% effective.

Recommended for:
- Persons aged 65 years or older.
- Impaired immunity.
  - Splenectomy, asplenia, or diseased spleen.
  - Alcoholics/cirrhosis of the liver.
  - HIV infection.
  - Chronic renal failure.
- Preexisting heart and lung disease.
  - Asthma, congenital heart disease, emphysema, others.
- Blood disorders.
  - Sickle cell anemia.
  - Hodgkin's lymphoma, multiple myeloma.

High-Risk Patients
- Repeat vaccine in 5 to 7 years (boosts antibodies):
  - If first dose was given before age of 65 years.
  - Asplenia, chronic renal failure (give at 19 years of age if asplenia, chronic renal disease).
  - Immunocompromised states.
  - Blood cancers: lymphoma, Hodgkin's disease, leukemia.

Atypical Pneumonia

An infection of the lungs by atypical bacteria. More common in children and young adults. Seasonal outbreaks (summer/fall). Highly contagious. Also known as "walking pneumonia."

Organisms
- *Mycoplasma pneumoniae* (atypical bacteria)
- *Chlamydia pneumoniae* (atypical bacteria)
- *Legionella pneumoniae* (atypical bacteria): Found in areas with moisture such as air conditioners (more severe with higher mortality)

Classic Case
A young adult complains of several weeks of fatigue that is accompanied by severe paroxysmal coughing that is mostly nonproductive. Gradual onset of symptoms. Illness may have started with cold-like symptoms (sore throat, clear rhinitis, and low-grade fever). Patient continues to go to work/school despite symptoms; may have coworkers with same symptoms.

Objective
- *Auscultation:* Wheezing and diffused crackles/rales.
- *Nose:* Clear mucus (may have rhinitis of clear mucus).
- *Throat:* Erythematous without pus or exudate.
- *Chest x-ray:* Diffuse interstitial infiltrates (up to 20% have pleural effusion).
- *CBC:* May have normal results.

Medications

- Macrolides:
    - Azithromycin (Z-Pack) × 5 days.
    - Clarithromycin (Biaxin) 500 mg BID × 10 to 14 days.
    - Erythromycin stearate 500 mg QID × 10 to 14 days.
- Antitussives (dextromethorphan, Tessalon Perles) as needed (PRN).
- Increase fluids and rest.

Acute Bronchitis

Acute viral (sometimes bacterial) infection of the bronchi causes inflammatory changes in the trachea, bronchi, and bronchioles, which results in increased reactivity of the upper airways. Usually self-limited. Also known as treacheobronchitis. Caused by adenovirus, influenza (winter/spring), coronavirus, respiratory syncytial virus, others.

Classic Case

Young adult complains of the sudden new onset of a cough that is keeping him awake at night. Cough is mainly dry, but it may become productive later with small amounts of sputum. The patient may have frequent paroxysms of coughing; may have low-grade fever, mild wheezing, and/or chest pain with cough.

Objective

- *Lungs:* Ranges from clear to severe wheezing (prolonged expiratory phase), rhonchi.
- *Percussion:* Resonant.
- *Chest x-ray:* Normal.
- Afebrile to low-grade fever.

Treatment Plan

- Treatment is symptomatic. Increase fluids and rest. Stop smoking (if smoker).
- Dextromethorphan BID to QID, Tessalon Perles (benzonatate) TID PRN (antitussives).
- Guaifenesin PRN (expectorant/mucolytic).
- For wheezing, albuterol inhaler (Ventolin) QID or nebulized treatment PRN.
- For severe wheezing, consider short-term oral steroid (Medrol Dose Pack).

Complications

- Exacerbation of asthma (increased risk of status asthmaticus).
- Pneumonia from secondary bacterial infection (pneumococcus, mycoplasma, others).

Pertussis

Also known as whooping cough. Caused by *Bordetella pertussis* bacteria (gram-negative).

A coughing illness of at least 14 days' duration with one of the following findings: paroxysmal coughing, inspiratory whooping (or post-tussive vomiting) without apparent cause. Illness can last from a few weeks to months. Pertussis has three stages (catarrhal, paroxysmal, and convalescent). Most infectious period is early in the disease (catarrhal stage) up to 21 days of cough (if not treated with appropriate antibiotic).

Classic Case

Suspect pertussis in previously "healthy" patient with a severe hacking cough of greater than 2 weeks' duration. Initial symptoms are low-grade fever and rhinorrhea with a mild cough (catarrhal stage). Cough becomes severe with inspiratory "whooping" sound.

The patient may vomit afterward (paroxysmal stage). Cough becomes less severe and less frequent and finally resolves (convalescent stage).

Labs

- Nasopharyngeal swab for culture and polymerase chain reaction (PCR).
- Pertussis antibodies by ELISA (enzyme-linked immunosorbent assay).
- *CBC:* Elevated WBCs and marked lymphocytosis (up to 80% lymphocytes in WBC differential). Chest x-ray should be negative. If positive, due to secondary bacterial infection.

Treatment Plan (Adolescents to Adults)

- First line: macrolides.
  - Azithromycin (Z-Pack) 500 mg on day 1, then 250 mg daily from day 2 to day 5.
  - Clarithromycin (Biaxin) BID × 7 days.
- Chemoprophylaxis for close contacts. Respiratory droplet precautions.
- Antitussives, mucolytics, rest, and hydration. Frequent small meals.

Tdap Booster

- Aged 11 to 18 years (and 18 years to adulthood): CDC recommends using Tdap (instead of Td).

Complications

- Sinusitis, otitis media, pneumonia, fainting, rib fractures, and others.

✍ EXAM TIPS

Classic findings: Respiratory infections
- Recognize presentation of bacterial pneumonia versus atypical pneumonia.
- The No. 1 bacterium in CAP is *Streptococcus pneumoniae* (and No. 2 is *Haemophilus influenzae*). Phlegm is rust-colored or blood-tinged.
- The No. 1 bacterium in atypical pneumonia is *Mycoplasma pneumoniae*.
- COPD: First-time treatment, start with Atrovent. Add salmeterol if poorly controlled.
- COPD/smoker with pneumonia: More likely to have *H. influenzae* bacteria.
- Know the drug classes of the meds used to treat acute bronchitis (such as antitussives, mucolytics, and so on).
- Presentation and treatment of pertussis (whooping cough).
- Symptomatic treatment for acute bronchitis. Do not pick antibiotics as a treatment option for acute bronchitis.

🗎 CLINICAL TIPS

- Depending on the stage of the disease and hydration status, the CXR result may be "normal" during the early phase of bacterial pneumonia (lobar pneumonia).
- Suspect pertussis in a "healthy" adult with no fever who has been coughing for more than 2 to 3 weeks, especially if previously treated with an antibiotic (that was not a macrolide) and is getting worse (rule out pneumonia first).
- Give Tdap (instead of Td) vaccine if patient is age 11 years or older.
- Emphasize importance of adequate fluid intake (best mucolytic, thins out mucus).
- Lung cancer can present as recurrent pneumonia (due to mass blocking bronchioles).

Common Cold (Viral Upper Respiratory Infection)

Self-limiting infection (range of 4–10 days). Most contagious from day 2 to day 3. More common in crowded areas and in small children. Transmission is by respiratory droplets and fomites. Highly contagious. Most cases occur in the winter months.

Classic Case

Acute onset of fever, sore throat. Frequent sneezing in early phase. Accompanied by nasal congestion, runny eyes, and rhinorrhea of clear mucus (coryza). The patient may complain of headache.

Objective

- *Nasal turbinates:* Swollen with clear mucus (may also have blocked tympanic membrane).
- *Anterior pharynx:* Reddened.
- *Cervical nodes:* Smooth, mobile, and small or "shotty" nodes (0.5 cm size or less) in the submandibular and anterior cervical chain.
- *Lungs:* Clear.

Treatment Plan

- Symptomatic treatment. Increase fluids and rest. Frequent handwashing.
- Analgesics (acetaminophen) or nonsteroidal anti-inflammatory drugs (NSAIDs) (ibuprofen) for fever and aches PRN.
- Oral decongestants (i.e., pseudoephedrine/Sudafed) PRN.
- Topical nasal decongestants (i.e., Afrin) can be used BID up to 3 days PRN only. Do not use for more than 3 days due to risk of rebound nasal congestion (rhinitis medicamentosa).
- Antitussives (i.e., dextromethorphan/Robitussin) PRN.
- Antihistamines (i.e., diphenhydramine/Benadryl) for nasal congestion PRN.

Complications

- Acute sinusitis.
- Acute otitis media.

Tuberculosis (TB)

An infection caused by *Mycobacterium tuberculosis* bacteria. Most common site of infection is the lungs (85%). Other sites include the kidneys, brain, lymph nodes, adrenals, and bone.

Most contagious forms are pulmonary TB, pleural TB, and laryngeal TB (coughing spreads aerosol droplets). CXR (reactivated TB) will show cavitations and adenopathy and granulomas on the hila of the lungs.

High-Risk Populations

Immigrants (from high-prevalence countries), migrant farm workers, illegal drug users, homeless, inmates of jails and nursing homes, HIV-infected, immunocompromised.

Latent TB Infection (LTBI)

An intact immune system causes macrophages to sequester the bacteria in the lymph nodes (mediastinum) in the form of granulomas. Not infectious.

Prior BCG (Bacille-Calmette-Guerin) Vaccine*

- History of BCG vaccine is not a contraindication for tuberculin testing.
- If more than 5 years have elapsed since last BCG vaccine, a positive TB skin test is most likely caused by a TB infection.

Miliary TB

Also known as *disseminated TB disease*. Infects multiple organ systems. More common in younger children (below the age of 5) and the elderly. CXR will show classic "milia seed" pattern.

Multidrug-Resistant TB (Or XDR TB)

Bacteria resistant to at least two of the best anti-TB drugs, isoniazid and rifampicin (these drugs are considered first-line drugs).

DOT (Direct Observed Treatment)

Mandatory for noncompliant patients. Success dependent on medication compliance.

- *How:* Patient is observed by a nurse when he or she takes the medications. Mouth, cheek, and area under the tongue checked to make sure the pill was swallowed adequately.

Reactivated TB Infection or Active TB Disease (Infectious)

Latent bacteria become reactivated due to depressed immune system. The majority of TB cases (90%) of active disease in the United States are reactivated infections.

Treatment Plan

- Report TB to local health department for contact tracing ASAP. A reportable disease.
- All active TB patients should be tested for HIV infection.
- Initial regimen for suspected TB before C&S results are available. Use four drugs: isonicotinylhydrazine (INH) 300 mg daily for adults, rifampin, ethambutal, and pyrazidamide three times a week.
- Narrow down number of medications after C&S results reveal most effective drugs.
- Several treatment regimens are available. Check TB website (www.cdc.gove/TB/).

Classic Case

Adult patient (from high-risk population) complains of fever, anorexia, fatigue, and night sweats along with a mild nonproductive cough (early phase). Aggressive infections (later sign) will have productive cough with blood-stained sputum (hemoptysis) along with weight loss (late sign).

Warning

Ethambutal causes optic neuritis. Avoid if patient has abnormal vision (i.e., blindness, retinal vein occlusion, and so forth).

Recent PPD Converters and Preventive Treatment and/or Latent TB Infection

Recent PPD converter is defined as person with history of negative PPD results who then converts to a positive PPD. Higher risk of active TB disease (up to 10%) within first 1 to 2 years after seroconversion.

- Assess for signs and symptoms of TB (cough, night sweats, weight loss).
- Order CXR (make sure has no hilar cavitations and mediastinal adenopathy).
- HIV-negative: INH 300 mg/day for 9 months.
- HIV-positive: INH 300 mg/day for at least 12 months.
- Check baseline liver function tests and monitor.

---

* Adapted from CDC Tuberculosis Fact Sheet (www.cdc.gov/TB/).

Generally, preventive treatment for latent TB infection is encouraged for those less than 35 years of age. After age of 35 years, much higher risk of liver damage from INH chemoprophylaxis. Assess risk versus benefits and discuss with the patient.

TB Skin Test (Mantoux Test or PPD) (Table 8.3)

Look for an induration (feels harder). The red color is not as important. If a PPD result is a bright red color but is not indurated (skin feels soft), it is a negative result.

- Less than or equal to 5 mm:
  - HIV (+).
  - Recent contact with infectious TB cases.
  - CXR with fibrotic changes consistent with previous TB disease.
  - Any child who had close contact or TB symptoms (before age of 5 years).
  - Immunocompromised (i.e., organ transplant, bone marrow transplant, renal failure, patients on biologic drugs, others).
- Greater than or equal to 10 mm:
  - Recent immigrants (within last 5 years) from high-prevalence countries (Latin America, Asia, Africa, India, Pacific islands).
  - Child less than 4 years of age or children/adolescents exposed to high-risk adult.
  - Intravenous drug user, health care worker, homeless.
  - Employees or residents from high-risk congregate settings (jails, nursing homes).
- Greater than 15 mm:
  - Persons with no known risk factors for TB.

Labs

TB Skin Test (TST)

- *Mantoux test/TST:* Inject 0.1 ml of 5TU-PPD subdermally. Do not use the Tine Test (has not been used for many years).

Blood Tests for TB

- *QuantiFERON-TB Gold or the T-SPOT TB test* (also known as interferon-γ release assays or IGRAs): Blood tests that measure γ-interferon (from lymphocytes).
- *IGRA test results:* Available within 24 hours (only one visit required). If history of previous BCG vaccination, IGRA blood tests preferred.

Table 8.3 TB Skin Test Results (Mantoux or the PPD)

Size	Test Results
≥ to 5 mm	HIV (+) Recent contact with infectious TB cases CXR with fibrotic changes consistent with previous TB disease Any child who had close contact or has TB symptoms (before age of 5 years) Immunocompromised (i.e., organ transplant, bone marrow transplant, renal failure, patients on biologic drugs, others)
≥ to 10 mm	Recent immigrants (within last 5 years) from high-prevalence countries (Latin America, Asia, Africa, India, Pacific islands) Child less than 4 years of age or children/adolescents exposed to high-risk adult Intravenous drug user (IDU), health care worker, homeless Employees or residents from high-risk congregate settings (jails, nursing homes)
≥ 15 mm	Persons with no risk factors for TB

CXR, chest x-ray; TB, tuberculosis.

Sputum Tests for TB

- *Sputum for PCR* (detects less than 10 organisms/mL versus > 10,000 organisms for acid fast bacillus [AFB]).
- Sputum C&S and AFB: takes from 3 to 6 weeks.
- Per the CDC: The interferon-γ release assay blood tests can be used in place of the TB skin test.

Booster Phenomenon (Latent TB Infection)

A person with latent TB infection (LTBI) can have a false negative reaction to the tuberculin skin test (TST) or the PPD if they have not been tested for many years.

- Two-step tuberculin skin testing is recommended by the CDC.

Explanation

- A person is negative after many years of no PPD testing.
- When the TST/PPD is done again (first time), there is no reaction (false negative).
- If PPD repeated in 1 to 3 weeks, it will be positive (the booster phenomenon). Otherwise, if still negative, more likely to be a true negative result.

Anergy Testing

Used for patients suspected of being immunocompromised (HIV infection) to rule out false-negative result. Per CDC, usefulness of anergy testing for HIV-infected persons has not been demonstrated.

Procedure

- The PPD is administered on the volar aspect of the left lower arm (as usual) and the "control" antigen is given on the right lower arm. Do not mix the PPD with the control.
- "Control" agents used are tetanus, *Candida*, or mumps antigens. Administer with tuberculin syringe subdermally.
- If control side is negative, it means that patient is immunocompromised (i.e., PPD will not work).
- Consider other methods for detecting infection (i.e., bronchoscopy).

✍ EXAM TIPS

- A PPD result may be listed as 9.5 mm. If the patient falls under the 10-mm group, then it is negative (by definition) unless the patient has the signs/symptoms and/or CXR findings suggestive of TB.
- Memorize the criteria for the 5-mm and 10-mm results.
- Small children exposed to active TB have a high chance of coming down with the disease.

🗎 CLINICAL TIPS

- The QuantiFERON-TB Gold and the T-SPOT TB tests are available at public health clinics. They only require one visit for the patient to be tested (1 vial of blood).
- Never treat TB with fewer than two or three drugs.
- According to the CDC, on the average, about 10 contacts are listed for each index person with infectious TB.

(Continued)

- Persons with HIV infection with CD4 less than 500 or patients who are taking tumor necrosis factor antagonists (or biologics) are at very high risk for active TB disease after initial exposure (primary TB).

Asthma

Reversible airway obstruction caused by chronic inflammation of the bronchial tree. Results in increased airway responsiveness to stimuli (internal or external). Genetic predisposition with positive family history of allergies, eczema, and allergic rhinitis (atopy or atopic history). Exacerbations can be life-threatening (status asthmaticus).

Treatment Plan

- Can perform usual "normal" activities with no limitations (can attend school full time, play "normally," go to work full time, no job absence due to asthmatic symptoms).
- Minimal to no exacerbations (daytime and nighttime).
- Minimal use of rescue medicine (less than 2 days a week albuterol use).
- Avoid ED visits/hospitalization.
- Maintain near normal pulmonary function (reduce permanent lung damage).

Classic Case

Young adult patient with asthma complains of worsening symptoms after a recent bout of a viral upper respiratory infection. The patient is using her albuterol inhaler more than normal (about 4 to 6 times/day) to treat the symptoms; complains of shortness of breath, wheezing, and chest tightness that is sometimes accompanied by a dry cough in the night and early morning (e.g., 3 a.m.) that awakens her from sleep.

Trigger Factors for Asthma
Viral URIs, Airborne Allergens

- Food allergies: sulfites, red and yellow dye, seafood.
- Cold air or cold weather and fumes from chemicals or smoke.
- Emotional stress and exercise (exercise-induced asthma).
- GERD (reflux of acidic gastric contents irritates airways).
- ASA or NSAIDs (patients with nasal polyps are more sensitive to ASA and NSAIDs).

Objective

- *Lungs:* Wheezing with prolonged expiratory phase. As asthma worsens, the wheezing occurs during both inspiration and expiration.
- *CV:* Tachycardia, rapid pulse.

Asthma Medications
"Rescue" Medicine

Only one drug class used for rescue: short-acting B2 agonists.

- Short-acting B2 agonists metered-dose inhalers (MDI) or by nebulizer.
  - Albuterol [(Ventolin HFA) or pirbuterol (Maxair)] 2 inhalations every 4 to 6 hours PRN.
  - Levalbuterol (Xopenex HFA): 2 inhalations every 4 to 6 hours PRN.
- Quick onset (15 to 30 minutes) and lasts about 4 to 6 hours.
  - Used for quick relief (of wheezing), but does not treat underlying inflammation.

Long-Term Control Medications (Table 8.4)
- These drugs act as anti-inflammatories. Must be taken every day to be effective.
- Long-acting B2 agonists (LABAs) are *not* rescue drugs. Must be taken BID.
- LABAs increase the risk of death from asthma.

Sustained-Release Theophylline (Theo-24)
- *Drug class:* Methylxanthine. Used as an adjunct drug. Acts as a bronchodilator.
- Monitor levels to reduce risk of toxicity. The drug has multiple drug interactions such as the following:
  - Macrolides, quinolones
  - Cimetidine
  - Anticonvulsants such as phenytoin, carbamazepine (Tegretol).
  - Check blood levels: normal is 12 to 15 mg/dL.

Spacers or Chambers
Use of "spacer" or "chamber" (Aerochamber) is encouraged. It will increase delivery of the aerosolized drug to the lungs and minimize oral thrush (for inhaled steroids).

Stepwise Treatment for Managing Asthma (Age 12 Years to Adults)[*,**]
Asthma is diagnosed based on the history, symptoms (Wheeze, dyspnea, cough) and reversible expiratory airflow obstruction (spirometry pulmonary function tests.)

Table 8.4 Asthma: Long-Term Control Medications

Drug class	Brand Name	Side Effects/Adverse Effects
Inhaled corticosteriods	Triamcinolone (Azmacort) BID Fluticasone (Flovent HFA) BID	Oral thrush (gargle or drink water after use). HPA axis suppression, glaucoma, others.
Long-acting B2 antagonist (LABA) combination	Salmeterol (Serevent) BID Formeterol (Foradil) BID Salmeterol + fluticasone (Advair) BID	Warn patients of increased risk of asthma deaths Warn patient that LABAs are not to be used as rescue drugs.
Leukotriene inhibitors	Montelukast (Singulair) daily Zileuton (Zyflo) daily	Neuropsychological effects (agitation, aggression, depression, others) Monitor LFTs (zileuton)
Mast cell stabilizers	Cromolyn sodium (Intal) QID Nedocromil sodium (Tilade) QID	Works better with children Cough, sneezing
Methylxanthines	Theophylline (not used often) Theo-24 capsules daily to BID Starting dose 300 mg/day BID	Sympathomimetic. Avoid with seizures, hypertension, stroke Several drug interactions
Immunomodulators	Omalizumab (anti-IgE) monoclonal antibody	Be equipped and prepared to treat anaphylaxis when starting this drug

BID, twice a day; CVA, cerebrovascular accidents; HPA, hypothalamic-pituitary-adrenal; IgE, immunoglobulin E; LFT, liver function test; QID, four times a day.

---

[*] All asthmatics need short-acting B2 agonists (the "rescue" drug).
[**] Adapted from the Expert Panel Report 3: Guidelines for the Diagnosis and Management of Asthma, August 2007.

Step 1
- Mild Intermittent (FEV1/PEF > 80% predicted. Symptoms < 2 days/week)
  - Albuterol (Ventolin) metered-dose inhaler as needed.

Step 2
- Mild Persistent Asthma (FEV1/PEF > 80% predicted. Symptoms > 2 days/week)
  - Albuterol (Ventolin) metered-dose inhaler as needed.
- PLUS
  - Low-dose inhaled corticosteroid (ICS) is preferred
  - Alternative: Cromolyn, montelukast, nedocromil, or theophylline.

Step 3
- Moderate persistent asthma (FEV1 or PEF 60%–80% of predicted daily symptoms)
  - Albuterol metered dose inhaler as needed.
- PLUS
  - Low-dose ICS with salmeterol (Advair) OR medium-dose ICS is preferred.
  - Alternative: Low-dosed ICS plus leukotriene inhibitor (Singulair), theophylline, or zileuton.

Step 4
- Severe persistent asthma (FEV1/PEF < 60% predicted. Symptoms most of the day)
- High-dose ICS plus long-acting B2 agonist plus oral steroid daily is the preferred treatment.
- Requires oral corticosteroid (prednisone) daily.
  - Albuterol metered-dose inhaler.

Lab Monitoring
- Theophylline requires serum concentration monitoring.
- Zileuton (Zyflo); must monitor liver function.

Exercise-Induced Asthma (Exercise-Induced Bronchospasm)
Premedicate 10 to 15 minutes before the activity with two puffs of a short-acting B2 agonist or SABA (albuterol/Ventolin, levalbuterol/Xopenex, pirbuterol/Maxair). Effect will last up to 4 hours.

ASTHMA TREATMENT: IN A NUTSHELL...

- Every patient should be on a short-acting B2 agonist (albuterol) PRN.
- Next step is inhaled corticosteroids. Dose depends on class of asthma.
- Then add long-acting B2 agonists (salmeterol) or use combination drug (Advair).
- Add leukotriene inhibitors, sustained-release theophylline, or mast cell stabilizer.

Asthmatic Exacerbation
- Respiratory distress: Tachypnea, using accessory muscles (intercostals, abdominal) to breathe, talks in brief/fragmented sentences, severe diaphoresis, fatigue, agitation.
- Lungs: Minimal to no breath sounds audible during lung auscultation. PEF < 40%. Lips/skin blue-tinged (cyanosis).
- Give nebulizer treatment: Albuterol or levalbuterol/saline solution by nebulizer. May repeat every 20 minutes (for three doses). If unable to use inhaled bronchodilators, give epinephrine IM.

- After nebulizer treatment(s):
  - Listen for breath sounds. If inspiratory and expiratory wheezing is present, a good sign (signals opening up of airways). If there is a lack of breath sounds or wheezing after a nebulizer treatment, a bad sign (patient is not responding). Call 911.
- Discharge
  - Medrol Dose Pack or prednisone tabs 40 mg per day × 4 days (no weaning necessary if 4 days or less). Continue medications and increase dose (or add another controller drug).
- Referral to ED (call 911):
  - Poor to no response to nebulizer treatment (peak expiratory flow [PEF] less than 40% of expected).
  - Impending respiratory arrest: give Epi-Pen STAT. Call 911.

Peak Expiratory Flow Rate: PEFR or PEF

Measures effectiveness of treatment, worsening symptoms, and exacerbations. During expiration, patient is instructed to blow hard using the spirometer (3 times). The highest value is recorded (personal best).
- PEF is based on height (H), age (A), and gender (G), or HAG.
- Mnemonic: HAG (height, age, gender)

Spirometer Parameters

- *Green Zone:* 80% to 100% of expected volume
  - Maintain or reduce medications.
- *Yellow Zone:* 50% to 80% of expected volume
  - Maintenance therapy needs to be increased or patient is having an acute exacerbation.
- *Red Zone:* Below 50% of expected
  - If after treatment patient's PEFR is still below 50% expected, call 911. If in respiratory distress, give epinephrine injection. Call 911.

✎ EXAM TIPS

- Memorize factors needed to figure out PERF (use HAG mnemonic).
- Do not confuse asthma "rescue" drugs with "long-term control or maintenance" drugs.
- Remember that all asthmatics need a short-acting B2 agonist (i.e., albuterol).
- Chronic use of high-dose inhaled steroids can cause osteoporosis, mild growth retardation in children, glaucoma, cataracts, immune suppression, hypothalamic-pituitary-adrenal suppression, and other effects.
- Recognize respiratory failure. Severe respiratory distress: tachypnea, disappearance of or lack of wheezing, accessory muscle use, diaphoresis, and exhaustion.
- First-line treatment for severe asthmatic exacerbation or respiratory distress is an adrenaline injection.

📋 CLINICAL TIPS

- If you suspect that the patient has allergic asthma, check serum immunogobulin G allergy panels (mold allergy, grass allergy panels, others). Refer to allergist for scratch testing and treatment.
- Consider supplementing with calcium with vitamin D 1500 mg tabs QD for menopausal women and other high-risk patients (for osteoporosis) who are on medium- to high-dose inhaled steroids long term.
- Consider bone density testing (in males or females) who are on chronic steroids.
- Annual eye exams if on long-term steroids since higher risk of cataracts and glaucoma.

9

Endocrine System Review

Severe Hypoglycemia

Blood glucose is less than 50 mg/dL. Complains of weakness, "feel like passing out," headache, clammy hands, and anxiety. Difficulty concentrating and thinking. If severe hypoglycemia is uncorrected, it will progress to coma.

Type 1 Diabetes Mellitus

School-aged child with recent history of viral illness complains of excessive hunger and thirst. Urinating more than normal (polyuria). Starts losing weight despite eating a large amount of food. Breath has a "fruity" odor. Large amount of ketones in urine.

Thyroid Cancer

A single large nodule (greater than 2.5 cm) on one lobe of the thyroid gland, size greater than 2.5 cm. The 24-hour radioactive iodine uptake (RAIU) test will show a "cold" nodule. Positive family history of thyroid cancer. May have a history of facial, neck, or chest radiation therapy.

Pheochromocytoma

Random episodes of severe hypertension (systolic BP greater than 200 mm Hg or diastolic BP greater than 110 mm Hg) associated with abrupt onset of severe headache, tachycardia, and anxiety. Episodes resolve spontaneously, but occur at random. In between the attacks, patient's vital signs are normal.

Hyperprolactinemia

Can be a sign of a pituitary adenoma. Slow onset. When tumor is large enough to cause a mass effect, the patient will complain of headaches.

☑ **NORMAL FINDINGS**

- The endocrine system works as a "negative feedback" system. If a low level of "active" hormone occurs, it stimulates production. Inversely, high levels of hormones stop production.

- The hypothalamus stimulates the anterior pituitary gland into producing the "stimulating hormones" (such as follicle-stimulating hormone [FSH], luteinizing hormone [LH], thyroid-stimulating hormone [TSH]).
- These "stimulating hormones" tell the target organs (ovaries, thyroid, etc.) to produce "active" hormones (estrogen, thyroid hormone, etc.).
- High levels of these "active" hormones work in reverse. The hypothalamus directs the anterior pituitary into stopping production of the stimulating hormones (TSH, LH, FSH, etc).

ENDOCRINE GLANDS (FIGURE 9.1)

Both glands interact to form the "hypothalamic-pituitary axis."

Hypothalamus ("Master Gland")

The master gland. Coordinates the endocrine system by sending signals to the pituitary gland. Directly produces oxytocin, the hormone responsible for uterine stimulation in labor and milk production.

Pituitary Gland

Located at the sella turcica (base of the brain). Stimulated by the hypothalamus into producing the "stimulating hormones" such as FSH, LH, TSH, adrenocorticotropin hormone (ACTH), and growth hormone.

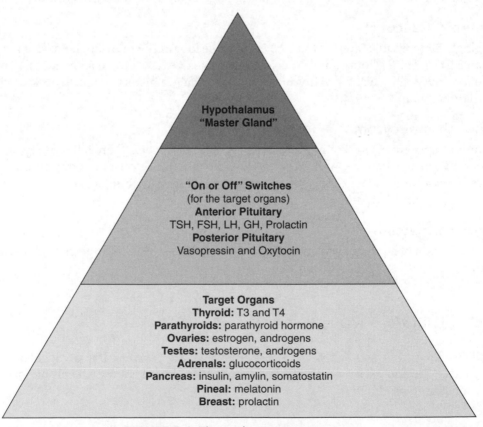

FIGURE 9.1 The endocrine system.

Anterior Pituitary Gland (Adenohypophysis)

Produces hormones that directly regulate the target organs (ovary, thyroid, etc.).

- FSH
  - Stimulates the ovaries enabling growth of follicles (or eggs).
  - Production of estrogen.
- LH
  - Stimulates the ovaries to ovulate.
  - Production of progesterone (by corpus lutea).
  - In males, LH stimulates the testicles (Leydig cells) to produce testosterone.
- TSH
  - Stimulates thyroid gland.
  - Production of thyroid hormones.
- Growth hormone
  - Stimulates somatic growth of the body.
- ACTH
  - Stimulates the adrenal glands (two portions of gland—medulla and cortex).
  - Production of glucocorticoids (cortisol) and mineralocorticoids (aldosterone).
- Prolactin
  - Affects lactation and milk production.

Posterior Pituitary Gland

Secretes vasopressin (antidiuretic hormone) and oxytocin, which are made by the hypothalamus but stored and secreted by the posterior pituitary.

Parathyroid Gland

Located behind the thyroid glands and produces parathyroid hormone (PTH).

PTH is responsible for the calcium balance of the body by regulating the calcium loss/gain from the bones, kidneys, and GI tract (calcium absorption).

☰ DISEASE REVIEW

Hyperthyroidism

The classic finding is a very low (or undetectable) TSH with elevations in both serum-free T4 (thyroxine) and T3 (triiodothyronine) levels. The most common cause for hyperthyroidism (60% to 80%) in the United States is a chronic autoimmune disorder called Grave's disease.

Grave's Disease (Thyrotoxicosis, Toxic Diffuse Goiter)

An autoimmune disorder causing hyperfunction and production of excess thyroid hormones (T3 and T4). Higher incidence in women (8:1 ratio). These women are also at higher risk for other autoimmune diseases such as rheumatoid arthritis and pernicious anemia and for osteoporosis.

Classic Case

Middle-aged female loses a large amount of weight rapidly, becomes irritable, anxious, and hyperactive. Insomnia with more frequent bowel movements (looser stools). Amenorrhea and heat intolerance. Enlarged thyroid (goiter) present. May present with hypertension.

Objective

- *Goiter:* Diffusely enlarged gland without nodules. May be tender to palpation or asymptomatic.
- *Hands/fingers:* Fine tremors on both hands, sweaty palms.
- *Eyes:* Exophthalmos in later stages.
- *Cardiac:* Tachycardia, atrial fibrillation, congestive heart failure.

Labs

- Look for very low TSH (less than 0.01) with elevated serum free T4 and T3. If Grave's disease, it will have positive thyroid-stimulating immunoglobulin.
- *Workup as follows:* Check TSH. If low, order serum free T3 and T4 (will be high). Next step is to order antibody tests to confirm whether Grave's disease (thyroid-stimulating immunoglobulin).
- If thyroid mass/nodule, order thyroid ultrasound. Refer to endocrinologist for management.
- *Imaging studies:* 24-hour RAIU shows homogenous uptake.

Medications

- *Propylthiouracil (PTU):* Shrinks thyroid gland/decreases hormone production.
- *Methimazole (Tapazole):* Shrinks thyroid gland/decreases hormone production.
- *Side effects:* Skin rash, granulocytopenia, hepatic necrosis (monitor CBC, LFTs).

Adjunctive Treatment

Given before thyroid under control to alleviate the symptoms of hyperstimulation (i.e., anxiety, tachycardia, palpitations). Beta-blockers are effective (i.e., propranolol or atenolol 25 mg/day).

Radioactive Iodine

Contraindicated during pregnancy/lactation. Permanent destruction of thyroid gland results in hypothyroidism for life. These patients need thyroid supplementation for life after thyroid is destroyed.

- *Pregnancy:* Hyperthyroidism.
- PTU is preferred treatment. Give lowest effective dose possible.

Complications

Thyroid storm (thyrotoxicosis): Acute worsening of symptoms due to stress or infection. Look for decreased LOC, fever, abdominal pain. Life-threatening. Immediate hospitalization needed.

Thyroid Gland Tests

- *Thyroid gland ultrasounds:* Used to detect goiter (generalized enlargement of gland), multinodular goiter, single nodule, and solid versus cystic masses.
- *Thyroid cancer:* Single painless nodule greater than 2.5 cm, history of neck irradiation in childhood.
- *Thyroid scan* (24-hour thyroid scan with RAIU): Shows metabolic activity of thyroid gland.
- *Cold spot:* Not metabolically active (more worrisome; rule out thyroid cancer). Biopsy.
- *Hot spot:* Metabolically active nodule with homogeneous uptake and is usually benign.

Laboratory Findings of Thyroid Disease

- TSH (thyroid-stimulating hormone or thyrotropin):
  - *Normal range:* 0.01 to 6.0 norm mIU/L (third-generation test)
  - TSH is used for both screening and monitoring response to treatment. If TSH is abnormal, next step is to order the full thyroid panel. Serum free T3 and T4 are high (free form of T3 and T4) and the TSH is very low (usually <0.05 mU/L). Check TSH every 6 to 8 weeks until thyroid is under control.
- Drug-induced thyroid disease: lithium, amiodarone, interferon-alfa, dopamine. Monitor thyroid function by periodically checking the TSH.

Hypothyroidism

The classic lab finding for hypothyroidism is a high TSH with low free T4 levels (do not confuse with total T4).

Some of the most common causes are Hashimoto's thyroiditis, postpartum thyroiditis, and thyroid ablation with radioactive iodine (to treat hyperthyroidism). Hashimoto's thyroiditis is the most common cause of hypothyroidism in the United States.

Hashimoto's Thyroiditis

A chronic autoimmune disorder of the thyroid gland. The body produces destructive antibodies (antimicrosomal antibodies) against the thyroid glands that gradually destroy it. Almost all patients (90%) with Hashimoto's thyroiditis have elevated antimicrosomal antibody titers. Most patients have developed a goiter.

Classic Case

Middle-aged to older woman who is overweight complains of fatigue, weight gain, cold intolerance, constipation, and menstrual abnormalities. Some elderly patients may present with atrial fibrillation. May have a history of another autoimmune disorder.

Severe hypothyroidism (myxedema) may present with puffy face, hands, and feet. There is thickening of the skin, thinning of the outer one-third of the eyebrows, and cognitive symptoms such as slowed thinking, poor short-term memory, and depression (or dementia).

Labs

- TSH elevated (greater than 6.0 mIU/L) with low levels of serum free T4.
- Antimicrosomal antibodies: elevated ("gold standard" test for diagnosing Hashimoto's thyroiditis).
  - Work-up: Order TSH first. If elevated, order thyroid panel. Next step is to order TSH-receptor antibodies to confirm Hashimoto's thyroiditis.

Treatment Plan

- Starting dose of levothyroxine (Synthroid) is 25 to 50 mcg per day.
- Start with lowest dose (Synthroid 25 mcg) for elderly or patients with history of heart disease (watch for angina, acute myocardial infarction, atrial fibrillation).
- Increase Synthroid dose by 25 mcg every few weeks until TSH is normalized.
- Re-check TSH every 6 to 8 weeks until TSH is normalized (less than 6 mIU/L).
- Advise patient to report if palpitations, nervousness, or tremors because this means that Synthroid dose is too high (decrease dose until symptoms are gone and TSH in normal range).

✍ EXAM TIPS

- If patient has elevated TSH (or very low TSH), next step is to order free T3 and T4 (free T4 is low in hypothyroidism).
- Starting dose of levothyroxine (Synthroid) is 25 mcg/day.
- Check TSH every 6 to 8 weeks (do not order earlier than 6 weeks) to monitor treatment response.
- Radioactive iodine treatment results in hypothyroidism for life. Supplemented with thyroid hormone (i.e., Synthroid) for life.
- PTU preferred for pregnant women.
- Thyroid cancer risk factors (history of neck irradiation in childhood or a painless nodule larger than 2.5 cm).
- Chronic amenorrhea and hypermetabolism results in osteoporosis. Supplement: calcium with vitamin D, weight-bearing exercises.

📋 CLINICAL TIPS

- Hashimoto's thyroiditis can present with signs and symptoms of hyperthyroidism during the acute phase.
- Subclinical hypothyroidism is defined as an elevated TSH with normal serum-free T4.

DIABETES MELLITUS

A chronic metabolic disorder affecting the body's metabolism of carbohydrates and fat. The result is microvascular and macrovascular damage, neuropathy, and immune system effects.

- *Microvascular damage:* Retinopathy, nephropathy, and neuropathy.
- *Macrovascular damage:* Atherosclerosis, heart disease (coronary artery disease, MI).
- *Target organs:* Eyes, kidneys, heart/vascular system, peripheral nerves, especially in the feet. Diabetes is the most common reason for chronic renal failure requiring dialysis and lower limb amputations in the United States.

Type 1 Diabetes

The massive destruction of B-cells in the islets of Langerhans results in an abrupt cessation of insulin production. If uncorrected, body fat will be used for fuel. Ketones, the metabolic product of fat breakdown, build up in the body until the result is diabetic ketotic acidosis and coma. Most patients are juveniles; occasionally adults (maturity onset diabetes of the young or MODY).

Type 2 Diabetes

Progressive decreased secretion of insulin (with peripheral insulin resistance) resulting in a chronic state of hyperglycemia and hyperinsulinemia. Has strong genetic component.

Type 2 diabetes mellitus represents 85% to 90% of U.S. cases. Obesity epidemic increasing rates of type 2 diabetes in younger ages.

Risk Factors for Type 2 Diabetes (Screen These Patients)

- Overweight or obese (body mass index [BMI] 30 or greater).
- Abdominal obesity; sedentary lifestyle.
- Metabolic syndrome.
- Hispanic, African American, Asian, or American Indian, or positive family history.

- History of gestational diabetes or infant weighing greater than 9 lbs at birth.
- Impaired fasting blood sugar (IFG) or impaired glucose tolerance (IGT) considered at higher risk for type 2 diabetes (prediabetes).

Metabolic Syndrome

- Obesity, hypertension, hyperglycemia, and dyslipidemia.
- Other names are insulin-resistance syndrome or Syndrome X.
- Higher risk for type 2 diabetes and cardiovascular disease.

Increased Risk of Diabetes (Prediabetes)

- A1C between 5.7% and 6.4%
  OR
- Fasting glucose of 100 to 125 mg/dL (impaired fasting plasma glucose)
  OR
- 2-hour OGTT (75 g load) of 140 to 199 mg/dL

Diagnostic Criteria for Diabetes

- A1c (was known as HbA1c) of equal to or > 6.5%
  OR
- Fasting plasma glucose (FPG) equal to or >126 mg/dL (fasting is no caloric intake for at least 8 hr).
  OR
- Symptoms of hyperglycemia (polyuria, polydipsia, polyphagia) plus random blood glucose equal to or > 200 mg/dL
  OR
- Two-hour plasma glucose greater than or equal to 200 mg/dL during an OGTT with a 75 g glucose load.

Serum Blood Glucose Norms (Nondiabetic Adults; Table 9.1)

- Fasting plasma glucose (FPG): 70 to 100 mg/dL
- Peak postprandial plasma glucose: Less than 180 mg/dL.
- Glycosylated hemoglobin (A1C): <6.0%
  - HbA1c or A1c: Defined as the average blood glucose levels over previous 3 months. No fasting required. Test measures excess glucose that attaches to the hemoglobin of the red blood cells.
  - A1c test must be certified by the NGSP (National Glycohemoglobin Standardization Program) and standardized to the DCCT (Diabetes Control and Complications Trial) assay.

Table 9.1 Recommendations for Nonpregnant Adult Diabetics

Test	Goal
Blood pressure	<140/80 mm Hg
LDL cholesterol	<100 mg/dL
A1c	<7% (exceptions exist)
Preprandial capillary plasma glucose (fasting)	70 to 130 mg/dL
Peak postprandial capillary plasma glucose (2 hours after meal)	<180 mg/dL

Source: Diabetes Mellitus: Diagnosis Guidelines (ADA, 2013).

- If tolerate A1c goal of 6% (especially younger diabetics), continue with the same goal.
- Less stringent goals acceptable for some (frail elderly, history of severe hypoglycemia, extensive comorbidity, limited life expectancy).
  - A1c goal of up to 8% is acceptable.

Labs
- Newly diagnosed diabetics: Check A1c every 3 months until blood glucose controlled or when changing therapy, then check twice a year (every 6 months).
- Lipid profile at least once a year (or more if elevated) with 9 to 12 hour fasting.
- Random or "on spot" urine for microalbuminuria at least once a year.
  - Urine albumin-to-creatinine ratio better than microalbumin test (spot urine sample) for evaluating microalbumin (the earliest sign of diabetic renal disease).
  - If positive, order 24-hour urine for protein and creatinine.
- ACEI or ARBs with tighter control of blood glucose/A1c may help renal disease.
- Check electrolytes (potassium, magnesium, sodium), liver function panel, TSH.

Treatment Plan
- *Every visit:* Check BP, feet, weight and BMI, blood sugar diary.
- *Check feet:*
  - Check for vibration sense (128-Hz tuning fork). Place on bony prominence of the big toe (MTP joint).
  - Light and deep touch, numbness. Place at right angle on plantar surface, push into skin until it buckles slightly (monofilament tool).
  - Check pedal pulses, ankle reflexes, skin.

Recommendations: Preventive Care
- Flu shot every year.
- Pneumococcal polysaccharide vaccine. If vaccinated <65 years of age, give one-time revaccination in 5 years. If 65 years, give one dose of the vaccine only.
- Aspirin 81 mg if high risk for MI, stroke (if <30 years old, not recommended).
- *Ophthalmologist:* Yearly dilated eye exam. If type 2: eye exam at diagnosis. If type 1: first eye exam 5 years after diagnosis.
- *Podiatrist:* Once to twice a year, especially with older diabetics.
- *BP goal:* 130/80 mm Hg.
- *Dental/tooth care:* Important (poor oral health associated with heart disease).

Dietary and Nutrition Recommendations (Or Macronutrients)
- Alcohol: For females one drink per day and for males two drinks per day.
- Monitor carbohydrate intake (i.e., carbohydrate counting).
- Saturated fat (animal fats, beef fat) intake should be <7% of total calories.
- Reduce intake of trans fat (will lower LDL and increase HDL) such as most fried foods, and "junk foods."
- Refer patient to a dietician at least once or more often if problems with diet.
- Routine vitamin supplementation of antioxidants is not yet advised.

Hypoglycemia
- *High risk:* 50 mg/dL or less.
- *Look for:* Sweaty palms, tiredness, dizziness, rapid pulse, strange behavior, confusion, and weakness. If patient on beta blockers, the hypoglycemic response can be blunted or blocked.

Treatment Plan

- Glucose (15 to 20 g) is preferred treatment for conscious patients. Other options are 4 oz orange juice, regular soft drink, hard candy. Recheck blood glucose 15 minutes after treatment. When blood glucose is normalized, eat a meal or snack afterward (complex carbs, protein).
- Glucagon: Prescribe for patients at significant risk of severe hypoglycemia.

Illness and Surgery

- Do not stop taking antidiabetic medicine. Keep taking insulin or oral meds as scheduled unless fasting blood glucose (FBG) lower than normal.
- Frequent self-monitoring of blood glucose.
- Eat small amounts of food every 3 to 4 hours to keep FBG as normal as possible.
- *Contact health care provider if:* Dehydrated, vomiting, or diarrhea for several hours, blood glucose greater than 300 mg/dL, changes in LOC (feel sleepier than normal/cannot think clearly).

Exercise

- Increases glucose utilization by the muscles. Patients may need to reduce their usual dose of medicine (or eat snacks before the activity and afterward to compensate).
- If patient does not compensate (reducing the dose of insulin, increasing caloric intake, snacking before and after), there is an increased risk of hypoglycemia within a few hours.
- *Example:* If patient exercises in the afternoon, high risk of hypoglycemia at night/bedtime if doesn't compensate by eating snacks, eating more food at dinner, or lowering insulin dose.

Snacks for Exercise

- Simple carbohydrates (candy, juices) before or during exercise.
- Complex carbohydrates (granola bars) after exercise (avoids post-exercise hypoglycemia).

Other Diabetic Issues

Dawn Phenomenon

This is a normal physiologic event. An elevation in the FBG occurs daily early in the morning. This is due to an increase in insulin resistance between 4 and 8 a.m. caused by the physiologic spike in growth hormone (anterior pituitary), glucagon (beta cells pancreas), epinephrine, and cortisol (adrenals).

Somogyi Effect (Rebound Hyperglycemia)

Severe nocturnal hypoglycemia stimulates counterregulatory hormones such as glucagon to be released from the liver. The high levels of glucagon in the systemic circulation result in high fasting blood glucose by 7:00 a.m. The condition is due to overtreatment with the evening and/or bedtime insulin (dose is too high). More common in type 1 diabetics.

- *Diagnosis:* Check blood glucose very early in the morning (3 a.m.) for 1 to 2 weeks.
- *Treatment:* Snack before bedtime, or eliminate dinnertime intermediate-acting insulin (NPH) dose or lower the bedtime dose for both NPH and regular insulin.

Diabetic Retinopathy: Specific Eye Findings

- Microaneurysms due to neovascularization. Cotton wool exudates.
- Neovascularization (growth of fragile small arterioles in retina rupture easily, causing bleeding and scarring on the retina).

Diabetic Foot Care

Patients with peripheral neuropathy should avoid excessive running or walking to minimize the risk of foot injury.

- Never go barefoot.
- Wear shoes that fit properly.
- Check feet daily, especially the soles of the feet (use mirror).
- Trim nails squarely (not rounded) to prevent ingrown toenails.
- Report redness, skin breakdown, or trauma to health care provider immediately (main cause of lower leg amputations in the United States).

Diabetic Medications (Table 9.2)

- *First line:* Biguanides
  - Metformin (glucophage).
  - Decreases gluconeogenesis and decreases peripheral insulin resistance. Very rarely may cause hypoglycemia. In addition to diet and exercise (lifestyle), metformin is the first-line drug.
- Preferred for obese patients (promotes weight loss).
- *Contraindications:*
  - Renal disease, hepatic disease acidosis, alcoholics, hypoxia.
  - Labs: monitor renal function (serum creatinine, GFR, UA) and LFTs.
- Increased risk of lactic acidosis (pH less than 7.25):
  - During hypoxia, hypoperfusion, renal insufficiency.
- *IV contrast dye testing:* Hold metformin on day of procedure and 48 hours after. Check baseline creatinine and recheck after procedure. If serum creatinine remains

Table 9.2 Types of Insulin

Insulin Type	Onset (Starts at)	Peak	Duration (Mean)
Rapid-acting Insulin lispro	15 minutes	30 minutes to 2½ hours	About 4½ hours
Short-acting Regular insulin	30 minutes	1 to 5 hours	6 to 8 hours
Intermediate NPH	1 hour	6 to 14 hours	18 to 24 hours
Basal insulin Lantus	1 hour	None	24 hours
Mixture 70/30 Humulin 70/30	30 minutes	4.4 hours	About 24 hours

Times are based on broad estimates and are designed for use only for the nurse practitioner certification exams. Do not use for clinical practice.

elevated after the procedure, do not restart metformin. Serum creatinine must be normalized before drug can be resumed.

Sulfonylureas

- Stimulates the beta cells of the pancreas to secrete more insulin.
- *First generation:* Chlorpropamide (Diabenase) daily or BID.
  - Long half-life (12 hours). Not commonly used due to high risk of severe hypoglycemia.
- *Second generation:* Glipizide (Glucotrol, Glucotrol XL) maximum dose 40 mg/day, glyburide (Diabeta) maximum dose 20 mg/day, glimepiride (Amaryl) maximum. dose 8 mg/day.

Adverse Effects

- Hypoglycemia (diaphoresis, pallor, sweating, tremor); increased risk of photosensitivity (use sunscreen).
- Blood dyscrasias (monitor CBC).
- Avoid if impaired hepatic or renal function (monitor LFTs, creatinine, urinalysis).
- Causes weight gain (monitor weight and BMI).

Thiazolidinediones (TZDs)

- Rosiglitazone (Avandia), pioglitazone (Actos).
  - Enhance insulin sensitivity in muscle tissue (decreases peripheral tissue resistance) and reduce hepatic glucagon production (gluconeogenesis). Take daily at breakfast with a meal.
- *Contraindications:*
  - Avoid with NYHA Class III and Class IV heart disease, heart failure (CHF).
  - Cause water retention and edema (aggravates or will precipitate heart failure (CHF)).
  - Actos is associated with a rare risk of bladder cancer (UA, urine cytology).
  - Cause weight gain (monitor weight and BMI).

Bile-Acid Sequestrants

- Cholestyramine (Questran), colesevelam (Welchol), colebystipol (Colestid).
- Reduce hepatic glucose production and may reduce intestinal absorption of glucose.
- Take with meals. Lowers LDL.
  - Side effect is GI related, such as nausea, bloating, constipation, increased triglycerides.
  - Common reason for noncompliance. Start patient on a low dose and titrate up slowly.
  - Kidney and liver effects (check serum creatinine, GFR, LFTs).

Meglitinide

- Repaglinide (Prandin), nateglinide (Starlix).
- Stimulates pancreatic secretion of insulin. Indicated for type 2 diabetics with postprandial hyperglycemia. Not recommended for monotherapy. Weight-neutral.
  - Rapid-acting with a very short half-life (less than 1 hour).
  - Take before meals or up to 30 minutes after a meal.
  - Hold dose if skipping a meal.
  - Side effects are bloating, abdominal cramps, diarrhea, flatulence.

Diabetic Medications: Subcutaneous Route

This is not an inclusive list.

Rapid-Acting Insulin
- Humalog (insulin lispro)
  - *Onset:* 15 to 30 minutes
  - *Peak:* 30 minutes to 2½ hours
  - *Duration:* 3 to 6½ hours

Short-Acting Insulin (Regular)
- Humulin R
  - *Onset:* 30 to 60 minutes
  - *Peak:* 1 to 5 hours
  - *Duration:* 6 to 8 hours

NPH
- Humulin N
  - *Onset:* 1 to 2 hours
  - *Peak:* 6 to 14 hours
  - *Duration:* 18 to 24 hours
- Lantus (insulin glargine), Levimir (insulin detimir)
  Considered a "basal insulin" (has no "peaks")
  - *Onset:* 1 hour
  - *Peak:* No pronounced peaks
  - *Duration:* 24 hours
  Give once a day at the same time.

Insulin Mixtures
- Humulin 70/30 (70% NPH insulin, 30% regular insulin)
  - *Onset:* Usually within 30 minutes
  - *Peak:* Mean peak of 4.4 hours
  - *Duration:* About 24 hours
- *American Diabetes Association (ADA) Guidelines for Mixed Insulins (2011)*
  - Premixed insulin is not recommended for type 1 diabetics.
  - After mixing NPH and regular insulin, use the mixture immediately.
  - Rapid-acting insulin can be mixed with NPH, but it should be used 15 minutes before a meal.

Incretin Mimetic or Glucagon-Like Peptide 1 (GLP-1) Mimetic
- Exenatide (Byetta) BID or Victoza once-a-day injections (SC).
- Stimulates GLP-1, causing an increase in insulin production and inhibits postprandial glucagon release (will decrease postprandial hyperglycemia).
- Causes weight loss.
- May cause pancreatitis and pancreatic duct metaplasia (precancerous changes). Monitor amylase/lipase.
- Incretin enhancer (Januvia, Onglyza).
- Januvia may cause acute pancreatitis (monitor amylase/lipase).

> **Note**
>
> Do not combine incretin mimetics (Byetta, Victoza) with any incretin enhancers (Januvia, Onglyza). Both act on incretin.

Amylin Analog (Symlin)

■ Slows gastric emptying; leads to feeling early satiety. Causes weight loss.

SUGGESTIONS FOR SOLVING AN INSULIN-RELATED QUESTION

The nurse practitioner certification exams are based on the primary care model of care. In general, it is not necessary to memorize specific doses. There is usually only one question about an insulin regimen. Keep in mind some broad concepts such as the peak and duration of each type of insulin. For example:

- Rapid-acting insulin covers "one meal at a time."
- Regular insulin lasts "from meal to meal."
- NPH insulin lasts "from breakfast to dinner."
- Lantus is "once a day."

Case Scenario

A type 1 diabetic patient is on regular insulin and NPH insulin (not premixed, but separate) injected twice a day. The first dose is injected before breakfast and the second dose is injected at bedtime. The blood sugar results from the patient's diary (fasting, before lunch, dinner, and bedtime) show that the lunchtime values are higher than normal. *Which insulin dose should be increased or decreased?*

In this case, the NPH component of the morning dose should be increased. Regular insulin peaks between breakfast and lunch (most of it is gone by lunchtime). In contrast, NPH insulin peaks between 6 and 14 hours. Therefore, it will cover the postprandial spike after lunch.

CLINICAL INFORMATION

■ Rapid-acting insulins (insulin lispro) are used mostly by type 1 diabetics before each meal.
■ Premixed insulins are used mostly by type 2 diabetics. The ADA does not recommend premixed insulin for type 1 diabetics.
■ Intermediate-acting insulin (NPH) can be used once to twice a day.

Summary of Prescribing Medications for Type 2 Diabetics

■ In addition to lifestyle, metformin is first-line treatment for most type 2 diabetics. Start on metformin 500 mg daily to BID (maximum dose is 2,550 mg/dL).
■ If metformin dose is at maximum (and blood sugar/A1c is still high), add a sulfonylurea (i.e., Glucotrol XL 20 mg per day).
OR
■ If patient is on a sulfonylurea at the maximum dose (i.e., Glucotrol XL 40 mg/day) and blood sugar/A1c is still elevated, then add metformin.
■ If blood sugar or A1c is still elevated and patient is on both metformin and sulfonylurea, consider starting patient on a basal insulin (Lantus SC once a day).
■ If patient refuses insulin, other options are thioglitazones (Avandia, Actos), Byetta, others. Keep in mind the contraindications for each drug class.

Antidiabetic Medications: Effect on Weight

- *Causes weight loss:* Metformin and incretin mimetic (Byetta), amylin analog (Symlin).
- *Causes weight gain:* Sulfonylureas, TZDs (Actos, Avandia), insulin.
- *Weight-neutral:* Meglitanides (Starlix, Prandin), bile-acid sequestrants (Wellchol).

Diabetes Mellitus: Management

- Lifestyle changes are first-line treatment along with oral antidiabetics.
- Weight loss improves metabolic control in type 2 diabetics.
- Eat more fiber and whole grains (brown rice, whole wheat).
- Exercise increases cellular glucose uptake in the body.
- Type 2 diabetics not well controlled on multiple oral agents; diet and lifestyle changes are good candidates for basal insulin therapy.

Diabetes: Possible Complications

- *Eyes:* Cataracts, diabetic retinopathy, blindness
- *Cardiovascular:* Hyperlipidemia, CAD, MI, hypertension
- *Kidneys:* Renal disease, renal failure
- *Feet:* Foot ulcers, skin infections, peripheral neuropathy, amputation
- *Gyn/GU:* Balanitis (candidal infection of the glans penis), candidal vaginitis

Primary Prevention

For individuals at high risk of type 2 diabetes: Encourage weight loss (7% of body weight) and regular physical activity (150 min/week). Increase dietary fiber and foods with whole grains.

✍ EXAM TIPS

- Do not use any oral antidiabetic drugs on type 1 diabetics.
- Memorize the specific key findings of diabetes versus hypertension.
- Moderate to severe heart disease or heart failure is a contraindication to glitizone drugs such as Avandia or Actos because they cause water retention, which may precipitate CHF.
- Mild type 2 diabetics do not need drug therapy if able to control blood glucose by diet and exercise alone.

📋 CLINICAL TIP

- Diabetics are at higher risk for cataracts and glaucoma.

Pharmacology*

- *Biguanindes:* Metformin (Glucophage).
  - Decreases gluconeogenesis and decreases peripheral insulin resistance.
- *Sulfonylureas:* Glucotrol XL, Diabeta, Amaryl.
  - Stimulates the beta cells of the pancreas to secrete more insulin.

---

* Adapted from the ADA Standards of Medical Care in Diabetes, 2012.

- *Thiazolidinediones:* Rosiglitazone (Avandia), pioglitazone (Actos).
  - Enhances insulin sensitivity in muscle tissue (decreases peripheral tissue resistance) and reduces hepatic glucagon production (gluconeogenesis).
- *Bile-acid sequestrant:* Colesevelam (Welchol).
  - Reduces hepatic glucose production and may reduce intestinal absorption of glucose.
- *Meglitinide:* Repaglinide (Prandin), nateglinide (Starlix).
  - Stimulates pancreatic secretion of insulin. Indicated for type 2 diabetics with postprandial hyperglycemia.
- Incretin mimetic or GLP-1 drug: Byetta BID or Victoza once-a-day injections (subcutaneous).
  - Stimulates GLP-1 causing an increase in insulin production and inhibiting postprandial glucagon release (will decrease postprandial hyperglycemia).

10

Gastrointestinal System Review

⚠ DANGER SIGNALS

Acute Pancreatitis

Adult patient complains of the acute onset of fever, nausea, and vomiting that is associated with rapid onset of abdominal pain that radiates to the midback ("boring") located in the epigastric region. Abdominal exam reveals guarding and tenderness over the epigastric area or the upper abdomen. Positive Cullen's sign (blue discoloration around umbilicus) and Grey–Turner's sign (blue discoloration on the flanks). The patient may have ileus, signs, and symptoms of shock. Refer to emergency department (ED).

Acute Diverticulitis

Elderly patient with acute onset of high fever, anorexia, nausea/vomiting, and left lower quadrant abdominal pain. Signs of acute abdomen such as rebound, positive Rovsing's sign, boardlike abdomen. CBC will show leukocytosis with neutrophilia and shift to the left. The presence of band forms signals severe bacterial infection (bands are immature neutrophils). May cause sepsis, ileus, and hemorrhage. May be life threatening.

Acute Appendicitis

Patient who is a young adult complains of an acute onset of periumbilical pain that is steadily getting worse. Over a time period of 12 to 24 hours, the pain starts to localize at McBurney's point. The patient has no appetite (anorexia).

When the appendix ruptures, clinical signs of acute abdomen present, such as involuntary guarding, rebound, and a boardlike abdomen. The psoas and obturator signs are positive.

Acute Cholecystitis

Overweight female complains of severe right upper quadrant or epigastric pain that occurs within 1 hour (or more) after eating a fatty meal. Pain may radiate to the right shoulder. Accompanied by nausea/vomiting and anorexia. If left untreated, may develop gangrene of the gall bladder (20%). Requires hospitalization.

Colon Cancer

Very gradual (years) with vague GI symptoms. Tumor may bleed intermittently and patient may have iron-deficiency anemia. Changes in bowel habits, stool, or bloody stool. Heme-positive stool, dark tarry stool, mass on abdominal palpation. Older patient (greater than 50 years of age), especially if history of multiple polyps or Crohn's disease.

Zollinger–Ellison Syndrome

A gastrinoma located on the pancreas or the stomach; secretes gastrin, which stimulates high levels of acid production in the stomach. The end result is the development of multiple and severe ulcers in the stomach and duodenum. Complains of epigastric to mid-abdominal pain. Stools may be a tarry color. Screening by serum fasting gastrin level.

Crohn's Disease

Right lower quadrant intermittent abdominal pain. Lower abdominal pain 1 hour after eating. Diarrhea with mucus. Fever, malaise, and mild weight loss. Abnormal liquid stools. Patients with Crohn's disease at higher risk for colon cancer.

Clostridium difficile Colitis (CDI)

Severe watery diarrhea from 10 to 15 stools a day that is accompanied by lower abdominal pain with cramping and fever. Symptoms usually appear within 5 to 10 days after initiation of antibiotics. Antibiotics such as clindamycin (Cleocin), fluoroquinolones, cephalosporins, and penicillins have been implicated as more likely to cause *C. difficile* infection. Most cases occur in hospitalized patients.

☑ NORMAL FINDINGS

Route of Food or Drink From the Mouth

Esophagus → stomach (hydrochloric acid, intrinsic factor) → duodenum (bile, amylase, lipase) → jejunum → ileum → colon → cecum → rectum → anus

Abdominal Contents

Right upper quadrant: Liver, gallbladder, ascending colon, kidney (right), pancreas (small portion). Right kidney is lower than the left because of displacement by the liver.

- *Left upper quadrant:* Stomach, pancreas, descending colon, kidney (left)
- *Right lower quadrant:* Appendix, ileum, cecum, ovary (right)
- *Left lower quadrant:* Sigmoid colon, ovary (left)
- *Suprapubic area:* Bladder, uterus, rectum

Benign Variants

The appendix can be located in any quadrant of the abdomen.

ABDOMINAL MANEUVERS

Acute Abdomen or Peritonitis

Psoas/Illiopsoas (Supine Position)
Used for acute appendicitis or any suspected retroperitoneal area acute process (i.e., ruptured ectopic pregnancy). Flex hip 90 degrees, ask patient to push against resistance (examiner's hand) and to straighten the leg.

Obturator Sign (Supine Position)
Used for acute appendicitis or any suspected retroperitoneal area acute process (i.e., ruptured ectopic pregnancy). Rotate right hip through full range of motion. Positive sign if pain with the movement or flexion of the hip.

Rovsing's Sign (Supine Position)

Deep palpation of the left lower quadrant of the abdomen results in referred pain to the right lower quadrant.

McBurney's Point

Area located between the superior iliac crest and umbilicus in the right lower quadrant. Tenderness or pain is a sign of possible acute appendicitis.

Markle Test (Heel Jar)

Instruct patient to raise heels, and then drop them suddenly. An alternative is to ask the patient to jump in place. Positive if pain is elicited or if patient refuses to perform because of pain.

Involuntary Guarding

With abdominal palpation, the abdominal muscles reflexively become tense or boardlike.

Rebound Tenderness

Patient complains that the abdominal pain is worse when the palpating hand is released compared to the pain felt during deep palpation.

Murphy's Maneuver (Figure 10.1)

Press deeply on the right upper quadrant under the costal border during inspiration. Mid-inspiratory arrest is a positive finding (Murphy's sign).

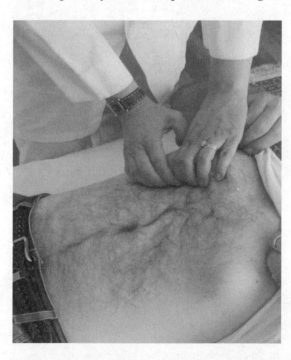

FIGURE 10.1 Murphy's sign.

:≡ DISEASE REVIEW

Gastroesophageal Reflux Disease (GERD)

Acidic gastric contents regurgitate from the stomach into the esophagus. Chronic GERD causes damage to squalors epithelium of the esophagus and may result in Barrett's esophagus (a precancer), which increases risk of squalors cell cancer (cancer of the esophagus).

Classic Case

Middle-aged to older adult complains of chronic heartburn of many years' duration. Symptoms associated with large and/or fatty meals and worsened when supine. Long-term history of self-medication with over-the-counter (OTC) antacids and H2 blockers. May be on chronic nonsteroidal anti-inflammatory drugs (NSAIDs), aspirin, or alcohol.

Objective

- Acidic or sour odor to breath.
- Reflux of sour acidic stomach contents, especially with overeating.
- Thinning tooth enamel due to increased hydrochloric acid.
- Chronic sore red throat (not associated with a cold).
- Chronic coughing.

Labs

Gold standard: Esophageal motility studies.

Treatment Plan

First line is lifestyle changes. Avoid large or high-fat meals especially 3 to 4 hours before bedtime; lose weight; avoid mints (relaxes gastric sphincter); avoid caffeine, alcohol, aspirin, NSAIDs, and aggravating foods. After lifestyle change and OTC antacids/H2 blockers, next step is to prescribe medications.

Medications

- H2 blockers (ranitidine) or proton pump inhibitor (omeprazole [Prilosec]) × 4 to 6 weeks.
- Usually on long-term proton pump inhibitor (PPI) therapy. PPIs irreversibly bind the proton pump.
- If no relief, high risk for Barrett's esophagus (long-term GERD, White male greater than 50 years) or worrisome symptoms, refer to GI specialist for upper endoscopy/biopsy (gold standard).
- *Worrisome symptoms:* Progressive dysphagia (difficulty swallowing that is getting worse), iron-deficiency anemia (blood loss), weight loss, hemoccult positive.

Complications

- Barrett's esophagus (a precancer for esophageal cancer)
- Esophageal cancer

✍ EXAM TIPS

- Barrett's esophagus is a precancer (esophageal cancer). Diagnosed by upper endoscopy with biopsy.
- Lifestyle factors to teach patient (no mints, avoid caffeine, etc.).
- Cullen's and Grey–Turner's sign.
- Acute pancreatitis classic pain (severe midepigastric radiates to midback).
- Rovsing's sign.
- Acute appendicitis presentation.
- Psoas and obturator signs positive for acute appendicitis.
- How to perform psoas maneuver.

📋 CLINICAL TIP

Any patient with at least a decade or more history of chronic heartburn should be referred to a gastroenterologist for an endoscopy to rule out Barrett's esophagus.

Irritable Bowel Syndrome (IBS)

A chronic functional disorder of the colon (normal colonic tissue) marked by exacerbations and remissions. Spontaneous remissions. Commonly exacerbated by excess stress.

Classic Case

A young adult to middle-aged female complains of intermittent episodes of moderate to severe cramping pain in the lower abdomen, especially on the left lower quadrant. Bloating with flatulence. Relief obtained after defecation. Stools range from diarrhea to constipation or both types with increased frequency of bowel movements.

Objective

- *Abdominal exam:* Tenderness in lower quadrants during an exacerbation. Otherwise the exam is normal.
- *Rectal exam:* Normal with no blood or pus.
  - Heme-negative stools.

Treatment Plan

- Increase dietary fiber. Supplement fiber with Metamucil (psyllium).
- Antispasmodics (i.e., Bentyl) as needed. Decrease life stress.
- *Rule out:* Amoebic, parasitic, or bacterial infections; inflammatory disease of the GI tract; and so forth. Check stool for ova and parasites (especially diarrheal stools) with culture.

PEPTIC ULCER DISEASE (PUD)

Gastric Ulcer and Duodenal Ulcer Disease

Duodenal ulcers are more common than gastric ulcers. Gastric ulcers have higher risk for malignancy (up to 10%) compared to duodenal ulcers, which are mostly benign. *Helicobacter pylori* is a common cause for both duodenal and gastric ulcers.

Etiology

- *H. pylori* (gram-negative bacteria)
- Chronic NSAID use, which disrupts prostaglandin production. Results in reduction of GI blood flow with reduction of protective mucus layer
- Bisphosphonates (Fosamax, Actonel)
- *Worrisome symptoms:* Early satiety, anorexia, anemia (bleeding), recurrent vomiting, hematemesis, weight loss

Classic Case

Middle-aged to older adult complains of episodic epigastric pain, burning/gnawing pain, or ache (80%). Pain relieved by food and/or antacids (50%) with recurrence 2 to 4 hours after a meal. Self-medicating with over-the-counter antacids. May be taking NSAIDs or aspirin.

Objective
■ *Abdominal exam:* Normal or mildly tender epigastric area during flare-ups.
■ Hemoccult can be positive if actively bleeding.

Labs
■ CBC (iron-deficiency anemia means bleeding), fecal occult blood test (FOBT).
■ If positive, refer to gastroenterologist.
　– *Serology (titers):* H. pylori immunoglobulin (IgG) levels elevated.
　– *Urea breath test:* Indicative of active H. pylori infection and is commonly used to document eradication of H. pylori after treatment. More sensitive for active infection than serology/titers.
　– *Gold standard:* Upper endoscopy and biopsy of gastric and/or duodenal tissue.
　– *Multiple severe ulcers:* Fasting gastrin levels to rule out Zollinger–Ellison syndrome as needed.

Treatment Plan
Treatment for H. pylori Negative Ulcers
■ Combine lifestyle changes with PPIs or H2 blockers. Use PPIs or H2 blockers × 4 to 8 weeks.
■ H2 blockers (or H2 antagonists)
　– Ranitidine (Zantac) 150 mg daily.
　– Cimetidine (Tagamet) 400 mg BID.
■ PPIs
　– Omeprazole (Prilosec) 20 mg daily.
　– Esomeprazole (Nexium) 40 mg daily.

Treatment for H. pylori Positive Ulcers
■ Triple therapy
　– Clarithromycin (Biaxin) BID PLUS amoxicillin 1 g BID × 14 days
　– PLUS PPI BID for 6 to 8 weeks to allow ulcer to heal
■ Quadruple therapy
　– Bismuth subsalicylate tab 600 mg four times a day (QID) PLUS
　– Metronidazole tab 250 mg QID PLUS
　– Tetracycline 500-mg caps QID × 2 weeks
　– PLUS PPI daily × 4 to 6 weeks after or longer

✍ EXAM TIPS

■ Distinguish whether question is about *H. pylori* negative ulcers or *H. pylori* positive ulcers.
■ Both treatment regimens have appeared on the exams before.
■ Barrett's esophagus is a precursor for esophageal cancer.
■ Worrisome symptoms of esophageal cancer and PUD.
■ *H. pylori* serology IgG positive plus symptoms of PUD: Treat with antibiotics plus PPI.
■ Treatment as for acute diverticulitis.
■ IBS: Increase fiber intake.

📋 CLINICAL TIPS

■ Triple therapy was first-line treatment before 2012 but due to high rates of clarithromycin resistance (42%), quadruple therapy is now the preferred treatment for *H. pylori* infections.

- *H. pylori* is resistant to clarithromycin (42%) and metronidazole (20%).
- PPIs cure ulcers faster than H2 blockers.

Diverticulitis

- Diverticula are small pouchlike herniations on the external surface of the colon secondary to a chronic lack of dietary fiber. Higher incidence in Western societies.
- Diverticulitis is infected diverticula. High risk of rupture and bleeding. Can be life-threatening.
- *Hospitalize if:* Elderly, high fever, leukocytosis, comorbidities, immunocompromised.

Classic Case

Elderly patient presents with acute onset of fever with left lower quadrant abdominal pain with anorexia, nausea, and/or vomiting. Abdominal palpation reveals tenderness on the left lower quadrant. Hematochezia (bloody stool) and anemia if hemorrhaging.

Objective

- *Acute diverticulitis:* If acute abdomen, positive for rebound, positive Rovsing's sign, and boardlike abdomen.
- *Diverticulosis:* Physical exam normal. No palpable mass. No tenderness.

Labs

- CBC with leukocytosis, neutrophilia greater than 70% and shift to the left (band forms). The presence of band forms signals severe bacterial infection. Bands are immature neutrophils. Refer to ED.
- FOBT positive if bleeding.
- Reticulocytosis if acute bleeding and low hemoglobin/hematocrit.

Treatment Plan

Uncomplicated cases of diverticulitis can usually be treated in the outpatient setting.
- Ciprofloxacin 500 mg BID PLUS metronidazole (Flagyl) 500 mg three times a day (TID) × 10 to 14 days.
- Close follow up. If no response in 48 to 72 hours or worsens (high fever, toxic), refer to ED. Moderate to severe cases: hospitalize.

Chronic Therapy for Diverticulosis

- High-fiber diet with fiber supplementation such as psyllium (Metamucil) or methyl-cellulose (Citrucel). Avoidance of nuts and seeds is not necessary.

Complications

- Abscess, perforation with peritonitis.
- Ileus, sepsis, death.

Acute Pancreatitis

- Acute inflammation of the pancreas secondary to many factors such as alcohol abuse, gallstones (cholelithiasis), elevated triglyceride levels, infections.
- Pancreatic enzymes become activated inside pancreas causing autodigestion.
- Varies in severity from mild to life-threatening/death.
- Elevated triglycerides (greater than 800 mg/dL) at very high risk of acute pancreatitis.

Classic Case

Adult patient complains of the acute onset of fever, nausea, and vomiting that is associated with rapid onset of abdominal pain that radiates to the midback, located in the epigastric region. Abdominal exam reveals guarding and tenderness over the epigastric area or the upper abdomen. Positive Cullen's and Grey–Turner's sign. May have ileus, signs, and symptoms of shock. Refer patient to ED.

Objective
- *Cullen's sign:* Bluish discoloration around umbilicus (hemorrhagic pancreatitis)
- *Grey–Turner's sign:* Bluish discoloration on the flank area (hemorrhagic pancreatitis)
- Hypoactive bowel sounds (ileus), jaundice, guarding, and boardlike upper abdomen if peritonitis

Labs
- Elevated pancreatic enzymes such as serum amylase, lipase, and trypsin.
- Elevated aspartate aminotransferase (AST), alanine aminotransferase (ALT), gamma glutamyl transferase (GGT), bilirubin, leukocytosis, and so forth.
- Abdominal ultrasound and computed tomography.

Complications
- Multiple serious complications such as ileus, sepsis, shock, multiorgan failure, death.
- May cause diabetes.

Clostridium difficile Colitis

The classic symptom is watery diarrhea a few days after starting antibiotic treatment due to changes in intestinal flora caused by antibiotics. Antibiotics such as clindamycin (Cleocin), fluoroquinolones, cephalosporins, and penicillins are more likely to cause *C. difficile* infection. Most cases occur in hospitalized patients. *C. difficile* is a gram-negative anaerobic bacteria.

Classic Case
Severe watery diarrhea from 10 to 15 stools a day accompanied by lower abdominal pain with cramping and fever. Patient is currently on antibiotics or recently completed a course of antibiotics. Symptoms usually appear within 5 to 10 days after initiation of antibiotics.

Labs
- CBC with leukocytosis (greater than 15,000 cells/μL).
- Stool assay (by enzyme-linked immunosorbent assay) for *C. difficile* toxins.
- Treatment (for nonsevere CDI)
  - Metronidazole (Flagyl) TID for 10 to 14 days.
  - Avoid antimotility agents (loperamide) or opiates because they can worsen and prolong disorder.
  - Probiotic use is controversial.
  - Increase fluid intake. Eat food as tolerated.

HEPATITIS

Hepatitis Serology
IgG Anti-HAV (Hepatitis A Antibody IgG Type) Positive
- Antibodies present (immune).
- No virus present and not infectious.

- *How:* History of native hepatitis A infection or vaccination with hepatitis A vaccine (Havrix).

IgM Anti-HAV (Hepatitis A Antibody IgM Type) Positive
- Acute infection. Patient is contagious.
- Hepatitis A virus still present (infectious). No immunity yet.

HBsAg (Hepatitis B Surface Antigen)
- Screening test for hepatitis B.
- If positive, patient has the virus and is infectious.
- *How:* Presence of antigen means either an acute infection or chronic hepatitis B infection.

Anti-HBs (Hepatitis B Surface Antibody) Positive
- Antibodies present and is immune.
- Presence may be due to either a past infection or vaccination with hepatitis B vaccine.

HbeAg (Hepatitis B "e" Antigen)
- Indicates active viral replication. May be highly infectious.
- Persistence of the "e" antigen indicates chronic hepatitis B.

Chronic Hepatitis Infection: Two Types
- Chronic infection with mildly elevated liver function tests (LFTs).
- Chronic and active infection with elevated LFTs (active viral replication).
- Patient is at higher risk of cirrhosis, liver failure, and liver cancer.

Anti-HCV (Antibody Hepatitis C Virus)
- Screening test for hepatitis C.
- Up to 85% of cases become carriers.
- Unlike hepatitis A and B, a positive anti-HCV (antibody) does not always mean that the patient has recovered from the infection and has developed immunity. It may instead indicate current infection because up to 85% of cases become carriers.
- *If this test is positive:*
  - Order HCV RNA or HCV polymerase chain reaction (PCR) to rule out chronic infection.
  - If positive, then patient has hepatitis C. Refer to GI specialist for liver biopsy/treatment.

Hepatitis D (Delta Virus)
- Requires the presence of hepatitis B to get the infection. Can be an acute or a chronic infection.
- Infection with both hepatitis B and hepatitis D increases the risk of fulminant hepatitis, cirrhosis, and severe liver damage. Low prevalence in the United States.

Liver Function Tests (LFTs)
Serum AST
- Also known as serum glutamic oxaloacetic transaminase (SGOT).
- *Normal:* 0 to 45 mg/dL.

- Present in the liver, heart muscle, skeletal muscle, kidney, and lung.
- Not specific for liver injury since it is also elevated in other conditions (i.e., acute myocardial infarction).

Serum ALT

- Also known as serum glutamic pyruvic transaminase (SGPT).
- *Normal:* 0 to 40 mg/dL.
- This enzyme is found mainly in the liver. A positive finding indicates liver inflammation.
- More specific for hepatic inflammation than AST.

AST/ALT Ratio (or SGOT/SGPT Ratio)

- A ratio of 2.0 or higher may be indicative of alcohol abuse.

Serum GGT

- Sensitive indicator of alcohol abuse. May be a "lone" elevation.
- Elevated in liver disease and acute pancreatitis.

Alkaline Phosphatase

- An enzyme derived from bone, liver, gallbladder, kidneys, GI tract, and placenta.
- Higher levels seen during growth spurts in children and teens.
- Also may be elevated with healing fractures, osteomalacia, malignancy, others.

Viral Hepatitis

Laboratory Tests

Hepatitis A, B, C

Hepatitis A

- No chronic or carrier state exists for hepatitis A.
- *Transmission:* Fecal and oral route from contaminated food or drink.
- Self-limiting infection. Treatment is symptomatic. Vaccine available (Havrix) and recommended for travelers to areas where hepatitis A is endemic.

Hepatitis B

- *Transmission:* Sexual (semen, vaginal secretions, and saliva), blood, blood products, organs.
- Vertical transmission from mother to infant. Hepatitis B can either be acute and self-limiting or it can be a chronic infection.

Hepatitis C

- *Transmission:* Intravenous drug use (50%), blood or blood products, sexual intercourse. In 40% of cases, the mode is unknown.
- *High-risk groups:* IV drug users, hemophiliacs, or anyone with history of frequent transfusions.
- Highest risk for chronic hepatitis infection and cirrhosis (30%). Cirrhosis markedly increases the risk for liver cancer or liver failure. Refer to GI for management.

- *Treatment:* Alpha-interferon injections and ribavirin. Liver biopsy to stage disease.

Acute Hepatitis

An acute liver inflammation with multiple causes. Examples include viral infection, hepatotoxic drugs (i.e., statins), excessive alcohol intake, and toxins.

Classic Case

Sexually active adult complains of a new onset of fatigue, nausea, and dark-colored urine for several days. New sexual partner (less than 3 months).

Objective

- Skin and sclera have a yellow tinge (jaundiced or icteric).
- *Liver:* Tenderness over the liver from percussion and deep palpation.

Labs

- *ALT and AST:* Elevated up to 10x normal during the acute phase of the illness.
- Other liver function tests may be elevated, such as the serum bilirubin and GGT.

Treatment Plan

Remove and treat the cause (if possible). Avoid hepatotoxic agents such as alcoholic drinks, acetaminophen, and statins (i.e., pravastatin or Pravachol). Treatment is supportive.

Case Studies for Viral Hepatitis

Patient A

- HBsAg: negative
- Anti-HBs: positive
- HBeAg: negative
- *Results:* Patient A indicative of either:
  - History of old hepatitis B infection. Has antibodies for hepatitis B (anti-HBs positive) or history of vaccination against hepatitis B.
  - Not a carrier of hepatitis B (HBeAg negative).

Patient B

- HBsAg: positive
- HBeAg: positive
- Anti-HBs: negative
- Anti-HAV: positive
- Anti-HCV: negative
- *Results:* Patient B indicative of:
  - Current hepatitis B infection (HBsAg positive).
  - Chronic carrier of hepatitis B (both HBsAg and HBeAg are positive).
  - Presence of antibodies to hepatitis A (anti-HAV). Patient either had a previous hepatitis A infection or had received the hepatitis A vaccine.
- This patient is an infectious carrier of the hepatitis B virus. If the HBeAg is positive, it means that the patient is a carrier (either lowly or highly contagious).

🖉 EXAM TIPS

- There will be a serology question (as just shown). You will have to figure out what type of viral hepatitis the patient has (A, B, or C). It is usually a patient with hepatitis B.
- PCR tests are not antibody tests. They test for presence of viral RNA. A positive result means that the virus is present.
- Hepatitis C has highest risk of cirrhosis and liver cancer.
- A lone elevation in the GGT is a sensitive indicator of possible alcoholism.
- The alkaline phosphatase is normally elevated during the teen years.
- A person must have hepatitis B to become infected with hepatitis D.
- ALT more sensitive to liver damage than AST.
- GERD and treatment.

11

Renal System Review

Acute Pyelonephritis

Patient presents with acute onset of high fevers, chills, dysuria, frequency, and unilateral flank pain. The flank pain is described as a deep ache. May complain of nausea (with/without vomiting). May have recent history of urinary tract infection (UTI).

Acute Renal Failure

Patient presents with the abrupt onset of oliguria, edema, and weight gain (fluid retention). Complains of lethargy, nausea, and loss of appetite.

Rapid decrease in renal function. Elevated urinary and serum creatinine. During the early stages of severe acute renal failure, the serum creatinine and the estimated glomerular filtration rate (GFR) may not accurately reflect true renal function.

☑ NORMAL FINDINGS

Kidneys

The kidneys are located in the retroperitoneal area. The right kidney is lower than the left kidney due to displacement by the liver.

The basic functional units of the kidney are the nephrons, which contain the glomeruli.

Function

Kidneys are the body's regulators of electrolytes and fluids. Water is reabsorbed back into the body by the action of antidiuretic hormone and aldosterone. Kidneys excrete water-soluble waste products of metabolism (i.e., creatinine, urea, uric acid) into the urine. They also produce the hormone erythropoietin, which stimulates bone marrow into producing more red blood cells. The average daily urine output is 1,500 mL. Oliguria is defined as a urinary output of less than 400 mL per day (adults). Kidneys also secrete several hormones such as erythropoietin (RBC production), renin and bradykinin (blood pressure), prostaglandins (renal perfusion), and calcitriol/vitamin D3 (bone).

⚗ LABORATORY TESTING

Serum Creatinine

- *Male:* 0.7 to 1.3 mg/dL
- *Female:* 0.6 to 1.1 mg/dL

When renal function decreases, the creatinine level will increase. Creatinine is the end product of creatine metabolism, which comes mostly from muscle. Serum creatinine may be falsely decreased in people with low muscle volume (elderly). Elevated values are seen with renal damage or failure, nephrotoxic drugs, etc. Factors that affect the serum creatinine are gender (males have higher levels), race (African Americans have more muscle mass), and muscle mass.

Creatinine Clearance (24-Hour Urine)

When renal function decreases, the creatinine clearance also decreases. This test is ordered to evaluate patients with proteinuria, albuminuria, and microalbuminuria. It is a more sensitive test than the serum creatinine alone because it reflects the renal function within a 24-hour period. Creatinine clearance is relatively constant and is not affected by fluid status, diet, or exercise. Creatinine clearance is doubled for every 50% reduction of the GFR.

Estimated Glomerular Filtration Rate (eGFR)

- *Normal*: eGFR greater than 90 mL/min.
- *Renal failure*: eGFR less than 15 mL/min (stage 5 chronic kidney disease).

The "estimated GFR" or the eGFR is the number that is derived by using the serum creatinine in a prediction equation (i.e., Cockcroft–Gault). The more damaged the kidneys, the lower the eGFR value. The GFR is the amount of fluid filtered by the glomerulus within a certain unit of time. It is used to evaluate renal function and to stage chronic kidney disease.

- Best if patient does not eat meat 12 hours before the blood test.
- GFR less reliable (interpret with care): drastic increase/reduction muscle mass (bodybuilders, amputees, wasting disorders), pregnancy, and acute renal failure.

Blood Urea Nitrogen (BUN)

The BUN is not as sensitive as the serum creatinine or the GFR. A high BUN may be caused by acute renal failure, high-protein diet, hemolysis, congestive heart failure, or drugs. If a patient has an abnormal BUN level, check the GFR. If the GFR is normal, the renal function is probably normal. The BUN is a measure of the kidney's ability to excrete urea (waste product of protein metabolism).

BUN-to-Creatinine Ratio

The ratio between the BUN and serum creatinine (BUN:Cr). It is used to help evaluate dehydration, hypovolemia, acute renal failure, and it is useful for classifying the type of renal failure (renal, infrarenal, or postrenal).

Urinalysis

Epithelial Cells

- Large amounts in a urine sample indicate contamination.
- A few epithelial cells are considered normal.

Leukocytes

- *Normal white blood cells (WBCs) in urine*: Less than or equal to 10 WBCs/mL.
- Called leukocyte esterase with dipstick strips.
- Presence of leukocytes in urine (pyuria) is always abnormal in males (infection).
- The urinalysis is a more sensitive test for infection in males than females.

Urine for Culture and Sensitivity

- Greater than or equal to 10^5 CFU/mL of bacteria (CFU or "colony-forming units") of one dominant bacteria (usually *Escherichia coli*) is indicative of a UTI.
- If multiple bacteria are present, it is considered a contaminated sample.
- Lower values indicative of bacteriuria.

Red Blood Cells (RBCs)

- Few RBCs (less than 5 cells) considered normal.
- Hematuria is seen with kidney stones, pyelonephritis, and sometimes in cystitis.
- Can be contaminated by menses or hemorrhoids.

Protein

- Indicates kidney damage (chronic kidney disease).
- May be present in acute pyelonephritis (resolves after treatment).
- Urine dipsticks only pick up albumin, not microalbumin (Bence–Jones proteins).
- Order 24-hour urine for protein and creatinine clearance.

Nitrites

- Indicative of infection with *E. coli*.
- Due to breakdown of nitrates to nitrites by certain bacteria.

Casts

- Casts are shaped like cylinders because they are formed in the renal tubules.
- Hyaline casts are "normal" and may be seen in concentrated urine.
- WBC cast may be seen with infections (UTI, pyelonephritis).
- RBC casts and proteinuria are diagnostic for glomerulonephritis.

⊟ DISEASE REVIEW

Urinary Tract Infections

Cystitis (urinary bladder inflammation) can be uncomplicated, recurrent, a reinfection, or relapse. The majority of infections are caused by *E. coli*. Others are *Staphylococcus saprophyticus*, *Proteus mirabilis*, and *Klebsiella pneumoniae*. UTIs in children younger than age 3 and pregnant women (20% to 40% chance) are more likely to progress to pyelonephritis.

- *Infancy*: UTIs are common in boys (usually due to anatomic abnormality).
- *Females:* Highest incidence is during the reproductive-age years.

Risk Factors

- Female gender; pregnancy.
- History of a recent UTI or history of recurrent infections.
- Diabetes mellitus (or immunocompromised).
- Failure to void after sex or increased sexual intercourse (i.e., honeymoon bladder).
- Spermicide use within past year (alone or with diaphragm).
- Other risk factors: Infected renal calculi, low fluid intake, poor hygiene, catheterization.

Classic Case

A sexually active female complains of new onset of dysuria, frequency, frequent urge to urinate, and nocturia. May also complain of suprapubic discomfort. Not associated with fever. Urine dipstick will show a moderate to large amount of leukocytes and will be positive for nitrites. May show a few RBCs (due to inflammation), negative for ketones (unless fasting), and protein.

Labs

Urinalysis (mid-stream sample): Leukocyte positive (WBCs greater than or equal to 10/mcL).

- Positive nitrites (*E. coli* converts urinary nitrate to nitrite).
- *Sometimes*: Hematuria (greater than 5 RBCs) and/or a few WBC casts.
- *Urine C&S*: Definitions.
- *UTI infection*: 100,000 CFU/mL (or 10^5 CFU/mL) with pyuria.
- *Urine culture with multiple bacteria*: A contaminated sample.
- *Bacteriuria* (with/without indwelling catheter): >100,000 CFU/mL.

Bacteriuria

Symptomatic bacteriuria (leukocytosis, fever, chills, malaise) is treated as a UTI.

Medications

Uncomplicated UTIs

- Healthy females aged 18 years or older can have the "3-day" treatment regimen (below agents are used for 7 to 10 days for complicated UTIs). Routine urine C&S before/after treatment is not recommended for this population. Increase fluid intake.
  - Trimethoprim/sulfamethoxazole (Bactrim, Septra) twice a day (BID) × 3 days.
  - Sulfa-allergic: Nitrofurantoin BID × 3 days, Augmentin BID × 3 days.
  - Ciprofloxacin (Cipro) or ofloxacin (Floxin) BID (age 18 years or older) × 3 days.
  - Phenazopyridine (Pyridium) by mouth BID × 2 days PRN (over the counter as Uristat, AZO).
  - Orange color to urine. Will stain contact lenses. Avoid if liver or renal disease, G6PD anemia.

Note

If clinical symptoms persist 48 to 72 hours after initiating antibiotics, order urine C&S and urinalysis. Rule out pyelonephritis. Switch to another antibiotic drug class (ciprofloxacin, ofloxacin) and treat for 7 to 10 days.

Complicated UTIs

- Must treat these patients for a minimum of 7 days or longer.
  - Males
  - Diabetics
  - Pregnant women
  - Children or elderly
  - Immunocompromised
  - Recurrent UTIs or reinfections
  - Anatomic abnormalities of the kidneys or ureters (including kidney stones)

Labs

- Urinalysis and urine C&S before and after treatment (to document resolution).
- *UTIs*: Special categories.

Elderly

- *Chronic indwelling Foley catheters*: Antibiotic prophylaxis and treatment is discouraged for asymptomatic bacteriuria unless symptomatic (leukocytosis, fever, chills, malaise, altered mental status, etc.). If symptomatic, treat with antibiotics.

Males

- UTIs are never "normal" in males. Rule out ureteral stricture, infected kidney stones, anatomic abnormality, acute prostatitis, sexually transmitted diseases, and so forth. Must be evaluated further. Refer to urologist.

Recurrent UTIs (In Women)

- Three or more UTIs in 1 year or two infections within 6 months. Never normal in males.
- *Rule out urologic abnormality*: Infected stones, reflux, fistulas, ureteral stenosis, and so forth.

Medications

- *Postcoital UTIs*: Bactrim or Bactrim DS one tablet after sex (or low-dosed nitrofurantoin, Cipro, Keflex). Increase fluids before and after sex.
- *Antimicrobial prophylaxis*: Bactrim one tablet at HS for 6 to 12 months.
- *Sulfa allergy*: Cephalexin (Keflex), Ceclor, Cipro (greater than 18 years). Consider prophylactic antibiotics for 6 months or longer (after ruling out pathology).

> **Note**
>
> Long-term use of nitrofurantoin associated with lung problems, chronic hepatitis, and neuropathy. Nitrofurantoin is contraindicated with renal insufficiency.

Acute Pyelonephritis

Acute bacterial infection of the kidney(s) most commonly due to gram-negative bacteria such as *E. coli* (75% to 95%), *Proteus mirabilis*, and *Klebsiella pneumoniae* (gram-negative anaerobe). Outpatient treatment is only for milder cases that are uncomplicated (immunocompetent adult female with normal urinary/renal systems without comorbidities) and compliant patients.

Classic Case

Adult patient presents with acute onset of high fever, chills, nausea/vomiting, and one-sided flank pain. Some patients may also have symptoms of cystitis such as dysuria, frequency, and urgency.

Physical Exam

- Fever equal or greater than 38°C (100.4°F).
- Costovertebral angle tenderness on one kidney.
- *Urine dipstick*: Large amount of leukocytes, hematuria, WBC casts, and proteinuria (albuminuria).
- *Urine C&S*: Presence of 10^5 CFU/mL of one organism.

- *CBC*: Leukocytosis (WBC greater than 11.0), neutrophilia (greater than 80%) with shift to the left.
- *Shift to the left*: Presence of bands or stabs (immature neutrophils) means serious infection.
- Chemistry profile (serum creatinine, others).

Treatment Plan

- May treat mild uncomplicated cases as outpatients with close follow-up (or refer to physician). Moderate to severe (or complicated) cases, hospitalization is required.
- Ceftriaxone (Rocephin) intramuscular injection during office visit.
- Ciprofloxacin (Cipro) BID × 14 days or levofloxacin (Levaquin) daily × 14 days.
- Trimethoprim/sulfamethoxazole (Bactrim, Septra) BID × 14 days.
- Close follow-up: 12 to 24 hours.
- Coexisting condition that compromises immune system or is toxic: Refer or hospitalize.
- *Refer*: Pregnant women, children/elderly, anatomic abnormalities, diabetics, others.
- *Complicated cases*: Gram-negative septicemia, shock, multi-organ dysfunction, renal failure.

✍ EXAM TIPS

- Memorize definition of UTI (greater than 10,000 CFU/mL of one organism).
- Recognize classic case of UTI and acute pyelonephritis.
- Can use 3-day treatment for healthy women with uncomplicated UTIs.
- WBC casts with proteinuria associated with pyelonephritis.
- Become familiar with urinalysis results of UTIs.
- Serum creatinine better measure of renal function compared with the BUN or BUN:creatinine ratio. The eGFR is considered a good measure of renal function in primary care.
- Right kidney sits lower than the left kidney because of displacement by the liver.
- Large numbers of epithelial cells in the urine mean contamination.
- Memorize the normal WBC count (10.5) and the neutrophil or segs (greater than 80%).
- Neutrophils make up from 50% to 75% of all the WBCs in a sample.
- If band forms (immature WBCs) are seen, it is indicative of a serious bacterial infection.
- The serum creatinine and the GFR are preferred to BUN when checking renal function.

📋 CLINICAL TIPS

- A study showed that some women with the classic symptoms of acute UTI may have lower counts of bacteria (less than 10,000 CFU/mL). Of these women, 88% had a UTI.
- Avoid long-term use of nitrofurantoin, if possible (associated with lung problems, chronic hepatitis and neuropathy).

Nephrolithiasis (Kidney Stones)

The majority of kidney stones are made up of calcium oxalate. The location and the size of the stone determine the pain. For example, stones located in the upper urethra or renal pelvis cause flank pain and tenderness, whereas stones on the lower urethra causes pain that radiates to the testicle or the labia of the vagina. Both can cause abdominal pain.

Risk Factors

- Family history of stones, low fluid intake, gout.
- Bariatric surgery (excrete higher levels of oxalate).

Classic Case

Adult with acute onset of severe colicky flank pain on one side that comes in waves. The pain builds up in intensity, then lessens and disappears (until the stone moves again). For some, the pain can be extreme and associated with nausea and vomiting. It may take a stone several hours, days, or weeks to pass. Majority have hematuria. Urine may be pink color from blood.

Labs

- Instruct patient to strain urine for several days and to bring kidney stone to office (if passed) for analysis by laboratory.
- Order renal ultrasound to determine location and stone size.
- Urinalysis until the episode resolves.
- Refer to urology: Large stone, inability to pass stone, acute renal failure.
- Refer to emergency department: High fever (possible urosepsis), extreme pain, acute renal failure.

Diet

- Increase fluid intake up to 2 liters/day (if tolerated). If calcium oxalate stones, dietary modifications to be advised.
- Avoid high oxalate foods: rhubarb, spinach, beets, chocolate, tea, and meats.

12

Nervous System Review

::= DISEASE REVIEW

Dangerous Headaches

- Abrupt onset of severe headache ("thunderclap" headache).
- "Worst headache of my life."
- First onset of headache age 50 years.
- Sudden onset of headache after coughing, exertion, straining, or sex (exertional headache).
- Sudden change in level of consciousness.
- Focal neurological signs (such as unequal pupil size).
- Headache with papilledema (increased intracranial pressure [ICP] secondary to any of above).
- "Worse-case" scenario of headaches (rule out) includes the following:
  - Subarachnoid hemorrhage (SAH) or acute subdural hemorrhage
  - Leaking aneurysm
  - Bacterial meningitis
  - Increased ICP
  - Brain abscess
  - Brain tumor

Acute Bacterial Meningitis

Acute onset of high fever, severe headache, and stiff neck and meningismus. Meningococcal disease (discussed under "Danger Signals" section in Chapter 6: Skin and Integumentary Review). Classic purple-colored petechial rashes. Accompanied by nausea, vomiting, and photophobia. Rapid worsening of symptoms progressing to lethargy, confusion, and finally coma. If not treated, fatal. Reportable disease.

Temporal Arteritis (Giant Cell Arteritis)

Acute onset of headache that is located on one temple on an older patient. The affected temple has an indurated, reddened, and cordlike temporal artery (tender to touch) that is accompanied by scalp tenderness. Abrupt onset of visual disturbances and/or transient blindness of affected eye (amaurosis fugax). Some may complain of jaw pain or jaw claudication (caused by artery obstruction). Markedly elevated sedimentation rate (ESR) and C-reactive protein (CRP). Patients with polymyalgia rheumatica (PMR) are at very high risk of developing temporal arteritis (up to 30%).

Acute/Narrow Angle-Closure Glaucoma

Acute onset of headaches behind an eye or around one eye accompanied by eye pain, blurred vision, and nausea and/or vomiting. The cornea looks hazy and the affected pupil is dilated midway. More common in older adults. Refer to ED.

Stroke (CVA)

Classified as either embolic (80%) or hemorrhagic (20%). A patient who has risk factor(s) for embolization (i.e., atrial fibrillation, prolonged immobilization) presents with acute onset of stuttering/speech disturbance, one-sided facial weakness and weakness of the arms and/or legs (hemiparesis). Patients who have hemorrhagic stroke often have poorly controlled hypertension and present with the abrupt onset of a severe headache, nausea/vomiting, and nuchal rigidity (subarachnoid bleed). Call 911.

Chronic Subdural Hematoma (SDH)

Chronic SDH presents gradually and symptoms may not show until a few weeks after the injury. Patient with a history of head trauma (falls, accidents) presents with a history of headaches and gradual cognitive impairment (apathy, somnolence, confusion). More common in the elderly and those who are on anticoagulation or aspirin therapy. The area of bleeding is between the dura and subarachnoid membranes of the brain.

Subarachnoid Hemorrhage (SAH)

Sudden onset of severe headache described as "the worst headache of my life" accompanied by photophobia, nausea/vomiting, meningeal irritation (stiff neck, positive Brudzinski and Kernig signs) with a rapid decline in level of consciousness. In the elderly, the most common cause is head trauma during a fall; among younger patients, it is motor vehicle accidents. Some suffer a "sentinel headache" or the sudden onset of a severe headache (caused by a minor leak) that resolves before the major hemorrhage happens. Sentinel headaches can occur from a few days up to 20 days before the event. Call 911.

NEUROLOGICAL TESTING

Neurological Exam

Mental Status (Frontal Lobes)
- Mini-Mental Exam (MME)
- Cranial nerve exam

MME (Mini-Mental Exam)
- Orientation (name, age, address, job, time/date/season).
- Registration (Recite three unrelated words. Distract patient for 5 minutes, then ask the patient to repeat the words).
- Attention and calculation.
- Spell "world" backward or serial 7s (subtract 7 starting at 100).
- Language.
- While speaking to patient, look for aphasia (impairment in language resulting in difficulty speaking).

Cerebellar System

- *Romberg test*: Tell patient to stand with arms/hands straight on each side and with the feet together. Then instruct patient to close both eyes while standing in the same position. Observe.
  - *Romberg positive*: Excessive swaying, falls down, keeps feet far apart to maintain balance.
  - Next tell patient to hold arms straight forward and close eyes. Observe.
- *Tandem gait*: Tell patient to walk a straight line in normal gait. Then instruct patient to walk in a straight line with one foot in front of the other.
  - *Positive*: Unable to perform tandem walking, losing balance, and falling.

Cerebellar Testing

Coordination (Diadochokinesia)

- *Rapid alternative movements*: Tell patient to place lower arms on top of each thigh and to move them by alternating between supination and pronation positions.
- *Heel-to-shin testing*: Patient is in a supine position with extended legs. Tell patient to place the left heel on the right knee and then move it down the shin (repeat with right heel on left knee).

Sensory System (Tell Patient to Close Eyes for These Tests)

- *Vibration sense*: Use 128-Hz tuning fork and tap lightly, then place one end into the distal joint of each thumb. Patient should have eyes closed.
- *Sharp-dull touch*: Use the sharp end of a safety pin for sharp touch and other end for dull.
- *Temperature*: Hot or cold.

Stereognosis (Ability to Recognize Familiar Object Through Sense of Touch Only)

- Place a familiar object (i.e., coin, key, pen) on the patient's palm and tell the patient to identify the object with the eyes closed.

Graphesthesia (Ability to Identify Figures "Written" on Skin)

- "Write" a large letter or number on the patient's palms using fingers (patient's eyes are closed).

Motor Exam

- *Gait*: Observe the patient's "normal gait." Check quadriceps and other leg muscles for atrophy.
- *Pronator drift test*:
  - Have patient stretch out the arms with palms facing up, then close eyes.
  - Wait for 5 to 10 seconds. Positive if one arm goes downward or drifts.
- Gross (legs) and fine motor movements (hands). Walking, using hands for manipulation/pincer grasp, jumping, and so forth.

Reflexes

- Both sides should be compared to each other and should be equal.

Grading Reflexes

0   No response
1+ Low response
2+ Normal or average response

3+ Brisker than average

4+ Very brisk response (sustained clonus)

Reflex Testing

Quadriceps Reflex (Knee-Jerk Response)

- Reflex center at L2 to L4. Tap patellar tendon briskly on each side.

Achilles Reflex (Ankle-Jerk Response)

- Reflex center at L5 to S2 (tibial nerve). With patient's legs dangling off the exam table, hold the foot in slight dorsiflexion and briskly tap the Achilles tendon.

Plantar Reflex (Babinski's Sign)

- Reflex center L4 to S2. Stroke plantar surface of foot on the lateral border from heel toward the big toe (plantar flexion is normal response). Babinski's sign positive if toes spread like a fan.

NEUROLOGICAL MANEUVERS

These tests are used to assess for meningeal irritation. All of these tests are done with the patient in a supine position. In general, these are more sensitive tests in children compared with adults.

Kernig's Sign

- Flex patient's hips one at a time, then attempt to straighten the leg while keeping the hip flexed at 90 degrees.
- *Positive*: Resistance to leg straightening because of painful hamstrings (due to inflammation on lumbar nerve roots) and/or complains of back pain.

Brudzinski's Sign (Figure 12.1)

- Passively flex/bend the patient's neck toward the chest.
- *Positive*: Patient reflexively flexes the hips and knee to relieve pressure and pain (due to inflammation of lumbar nerve roots).

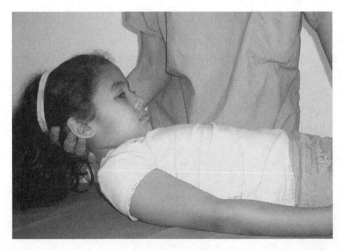

FIGURE 12.1 Brudzinski's test.

Nuchal Rigidity

■ Tell patient to touch chest with the chin. Inability to touch the chest secondary to pain is a positive finding.

Cranial Nerve (CN) Testing

■ *Mnemonic*: "On Old Olympus' Towering Tops, A Finn and German Viewed Some Hops." The first letter stands for the name of the cranial nerve. The word order corresponds to the sequential numbering of the cranial nerves.

CN 1:   On (olfactory)
CN 2:   Old (optic)
CN 3:   Olympus' (oculomotor)
CN 4:   Towering (trochlear)
CN 5:   Tops (trigeminal)
CN 6:   A (abducens)
CN 7:   Finn (facial)
CN 8:   And (acoustic)
CN 9:   German (glossopharyngeal)
CN 10: Viewed (vagus)
CN 11: Some (spinal accessory)
CN 12: Hops (hypoglossal)

✍ EXAM TIPS

■ Memorization tips on cranial nerves:
   CN 1: You have one nose
   CN 2: You have two eyes
   CN 8: The number 8 stands for two ears sitting on top of each other
   CN 11: The number reminds you of the shoulders shrugging together
■ Because cranial nerves are listed only by number on the test (not by name), the correct chronological order is important. Memorize the mnemonic to guide you.
■ Herpes zoster infection (shingles) of CN 5 ophthalmic branch can result in corneal blindness.
■ Rash at tip of nose and the temple area: Rule out shingles infection of the trigeminal nerve.
■ Cranial nerves are listed by number only.
■ Write down on scratch paper with corresponding cranial nerve "numbers."

☰ DISEASE REVIEW

Acute Bacterial Meningitis

A serious acute bacterial infection of the leptomeninges that cover the brain and the spinal cord. The most common pathogen for adults is *Streptococcus pneumonia, Neisseria meningitides,* and *Haemophilus influenzae* (both gram-negative).

Classic Case

Acute onset of high fever, severe headache, stiff neck (nuchal rigidity), and rapid changes in mental status and LOC. Up to 78% of patients have mental status changes (confusion, lethargy, stupor). Other symptoms include photophobia and nausea/vomiting. Some patients may not present with all three symptoms (triad of fever, nuchal rigidity, and change in LOC).

Labs
- Lumbar puncture: CSF contains large numbers of WBCs (CSF cloudy).
- Elevated opening pressure. CT or MRI scan. Laboratory tests such as the CBC, etc.
- Gram stain and C&S of the CSF fluid and the blood (before antibiotics).

Medications (IV)
- *Infants*: Ampicillin or third-generation cephalosporin
- *Adults*: Third-generation cephalosporin plus chloramphenicol
- *Older than age 50 years*: Amoxicillin plus third-generation cephalosporin
- Prophylaxis of close contacts with rifampin or ceftriaxone. Reportable disease

Complications
Patients who recover usually have permanent neurologic sequelae.

Migraine Headaches (With or Without Aura)
Migraine headache with aura (precedes the migraine headache) may present as scotomas (blind spots on visual field) or flashing lights that precede the headache. A positive family history and being female puts one at higher risk (3:1). Migraine headaches can present as abdominal pains in small children.

Classic Case
Adult female complains of the gradual onset of a bad throbbing headache behind one eye that gradually worsened over several hours. Reports sensitivity to bright light (photophobia) and to noise (phonophobia). Frequently accompanied by nausea and/or vomiting, which can be severe. Migraines can last from 2 to 3 days and may become bilateral if it is not treated.

Treatment Plan
- Neurological exam will be normal.
- Rest in a quiet and darkened room with an ice pack to forehead.
- *Nausea*: Drink ginger ale or chew dry toast.
- Avoid heavy fatty meals.
- Avoid precipitating foods or activities such as:
  - Monosodium glutamate (MSG) in Chinese food, chocolate
  - Red wines, beer, caffeine
  - Sleep changes, drinks, stress

Abortive Treatment
- 5-HT-1 agonists: sumatriptan (Imitrex):
  - First, rule out cardiovascular disease. Do not use if history or signs of ischemic heart disease (MI, angina), CVA, transient ischemic attacks (TIAs), uncontrolled hypertension, hemiplegic migraine.
  - Warn patient of possible flushing, tingling, chest/neck/sinus/jaw discomfort, etc.
  - Supervise first dose, especially if patient has risk factors for CV disease (diabetics, obese, males more than 40 years, high lipids, etc.). Give first dose in office (theoretical risk of an acute MI).
  - Consider EKG monitoring if patient at high risk for heart disease.
  - Higher risk of serotonin syndrome if combined with SSRIs or SNRIs (duloxetine or Cymbalta, venlafaxine or Effexor). Do not start within 2 weeks of MAOI use.
  - Do not combine with ergots or within 24 hours (i.e., ergotamine/caffeine or Cafergot).
- NSAIDs, analgesics (i.e., Extra Strength Tylenol), or narcotics (i.e., codeine, hydrocodone).

Table 12.1 Classic Signs and Symptoms: Headaches

Headache	Symptoms	Aggravating Factors
Migraine without aura	Throbbing pain behind one eye Photophobia, phonophobia Nausea/vomiting	Red wine, MSG, aspartame, menstruation, stress, etc.
Migraine with aura	Above plus scotoma, scintillating lights, halos, etc.	Foods high in tryptans Teenage to middle-age females
Trigeminal neuralgia (CN 5)	Intense and very brief; sharp stabbing pain; one cheek (2nd branch CN 5)	Cold food, cold air, talking, touch, chewing Older adults and elderly
Cluster	Severe "ice-pick" piercing pain behind one eye and temple. With tearing, rhinorrhea, ptosis, and miosis on one side (Horner's syndrome)	Occurs at same time daily in clusters for weeks to months Middle-aged males
Temporal arteritis (also known as giant cell arteritis)	Unilateral pain, temporal area with scalp tenderness. Skin over artery is indurated, tender, warm, and reddened. Amaurosis fugax (temporary blindness) may occur	Polymyalgia rheumatica common in these patients (up to 50%) Medical urgency Older adults and elderly
Muscle tension	Bilateral "bandlike" pain, continous dull pain, may last days. May be accompanied by spasms of the trapezius muscles	Stress Adolescents, adults

- Ergotamine/caffeine (Cafergot):
  - Potent vasoconstrictor.
  - Do not mix with other vasoconstrictors (triptans, decongestants, etc.).
  - Common side effect is nausea.
- Antiemetics:
  - Trimethobenzamide (Tigan) IM, suppository, PO.
  - Metoclopramide (Reglan) increases peristalsis in the duodenum and jejunum.

Prophylactic Treatment
- *Beta-blockers*: Propranolol (Inderal) daily or BID (other beta-blockers can also be used)
- *Tricyclic antidepressants (TCAs)*: Amitriptyline (Elavil) at bedtime (HS)
- *Other TCAs*: Desipramine (Norpramin), imipramine (Tofranil), nortriptyline (Pamelor)
- *Other drug classes*: Anticonvulsants (valproate, topiramate), gabapentin (Neurontin)

Contraindications (Vasoconstricting Drugs)
- Suspected or known cardiovascular disease (angina, MI, peripheral arterial disease)
- Suspected or known CVA and/or TIAs
- Hyperlipidemia, males more than 40 years, menopausal females
- Uncontrolled hypertension
- Complex migraine (i.e., basilar/hemiplegic migraine)

Basilar or Hemiplegic Migraines
Focal neurological findings (i.e., cranial nerve exam) with stroke-like signs and symptoms. Resembles a TIA. These patients are at higher risk of stroke. Avoid giving estrogens or any agents promoting clot formation.

✍ EXAM TIPS

- Distinguish the drugs used for abortive treatment versus chronic prophylaxis.
- Answer options may list the drug class instead of the generic name.

Temporal Arteritis (Giant Cell Arteritis)

Acute onset of a unilateral headache that is located on the temple and is associated with temporal artery inflammation. A systemic inflammatory disorder (vasculitis) of the medium and large arteries of the body. Mean age of diagnosis is 72 years of age. Visual loss is not uncommon and occurs in 15% to 20% of patients (despite availability of steroids).

Classic Case

An older male complains of headache on his temple along with marked scalp tenderness on the same side. Presence of an indurated cordlike temporal artery that is warm and tender. Sometimes accompanied by jaw claudication (pain with chewing that is relieved when he stops chewing).

Complains of visual symptoms such as amaurosis fugax (transient monocular loss of vision or partial visual field defect) or blindness. Can be accompanied by systemic symptoms such as low-grade fever and fatigue. Sedimentation rate is markedly elevated.

Labs

- Check erythrocyte sedimentation rate (ESR)/sed rate (often reaches 100 mm/hour or more)
- Normal range is between 0 to 22 mm/hour (men) and 0 to 29 mm/hour (women)
- Check both the ESR and CRP

Treatment Plan

- Refer to ophthalmologist or refer to ED STAT.
- Temporal artery biopsy is definitive test (gold standard) and is done by an ophthalmologist.
- High-dosed steroids are part of first-line treatment (prednisone 40 to 60 mg PO daily).

Complications

- Permanent blindness of one (or both eyes) if not diagnosed early (ischemic optic neuropathy).

✍ EXAM TIPS

- Temporal arteritis is treated with high-dosed prednisone × several weeks.
- Sedimentation rate is screening test for temporal arteritis (elevated).

Polymyalgia Rheumatica (PMR)

- PMR patients are at very high risk (up to 40% to 50%) for developing temporal arteritis. PMR patients are educated on how to recognize temporal arteritis.
- *Signs/symptoms*: Bilateral morning stiffness and aching (lasting 30 minutes or longer) located in the shoulders, neck, hips, and torso (difficulty putting on clothes/bra). Mostly females are affected (50 years or above). Symptoms usually respond quickly to oral steroids (i.e., prednisone daily).

📋 CLINICAL TIPS

- A high index of suspicion is necessary since 15% to 20% of patients become blind (one or both eyes). If history and physical exam suggestive, treat as soon as possible. Order the sed rate and CRP STAT. Start treatment in office if unable to see ophthalmologist ASAP or refuses to go to the ED.
- CRP is similar to the sed rate and will also be elevated (it is elevated about 1 week earlier than the sed rate).

Trigeminal Neuralgia (Tic Douloureux)

The trigeminal nerve (CN 5) has three divisions. They are the ophthalmic (V1), maxillary (V2), and the mandibular (V3) branches. Most cases are caused by compression of the nerve root by an artery or tumor, causing a unilateral headache that follows one of the branches of the trigeminal nerve. The pain is usually located close to the nasal border and the cheeks. Peaks in the 60s.

Classic Case

Older female complains of the sudden onset of severe and sharp shooting pains on one side of her face or around the nose that are triggered by chewing, eating cold foods, and cold air. The severe lacerating pain (piercing knifelike pain) lasts a few seconds. The patient may stop chewing or speaking momentarily (few seconds) if it causes the pain.

Treatment Plan

High doses of anticonvulsants such as carbamazepine (Tegretol) or phenytoin (Dilantin). MRI or CT scan if young, bilateral involvement, or numbness (rule out tumor/artery pressing on nerve).

Bell's Palsy

Abrupt onset of unilateral facial paralysis due to dysfunction of the motor branch of the facial nerve (CN 7). Facial paralysis can progress rapidly within 24 hours. Skin sensation remains intact, but tear production on the affected side may stop. Most cases spontaneously resolve. Etiology ranges from viral infection, an autoimmune process, or pressure from a tumor or blood vessel.

Classic Case

An older adult reports waking up that morning with one side of his face paralyzed. Complains of difficulty chewing and swallowing food on the same side. Unable to fully close eyelids.

Treatment Plan

- Rule out stroke, TIA, mastoid infections, bone fracture, Lyme disease, and tumor.
- Corticosteroids at high doses × 10 days (wean).
- Acyclovir (Zovirax) if herpes simplex suspected.
- Protect cornea from drying and ulceration with applications of an eye lubricant (a.m.) and lubricating ointment at bedtime. Patch eye if patient is unable to fully close the eyelid.

Complications

Corneal ulceration. Prolonged cases (several weeks) may leave permanent neurological sequelae such as permanent facial weakness in up to 10%.

Cluster Headache

An idiopathic and severe one-sided headache that is marked by recurrent episodes of brief "ice-pick" (lacerating pain) located behind one eye that is accompanied by tearing and clear rhinitis.

- Abrupt onset. The attacks happen several times a day (cluster). Resolves spontaneously, but may return in the future in some patients. More common in adult males in their 30s to 40s.

Classic Case

A 35-year-old male complains of the abrupt onset of recurrent episodes of brief "ice-pick" (lacerating pain) headaches behind one eye that are accompanied by autonomic symptoms such as tearing and clear nasal discharge (rhinitis). Some may have drooping eyelid (ptosis).

Treatment Plan
Acute Treatment

- High-dose oxygen may relieve headache (100% oxygen at least 12 L/min by mask). Continue oxygen treatment for 15 minutes. Do not use this treatment if a patient has COPD.
- Sumatriptan (Imitrex) by injection or intranasal route.
- *Prophylaxis:* If chronic, verapamil PO daily is effective for use as prophylaxis.

Complications

- Higher risk of suicide (males) compared with the other types of chronic headaches.

Muscle Tension Headache

Emotional/psychic stress in some people causes the muscles of the scalp and the neck to become chronically tense (or in contraction). It is a bilateral headache.

Classic Case

An adult patient complains of a headache that is "bandlike" and feels like "someone is squeezing my head." The pain is described as dull and constant. Often accompanied by tensing of the neck muscles. The headache may last several days. Reports recent increased life stressor(s).

Treatment Plan

- NSAIDs such as naproxen sodium (Anaprox DS) BID or ibuprofen 800 mg (Motrin) PO QID. Analgesics (acetaminophen QID) or aspirin as needed (PRN).
- Narcotics and butalbital are habit-forming and increase the risk of rebound headaches.
- Combination OTC medications of analgesics/aspirin plus caffeine (Anaxin, Excedrin, others).
- Stress reduction and relaxation: Yoga, Tai-Chi exercises. Exercise several times per week. Gradually reduce and stop caffeine intake. Regular eating/sleep schedule. Counseling with therapist.

Rebound Headache

Patient complains of daily headaches (or almost daily headaches). May be accompanied by irritability, depression, and insomnia. Caused by overuse of abortive medicines such as analgesics, NSAIDs, aspirin, or narcotics. Treatment is to discontinue the medicine immediately (if not contraindicated) or to gradually taper the dose and/or reduce frequency.

Stroke (CVA)

Stroke is also called a "brain attack." Ischemic cerebral infarction (embolism, thrombosis) make up 80% of all strokes and hemorrhagic strokes (aneurysms) accounts for 20%. Signs and symptoms depend on the severity and the area of the brain that is damaged.

- *Risk factors*: Hypertension, atrial fibrillation, stimulants (cocaine), aneurysms.

Transient Ischemic Attack (TIA)

Resembles a stroke and usually resolves within 24 hours. Symptoms usually resolve for most, but some patients may have minor neurologic deficits.

Classic

A patient with embolic stroke presents with the abrupt onset of difficulty speaking, unilateral hemiparesis, and weakness of the arms or legs (or both). Patients with hemorrhagic stroke often initially present with severe headache, nausea/vomiting, photophobia, and nuchal rigidity that is accompanied by hemiparesis and difficulty speaking.

Treatment Plan

Call 911. Give oxygen as soon as possible.

Long-Term Management

- Remove or treat the cause of the emboli (i.e., atrial fibrillation). Control hypertension.
- For embolic strokes: Anticoagulation with warfarin (Coumadin). Keep INR between 2.0 and 3.0.
- For hemorrhagic strokes: Avoid heparin, Coumadin, aspirin.

Common Drugs: Headache Treatment (Table 12.2)

Acute Treatment (PRN Only)

NSAIDs

- Naproxen sodium (Naprosyn, Aleve) BID or ibuprofen (Advil, Motrin) TID to QID
- *Side effects*: GI pain/bleeding/ulceration, renal damage, increased BP in HTN

Table 12.2 Treatment of Headaches

Headache	Acute Treatment	Prophylaxis/Other
Migraine	Ice pack on forehead. Rest in quiet and darkened room Rx: Triptans (Imitrex), Tigan suppositories (for nausea) Ultram, NSAIDs, analgesics, narcotics	Tricyclics (TCAs) Beta-blockers
Temporal arteritis	Refer to ED or ophthalmologist STAT. Lab: ESR ↑ (sed rate) (screening lab test) Rx: High-dose steroids	Permanent blindness can result. Temporal artery biopsy is the gold standard.
Cluster	100% oxygen at 7–10 L/minute. Use mask. Intranasal 4% lidocaine	May become suicidal Spontaneous resolution; can recur
Trigeminal neuralgia	Carbamazepine (Tegretol) or phenytoin (Dilantin). Check serum levels	Tegretol or Dilantin for several weeks to months. Watch for drug interactions
Muscle tension	NSAIDs, Tylenol, hot bath/ shower, massage, etc.	Stress reduction, yoga, massage, biofeedback

Triptans
- Sumatriptan (Imitrex) injection, nasal, PO tabs, or sublingual
- *Side effects:* Nausea, acute MI, etc.

Analgesics
- Acetaminophen (Tylenol) QID PRN
- *Side effects:* Hepatic damage, etc.
- Prophylaxis (must be taken daily to work)

Prophylaxis
Tricyclic Antidepressants (TCAs)
- Amitriptyline (Elavil) at HS or imipramine (Tofranil) at HS
- *Side effects:* Sedation, dry mouth, confusion in elderly, etc.

Beta-Blockers
- Propranolol (Inderal LA) or atenolol (Tenormin) daily
- *Contraindications:* Second- or third-degree AV block, asthma, COPD, bradycardia, etc.

Carpal Tunnel Syndrome (CTS)

Commonly caused by activities that require repetitive wrist/hand motion. Both hands affected in 50% of patients. Median nerve (Figure 12.2) compression due to swelling of the carpal tunnel. Other factors that increase risk are hypothyroidism, pregnancy, and obesity.

Classic Case

Adult patient who uses hands frequently for job (i.e., computer typing) complains of gradual onset (over weeks to months) of numbness and tingling (paresthesias) on the thumb, index finger, and middle finger areas. Hand grip of affected hand(s) weaker. May complain of problems lifting heavy objects with the affected hand. Chronic severe cases involve atrophy of the thenar eminence (the group of muscles on the palm of the hand at the base of the thumb), which is a late sign. History of an occupation or hobby that involves frequent wrist/hand movements.

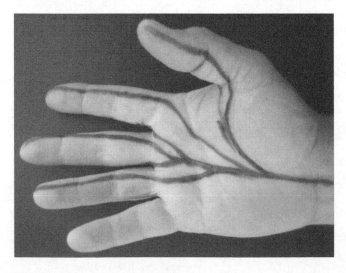

FIGURE 12.2 Median nerve.

Tinel's Sign (Figure 12.3)

- Tap anterior wrist briskly.
- *Positive finding*: Reports "pins and needles" sensation of the median nerve over the hand after lightly percussing the wrist.

Phalen's Sign (Figure 12.4)

- Full flexion of wrist for 60 seconds.
- *Positive finding*: Tingling sensation of the median nerve over the hand evoked by passive flexion of the wrist for 1 minute.

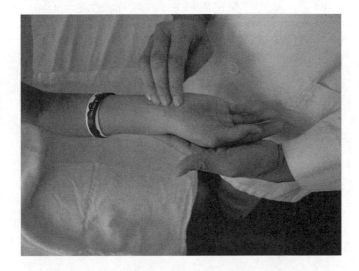

FIGURE 12.3 Tinel's sign.

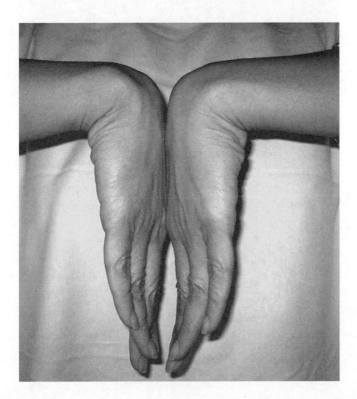

FIGURE 12.4 Phalen's sign.

✍ EXAM TIPS

- Recognize both Tinel's and Phalen's signs.
- Learn classic presentation of CTS.
- Headache treated with high-dosed oxygen is cluster headache.
- Headache treated with high-dosed anticonvulsants is trigeminal neuralgia.
- With the exception of muscle tension headaches, which are bilateral, all of the headaches seen on the exam (and notes) are unilateral.
- Muscle tension: Bandlike head pain; may last for days.
- Migraine: Throbbing, nausea, photophobia, phonophobia.
- Trigeminal neuralgia (tic douloureux): Pain on one side of face/cheek is precipitated by talking, chewing, cold food, or cold air on affected area.
- Temporal arteritis: Indurated temporal artery, pain behind eye/scalp.
- Cluster: Only HA accompanied by tearing and nasal congestion; severe pain is behind one eye/one side of head. Occurs several times a day. Spontaneously resolves. Seen more in middle-aged males.

13

Hematological System Review

⚠ DANGER SIGNALS

Acute Hemorrhage

Blood loss of 15% or higher results in orthostatic hypotension (systolic BP drop more than 20 mm Hg). Look for signs and symptoms of shock. When checking the CBC, be aware that the initial hemoglobin value (during active bleeding) may be in the normal range. The correct hemoglobin value will not show up until about 24 hours after onset of the hemorrhage.

Neutropenia

- Frequent infections (especially bacterial). Fever, sore throat, oral thrush, and so forth.
- Defined as an absolute neutrophil count (ANC) of less than $1,500/mm^3$.
- African Americans may have a lower ANC count that is "benign" (bone marrow aspirate normal).

Vitamin B12 Deficiency

Gradual onset of symmetrical peripheral neuropathy starting in the feet and/or arms. Other neurological signs are numbness, ataxia (positive Romberg test), loss of vibration and position sense, impaired memory, and dementia (severe cases). Peripheral smear shows macroovalocytes, some megaloblasts, and multisegmented neutrophils (more than 5 to 6 lobes).

Hodgkin's Lymphoma

A cancer of the beta lymphocytes (B cells). Night sweats, fevers, and pain with ingestion of alcoholic drinks. Generalized pruritus with painless enlarged lymph nodes (neck). Anorexia and weight loss. Higher incidence among young adults (20 to 40 years) or older adults (more than 60 years), males, and Whites.

Non-Hodgkin's Lymphoma

A cancer of the lymphocytes (usually B cells) and killer cells. Older adult (more than 65 years) with night sweats, fever, weight loss, generalized lymphadenopathy (painless). Poor prognosis.

Multiple Myeloma

A cancer of the plasma cells. Fatigue, weakness, and bone pain that is usually located in the back or chest. Proteinuria with Bence-Jones proteins; hypercalcemia; normocytic anemia. More common in older adults.

Thrombocytopenia

Thrombocytopenia is defined as a platelet count of less than 150,000/μL. Symptoms usually do not show until the platelet count is less than 100,000/μL. Look for easy bruising (ecchymoses, petechiae), bleeding gums, spontaneous nosebleeds, hematuria, and so forth.

- Normal platelet count: Ranges between 150,000 and 450,000/μL.

Easy Bruising

Bruising on the distal lower and upper extremities is usually related to physical activities. Children commonly have bruises on the anterior shin area. The presence of petechiae and/or purpura, large hematomas (from mild trauma) not accompanied by other symptoms (fever, headaches, infection) is suspicious. Check medications (ASA, NSAIDs, heparin, warfarin, SSRIs, steroids, etc.). Evaluate patient for a possible coagulation disorder (von Willebrand disease, vitamin C deficiency or scurvy, etc.). Initial labs to order are CBC, prothrombin time (PT), and partial thromboplastin time (PTT).

Platelet count greater than 150,000/μL is normal (rules out thrombocytopenia).

LABORATORY TESTING

Laboratory Norms

Hemoglobin (Hgb)

- *Males*: 14.0 to 18.0 g/dL
- *Females*: 12.0 to 16.0 g/dL
- *Long-term high-altitude (mountain)/chronic hypoxia*: Elevated (secondary polycythemia)

Hematocrit

- The proportion of red blood cells (RBCs) in 1 mL of plasma.
- *Males*: 42% to 52%
- *Females*: 37% to 47%

Mean Corpuscular Volume (MCV)

- *Normal:* 80 to 100 fL (femoliters)
- A measure of the average size of the RBCs in a sample of blood.
  - MCV less than 80 with microcytic anemia.
  - MCV between 80 and 100 with normocytic anemia.
  - MCV more than 100 with macrocytic anemia.

Mean Corpuscular Hgb Concentration (MCHC)

- A measure of the average color of the RBCs in a sample of blood.
- Decreased in iron-deficiency anemia and thalassemia. Normal in macrocytic anemias.
- *Normal*: 31.0 to 37.0 g/dL

Mean Corpuscular Hemoglobin (MCH)

- Indirect measure of the color of RBCs. Decreased values means pale or hypochromic RBCs. Decreased in iron-deficiency anemia and thalassemia. Normal with the macrocytic anemias.
- *Normal*: 25.0 to 35.0 pg/cell

Total Iron-Binding Capacity (TIBC)

- A measure of available transferrin that is left unbound (to iron). Transferrin is used to transport iron in the body. Elevated if there is not enough iron to

transport (as seen with iron-deficiency anemia). Normal TIBC seen with thalassemia, B12-deficiency, and folate-deficiency anemia (because iron levels are normal).
- *Normal*: 250 to 410 mcg/dL

Serum Ferritin
- The storage form of iron. Produced in the intestines. Stored in body tissue such as the spleen, liver, and bone marrow. Correlates with iron storage status in a healthy adult. Most sensitive test for iron-deficiency anemia.
- *Iron-deficiency anemia*: Markedly decreased.
- *Thalassemia trait*: Normal to high. May be high if patient was misdiagnosed with iron-deficiency anemia and erroneously given iron supplementation.
- *Normal*: 20 to 400 ng/mL

Serum Iron
- Decreased in iron-deficiency anemia. Normal to high in thalassemia and the macrocytic anemias. Not as sensitive as ferritin. Affected by recent blood transfusions. Avoid iron supplements 24 hours before testing the serum ferritin level.
- *Normal*: 50 to 175 mcg/dL

Red Cell Distribution Width (RDW)
- A measure of the variability of the size of RBCs in a given sample. Elevated in iron-deficiency anemia and thalassemia.

Reticulocytes (Also Called Stabs)
- Immature RBCs that still have their nuclei. After 24 hours in circulation, reticulocytes lose their nuclei and mature into RBCs (no nuclei). The bone marrow normally will release small amounts to replace damaged RBCs. RBCs survive 120 days before being sequestered by the spleen and broken down by the liver into iron and globulin (recycled) and bilirubin (bile).
- *Normal*: 0.5% to 2.5% (of total red cell count)

Reticulocytosis (More Than 2.5% of Total RBC Count)
- An elevation of reticulocytes is seen when the bone marrow is stimulated into producing RBCs. It is elevated with supplementation of iron, folate, or B12 (after deficiency), after acute bleeding episodes, hemolysis, leukemia, and with erythropoietin (EPO) treatment. Chronic bleeding does not cause elevation of the reticulocytes due to compensation.
- If no reticulocytosis after an acute bleeding episode (after 3 to 4 days), hemolysis, or after appropriate supplementation of deficient mineral (iron, folate, or B12), or with EPO, rule out bone marrow failure (i.e., aplastic anemia). Diagnosed by bone marrow biopsy.

Poikilocytosis (Peripheral Smear)
- Seen with severe iron-deficiency anemia. RBCs abnormal with variable shapes seen in the peripheral smear. May be accompanied by anisocytosis (variable sizes of RBCs).

Serum Folate and B12
- Low values if deficiency exists. Deficiency will cause a macrocytic anemia.
- *Normal folate level*: 3.1 to 17.5 ng/mL
- *Normal B12 level*: more than 250 pg/mL

White Blood Cells (WBCs) With Differential

- *White cell differential*: Percentage of each type of leukocyte in a sample of blood. The differential for each type of WBC should add up to a total of 100%.
- *Normal WBC count (child more than 2 years to adults)*: 5.0 to 10.0 × 10^9 (5,000 to 10,000/10 mm^3).
  - *Neutrophils or segs (segmented neutrophils)*: 55% to 70%
  - *Band forms or stabs (immature neutrophils)*: 0% to 5%
  - *Lymphocytes*: 20% to 40%
  - *Monocytes*: 2% to 8%
  - *Eosinophils*: 1% to 4%
  - *Basophils*: 0.5% to 1%

HEMOGLOBIN

Hemoglobin Electrophoresis

The "gold standard" test to diagnose hemoglobinopathies such as sickle cell anemia, the thalassemias, and many others. Normal hemoglobin contains two alpha and two beta-chains.

- *Adult norms*: 97% is hemoglobin A (HbA) and 2.5% is hemoglobin A2 (HbA2). An extremely small amount (less than 1%) of total hemoglobin is fetal hemoglobin (HbF), which is a normal finding.

Secondary Polycythemia

Chronic smokers, long-term COPD, long-term residence at high altitudes, or EPO treatment have a higher incidence of secondary polycythemia (vs. primary polycythemia vera).

- Polycythemia is defined as:
  - Hematocrit in adults of more than 48% (women) and more than 52% (men)
  - Hemoglobin in adults of more than 16.5 (women) and more than 18.5% (men)

High-Altitude Stress

Lower barometric pressure causes a reduction in the arterial PO2. Patients with CAD, CHF, or sickle cell anemia are at higher risk of complications.

☷ DISEASE REVIEW

ANEMIAS

Anemia is simply defined as a decrease in the hemoglobin/hematocrit value below the norm for the patient's age and gender.

Iron-Deficiency Anemia

Microcytic and hypochromic anemia (small and pale RBCs) are caused by deficiency in iron. The most common type of anemia in the world for all races, ages, and gender.

Classic Case

Pallor of the skin, conjunctiva, and nail beds. Complaints of daily fatigue and exertional dyspnea. May have glossitis (sore and shiny red tongue) and angular chelitis (irritated skin or fissures at the corners of the mouth). Cravings for nonfood items such as ice or dirt (pica). Severe anemia will cause spoon-shaped nails (koilonychia), systolic murmurs, tachycardia, or heart failure.

Etiology

Most common cause is blood loss (overt or occult). Reproductive-aged females (heavy periods, pregnancy), poor diet, GI blood loss, postgastrectomy, and increased physiologic requirement.

Infants: Rule out chronic intake of cow's milk before 12 months of age (causes GI bleeding)

Labs

Decreased:

- Hemoglobin and hematocrit
- MCV less than 80 fL
- MCHC (paler color)
- Ferritin and iron level

Table 13.1 Laboratory Findings: Anemia

Type of Anemia	Diagnostic Tests	Red Blood Cell Changes
Iron deficiency	**Ferritin/serum iron ↓** TIBC ↑ RDW ↑ (red cell distribution width)	MCV less than 80 (microcytic) MCHC ↓ (hypochromic) Poikilocytosis (variable shapes) Anisocytosis (variable sizes)
Thalassemia minor	**Hemoglobin electrophoresis**	Abnormal if beta-thalassemia Normal if alpha-thalassemia MCV less than 80 (microcytic) MCHC ↓ (hypochromic)
Pernicious anemia	**Antiparietal antibodies ↑** Most common cause of B12 deficiency anemia	MCV more than 100 (macrocytic) Megaloblastic RBCs Normal color (normochromic)
Folate deficiency	**Folate level ↓**	MCV more than 100 (macrocytic) Megaloblastic RBCs Normal color (normochromic)
B12 deficiency	**B12 level ↓** Hypersegmented neutrophils (More than 5 to 6 lobes)	MCV more than 100 (macrocytic) Megaloblastic RBCs Normal color (normochromic)
Normocytic anemia	**MCV between 80 and 100** History of chronic disease or inflammatory disease such as rheumatoid arthritis (RA)	MCV between 80 and 100 (normal-sized RBCs) Normochromic RBCs
Sickle cell anemia	**Hemoglobin electrophoresis** Hb S and Hb F both elevated Reticulocytosis A hemolytic anemia	Sickle-shaped RBCs with shortened lifespan of 10 to 20 days (norm is 120 days) Howell-Jolly bodies and target cells (peripheral smear) Normocytic/normochromic

Note: Boldfaced lab tests are diagnostic or the "gold standard" for the exams.

Increased:
- TIBC

Peripheral Smear:
- Anisocytosis (variations in size) and poikilocytosis (variations in shape).

Treatment Plan
- Identify cause of anemia and correct cause (if possible). Rule out GI malignancy.
- Ferrous sulfate 325 mg PO TID between meals (take with vitamin C, orange juice for better absorption). Treat iron-deficiency anemia from 3 to 6 months to restore ferritin stores.
- Increase fiber and fluids. Consider fiber supplements (psyllium, guar gum) for constipation.
- Iron-rich foods are red meat, some beans (e.g., black beans), and green leafy vegetables.
- *Common side effects of iron*: Constipation, black-colored stools, stomach upset.
- *Interactions*: Avoid taking iron supplement at the same time with antacids, dairy products, quinolones, or tetracyclines (inactivates iron).

Thalassemia Minor or Trait

A genetic disorder in which the bone marrow produces abnormal hemoglobin (defective alpha- or beta-globin chains). Normal hemoglobin contains two alpha- and two beta-chains. Results in a microcytic/hypochromic anemia.
- *Ethnic groups*: Mediterranean, North African, Middle Eastern, and Southeast Asians.
- Alpha thalassemia is more common in Southeast Asians (Chinese, Cambodian, Filipinos, Thai).

Classic Case
Vast majority are asymptomatic. Discovered incidentally because of abnormal CBC results, which reveal microcytic and hypochromic RBCs. Total RBC count may be mildly elevated. Ethnic background is either Mediterranean or Asian.

Treatment Plan
- "Gold standard" diagnostic test: Hemoglobin electrophoresis
  - In beta-thalassemia, abnormal (elevated Hgb, A2, Hgb F)
  - In iron-deficiency anemia, normal
- *Blood smear*: Microcytosis, anisocytosis, and poikilocytosis
- Serum ferritin and iron level normal (but low in iron deficiency anemia)
- Genetic counseling; educate about the possibility of having a child with the disease if partner also has trait (25% chance or 1 in 4 of their children).
- Thalassemia minor/trait does not need treatment (asymptomatic genetic disease).

✍ EXAM TIPS

- The screening test for all anemias is the CBC (hemoglobin/hematocrit).
- The diagnostic test for thalassemia and sickle cell anemia is the hemoglobin electrophoresis.
- Learn to differentiate the lab results of thalassemia from iron-deficiency anemia.
- If the ferritin level is low, the patient has iron-deficiency anemia.
- If the ferritin level is normal to high, the patient has thalassemia minor/trait.
- The ethnic background may not be "revealed" in a question about thalassemia.

■ Patients with chronic illness and/or autoimmune disease have higher risk of normocytic anemia.

CLINICAL PEARLS

■ Best absorbed form of iron supplementation (and cheapest) is ferrous sulfate (OTC).
■ If patient took an antacid, wait about 4 hours before taking iron pill (minimizes binding).
■ Failure to respond (if treatment compliant) may be a sign of continuing blood loss, misdiagnosis (has thalassemia instead of iron-deficiency anemia), malabsorption (i.e., celiac disease).
■ Iron poisoning in children (especially if age less than 6 years) may cause death. Advise patient to store iron supplements in an area that is not accessible to children (or to grandchildren).

Aplastic Anemia

Aplastic anemia is caused by destruction of the pluripotent stem cells inside the bone marrow. Multiple causes (radiation, adverse effect of a drug, viral infection, others). Bone marrow production slows or stops—all the cell lines are affected. The result is pancytopenia (leukopenia, anemia, thrombocytopenia).

Classic Case

Patient with severe case of anemia presents with fatigue and weakness. Skin and mucosa are a pale color. Tachycardia and systolic flow murmur are present. Neutropenia results in bacterial and fungal infections. Thrombocytopenia results in large bruises from trauma and bleeding. Signs and symptoms depend on the severity of the aplastic anemia.

Labs

■ CBC with differential
■ Platelet count
■ Gold standard is the bone marrow biopsy.

Treatment Plan

■ Refer to hematologist as soon as possible. If septic, refer to the ED.

Macrocytic/Megaloblastic Anemias

Vitamin B12-Deficiency Anemia

Caused by a deficiency in vitamin B12, which is necessary for the health of the neurons and the brain, and for normal DNA production of the RBCs. Total body supply of B12 lasts from 3 to 4 years. Chronic B12 deficiency causes nerve damage (i.e., peripheral neuropathy, paraplegia) and brain damage (dementia if severe). Neurologic damage may not be reversible. Highest incidence in older women. Most common cause is pernicious anemia.

Pernicious Anemia

An autoimmune disorder caused by the destruction of parietal cells in the fundus (by antiparietal antibodies) resulting in cessation of intrinsic factor production. Intrinsic factor is necessary in order to absorb vitamin B12 from the small intestine.

■ *Other causes of B12 deficiency*: Gastrectomy, strict vegans, alcoholics, small bowel disease.
■ *Vitamin B12 sources*: All foods of animal origin (meat, poultry, eggs, milk, cheese).

Classic Case

Older to elderly female complains of gradual onset of paresthesias on her feet and/or hands that is slowly getting more severe. Pallor, pale conjunctiva, glossitis, and other signs of anemia.

Neuropathic symptoms may include any of the following:

- Tingling/numbness of hands and feet
- Neuropathy starts in peripheral nerves and migrates centrally
- Difficulty walking (gross motor)
- Difficulty in performing fine motor skills (hands)

Objective

Decreased reflexes in affected extremity. If the legs are involved, the ankle jerk (Achilles reflex) will be reduced ("+ 1" is sluggish and "0" is none). Normal reflex is grade "+2."

- *Motor tests*: Weak hand grip, decreased vibration sense, abnormal Romberg, and so forth.
- Inflamed tongue or glossitis (not a specific finding since it is found in other disorders).

Treatment Plan

B12 is also known as cobalamin. Check for both B12 level and folate level (both levels must always be checked together).

- Decreased B12 level (less than 200 pg/mL)
- *Antibody tests*: Antiparietal and anti-intrinsic factor (IF) antibody
- *24-hour urine for methylmalonic acid (MMA)*: Elevated
- *Homocysteine level*: Elevated in B12 (and folate) deficiency
- *Schilling test*: Not commonly used now. Positive if B12 (radioactive) excretion is normal after administration of intrinsic factor (but has poor excretion when given B12 alone).
- *Peripheral blood smear*: Macroovalocytes, hypersegmented neutrophils (more than 5 to 6 lobes)

Medications

- *Pernicious anemia*: Lifetime supplementation of B12 (monthly injections or nasal B12 spray, or high-dose oral B12 from 1 to 2 mg/day.

✍ EXAM TIPS

- Pernicious anemia (PA) results in:
  - B12-deficiency anemia.
  - Macrocytic/megaloblastic anemia.
  - Neurologic symptoms.
- A cheap screening test for sickle cell is the Sickledex™, but gold standard is hemoglobin electrophoresis.
- If the parietal antibody test (antiparietal antibody) and/or the intrinsic factor antibody test (anti-intrinsic factor) are elevated, the patient has pernicious anemia.

📋 CLINICAL TIPS

- Serum B12 levels may be normal in up to 5% of patients with B12 deficiency. Do not rely on B12 levels alone. Also check antibodies, urine methylmalonic acid (MMA), etc.
- Missing a diagnosis of B12 deficiency can result in irreversible neurological damage.

- Any patient complaining of neuropathy or with dementia should have B12 levels checked.
- Almost 1 out of every 500 African Americans in the United States has sickle cell anemia.

Folic Acid Deficiency Anemia

- Deficiency in folate results in damage to the DNA of RBCs, which causes macrocytosis (MCV greater than 100). The body supply of folate lasts 2 to 3 months. Does not cause neurologic damage.
- *Most common cause*: Inadequate dietary intake (elderly, infants, alcoholics, overcooking vegetables, low citrus intake)
- *Other causes*: Increased physiologic need (pregnancy), malabsorption (gluten-enteropathy)
- *Drugs (long-term)* that interfere with folate absorption: Phenytoin (Dilantin), trimethoprim-sulfa, methotrexate, zidovidine (Retrovir, AZT), others

Classic Case

Elderly patient and/or alcoholic older male complains of anemia signs/symptoms (tiredness, fatigue, pallor, and a reddened and sore tongue or glossitis). No neurological complaints. If anemia severe (applies to all anemias), may have tachycardia, palpitations, angina, or heart failure.

Treatment Plan

- *CBC*: Decreased hemoglobin and hematocrit, increased MCV
- *Peripheral smear*: Macroovalocytes, hypersegmented neutrophils (more than 5 to 6 lobes)
- *Folate level*: Low (if more than 4 ng/mL, rules out folate deficiency).
- *Food sources*: Leafy green vegetables (kale, collard greens), grains, beans, liver

Medications

- Correct primary cause. Improve diet. Stop overcooking vegetables.
- Folic acid PO 1 to 5 mg per day. Treat until RBC indicators and anemia are normal.

Sickle Cell Anemia

A genetic hemolytic anemia (autosomal recessive). Many forms ranging from sickle cell trait to various forms of full-blown disease. Persons with sickle cell have an increased resistance to malarial infection (*Plasmodium falciparum* from mosquito bite). Higher risk of death from infection with encapsulated bacteria (i.e., *Streptococcus pneumoniae*, *Haemophilus influenzae*, etc.) due to hyposplenia. Patients with splenectomy (for other causes) are also at higher risk of death.

In the United States, it is most commonly found in African Americans (1 in 500 have the disease and more than 2 million carry the trait). Higher prevalence in people from Africa, the Mediterranean, the Middle East, and some areas of India. Mean hemoglobin of about 8 g/dL and a shortened RBC lifespan (17 vs. 120 days).

- Sickledex is the screening test. Hemoglobin electrophoresis is the diagnostic test.
- *Hemoglobin electrophoresis:* 80% to 100% Hb S, elevated Hb F (no HbA)

Classic Case

Majority of sickle cell trait is usually asymptomatic. Patients who have the full-blown sickle cell disease are extremely anemic, have frequent sickling episodes, and have painful crises (of affected organ systems). Signs and symptoms include ischemic necrosis of bones or skin; renal and/or liver dysfunction; priapism; hemolytic episodes; hyposplenism; frequent infections; others.

Labs
- CBC is the screening test.
- Gold standard is the hemoglobin electrophoresis (Hb S).

Treatment Plan
- Refer patients with disease to hematologist.
- Almost all states in the United States screen newborns for sickle cell anemia.
- Sickle cell is an autosomal recessive pattern genetic disease. Genetic counseling if both partners are at risk. If each parent has the sickle cell trait, 1 child out of 4 will have the disease.

✍ EXAM TIPS

- Order both B12 and folate levels when evaluating MCV greater than 100 (even if no neurological symptoms).
- Pernicious anemia results in B12 deficiency.
- Pernicious anemia is a macrocytic anemia.
- Learn food groups for both folate and B12.
- RBC size is described in many ways, such as:
  - MCV less than 80: Microcytic and hypochromic RBCs, small and pale RBCs.
  - MCV greater than 100: Macrocytes or macroovalocytes, larger than normal RBCs, or RBCs with enlarged cytoplasms.
- Ethnic background may not be mentioned in a thalassemia problem, or it may be a distractor.
- Only B12-deficiency anemia has neurologic symptoms (tingling, numbness).

≣ SUMMARY: MICROCYTIC ANEMIAS

Iron-Deficiency Anemia Versus Thalassemia Trait

Ferritin Level
- Low in iron deficiency
- Normal to high in thalassemia

Serum Iron
- Decreased in iron deficiency
- Normal to high in thalassemia

TIBC
- Elevated in iron deficiency
- Normal or borderline thalassemia

MCHC or Color
- Decreased in iron deficiency
- Normal in thalassemia

Hgb Electrophoresis
- Normal in iron deficiency
- Abnormal in thalassemia

Ethnic Background
- Ethnicity or age does not matter in iron-deficiency anemia.
- Iron-deficiency anemia is the most common anemia overall in any age group, gender, or ethnicity.
- Thalassemia is seen in people from Southeast Asia (e.g., China), the Mediterranean (e.g., Italy), North Africa (e.g., Morocco), the Middle East (e.g., Libya), and Asia (e.g., India).

14

Musculoskeletal System Review

⚠ DANGER SIGNALS

Navicular Fracture (Scaphoid Bone Fracture; Figure 14.1)

Wrist pain on palpation of the anatomic snuffbox. Pain on axial loading of the thumb. History of falling forward with outstretched hand (hyperextension of the wrist) to break the fall. Initial x-ray of the wrist may be normal, but a repeat x-ray in 2 weeks will show the scaphoid fracture (due to callus bone formation). High risk of avascular necrosis and nonunion. Splint wrist (thumb spica splint) and refer to a hand surgeon.

Colles Fracture

Fracture of the distal radius (with or without ulnar fracture) of the forearm along with dorsal displacement of wrist. History of falling forward with outstretched hand (as in navicular fracture). This fracture is also known as the "dinner fork" fracture due to the appearance of arm and wrist after the fracture. The most common type of wrist fracture.

Hip Fracture

History of slipping or falling. Sudden onset of one-sided hip pain. Unable to walk and bear weight on affected hip. If mild fracture, may bear weight on affected hip. If displaced fracture, presence of severe hip pain with external rotation of the hip/leg (abduction) and leg shortening.

More common in elderly. Elderly have a 1-year mortality rate from 12% to 37%.

Pelvic Fracture

History of significant or high-energy trauma such as a motor vehicle or motorcycle accident. Signs and symptoms depend on degree of injury to the pelvic bones and other pelvic structures such as nerves, blood vessels, and pelvic organs. Look for ecchymosis and swelling in the lower abdomen, the hips, groin, and/or scrotum. May have bladder and/or fecal incontinence, vaginal or rectal bleeding, hematuria, numbness, etc. May cause internal hemorrhage, which can be life threatening. Check airway, breathing, and circulation first (the ABCs).

Cauda Equina Syndrome

Acute onset of saddle anesthesia, bladder incontinence (or retention of urine), and fecal incontinence. Accompanied by bilateral leg numbness and weakness. Pressure (most common cause is a bulging disc) on a sacral nerve root results in inflammatory and ischemic changes to the nerves. A surgical emergency. Needs spinal decompression. Refer to ED.

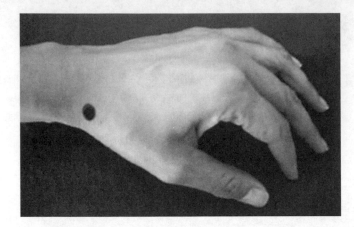

FIGURE 14.1 Navicular space.

Low Back Pain (From a Dissecting Abdominal Aneurysm)

Acute and sudden onset of "tearing" severe low back/abdominal pain. Presence of abdominal bruit with abdominal pulsation. Patient with signs and symptoms of shock. More common in elderly males, atherosclerosis, White race, and smokers.

☑ NORMAL FINDINGS

Joint Anatomy

- *Synovial fluid*: Thick serous clear fluid (sterile) that provides lubrication for the joint
  - Cloudy synovial fluid can be indicative of infection; order C&S.
- *Synovial space*: Space between two bones (the joint) filled with synovial fluid.
- *Articular cartilage*: The cartilage lining the open surfaces of bones in a joint.
- *Meniscus or menisci (plural)*: Crescent-shaped cartilage located in each knee. There are two menisci in each knee. Damage to menisci may cause locking of the knees and knee instability.
- *Tendons*: Connects muscles to the bone. Ligaments connect bone to bone.
- *Bursae*: Sac-like structures located on the anterior and posterior areas of a joint that act as padding. Filled with synovial fluid when inflamed (bursitis). Cloudy fluid is abnormal and is indicative of infection.

Joint Injections

Administering intra-articular/periarticular joint injections with steroids (e.g., triamcinolone) is a controversial treatment for osteoarthritis (OA). Some expert panels suggest about four injections per joint (such as a knee) in a lifetime. If high resistance is felt when pushing syringe, do not force. Withdraw needle slightly (do not remove from joint) and redirect.

- *Complications*: Tendon rupture, nerve damage, infection, bleeding, hypothalamic–pituitary–adrenal suppression, etc.

Radiography, Computed Tomography (CT) Scans, and Magnetic Resonance Imaging (MRI) Scans

- *Plain x-ray films (radiographs):* Show bone fractures, damaged bone (osteomyelitis, metastases), metal, and other dense objects. Not recommended for soft tissue structures such as tendons and ligaments.

- *MRI*: Gold standard for injuries of the cartilage, menisci, tendons, ligaments, or any joint of the body. The MRI uses a magnetic field and not radiation (compared with x-rays and CT scans).
  - *Contraindicated*: Metal implants, pacemakers, aneurysm clips, metallic joints.
- *CT scan*: Costs less than MRI. Uses radiation to view structures. Can be done with contrast. Detects bleeding, aneurysms, masses, pelvic and bone trauma, fractures. Uses x-ray images to form 3-D picture.

BENIGN VARIANTS

- *Genu recurvatum*: Hyperextension or backward curvature of the knees
- *Genu valgum*: Knock-knees
- *Genu varum*: Bowlegs

✍ EXAM TIP

- To remember valgum, think of "gum stuck between the knees" (knock knees). Opposite is varus or bowlegs.

EXERCISE AND INJURIES

- Within the first 48 hours, acutely inflamed joints should not be:
  - Exercised in any form (not even isometric exercises).
  - No heat of any form × 24–48 hours (i.e., hot showers or tub baths, hot packs).
  - No active range-of-motion (ROM) exercises. If done too early, they will cause more inflammation and damage to the affected joints.
- Avoid exacerbating activities. Protect joint.

RICE Mnemonic

Within the first 48 hours after musculoskeletal trauma, follow these rules:

- *Rest*: Avoid using injured joint or limb.
- *Ice*: Cold packs on injured area (i.e., 20 minutes on, 10 minutes off) for first 48 hours.
- *Compression*: Use an Ace bandage over joints to decrease swelling and provide support. Joints that are usually compressed are the ankles and the knees.
- *Elevation*: Prevents or decreases swelling. Avoid weight-bearing on affected joint.

Isometric Exercise

- Useful during the early phase of recovery before regular active exercise is performed.
- Defined as the controlled and sustained contraction and relaxation of a muscle group.
- Less stressful on joints than regular exercise.
- Usually done first before active exercise postinjury.
- Non-weight-bearing exercise:
  - Isometric exercises
  - Only weight-bearing exercises work for osteoporosis (e.g., walking, biking)

ORTHOPEDIC MANEUVERS

Test both extremities. Use the normal limb as the "baseline" for comparison.

Drawer Sign (Figure 14.2)

A test for knee stability. A diagnostic sign of a torn or ruptured ligament. The positive anterior drawer sign is the test for the anterior cruciate ligament (ACL). The posterior drawer sign is the test for the posterior cruciate ligament (PCL).

Finkelstein's Test (Figure 14.3)

De Quervain's tenosynovitis is caused by an inflammation of the tendon and its sheath, which is located at the base of the thumb. The screening test is Finkelstein's, which is positive if there is pain and tenderness on the wrist (thumb side) upon ulnar deviation (abductor pollicis longus and extensore pollicis brevis tendons).

McMurray's Test (Figure 14.4)

Knee pain and a "click" sound upon manipulation of the knee is positive. Suggests injury to the medial meniscus. Gold standard test for joint damage is the MRI.

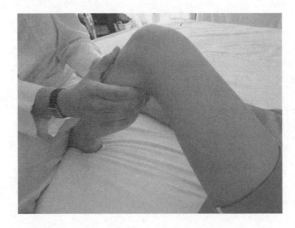

FIGURE 14.2 Drawer sign.

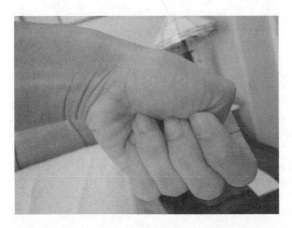

FIGURE 14.3 Finkelstein's test.

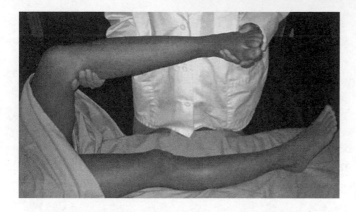

FIGURE 14.4 McMurray's test.

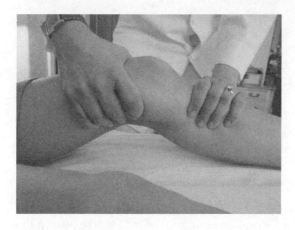

FIGURE 14.5 Lachman's sign.

Lachman's Sign (Figure 14.5)

Knee joint laxity is positive. Suggestive of ACL damage of the knee. More sensitive than the anterior drawer test for ACL damage.

Collateral Ligaments (Knees)

Positive finding is an increase in laxity of the damaged knee (ligament tear).
- Valgus stress test of the knee: A test for medial collateral ligament (MCL).
- Varus stress test of the knee: A test for the lateral collateral ligament (LCL).

MRI

- Best for soft tissue injuries such as tendons and cartilage.

X-Rays (Radiographs)

- Best for bone injuries such as fractures.

ORTHOPEDIC TERMS

Abduction and adduction:
- *Abduction (varus)*: Movement is going away from the body
- *Adduction (valgum)*: Movement is going toward the body

Hands and Feet
- *Carpal (carpo)*: Refers to the bones of the hands and the wrist
- *Phalanges*: The fingers and the toes. Singular form of the term is "phalanx"
- Tarsal (tarso): Refers to bones of the feet or the ankle

Proximal and Distal
- *Proximal*: Body part is located closer to the body (compared to distal)
- *Distal*: Body part is farther away from the center of the body

⠿ DISEASE REVIEW

Plantar Fasciitis

Acute or recurrent pain on the bottom of the feet that is aggravated by walking. Caused by microtears in the plantar fascia due to tightness of the Achilles tendon. Higher risk with obesity (body mass index [BMI] greater than 30), diabetics, aerobic exercise, flat feet, prolonged standing.

Classic Case
Middle-aged adult complains of plantar foot pain (either on one or both feet) that is worsened by walking and weight bearing. Complains that foot pain is worse during the first few steps in the morning. Worsened with prolonged walking.

Treatment Plan
- Nonsteroidal anti-inflammatory drugs (NSAIDs): Naproxen (Aleve) PO BID, ibuprofen (Advil) PO every 4 to 6 hours.
- Topical NSAID: Diclofenac gel (Voltaren Gel) applied to soles of feet BID.
- Use orthotic foot appliance at night × few weeks. Ice pack to affected foot.
- Stretching and massaging of the foot: Rolling a golf ball with soles of foot several times a day.
- Lose weight (if overweight).
- Consider x-ray to rule out fracture, heel spurs, complicated case. Refer to podiatry PRN.

Morton's Neuroma

Inflammation of the digital nerve of the foot between the third and fourth metatarsals. Increased risk with high-heeled shoes, tight shoes, obesity, dancers, runners.

Classic Case
Middle-aged adult female complains of many weeks of plantar foot pain that is worsened by walking, especially while wearing high heels or tight narrow shoes. The pain is described as burning and/or numbness and is located on the space between the third and fourth toes (metatarsals) on the forefoot. Physical exam of the foot may reveal a small

nodule on the space between the third and fourth toes. Some patients palpate the same nodule and report it as "pebble-like."

Mulder Test

A test for Morton's neuroma. Done by grasping the first and fifth metatarsals and squeezing the forefoot. Positive test is hearing a click along with a patient report of pain during compression. Pain is relieved when the compression is stopped.

Treatment Plan

- Avoid wearing tight narrow shoes and high heels. Use forefoot pad. Wear well-padded shoes.
- Diagnosed by clinical presentation and history. Refer to podiatrist.

Degenerative Joint Disease (Osteoarthritis)

Arthritis occurs when the cartilage covering the articular surface of joints becomes damaged. Large weight-bearing joints (hips and knees) and the hands are most commonly affected. *Risk factors*: Older age, overuse of joints, and positive family history.

Goal of Treatment

- Pain relief
- Preserve joint mobility and function
- Minimize disability and protect joint

Classic Case

Gradual onset (over years). Early-morning joint stiffness with inactivity. Shorter duration of joint stiffness (less than 15 minutes) compared to rheumatoid arthritis (RA). Pain aggravated by overuse of joint. During exacerbations, involved joint may be swollen and tender to palpation. May be one sided (e.g., right hip only). Absence of systemic symptoms (not a systemic inflammatory illness like RA).

- *Heberden's nodes*: Bony nodules on the distal interphalangeal joints (DIP).
- *Bouchard's nodes (Figure 14.6)*: Bony nodules on the proximal interphalangeal joints (PIP).

Nonpharmacologic Management

- Exercise (with care) at least three times a week. Lose weight. Stop smoking.
- Isometric exercises to strengthen quadriceps muscles (knee OA).

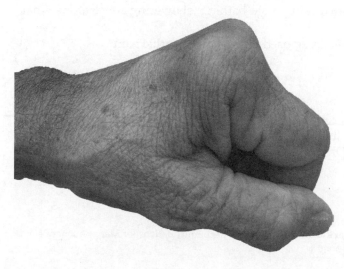

FIGURE 14.6 Bouchard's node.

- Exercise (swimming, walking, biking); resistance-band exercises.
- Avoid aggravating activities. Cold or warm packs. Ultrasound treatment.
- Walking aids. Patellar taping (reduces load on knees) by physical therapist.
- Alternative medicine: Glucosamine supplements, SAM-e, Tai-Chi exercises, acupuncture.
- Join Arthritis Self-Management Program (ASMP) with physical therapy.

Treatment Plan*

- First-line medication is acetaminophen 325 mg to 650 mg every 4 to 6 hours (maximum 4 g per day) PRN.

OR

- Tylenol Extra Strength 500 mg to 1,000 mg every 6 hours (maximum 6 tablets per day) PRN.
- If no relief with high-dosed acetaminophen, switch to a short-acting NSAID.
- Start with NSAIDs such as ibuprofen (Advil) 1 to 2 tablets every 4 to 6 hours or naproxen (Aleve) BID or Anaprox DS 1 tablet every 12 hours PRN.
- For added gastrointestinal (GI) protection, add a PPI (omeprazole) or misoprostol (Cytotec).
- If patient is at high risk for both GI bleeding and cardiovascular (CV) side effects, avoid NSAIDs.
- Age greater than 75 years: Use topical NSAIDs for treatment (versus oral form).
- Rule out osteoporosis. Order bone density testing.
  - GI bleed risk factors: History of uncomplicated ulcer, aspirin, Coumadin, PUD, platelet disorder.
  - Opioid analgesics: Avoid if possible (especially if patient is a recovering addict/alcoholic).

Topical Medicine

- *NSAID*: Diclofenac gel (Voltaren Gel); apply to painful area and massage well into skin BID.
- *Capsaicin cream*: Apply to painful area QID. Avoid contact with eyes/mucous membranes.
- Do not use on wounds/abraded skin. Avoid bathing/showering afterward (so that it is not washed off).
- Capsaicin is from chili peppers. Also used to treat neuropathic pain (e.g., postshingles).

NSAIDs

- Highest risk for GI bleeding: Ketorolac (Toradol) and piroxicam (Feldene)
- Lowest risk for GI bleeding: Ibuprofen, celecoxib (Celebrex)
- Highest risk for CV events: Diclofenac and celecoxib at higher doses
- Lowest CV risk: Naproxen

---

* Adapted from the American College of Rheumatology (2012), Recommendations for Management of Hand, Hip, and Knee OA. www.rheumatology.org

✍ EXAM TIPS

- Distinguish classic presentation differences between RA and OA. With RA, the joint stiffness lasts longer. It involves multiple joints and has a symmetrical distribution. RA is accompanied by systemic symptoms like fatigue, fever, normocytic anemia, etc.
- Heberden's and/or Bouchard's nodes have appeared many times on the exam. Memorize the location of each. The following may help:
  - Heberden's: The "-den" ending on the word is the letter "D" for DIP joint.
  - By the process of elimination, Bouchard's is on the PIP joint.
  - Another way to distinguish them is by using the alphabet. The letter "B" comes before the letter "H." Therefore, Bouchard's node comes before Heberden's nodes.
- Types of treatment methods used for DJD: Analgesics, NSAIDs (PO and topical), steroid injection on inflamed joints (NO systemic/oral steroids), surgery (i.e., joint replacement).
- Do not confuse OA treatment with treatment for RA.
- Treatment for RA includes all DJD treatment methods plus systemic steroids, antimalarials (Plaquenil), antimetabolites (methotrexate), biologics (Humira, Enbrel).

Systemic Lupus Erythematosus (SLE)

A multisystem autoimmune disease that is more common in women (9:1 ratio). Remissions and exacerbations. More common in African American and Hispanic women. Organ systems affected are the skin, kidneys, heart, and blood vessels. Milder form of lupus is called cutaneous lupus erythematosus.

Classic Case

Typical patient is a woman of age between 20 and 35 years. Classic rash is the maculo-papular butterfly-shaped rash on the middle of the face (malar rash). May have nonpruritic thick scaly red rashes on sun-exposed areas (discoid rash). Urinalysis positive for proteinuria.

Management

Refer to rheumatologist (topical and oral steroids, Plaquenil, methotrexate, biologics).

Patient Education

- Avoid sun 10 a.m. to 4 p.m. (causes rashes to break out).
- Cover skin with high SPF (UVA and UVB) sunblock.
- Sun-protective clothing such as hats with wide brims, long-sleeved shirts.
- More sensitive to indoor fluorescent lighting. Use non-fluorescent light bulbs.

Rheumatoid Arthritis

Systemic autoimmune disorder that is more common in women (8:1). Mainly manifested through multiple joint inflammation and damage. Patients are at higher risk for other autoimmune disorders, Grave's disease, pernicious anemia, and others.

Classic Case

Adult to middle-aged female complains of gradual onset of symptoms over months with daily fatigue, low-grade fever, generalized body aches, and myalgia. Complains of generalized aching joints, which usually involves the fingers/hands and wrist. Morning stiffness lasts longer than DJDs with painful, warm, and swollen joints. Swollen fingers with warm tender joints (PIP and DIP). Also called "sausage joints."

Objective

- Joint involvement is symmetrical with more joints involved compared to DJD.
- Most common joints affected: Hands, wrist, elbows, ankles, and shoulders.
- Swollen fingers with warm tender joints (PIP and DIP). Also called "sausage joints."
- Morning stiffness lasts longer than OA (DJD).
- Rheumatoid nodules present (chronic disease).
- Swan's neck deformity (50%): Flexion of the DIP joint with hyperextension of the PIP joint.
- Boutonniere deformity: Hyperextension of the DIP with flexion of the PIP joint.

Labs

- *Sedimentation rate*: Elevated
- *CBC*: Mild microcytic or normocytic anemia common
- *Rheumatoid factor (RF)*: Positive in 75% to 80% of patients
- *Radiographs:* Bony erosions, joint space narrowing, subluxations (or dislocation)

Treatment Plan

Refer to rheumatologist for early aggressive management to minimize joint damage.

Medications

- NSAIDs (i.e., ibuprofen, naproxen sodium) help to relieve inflammation and pain.
- Steroids: Systemic oral doses.
- Steroid joint injections (synovial space).
- Disease-modifying agent for rheumatoid disease (DMARD) such as methotrexate, sulfasalazine, cyclosporine, and hydroxychloroquine (an antimalarial drug).
- Gold salt compounds as intramuscular (IM) injections (i.e., Ridaura, Myochriysine).
- If poor response to DMARDs, use other options: antitumor necrosis factor (anti-TNF) drugs (Humira, Enbrel, Remicade), alkalating agents (i.e., Cytoxan, cyclosporine).
- Surgery: Joint replacement (hip, knees).
- Biologics or anti-TNF drugs are contraindicated (or should be stopped) if signs and symptoms of infection (fever, sore throat).

Complications

- Uveitis (ophthalmologist STAT).
- Scleritis, vasculitis, pericarditis, and so forth.
- Increased risk of certain malignancies.

✍ EXAM TIPS

- Uveitis: swelling of the uvea, the middle layer of the eye that supplies blood to the retina (refer to ophthalmologist). Patient treated with high-dose steroids for several weeks.
- Plaquenil is an antimalarial.
- Methotrexate is a DMARD.
- Presentation of RA, lab findings.

Gout

Deposition of uric acid crystals inside joints and tendons due to genetic excess production or low excretion of purine crystals (byproduct of protein metabolism). High levels of uric acid crystallize in joints with predisposition for first joint of large toe. More common in middle-aged males more than 30 years.

Classic Case

Middle-aged male presents with painful, hot, red, and swollen metatarsophalangeal joint of great toe (podagra). Patient is limping due to severe pain from weight bearing on affected toe. History of previous attacks on the same site. Precipitated by alcohol, meats, or seafood. Chronic gout has tophi (small white nodules full of urates on ears and joints).

Labs

- *Uric acid level*: Elevated (more than 7 mg/dL).
- *Acute phase*: First goal is to provide pain relief.
- Only two types of NSAIDs most effective (narcotics do not work as well).

Acute Phase

- Indomethacin (Indocin) BID or naproxen sodium (Anaprox DS) BID PRN.
- If no relief, combine with colchicine 0.5 mg 1 tab every hour until relief or diarrhea occurs.
- After acute phase is over, wait at least 4 to 6 weeks before initiating maintenance treatment.
- Stop allopurinol during acute phase. Restart 4 to 6 weeks after resolved.

Maintenance

- Allopurinol (Zyloprim) daily for years to lifetime. Check CBC (affects bone marrow).
- Probenecid (a uricosuric) lowers uric acid.
- Colchicine has anti-inflammatory effects and can be used during acute phase (with NSAIDs) and for maintenance phase.

Complication

- Joint destruction

Ankylosing Spondylitis

More common in males (2 to 3 times) and HLA-B27 positive. Average age of onset is the early 20s. Chronic inflammatory disorder (seronegative arthritis) that affects mainly the spine (axial skeleton) and the sacroiliac joints. Some other joints affected are the shoulders and hips.

Classic Case

Young adult male complains of a chronic case of back pain (more than 3 months) that is worse in the upper back (upper thoracic spine). Joint pain keeps him awake at night. Associated with generalized symptoms like low-grade fever and fatigue. May have chest pain with respiration (costochondritis). Long-term stiffness that improves with activity. Some have buttocks pain.

Objective Findings

- Marked loss of ROM of the spine such as forward bending, rotation, and lateral bending.
- Decreased respiratory excursion down to less than 2.5 cm (norm 5 cm). Some have lordosis.
- Uveitis (up to 40% patients): Complains of eye irritation, photosensitivity, and eye pain. Scleral injection and blurred vision. Refer to ophthalmologist as soon as possible (treated with steroids).

Labs

- Sedimentation rate and C-reactive protein slightly elevated. RF is negative.
- *Spinal radiograph*: Classic "bamboo spine."

Treatment Plan

- Referral to rheumatologist. Buy mattress with good support. Postural training.
- First-line treatment is NSAIDs (dramatic response).
- If high risk of bleeding, prescribe PPI with NSAIDs, or COX-2 inhibitor (celecoxib or Celebrex).
- For severe cases, treatment options are DMARDs, biologics (anti-TNF drugs), spinal fusion.

Complications

- Anterior uveitis.
- Aortitis (inflammation of the aorta).
- Fusing of the spine with significant loss of range of motion. Spinal stenosis.

Low-Back Pain

Very common disorder with a lifetime incidence of 85%. Usually due to soft tissue inflammation, sciatica, sprains, muscle spasms, or herniated discs (usually on L5 to S1). Rule out fracture and other etiology (see below).

Further Evaluation Is Recommended:

- History of significant trauma
- Suspect cancer metastases
- Suspect infection (osteomyelitis)
- Suspect spinal fracture (elderly with osteoporosis, chronic steroid use male/female)
- Patient age more than 50 with new onset of back pain (rule out cancer)
- Suspect spinal stenosis (rule out ankylosing spondylitis)
- Symptoms worsening despite usual treatment
- Herniated disc with symptoms: Common site is at L5 to S1 (buttock/leg pain)

Labs

- *MRI*: Best method for diagnosing a herniated disc

Treatment Plan

- Treatment depends on etiology. For uncomplicated back pain, use NSAIDs (naproxen sodium); warm packs if muscle spasms.
- Muscle relaxants if associated with muscle spasms (causes drowsiness; warn patient).
- Abdominal and core strengthening exercises after acute phase.
- Consider chiropractor for uncomplicated low-back pain.

Note

No bed rest except for severe cases since bed rest will cause deconditioning (loss of muscle tone and endurance) and increased risk of pneumonia.

Complications

Cauda Equina Syndrome

Acute pressure on a sacral nerve root results in inflammatory and ischemic changes to the nerve. Sacral nerves innervate pelvic structures such as the sphincters (anal and bladder). Considered a surgical emergency. Needs decompression. Refer to ED.

Signs
- Bowel incontinence
- Bladder incontinence
- Saddle anesthesia

✎ EXAM TIP

- Recognize signs and symptoms so you are able to diagnose it on the exam.

📋 CLINICAL TIPS

- The innervation of the bladder and anal sphincter comes from the sacral nerves.
- The name *cauda equina* means "horse tail." Sacral nerves when spread out straight appear like a horse's tail.

Acute Musculoskeletal Injuries

Treatment
RICE (Rest, Ice, Compression, Elevation)
- Cold is best first 48 hours postinjury:
  - 20 minutes per hour × several times/day (frequency varies).
- Rest and elevate affected joint to help decrease swelling.
- Compress joints as needed. Use Ace bandage (joints most commonly compressed are knees and ankles). Helps with swelling and provides stability.
- NSAIDs (naproxen BID, ibuprofen QID) for pain and swelling PRN.

Tendinitis (All Cases)

Microtears on a tendon(s) cause inflammation resulting in pain. Usually due to repetitive microtrauma, overuse, or strain. Gradual onset. Follow RICE mnemonic for acute injuries.

Supraspinatus Tendinitis
Common cause of shoulder pain. Also called cuff tendinitis. Due to inflammation of the supraspinatus tendon.

Classic Case
Complains of shoulder pain with certain movements. The movements that aggravate the pain are arm elevation and abduction (e.g., reaching to the back pocket). There is local point tenderness over the tendon located on the anterior area of the shoulder.

Epicondylitis

Common cause of elbow pain. Lateral epicondyle tendon pain (tennis elbow) or medial epicondyle tendon pain (golfer's elbow).

Lateral Epicondylitis (Tennis Elbow)
Classic Case
Gradual onset of pain on the outside of the elbow that sometimes radiates to the forearms. Pain worse with twisting or grasping movements (opening jaris, shaking hands).

Medial Epicondylitis (Golfer's Elbow)

Classic Case

Gradual onset of aching pain on the medial area of the elbow (the side of the elbow that is touching the body). Higher risk in baseball players, bowlers, golfers. Also called the "funny bone."

Complication:

Ulnar nerve neuropathy and/or palsy (long-term pressure/ damage). Complains of numbness/tingling on the little finger and the lateral side of the ring finger and weakness of the hand. Worse-case scenario is development of a permanent deformity called "claw hand."

Chronic neuropathy treated with TCAs, gabapentin, phenytoin, and pain medications.

SPRAINS

Ottawa Rules (of the Ankle)

- Used to determine whether a patient needs radiographs of the injured ankle in the ED.
- Mild to moderate sprains during acute phase, use RICE and Ace bandage.

Grade I Sprain

- Mild sprain (slight stretching and some damage to ligament fibers). Able to bear weight and ambulate.

Grade II Sprain

- Moderate sprain (partial tearing of ligament). Presence of ecchymoses, moderate swelling, and pain. Joint tender to palpation. Ambulation and weight-bearing painful. Mild to moderate joint instability. Consider x-ray, referral.

Grade III (Complete Rupture of Ligaments)

Referral to ED for ankle fracture. Ankle series (done in the ED) if:

- Inability to bear weight immediately after the injury.
- Inability to ambulate at least 4 steps.
- Tenderness over the posterior edge of the lateral or medial malleolus.

Other findings (not part of criteria) are: resists any foot motion, severe bruising, and severe pain.

Meniscus Tear (of Knees)

The meniscus is the cartilaginous lining between certain joints that is shaped like a crescent. Tears on the meniscus result from trauma and/or overuse.

Classic Case

- Complains of locking of the knee(s). Some patients are unable to fully extend affected knee.
- Patient may limp. Complains of knee pain and difficulty walking and bending the knee. Some complain of joint line pain. Decreased ROM.
- *Best test*: MRI (magnetic resonance imaging). Refer to orthopedic specialist for repair.

Ruptured Baker's Cyst (Bursitis)

A Baker's cyst is a type of bursitis that is located behind the knee (popliteal fossa). Sometimes when a joint is damaged and/or inflamed, synovial fluid production increases, causing the bursa to enlarge. Bursae are the protective synovial sacs that are located on certain on joints.

Classic Case

Physically active patient (jogs or runs) complains of ball-like mass behind one knee that is soft and smooth. Pressure pain or asymptomatic. If cyst ruptures, will cause an inflammatory reaction resembling cellulitis on the surrounding area (the calf) such as redness, swelling, and tenderness.

Labs

Diagnosed by clinical presentation and history. MRI if diagnosis is uncertain.
Rule out plain bursitis from bursitis with infection ("septic joint").

Treatment Plan

- RICE (rest, ice, compression, and elevation). Gentle compression with Ace bandage.
- NSAIDs as needed.
- Large bursa can be drained with syringe, 18-gauge needle if causing pain. Synovial fluid a clear golden color. If cloudy synovial fluid and red, swollen, and hot joint, order C&S to rule out septic joint infection.

📝 EXAM TIPS

- Baker's cyst presentation.
- Ankylosing spondilytis presentation.
- Anterior uveitis is complication of RA, ankylosing spondylitis.
- Presentation of cauda equina, refer to ED.
- X-ray of knee does not show meniscal injury or any joint cartilage.
- The gold standard test for assessing joint damage is the MRI.

📋 CLINICAL TIPS

- GI bleed and CV risk increases with higher doses of NSAIDs, long-acting forms, and longer duration.
- Do not forget that NSAIDs increase CV risk, renal damage, and GI bleeding.
- Experts state that dramatic response to NSAIDs is helpful with diagnosing ankylosing spondylitis.

15

Psychosocial Mental Health Review

Suicide Risk Factors

- Older people who have lost a spouse (due to death or divorce).
- Plan to use a gun or other lethal weapon.
- History of attempted suicide and/or family history of suicide.
- Mental illness such as depression, bipolar disorder.
- History of sexual, emotional, and/or physical abuse.
- Terminal illness, chronic illness, chronic pain.
- Alcohol abuse, substance abuse.
- Significant loss (divorce, boyfriend/girlfriend, job loss, death of someone close to the person).
- Females make more attempts compared to males, but males have a higher success rate.
- Bipolar disorder (also known as manic-depressive disorder).

A person with bipolar disorder is at higher risk of suicide during the depression phase of the illness. Look for signs and symptoms of depression and suicide warning signs. Moods cycle between mania and depression. Severe anxiety, rage, and chronic relationship difficulties. Classic manic symptoms include labile moods, euphoria, talkativeness, flight of ideas, grandiosity, and less need for sleep. There are two types of bipolar disorder: Type 1 (classic manic episodes) or type 2 (hypomanic episodes). Strong genetic component. Peak incidence of onset is in the 20s (ranges from age 14 to age 30 years).

Acute Serotonin Syndrome

Occurs from high levels of serotonin accumulating in the body due to the introduction of a new drug (drug interaction) and an increase in the dose. Acute onset with rapid progression. Signs and symptoms are sudden onset of high fever, muscular rigidity, mental status changes, hyperreflexia/clonus, and uncontrolled shivering. Look for dilated pupils (mydriasis). Higher risk if combining two drugs that both block serotonin (i.e., selective serotonin reuptake inhibitors [SSRIs], monoamine oxidase inhibitors [MAOIs], tricyclic antidepressants [TCAs], triptans, tryptophan). If switching to another drug affecting serotonin, wait a minimum of 2 weeks. Potentially life-threatening reaction.

Malignant Neuroleptic Syndrome

Rare life-threatening idiopathic reaction from typical and atypical antipsychotics. These drugs affect the dopaminergic system of the brain. Usually develops following initiation or an increase in dose. Signs and symptoms are sudden onset of high fever, muscular rigidity, mental status changes, fluctuating blood pressure, and urinary incontinence.

Look for a history of mental illness and prescription of an antipsychotic(s). Potentially life-threatening reaction.

The Baker Act

Allows 72 hours (3 days) of involuntary detention for evaluation and treatment of persons who are considered at very high risk for suicide and/or for hurting others.

Common Questionnaires in Mental Health

- Beck Depression Inventory
  - A multiple-choice self-report inventory for evaluating depression. Based on the theory that negative cognitions about the self and the world in general can cause depression.
- *Diagnostic and Statistical Manual of Mental Disorders*, Fifth Edition (*DSM-5*)
  - The diagnostic manual for mental and emotional disorders by the American Psychiatric Association.
- Minnesota Multiphasic Personality Inventory, Second Edition (MMPI-2)
  - A popular questionnaire that is used to assess for mental illness.
- Mini-Mental State Exam, Second Edition; Folstein Mini-Mental Exam (MMSE-2) (Table 15.1).
  - A questionnaire that is used to evaluate an individual for confusion and dementia (Alzheimer's, stroke, others).
- Geriatric Depression Scale (GDS)
  - A 30-item (yes/no response) questionnaire. Shorter version contains 15 items. Used to assess depression in the elderly. Self-assessment format.

Psychotropic Drugs (Table 15.2)

SSRIs

First-line treatment for:

- Major depression, obsessive-compulsive disorder.
- Generalized anxiety disorder, panic disorder, social anxiety disorder.
- Premenstrual dysphoric disorder.

Table 15.1 Folstein Mini-Mental State Exam (MMSE)

Cognitive Skill	Action Required
Orientation	What is the date today? (current day, month, year)
	Location (name the city, county, state)
Immediate recall	
Recall three objects	Instruct that you will be testing his/her memory. Say 3 unrelated words (pencil, apple, ball). Ask patient to repeat words
Attention and calculation	
Counting backward	Say "starting at 100, count backward and keep subtracting 7"
Backward spelling	Spell the word "WORLD" backward
Writing and copying	
Writing a sentence	Give person one blank paper and ask him/her to write a sentence
Copying a figure	Draw intersecting pentagons. Ask patient to copy the pentagons
Scoring	Maximum score is 30 correctly done. Impaired is a score of less than 19

Adapted from Folstein, Folstein, and McHugh (1975).

Table 15.2 Monitoring Psychiatric Medications

Drug Class	Adverse Effects	Monitor
Atypical Antipsychotics		
Olanzapine (Zyprexa) Rispiradone (Risperdal) Quetiapine (Seroquel)	Obesity Diabetes type 2	All can cause weight gain. Check BMI. Check weight every 3 months
Typical Antipsychotics		
Haloperidol (Haldol) Chlorpromazine	Elevates lipids/ triglycerides Malignant neuroleptic syndrome (rare)	Labs: Fasting blood glucose and lipid profile *Black Box Warning:* Frail elderly at higher risk of death from antipsychotics
Anticonvulsants		
Lamotragine (Lamictal) Carbamezapine (Tegretol) Valproate (Depakote)	Stevens–Johnson syndrome (Lamictal)	Advise patient to report rashes (Stevens–Johnson). Some anticonvulsants are also used as a mood stabilizer for Bipolar Disorder
SSRIs		
Sertraline (Zoloft) Paroxetine (Paxil) *Citalopram (Celexa) *Escitaprolam (Lexapro)	Anxiety Insomnia Sexual side effects Serotonin syndrome	*Black Box Warning:* Suicidal ideation/plans (less than 24 years of age) Do not discontinue Paxil abruptly. Wean gradually
Atypical Antidepressants		
Bupropion (Wellbutrin) Zyban for smoking cessation	Seizures	Contraindicated with seizures disorder, anorexia or bulimia
SNRI		
Venlafaxine (Effexor) Duloxetine (Cymbalta**)	Can precipitate acute narrow-angle glaucoma	Avoid with uncontrolled narrow-angle glaucoma
TCAs		
Amytriptiline (Elavil) Nortriptyline	Anticholinergic effects Category X	Do not combine with SSRIs or MAOI since it will increase risk of serotonin syndrome For bipolar disorder. "Ebstein's anomaly" is congenital heart defect caused by lithium. Check blood levels
Lithium		
Lithium carbonate (Eskalith)		Lithium is a metal

BMI, body mass index; SNRI, selective norepinephrine reuptake inhibitor; SSRIs, selective serotonin reuptake inhibitors; TCA, tricyclic antidepressant.
* Lowest number of drug interactions compared to other SSRIs.
** Cymbalta also used for neuropathic pain.

Common SSRIs

- Fluoxetine (Prozac): Longest half-life of all SSRIs (may last up to 4 weeks) and the first SSRI.
- Paroxetine (Paxil): Shortest half-life, but was reformulated to Paxil CR (to prolong half-life).
- Citalopram (Celexa): Has fewer drug interactions compared with other SSRIs.
- Escitaplopram (Lexapro): Compound derived from citalopram (Celexa).
- Duloxetine (Cymbalta): Can treat both depression and neuropathic pain.
- Other SSRIs: Sertraline (Zoloft), fluvoxamine (Luvox).

Side Effects

- Loss of libido, erectile dysfunctile (ED), women with sexual dysfunction, anorexia, insomnia.
- Avoid with anorexic patients and undernourished elderly (depresses appetite more).
- Paxil: Common side effect is ED.

Contraindications

- Avoid SSRIs within 14 days of taking an MAOI (serotonin syndrome).
- Can induce mania with bipolar patients.
- TCAs.
- Not considered first-line treatment for depression.
- Other uses: Post-herpetic neuralgia (chronic pain), stress urinary incontinence.
- Avoid if patient at high risk of suicide because may hoard pills and overdose (suicide attempt).
- Overdose will cause fatal cardiac (ventricular arrhythmia) and neurologic effects (seizures).
- *Example:* Imipramine (Tofranil), amitriptyline (Elavil), nortriptyline (Norpramine).

MAOIs

- Rarely used due to serious food (high tyramine content) and drug interactions.
- Phenelzine (Nardil), tranylcypromine (Parnate).

Contraindications

- Do not combine MAOI with SSRI or TCAs.
- Wait at least 2 weeks before initiating SSRI or TCA (high risk of serotonin syndrome).

High-Tyramine Foods and MAOIs

- Cause the tyramine pressor response (elevates blood pressure, risk of stroke). Avoid combining with fermented foods such as beer, chianti wine, some aged cheeses, fava beans, others.
- High-tyramine foods can also cause migraine headache in susceptible persons.

Benzodiazepines (Tranquilizers)

- Benzodiazepines are indicated for anxiety disorders, panic disorder, and insomnia.
- Diazepam (Valium) is also used for severe alcohol withdrawal and seizures.
- Do not discontinue abruptly because it increases risk of seizures. Wean slowly.
- *Example:*
  - Ultra-short acting: Midazolam IV only (Versed), triazolam (Halcion).
  - Medium-acting: Alprazolam (Xanax), lorazepam (Ativan).
  - Long-acting: Diazepam (Valium), chlordiazepoxide (Librium), temazepam (Restoril), and clonazepam (Klonopin). Avoid with elderly.

▤ DISEASE REVIEW

Major and Minor Depression

Also known as unipolar depression (vs. bipolar depression). Minor depression is a milder form. The criteria of signs and symptoms are the same as major depression except that there are fewer symptoms (at least two, but less than five). Attributed to dysfunction of the neurotransmitters serotonin and norepinephrine. Strong genetic component.

Symptoms of Depression

- *Mood*: Depressed mood most of the time. May become tearful.
- *Anhedonia*: Diminished interest or pleasure in all or most activities.
- *Energy*: Fatigued or loss of energy.
- *Sleep*: Insomnia or hypersomnia.
- *Guilt*: Feelings of worthlessness and inappropriate guilt.
- *Concentration*: Diminished concentration and difficulty making decisions.
- *Suicide*: Recurrent/obsessive thoughts of death and suicidal ideation.
- *Weight*: Weight loss (greater than 5% body weight) or weight gain.
- *Agitation*: Psychomotor agitation or retardation.

Immediate Goal: Assess for Suicidal and/or Homicidal Ideation or Plan

If patient is considered to be a real and present threat of harm to self or to others:

- Refer to a psychiatric hospital. Patient must be driven by a family member or a friend.
- If none are available, call 911 for police. The police can "Baker Act" the patient. A Baker Act proceeding is a means of providing emergency services for mental health treatment on a voluntary or involuntary basis.

Differential Diagnosis

Rule out organic causes such as hypothyroidism, anemia, autoimmune disorders, B12 deficiency.

SCREENING TOOLS FOR DEPRESSION

- Beck Depression Inventory: Contains 21 items.
- Beck Depression Inventory for Primary Care (99% specificity): Contains 7 items.
- Two-item question: Ask these two questions: 1) "During the past month, have you felt down, depressed, or hopeless?" 2) "During the past month, have you felt little interest or pleasure doing things?" If answered yes to either question (or both), positive finding.

Treatment Plan

- Rule out diseases such as anemia (CBC), diabetes, hypothyroid (thyroid-stimulating hormone [TSH]/thyroid panel), chemistry panel (low potassium for Addison's disease), and Vitamin B12 level (B12 anemia).
- First line: Selective SSRIs. Advise patients that antidepressant effect may take from 4 to 8 weeks (up to 12 weeks) to manifest.
- After initiation, follow up in 2 weeks to check for compliance and side effects.
- Wait for at least 4 to 8 weeks before changing medication.
- Continue SSRI therapy for at least 4 to 9 months after symptoms have resolved (usually on first episode). Frequent relapse means patient may need lifetime treatment.
- Second line: Tricyclic antidepressants or TCAs (amitryptiline/Elavil, nortriptyline/Pamelor).
- Prefer bedtime dosing due to sedation. Other uses are post-herpetic neuralgia, chronic pain, stress urinary incontinence.

- Refer for psychotherapy. Cognitive-behavioral therapy can reduce symptoms (comparable to an antidepressant medication) and is usually effective.
- Psychotherapy plus antidepressants works better than either method alone.

Special Considerations: Antidepressants
SSRIs

- *FDA Black Box Warnings*: Increased risk of suicidal thinking and behavior in children, adolescents, and young adults.
- *Elderly patients*: Consider using citalopram (Celexa) and escitalopram (Lexapro). Fewer drug interactions than other SSRIs. May prolong QT interval.
- *Patients with sexual dysfunction caused by an SSRI*: Consider adding bupropion (Wellbutrin) to the SSRI prescription.
- *Depressed patient who wants to quit smoking*: Consider bupropion (Zyban). Can be combined with nicotine products (patches, gum).
- *Depressed patient with peripheral neuropathy*: Consider duloxetine (Cymbalta), which is also indicated for neuropathic pain.
- Depressed patient with post-herpetic neuralgia and chronic pain: Consider TCAs.
- Depressed patient with stress urinary incontinence: Consider TCAs.

✎ EXAM TIPS

- Antipsychotics lead to an increased risk of obesity, type 2 diabetes, and hyperlipidemia, metabolic syndrome, and hypothyroidism.
- Learn how medication use should be monitored (see Table 15.2).
- FDA Black Box Warnings of SSRIs and antipsychotics.
- Diagnose bipolar disorder, depression, and anorexia.
- MAOI and high-tyramine foods to avoid.
- St. John's wort is used for depression, menopausal symptoms, and others. Herb-drug interactions of St. John's wort are indinavir (protease inhibitor), cyclosporine, oral contraceptives, SSRIs, TCAs, and others.
- Kava-kava and/or valerian root are both used for anxiety and insomnia. Do not mix with benzodiazepines, hypnotics, or any CNS depressants.
- In general, there are now more questions on alternative treatments.
- A question on the MMSE (or the MME) will describe an action (such as asking a patient to spell "world" backwards). The exam will ask you to indicate the name of the tool that is being used.
- Know how to diagnose minor depression and major depression.
- Psychotic symptoms include delusions and paranoia (disorganized speech and behavior). Hallucinations are common (usually auditory) with loss of ego boundaries. Flat and restricted affect with poor social skills. Executive function is very poor (ability to plan and organize day-to-day activities). Onset is usually around the second decade. Peak incidence is between 16 and 30 years of age.

Labs

- Rule out organic causes. CBC, chemistry profile, TSH, folate and B12 levels, urinalysis. Toxicology screen to rule out illicit drug use.

Treatment Plan

- Refer to psychiatrist for evaluation and treatment. If psychotic, refer to the ED.
- Psychotherapeutic drugs: Safety considerations.
- *FDA Black Box Warning*: Increased risk of death in elderly.

Table 15.3 Alternative Medicine for Depression

Name	Drug Interactions	Adverse Effects
St. John's wort	SSRIs (citalopram/Celexa, paroxetine/Paxil, etc) Tricyclics (amitriptyline/Elavil, imipramine/Tofranil, etc.) MAOIs, Xanax, protease inhibitors (indinavir), and many others	Decreases digoxin effectiveness Causes breakthrough bleeding that decreases effectiveness of birth control pills
Amino acid supplements such as 5-HTP (5-hydroxytryptophan) L-tryptophan	SSRIs and MAOIs Dextromethorphan Triptans (Imetrix, Zomig, others)	Serotonin syndrome Dextromethorphan increases risk of serotonin syndrome
Omega-3 fatty acids (cold-water fish oil such as salmon) Folate and B6 (pyridoxine) Exercise, yoga, massage, guided imagery, acupuncture, light therapy	No major drug interactions	High doses of omega-3 fish oil may increase risk of bleeding. Usually stopped about 1 week before surgery

MAOI, monoamine oxidase inhibitors; SSRIs, selective serotonin reuptake inhibitors.

Antipsychotics: Adverse Effects

- Extrapyramidal symptoms.
- Pill-rolling, shuffling gait, and bradykinesia. Caused by chronic use of antipsychotics.
- Akinesia (inability to initiate movement).
- Akathisia (a strong inner feeling to move, unable to stay still).
- Bradykinesia (slowness in movement) when initiating activities or actions that require successive steps such as buttoning a shirt.
- Tardive dyskinesia: Involuntary movements of the lips (smacking), tongue, face, trunk, and extremities (more common in schizophrenics).

Anticholinergics: Side Effects

- Many drug classes have strong anticholinergic effects such as antipsychotics, TCA, decongestants, and antihistamines (e.g., pseudoephedrine).
- Caution with: benign prostatic hypertrophy (BPH) (urinary retention), narrow-angle glaucoma, pre-existing heart disease.
- Use the "SAD CUB" mnemonic to help you remember anticholinergic side effects:
  - **S**edation
  - **A**norexia
  - **D**ry mouth
  - **C**onfusion and constipation
  - **U**rinary retention
  - **B**PH

ALCOHOLISM

Compulsive desire to drink alcohol despite personal, financial, and social consequences. With alcohol dependence, a patient experiences cognitive, behavioral, and physiologic symptoms that are generated from persistent and chronic use. Abrupt cessation causes withdrawal symptoms.

Alcohol abuse occurs when a maladaptive behavior pattern occurs from repeated alcohol use.

Definitions
- Elevated blood alcohol level greater than 0.08% is illegal for driving (blood alcohol or breathalyzer).
- Standard drink sizes for the United States (considered as "one drink"):
  - Beer: 12-ounce bottle.
  - Wine: 5 ounces.
  - Liquor/spirits: 1.5 ounces or a "shot" of 80-proof gin, vodka, rum, or whiskey.

Dietary Guidelines for Americans (Alcohol Limits)
- *Women*: One drink per day.
- *Men*: Two drinks per day.
- Binge drinking:
  - A pattern of alcohol consumption that brings the blood alcohol level to 0.08% or higher in one occasion (generally within 2 hours).
  - *Males*: At least five drinks or more on a single occasion.
  - *Women*: At least four drinks or more on a single occasion.
- Females metabolize alcohol (50%) more slowly than do males.

Alcohol Addiction (Alcoholism)
- Continued drinking despite repeated physical, psychological, interpersonal, and social problems. Strong craving for alcohol. Inability to limit drinking. Withdrawal symptoms if stop drinking.

Labs Results
Gamma Glutamyl Transaminase (GGT)
- Lone elevation (with/without alanine transaminase [ALT] and aspartate aminotransferase [AST]) is a possible sign of occult alcohol abuse.

AST/ALT Ratio (Liver Transaminases)
- Both AST and ALT are usually elevated (with or without elevated GGT) in alcoholism.
- Ratio of 2:1 with AST/ALT (AST level is double the level of ALT) is associated with alcohol abuse (alcoholic hepatitis).
- ALT is more specific for the liver than the AST because AST is also found in the liver, cardiac and skeletal muscle, kidneys, and lungs.

Mean Corpuscular Volume (MCV)
- Larger size of red blood cells (due to nutritional deficiencies) that resembles macrocytic anemia (MCV > 100 fl).

Quick Screening Tests for Identification of Alcohol Abuse/Alcoholism
CAGE Test
- Positive finding of at least two (out of four) highly suggestive of alcoholism:
  - **C:** Do you feel the need to *cut down*?
  - **A:** Are you *annoyed* when your spouse/friend comments about your drinking?
  - **G:** Do you feel *guilty* about your drinking?
  - **E:** Do you need to drink *early* in the morning? (an *eye-opener*).
- Examples of some quotes using CAGE:
  - **C:** "I would like to drink less on the weekends," "I only drink a lot on weekends."
  - **A:** "My wife nags me about my drinking," "My best friend thinks I drink too much."
  - **G:** "I feel bad that I don't spend enough time with the kids because of my drinking."
  - **E:** "I need a drink to feel better when I wake up in the morning."

Short Michigan Alcoholism Screening Test (SMAST) Questionnaire
- A 13-item questionnaire. A shorter version of the original MAST Questionnaire (contains 24 items).

Alcohol Use Disorders Identification Test (AUDIT)
- A 10-question tool that is used with women, minorities, and adolescents.

Acute Delirium Tremens
- Sudden onset of confusion, delusions, transient auditory, tactile or visual hallucinations, tachycardia, hypertension, hand tremors, disturbed psychomotor behavior (picking at clothes), and grand mal seizures.
- Considered a medical emergency. Refer to ED.

Treatment Plan
- Benzodiazepines (Librium, Valium), antipsychotics if needed (i.e., Haldol).
- Vitamins: Thiamine 100 mg IV, folate 1 mg PO/IV daily, and multivitamins with high-caloric diet.
- Refer to Alcoholics Anonymous (12-step program), therapist, and/or a recovery program.
- Avoid prescribing recovering alcoholic/addict drugs with abuse potential such as narcotics or any medication that contains alcohol (cough syrups).

Medications
- *Disulfiram (Antabuse):* Causes severe nausea/vomiting, headache, other unpleasant effects.
- *Naltrexone (Vivitrol):* Decreases alcohol cravings.

Korsakoff's Syndrome (Wernicke–Korsakoff Syndrome)
A complication from chronic alcohol abuse. A neurologic disorder with signs that include hypotension, visual impairment, and coma. Signs include mental confusion, ataxia, stupor, coma, and hypotension. Treated with high-dose parenteral vitamins, especially thiamine (vitamin B1).

Korsakoff's Amnesic Syndrome

A type of amnesia. Problems with acquiring (and learning) new information and retrieving older information. Symptoms include confabulation, disorientation, attention deficits, and visual impairment.

- Etiology: Chronic thiamine deficiency damages the brain permanently.

Alcoholic Anonymous (AA)

- One of the most successful methods for recovering alcoholics. Founded by Bill W. Person.
- Patient is paired with a mentor (a recovered alcoholic). Belief in a "higher power."
- Must follow a 12-step program and attend AA meetings (uses "chip" reward).
- Support group for family members and friends is called Al-Anon (Al-Anon Family Groups).
- Support group for teen children is called Alateen.

Insomnia (Sleep Disorder)

It is thought that 7 to 8 hours of sleep is the ideal. About 40 to 70 million Americans (20% of the population) suffer from either transient (less than 1 week), short-term (1–3 weeks), or chronic (greater than 3 weeks) insomnia. Insomnia in the aged occurs due to changes in sleep pattern, physical activity, health, and increased used of medications. Insomnia can manifest either as difficulty falling asleep (sleep-onset insomnia) or falling asleep but waking up during the night or too early and being unable to go back to sleep. Can have daytime drowsiness, fatigue, tension headache, irritability, and difficulty concentrating/focusing on tasks.

Risk Factors

Depression, severe anxiety, gastroesophageal reflux disease, female gender, illicit drug use, musculoskeletal illness, pain, chronic health problems, shift work, alcohol, caffeine, and nicotine. Certain medications (SSRIs, cardiac, blood pressure, allergy, steroids) can cause insomnia.

Etiology

Circadian rhythm disorders, psychic issues, mental illness, obstructive sleep apnea, restless leg syndrome, environmental factors, certain medications, idiopathic, and others.

Classifications

- *Primary insomnia (25%)*: Not caused by disease, mental illness, or environmental factors.
- *Secondary insomnia*: Caused by disease (physical, emotional, mental) or environmental factors.

Treatment Plan

- Sleep hygiene (maintain regular sleeping time, nighttime ritual, avoid caffeine/ tobacco/heavy meals before bedtime, get out of bed in 30 minutes if not asleep, use bed only for sleep and sex).
- Home or sleep lab monitoring (polysomnography) (needed to diagnose obstructive sleep apnea). After diagnosis, refer to ENT specialist (otolaryngologist).

Medications

- Over-the-counter antihistamine: Diphenhydramine (Benadryl) can cause excess sedation and confusion in the elderly. It is the most sedating antihistamine. Avoid with elderly.

Benzodiazepines/Hypnotics (Listed Under Psychotrophic Drugs)

- *Short-acting*: Alprazolam (Xanax), triazolam (Halcion), midazolam (Versed).
- *Intermediate-acting*: Lorazepam (Ativan), temazepam (Restoril).
- *Long-acting*: Diazepam (Valium), clonazepam (Klonopin), chlordiazepoxide (Librium).

Non-Benzodiazepine Hypnotics*

- Zolpidem (Ambien) for sleep-onset or inability to stay asleep.
- Eszopiclone (Lunesta) for sleep-onset or inability to stay asleep.
- Ramelteon (Rozerem) for sleep-onset insomnia (melatonin agonist).
- *Directions*: Do not take medication if unable to get from 7 to 8 hours of sleeping time.

Complementary Alternative Treatment for Insomnia

- Kava-kava (avoid mixing with alcohol, tranquilizers, hypnotics; will increase sedation). Do not give kava-kava, valerian root, or herbal supplements to children, lactating/pregnant women.
- Valerian root (sedating, also used for anxiety).
- Melatonin (also for circadian rhythm disorders such as shift work, jet lag).
- Chamomile tea.
- Meditation, yoga, Tai-Chi, acupuncture, regular exercise (avoid 4 hours before bedtime).

Smoking Cessation

- Tobacco use is the most common cause of preventable death.
- Discuss smoking cessation at every visit for patients who are smokers.
- Nicotine patches (also available as chewing gum, inhaler).
- Patient cannot smoke while on nicotine patches. Do not use with other nicotine products (e.g., gum, inhaler); patient will overdose with nicotine. Nicotine overdose can cause acute myocardial infarctions, hypertension, agitation in susceptible patients. Can be combined with bupropion (Zyban).
- Bupropion (Zyban) decreases cravings to smoke. Can be combined with nicotine products. Patients can still smoke while on bupropion. Eventually loses desire to smoke and finally quits.

✍ EXAM TIPS

- Lone GGT elevation can be a sign of occult alcohol abuse.
- AST/ALT ratio of 2.0 or higher more likely in alcoholism.
- Recognize Korsakoff's syndrome and that it is caused by chronic thiamine deficiency.
- Al-Anon is the support group for an alcoholic's family and friends.
- A person who drinks one glass of wine or one beer per day is not considered an alcoholic.
- Questions may be asked about who is most likely (or least likely) to become an alcoholic.
- Do not mix nicotine patches with nicotine gum. Do not smoke while on patches.
- Bupropion (Zyban) is for smoking cessation. Patients can smoke while on Zyban.
- Women are allowed one drink/day and men are allowed two drinks/day.

---

* Quick onset (15–30 minutes). Do not take if unable to get 7 to 8 hours of sleeping time. Adverse effects include agitation, hallucinations, nightmares, suicidal ideation. There have been cases in which a person wakes up and does their normal routines (sleep driving, eating, job) but is unable to recall the incident.

- Kava-kava and valerian root are natural supplements used for insomnia/anxiety. Do not mix with benzodiazepines or hypnotics.
- Discuss smoking cessation with patients (who are smokers) at every visit.

Anorexia Nervosa

Onset usually during adolescence. Irrational preoccupation with and intense fear of gaining weight (even if underweight). Patients tend to be secretive, perfectionistic, and self-absorbed. Marked weight loss (greater than 15% of body weight). Lanugo (face, back, and shoulders). Amenorrhea for 3 months or longer. If purging, dental enamel loss may be present. Severe food restriction or binge eating and purging. Some examples of purging are laxatives, vomiting, and excessive daily exercise.

Complications

- Osteopenia/osteoporosis: Due to prolonged estrogen depletion (from amenorrhea) and low calcium intake. Higher risk of stress fractures.
- Peripheral edema (low albumin from low protein intake).
- Cardiac complications, the most common cause of death (arrhythmias, cardiomyopathy, hypokalemia, etc.).

✍ EXAM TIPS

- Recognize how anorexic patients present (i.e., lanugo, peripheral edema, amenorrhea, weight loss greater than 10% of body weight).
- Anorexic patients are at higher risk of osteopenia/osteoporosis.
- Bupropion (Wellbutrin) is contraindicated for anorexic/bulimic patients. It increases the seizure threshold.
- Paroxetine (Paxil) has a common side effect of exectile dysfunction.
- Paroxetine has a short half-life (compared with the SSRIs) and patients need to be weaned. Do not discontinue abruptly. It is FDA Category D.
- Caution with: BPH (urinary retention), narrow-angle glaucoma, pre-existing heart disease.
- An elderly patient who is depressed (and has multiple medications) can be prescribed citalopram. Citalopram (Celexa) does have drug interactions, but less than the other SSRIs.
- TCAs: Herpetic neuralgia, migraine headache prophylaxis (not acute treatment).

📋 CLINICAL TIPS

- Patients starting to recover from depression may commit suicide (from increase in psychic energy). Monitor closely.
- If potentially suicidal, be careful when refilling or prescribing certain medications that may be fatal if patient overdoses (i.e., benzodiazepines, hypnotics, narcotics, amphetamines, TCAs, etc.). Give the smallest amount and lowest dose possible.

Abuse: All Types

Abusive behaviors are multifactorial. They may include physical, emotional, and sexual abuse, and/or neglect. They can happen at any age and during pregnancy (higher risk).

A common finding is a delay in seeking medical treatment for the injury. The pattern of the injuries is inconsistent with the history. Elderly who are most likely to be abused are those greater than 80 years old and/or frail. Children with mental, physical, or other disabilities, and stepchildren are more likely to be abused.

Types of abuse are: physical abuse, sexual abuse, emotional/psychological abuse, neglect, economic abuse, or material exploitation.

Risk Factors That Increase Likelihood of Abuse (All Types)
- Increased stress (partner/parent/caregiver).
- Alcohol/drug abuse.
- Personal history of abuse, positive family history of abuse.
- Major loss (financial, job loss, others).
- Social isolation.
- Pregnancy (domestic abuse).
- Elderly abuse.
- Frail elderly and those with dementia are more likely to be abused. About two-thirds of all elder abuse is perpetrated by family members (usually an adult child or a spouse). Most abused elderly suffer economic abuse. Only certain states have mandatory reporting of partner abuse. Be mindful of institutional abuse of elderly, children, and disabled.

Physical Exam: Abuse (All Types)
- Another health provider (witness) should be in the same room during the exam.
- Interview victim without abuser in the same room.
- Collect visual evidence of trauma via Polaroid or digital camera to document all injuries. Keep all evidence in a safe place.
- Look for spiral fractures (greenstick fracture), multiple healing fractures especially in rib area, burn marks with pattern, welts, and so forth.
- Look for signs of neglect (dirty clothes, inappropriately dressed for the weather, etc.).
- For partner abuse, focus on developing a plan for safety with the patient when appropriate. Give the patient the phone number of the crisis center and/or safe place.
- Sexually transmitted disease (STD) testing:
  - Chlamydial and GC cultures (must use cultures in addition to the Gen Probe).
  - HIV, hepatitis B, syphilis, herpes type 2.
  - Genital, throat, and anal area culture and testing must be done.
- Abused patient is very fearful and quiet when with the "abuser."

Treatment Plan
- Prophylactic treatment against several STDs (with parental consent for minors).
- Health care professionals must report actual or suspected child abuse.

Good Communication Concepts
- State things objectively. Do not be judgmental.
  Example: "You have bright red stripes on your back" instead of "It looks as if you have been whipped on the back."
- Open-ended questions are preferred.
  Example: "How can I help you?" instead of "What type of object was used to hurt your back?"
- Do not reassure patients (stops a patient from talking more about his/her problems).
  Example: "We will make sure you get help," instead of "Don't worry, everything will be fine."

- Let the patient vent his/her feelings. Do not discourage patient from talking.
  Example: "Please tell me why you feel so sad."
- Validate feelings.
  Example: "Yes, I understand your anger when someone hits you."

✎ EXAM TIPS

- Of all the SSRIs, Paxil is more likely to cause erectile dysfunction.
- There will always be a few questions on physical abuse. The questions may address physical abuse, child abuse, sexual abuse, and/or elder abuse.
- The abuser is described as a person who does not want the abused person out of sight or interviewed alone.
- The abuser typically answers all the questions for the patient and will exhibit "controlling" behaviors toward the abused patient.
- Abuse cases: Interview together and then separately.
- Any answer choice that reassures patients is always wrong.
- Delaying an action (i.e., waiting until the patient feels better, etc.) is always wrong.

Reproductive Review

III

Men's Health Review

Priapism

Male complains of a prolonged and painful erection of the penis for several hours (at least 2 to 4 hours). Males with sickle cell disease are at very high risk (6% to 45%). Other risk factors are high doses of erectile dysfunction drugs, cocaine, quadriplegia, and others. Several types of priapism. The ischemic form of priapism is a medical/surgical emergency.

Testicular Cancer

Teenage to young adult male complains of nodule, sensation of heaviness or aching, one larger testicle, and/or tenderness in one testicle. Testicular cancer can present as a new onset of a hydrocele (from tumor pressing on vessels). Usually painless and asymptomatic until metastasis. More common in White males age 15 to 30 years. Rare in African Americans.

Prostate Cancer

Older to elderly male complains of a new onset of low back pain, rectal area/perineal pain or discomfort accompanied by obstructive voiding symptoms such as weaker stream and nocturia. May be asymptomatic. More common in older males (greater than 50 years), obese males, men with a family history of prostate cancer (father, brother), and Black males.

Torsion of the Appendix Testis (Blue Dot Sign)

School-age boy complains of the abrupt onset of a blue-colored round mass located on the testicular surface. The mass resembles a "blue dot." The appendix testis is a round, small (0.03 cm), pedunculated polyp-like structure that is attached to the testicular surface (on the anterior superior area). The blue dot is caused by infarction and necrosis of the appendix testis due to torsion. More common during childhood. *Not* testicular torsion. Refer to ED.

Testicular Torsion

A 14-year-old male reports waking up at midnight or in the morning with abrupt onset of an extremely painful and swollen red scrotum. Frequently accompanied by nausea and vomiting. Affected testicle/scrotum is located higher and closer to the body than the unaffected testicle. Missing cremasteric reflex. Majority of cases (2/3) occur between the ages of 10 and 20 years.

☑ NORMAL FINDINGS

Spermatogenesis
- Ideal temperature (for sperm production) is from 1° to 2°C lower than core body temperature.
- Sperm production starts at puberty and continues for the entire lifetime of the male.
- Sperm are produced in seminiferous tubules of the testes.
- Sperm require 64 days (about 3 months) to mature.

Testes
- Cryptoorchidism (undescended testes) increases risk of testicular cancer.
- Production of testosterone/androgens is stimulated by release of luteinizing hormone.
- Spermatogenesis is stimulated by both testosterone and follicle-stimulating hormone.
- The left testicle usually hangs lower than the right.

Prostate Gland
- Heart-shaped gland that grows throughout the life cycle of the male.
- Produces prostate-specific antigen (PSA) and prostatic fluid.
- Prostatic fluid (alkaline pH) helps the sperm survive in the vagina (acidic pH).
- Up to 50% of 50-year-old males have benign prostatic hypertrophy (BPH).

Epididymis
- Coiled tubular organ that is located at the posterior aspect of the testis. Storage area for immature sperm (takes 3 months to mature). Resembles a "beret" on the upper pole of the testes.

Vas Deferens (Ductus Deferens)
- Tubular structures that transport sperm from the epididymis toward the urethra in preparation for ejaculation. These tubes are cut/clipped during a vasectomy procedure.

Cremasteric Reflex
- The testicle is elevated toward the body in response to stroking or lightly pinching the ipsilateral inner thigh (or the thigh on the same side as the testicle). Absent with testicular torsion.

Transillumination: Scrotum
- Useful for evaluating testicular swelling, mass, or bleeding.
- Direct a beam of light behind the scrotum.
- Serous fluid inside scrotum = brighter red glow (i.e., hydrocele).
- Blood or mass = dull glow to no glow (i.e., cancerous tumor).

☰ DISEASE REVIEW

Testicular Cancer

Most common tumor in males age 15 to 30 years. More common in White males.

Classic Case

Teenage to young adult male complains of nodule, sensation of heaviness or aching, one larger testicle, tenderness in one testicle. May present as a new onset of a hydrocele (from tumor pressing on vessels). Usually painless and asymptomatic until metastasis.

Objective

- Affected testicle feels "heavier" and more solid.
- May palpate a hard fixed nodule (most common site is the lower pole of the testes).
- 20% will have concomitant hydrocele.

Labs

- Ultrasound of the testicle reveals solid mass.
- *Gold standard of diagnosis:* Testicular biopsy.
- Refer to urologist for biopsy and management. Surgical removal (orchiectomy).

Testicular Torsion

When the spermatic cord becomes twisted, the testis's blood supply is interrupted. Permanent testicular damage results if not corrected within the first few hours (less than 6 hours). If not corrected within 24 hours, 100% of testicles become gangrenous and must be surgically removed. More common in males with the "bell clapper deformity." Most cases are idiopathic.

Classic Case

A 14-year-old male reports the sudden onset of severe testicular pain with an extremely swollen red scrotum. Some may have acute hydrocele (severe edema). Complains of severe nausea and vomiting. The affected testicle is higher than the normal testicle. Cremasteric reflex is missing.

Treatment Plan

- Call 911 as soon as possible.
- Preferred test in the ED is the Doppler ultrasound with color flow study.
- Treatment can be manual reduction or surgery with testicular fixation using sutures.

Prostate Cancer

Most common cancer in men (incidence). Average age of diagnosis is 71 years. Risk factors are age greater than 50 years, African American, obesity, and positive family history (first-degree relative will double the risk). Routine prostate cancer screening (digital rectal exam [DRE] with prostate specific antigen [PSA]) is not recommended (USPTF). Studies show that absolute risk reduction of prostate cancer deaths with screening is very small. Individualize, based on patient's risk factors and age.

Objective

Painless and hard fixed nodule (or indurated area) on the prostate gland on an older male that is detected by DRE.

- *Elevated PSA:* Greater than 4.0 ng/mL.
- *Diagnostic test:* Biopsy of prostatic tissue (obtained by transurethral ultrasound).

- *Screening test:* PSA level with DRE. If limited life span (less than 10 years), not recommended.

Treatment Plan

- Refer to urologist if PSA greater than 4.0 ng/mL, suspect or not sure if prostate cancer.
- Individualize screening based on risk factors. Discuss risk (bleeding, infection, impotence, procedures, and psychological trauma) versus benefits.
- Most cancers are not aggressive and are slow-growing. Watchful waiting/monitoring by urologist.
- Drug therapy with antiandrogens (Proscar), hormone blockers (i.e., Lupron), others.

BPH

Seen in 50% of males older than age 50 (up to 80% of males older than 70 years of age). Rarely seen in males younger than age 40. Rule out prostate cancer.

Classic Case

Older male complains of gradual development (years) of urinary obstructive symptoms such as weak urinary stream, postvoid dribbling, feelings of incomplete emptying, and occasional urinary retention. Nocturia very common.

Objective

- PSA is elevated (norm ranges from 0 to 4 ng/mL).
- Enlarged prostate that is symmetrical in texture and size (rubbery texture).

Medications

- *Alpha-adrenergic antagonist:* Terazosin (Hytrin) 5 mg or tamsulosin (Flomax).
- *5-Alpha-reductase inhibitors (blocks testerone):* Finasteride (Proscar).
- Duration of treatment ranges from a few months to daily for many years.
- *Avoid drugs that worsen symptoms:* Cold medications (antihistamines, decongestants), caffeine.
- *Herbal:* Saw palmetto (mild improvement for some). Does not work for everyone.
- Classify severity of BPH using the American Urological Association questionnaire.

✍ EXAM TIPS

- Proscar is an example of a 5-alpha reductase inhibitor.
- The prostate shrinks by 50% while on Proscar (so PSA has to be doubled).
- To determine effectiveness of Proscar, obtain PSA and multiply value by 2. That value should be below baseline.
- Proscar is a category X drug. Teratogenic. Should not be touched with bare hands if reproductive-aged female (adversely affects male fetus).
- Male with BPH and hypertension: Start with alpha-blocker (Hytrin) first. Works by relaxing smooth muscles on prostate gland and bladder neck.

Chronic Bacterial Prostatitis

Chronic (greater than 6 weeks) infection of the prostate. Some report a history of acute urinary tract infection (UTI) or of acute bacterial prostatitis. Some men are asymptomatic. More common in older males. Caused most commonly by *Escherichia coli* and *Proteus*. Nonbacterial prostatitis has same symptoms but is culture negative.

Classic Case

Elderly male with history of several weeks of suprapubic or perineal discomfort that is accompanied by irritative voiding symptoms such as dysuria, nocturia, and frequency.
Not accompanied by systemic symptoms. Some men are asymptomatic.

Objective

- Prostate may feel normal or slightly "boggy" to palpation. Not tender.
- *UA:* Normal (unless patient has cystitis).
- *Urine mixed with prostatic fluid:* Positive for *E. coli.*

Lab

Urine and prostatic fluid cultures. Uses three tubes: first, urethra; second, bladder; third, urine with prostatic fluid (obtained after prostatic massage). PSA will be elevated (inflammation).

Medications

- Trimethoprim-sulfamethoxazole (Bactrim) PO BID for 4 to 6 weeks (if sensitive).
- Some prefer ofloxacin (Floxin) BID or levofloxacin (Levaquin) daily for 4 to 6 weeks.

Acute Prostatitis

Acute infection of the prostate. Infection ascends into urinary tract. Most common non-sexually transmitted cause is *Enterobacter*. If condition occurs in a male under 35 years old, it is treated like gonococcal or chlamydial urethritis.

Classic Case

Adult to older male complains of sudden onset of high fever and chills with suprapubic and/or perineal pain/discomfort. Pain sometimes radiates to back or rectum. Acompanied by UTI symptoms such as dysuria, frequency, nocturia with cloudy urine. DRE reveals extremely tender prostate that is warm and boggy.

Objective

- Gently examine prostate. Prostate will be extremely tender and warm.
- *Warning:* Vigorous palpation and massage of an infected prostate can cause septicemia.

Labs

- *CBC:* Leukocytosis with shift to the left (presence of band cells).
- *UA:* Large amount of white blood cells (pyuria), hematuria.
- *Urine C&S* (if possible, also obtain urine after gentle prostatic massage).

Medications

- Based on age and presumptive organism:
  - Age < 35, treat with ceftriaxone 250 mg IM and doxycycline 100 mg BID x 10 days.
  - Age > 35 or unlikely sexual transmission, treatment with ciprofloxacin or ofloxacin PO twice a day (BID) or levofloxacin (Levaquin) PO daily for 4 to 6 weeks.
- *Others:* Levofloxacin (Levaquin) PO daily, Bactrim PO BID.
- Antipyretics, stool softener without laxative (Colace), sitz baths, hydration.
- Refer if septic or toxic.

✍ EXAM TIPS

- Become familiar with the duration of treatment for acute versus chronic bacterial prostatitis.
- Learn to distinguish between chronic prostatitis and acute prostatitis.
- Chronic: Gradual onset; prostate can feel normal (older males).
- Acute prostitis presents as: Sudden onset; prostate swollen and very tender (younger males).

Acute Bacterial Epididymitis

Bacteria ascends up the urethra (urethritis) and reaches epididymis, causing an infection. Also known as bacterial epididymo-orchitis. Rule out testicular torsion (can mimic condition).

- Sexually active males less than 35 years old.
  - More likely to be infected with a sexually transmitted disease (chlamydia, GC).
- Males more than 35 years old.
  - Usually due to gram-negative *E. coli.*

Classic Case

Adult to older male complains of acute onset of a swollen red scrotum that hurts. Accompanied by unilateral testicular tenderness with urethral discharge. Scrotum is swollen and erythematous with induration of the posterior epididymis. Sometimes may be accompanied by a hydrocele, and signs and symptoms of UTI. Some will have systemic symptoms such as fever.

- *Discharge:* Green-colored purulent or serous clear (chlamydia, viral, chemical, others).
- *Positive Prehn's sign:* Relief of pain with scrotal elevation.

Labs

- *CBC:* Leukocytosis.
- *UA:* Leukocytes (pyuria), blood (hematuria), nitrites.
- Urine C&S and urine for Gram stain.
- Testing for GC and chlamydia (urine or Gen-Probe).

Medications

- Age less than 35 years, give doxycycline PO BID × 10 days plus ceftriaxone 250 mg IM × one dose. Do not forget to treat sex partner.
- Older male (greater than 35 years), give ofloxacin (Floxin) 300 mg PO × 10 days or levofloxacin (Levaquin) 500 mg PO 7 to 10 days.
- Treat pain with NSAIDs (ibuprofen, naproxen) or acetaminophen with codeine (severe pain).
- Scrotal elevation and scrotal ice packs. Bed rest for few days.
- Stool softeners (i.e., docusate sodium or Colace) if constipated.
- Refer to ED if septic, severe intractable pain, abscessed, others.

Erectile Dysfunction

Inability to produce an erection firm enough to perform sexual intercourse. Vascular insufficiency, neuropathy (diabetics), medications (selective serotonin reuptake inhibitors, beta-blockers), smoking, alcohol, hypogonadism. May be psychic causation or mixture of both.

- *Organic cause:* inability to have an erection under any circumstance. Due to neurovascular or vascular damage.

- *Psychiatric cause:* Spontaneously has early morning erections or can achieve a firm erection with masturbation.

Medications
- *First line:* Phosphodiesterase type 5 inhibitors drug class.
- Take Viagra and Levitra on an empty stomach. Food and fats delays action.
- Sildenafil citrate (Viagra) 25/50/100 mg; take one dose 30 to 60 minutes before sex. Use only one dose every 24 hours.
- Vardenafil (Levitra); take one dose 30 to 60 minutes before sex. Duration 4 hours.
- Taladafil (Cialis) 5 to 20 mg; take 2 hours before sex. Duration up to 36 hours.
- *Adverse effects:* Headache, facial flushing, dizziness, hypotension, nasal congestion, priapism.
- *Other forms of treatment:* Intracavernous injections (alprostadil or Caverject).

Contraindications
- Concomitant nitrates. Caution with alpha-blockers, recent post-myocardial infarction, post-CVA, major surgery, or any condition where exertion is contraindicated.

Peyronie's Disease
- An inflammatory and localized disorder of the penis that results in fibrotic plaques on the tunica albuginea. Results in penile pain that primarily occurs during erection, palpable nodules, and penile deformity (crooked penile erections). May resolve spontaneously or worsen over time.

Labs
- None. Clinical diagnosis.

Plan
- Refer to urologist.

Other Conditions
Balanitis
- Candidal infection of the glans penis; more common in uncircumcised men, diabetics, and/or immunocompromised males. Treated with topical OTC azole creams. If partner has candidiasis, treat at the same time.

Cryptoorchidism
- Undescended testicles that remain in the abdominal cavity. Can affect both or only one testicle. Markedly increases the risk of testicular cancer. Usually corrected during infancy.

Phimosis
- Foreskin cannot be pushed back from the glans penis because of edema; usually seen in neonates.

Varicocele
- Varicose veins in scrotal sac (feels like "bag of worms"). New-onset varicocele can signal testicular tumor (20%) or a mass that is impeding venous drainage. Order an ultrasound of the scrotum.

17

Women's Health Review

⚠ DANGER SIGNALS

Ectopic Pregnancy

Sexually active female who has not had a period (or had period but light to scant bleeding) in 6 to 7 weeks complains of lower abdominal/pelvic pain or cramping (intermittent, persistent, or acute). Pain worsens when supine or with jarring. If ruptured, pelvic pain worsens and can be referred to the right shoulder. Medical history of pelvic inflammatory disease (PID), tubal ligation, or previous ectopic pregnancy. Leading cause of death for women in the United States in the first trimester of pregnancy.

Dominant Breast Mass/Breast Cancer

Middle-aged to older female with a dominant mass on one breast that feels hard and is irregular in shape. The mass is attached to the skin/surrounding breast tissue (or is immobile). Among the most common locations are the upper outer quadrants of the breast (the tail of Spence). Skin changes may be seen, such as the "peau d'orange" (localized area of skin that resembles an orange peel), dimpling, and retraction. Mass is painless or may be accompanied by serous or bloody discharge. The nipple may be displaced or become fixed.

Paget's Disease of the Breast (Ductal Carcinoma In Situ)

Older female reports a history of a chronic scaly red-colored rash resembling eczema on the nipple (or nipple and areola) that does not heal. Some women complain of itching. The skin lesion slowly enlarges and evolves to include crusting, ulceration, and/or bleeding on the nipple.

Inflammatory Breast Cancer

Recent or acute onset of a red, swollen, and warm area in the breast of a younger woman. Can mimic mastitis. Often, there is no distinct lump on the affected breast. Symptoms develop quickly (few weeks to months). The skin may be pitted (peau d'orange) or appear bruised. More common in African Americans. A rare but very aggressive form of breast cancer (1% to 5%).

Ovarian Cancer

Older women with complaints of vague symptoms such as abdominal bloating and discomfort, low-back pain, pelvic pain, urinary frequency, and constipation (e.g., frequently blamed on benign conditions). By the time it is diagnosed, the cancer has already metastasized. If metastases, symptoms depend on area affected. Symptoms may be bone pain, abdominal pain, headache, blurred vision, others. Ovarian cancer is rarely diagnosed during the early stage of the disease (before metastasis). It is the fifth most common cancer among women in the United States.

☑ NORMAL FINDINGS

Breasts

- Breast development starts in Tanner Stage II (breast buds) and ends at Stage V.
- During puberty, it is common for both girls and boys (gynecomastia) to have tender and asymmetrical breasts. One breast may be larger than the other breast.
- The upper outer quadrant of the breasts (called the "tail of Spence") is where the majority of breast cancer is located.
- Very high risks factors for breast cancer includes the *BRCA1* or *BRCA2* gene mutation or a history of radiation therapy to the chest between the ages of 10 and 30 years. (Risk factors for breast cancer in men are cryptorchidism, positive family history, others.)
- The diagnostic test for breast cancer (or any type of cancer) is the tissue biopsy.

Cervix

- A cervical ectropion is benign. Adolescents have large ectropion (immature cervix).
- An ectropion looks like bright red tissue with an irregular surface on top of the os.
- If an ectropion is present, it is important to sample the surface of the transformation zone area (or the transitional zone) when performing a Pap smear.
- The transformation zone (or the squamocolumnar junction) is an area where abnormal cells are more likely to develop (due to metaplasia).

Uterus

- Fibroids (uterine leiomyoma or myoma) can enlarge the uterus. The symptoms are heavy menstrual bleeding (menorrhagia), pelvic pain or cramping, and bleeding between periods.

Ovaries

- The ovaries produce estrogen, progesterone, and a small amount of testosterone (androgens).
- Females with polycystic ovarian syndrome (PCOS) have multiple cysts on their ovaries and high androgen levels (causes acne, hirsutism, oligomenorrhea).

BENIGN VARIANTS

- Supernumerary nipples form a V-shaped line on both sides of the chest down the abdomen and are symmetrically distributed.
- Fibroids (uterine leiomyoma/myoma) are usually benign. Can cause heavy menstrual bleeding and cramping, pelvic pain, and urgency (due to fibroid pressing on the bladder).
- On rare occasions, fibroids can be malignant and cause uterine cancer (leiomyosarcoma).

MENSTRUAL CYCLE

This example is based on a perfect 28-day menstrual cycle.

Follicular Phase (Days 1 to 14)

Estrogen is the predominant hormone during the first 2 weeks of the menstrual cycle. It stimulates the development and growth of the endometrial lining. Follicle-stimulating hormone (FSH) from the anterior pituitary stimulates the follicles (or the "eggs") into producing estrogen. Also known as the proliferative phase.

Midcycle (Day 14): Ovulatory Phase

Luteinizing hormone (LH) is secreted by the anterior pituitary gland, which induces ovulation of the dominant follicle.

Luteal Phase (Days 14 to 28)

Progesterone is the predominant hormone during the last 2 weeks of the cycle. It is produced by the corpus luteum. Helps to stabilize the endometrial lining.

Menstruation

If not pregnant, both estrogen and progesterone fall drastically, inducing menses. Low hormone levels stimulate the hypothalamus, then the anterior pituitary (FSH), and the cycle starts again.

Fertile Time Period

Starts about 5 days before and 1 to 2 days after ovulation (day 14 in a perfect 28-day cycle).

At this time of the menstrual cycle, there are copious amounts of clear mucus that feels thin and elastic in the vagina. It is a sign that is used in the cervical mucus method of birth control.

In contrast, the vaginal discharge is scant, whitish, and thick during the first week of the menstrual cycle.

LABORATORY PROCEDURES

Pap Smears and Liquid-Based Cervical Cytology

Both are used as screening tests. High false-negative rate of 20% to 45%. The liquid-based Pap smear (ThinPrep) is now more popular in the United States than the conventional Pap smear kit.

Diagnostic test for cervical cancer: Biopsy of the cervix (cervical biopsy).

Instructions
- Do not perform a Pap test or liquid-based cytology during the menstrual period.
- The best time to perform a Pap test is between 10 and 20 days after the last menses.
- About 2 days before the Pap test, tell patient to avoid douching and vaginal foams/medicines.

Liquid-Based Cervical Cytology (ThinPrep)

Insert the broom-shaped plastic brush into the cervical os and rotate a few times. Place the brush in the liquid medium and swish gently. Remove brush and cover with the plastic cap. The Pap is read by a computer and abnormals are reviewed by a cytologist and/or pathologist.

Conventional Pap Smear

Insert the brush into the cervical os and twist gently. Use wooden spatula to scrape cervical surface. Smear the glass slide with both samples. Spray the liquid fixative on the glass slide.

The Bethesda System

Baseline Pap at age 21 years and repeat every 3 years. Recent USPTF guidelines discourage Pap testing for females younger than age 21 years (even if sexually active). Cervical cancer is rare before the age of 21 years. Starting at age 30 through to age 65, another screening option is a Pap smear with HPV co-testing every 5 years. Women who had a hysterectomy with removal of the cervix (and no history of cervical cancer or high-grade lesion), can discontinue Pap testing (USPTF, March 2012).

- Satisfactory specimen only if both squamous epithelial cells and endocervical cells are present.
- If endocervical cells are missing, repeat Pap (incomplete).

Endometrial Cells

- If present, refer for endometrial biopsy to rule out endometrial cancer.

Atypical Squamous Cells of Undetermined Significance

- Age 20 years or younger: Repeat Pap smear in 12 months.
- Age 21 years or older: Order Pap smear with "reflex" HPV DNA testing. If Pap abnormal, HPV strain testing is done automatically by the lab (the "reflex").
- Oncogenic HPV types (#16 and #18): refer for colposcopy and cervical biopsy.

Atypical Glandular Cells of Undetermined Significance

- Refer for endometrial biopsy (endometrial and endocervical biopsy).

Low-Grade Squamous Intraepithelial Lesions and High-Grade Squamous Epithelial Lesions

- HPV testing (if not done). Refer for colposcopy and biopsy.

HPV DNA Test

- HPV types 16 and 18 together cause 70% of all cases of cervical cancer in the United States (National Cancer Institute, 2011).
- Gardasil and Cervarix are FDA-approved vaccines that are very effective in preventing persistent infections with the oncogenic HPV strains.

Potassium Hydroxide Slide

Useful for helping with the diagnosis of fungal infections (hair, nails, skin). Potassium hydroxide (KOH) works by causing lysis of the squamous cells, which makes it easier to see hyphae and spores.

Whiff Test

A test for bacterial vaginosis (BV). A positive result occurs when a strong, fishlike odor is released after one to two drops of KOH are added to the slide (or a cotton swab soaked with discharge).

Tzanck Smear

Used as an adjunct for evaluating herpetic infections (oral, genital, skin). A positive smear will show large abnormal nuclei in the squamous epithelial cells. Not commonly used.

Gram Stain

Time-consuming and rarely done in clinical area. Gram-stained white blood cells are examined for *Neisseria gonorrhoeae* (gram-negative bacteria) under high power.

ORAL CONTRACEPTIVES

Combined Oral Contraceptives

Dosed Monophasic Pills

- *Loestrin FE 1/20:* 21 consecutive days of estrogen/progesterone (same dose daily). For the last 7 days of the cycle, the placebo pills contain iron supplementation (7 days of iron pills).

Triphasic Pills

- *Ortho Tri-Cyclen:* Contains 21 days of active pills and 7 days of placebo pills. The dose of hormones varies weekly for 3 weeks ("tri-phasic"). Progestin used is norgestimate. Indicated for acne.

Extended-Cycle Pills

- *Seasonale:* Contains 84 consecutive days (3 months) of estrogen/progesterone with a 7-day pill-free interval. This method typically results in 4 periods per year although breakthrough bleeding is not uncommon.

Ethinyl Estradiol and Drospirenone

- *Yaz (24 active pills and 4 placebo pills)/Yasmin:* Uses drospirenone (a spironolactone analog) as the progestin component. Consider for women with acne, PCOS, hirsuitism, or premenstrual dysphoric disorder (PMDD). Higher risk of DVT and hyperkalemia.
- *Labs:* Check the potassium level if patient is on an angiotensin-converting enzyme inhibitor (ACEI), angiotensin receptor blocker (ARB), or potassium-sparing diuretics.

Progestin-Only Pills

Safe for breastfeeding women. Also known as the "minipill." Use on day 1 of menstrual cycle.

- *Micronor:* Take one pill daily at about the same time each day (each pack contains 28 pills). Start taking pill on day 1 of menstrual cycle.

Absolute Contraindications

- Any condition (past or present) that increases the risk of blood clotting
  - History of thrombophlebitis or thromboembolic disorders (i.e., DVT)
  - Genetic coagulation defects such as factor V Leiden disease
  - Major surgery with prolonged immobilization
- Smoker over the age of 35 years
  - Also considered a relative contraindication since women younger than 35 years who smoke can have the pill (if no other contraindications exist)

- Any condition that increases the risk of strokes
  - Headaches with focal neurological symptoms (i.e., basilar migraines)
  - History of CVA and transient ischemic attacks (TIAs)
  - Hypertension
  - Migraine headache with aura or with focal neurologic symptoms (basilar migraines)
- Inflammation and/or acute infections of the liver with elevated liver function tests (LFTs)
  - In acute infection or inflammation of the liver (i.e., mononucleosis) with elevated LFTs, estrogen is contraindicated.
  - When LFTs are back to normal, can go back on birth control pills
  - Hepatic adenomas or carcinomas
  - Cholestatic jaundice of pregnancy
- Known or suspected cardiovascular disease
  - Coronary artery disease (CAD)
  - Diabetes with vascular component
- Some reproductive system conditions or cancers
  - Known or suspected pregnancy
  - Undiagnosed genital bleeding
  - Breast, endometrial, or ovarian cancer (or any estrogen-dependent cancer)

Absolute Contraindications Mnemonic: "My CUPLETS"

My Migraines with focal neurologic aura
C   CAD or CVA
U   Undiagnosed genital bleeding
P   Pregnant or suspect pregnancy
L   Liver tumor or active liver disease
E   Estrogen-dependent tumor
T   Thrombus or emboli
S   Smoker age 35 or older

Relative Contraindications

- Migraine headaches
  - Migraine with or without aura is a relative contraindication
  - Migraines with focal neurological findings (basilar migraines mimic TIAs) are an absolute contraindication due to increased risk of stroke
- Smoker below age of 35 years
- Fracture or cast on lower extremities
- Severe depression
- Hyperlipidemia

Advantages of the Pill (After 5 or More Years of Use)

- Ovarian cancer and endometrial cancers (decreased by 40 to 50%)
- Decreased incidence of:
  - Dysmenorrhea and cramps (decrease in prostaglandins)
  - PID (due to thickened cervical mucus plug)
  - Iron-deficiency anemia (less blood loss from lighter periods)
  - Acne and hirsutism (lower levels of androgenic hormones)
  - Ovarian cysts (due to suppression of ovulation)
  - Heavy and/or irregular periods (due to suppression of ovaries)

New Prescriptions

- There are two methods of starting the first pill pack (rule out pregnancy first).
- All patients should be instructed to use "back-up" (condoms) in the first 2 weeks during the first pill pack.
  - "Sunday Start": Take first pill on the first Sunday during the menstrual period.
  - "Day One Start": Take the first pill during the first day of the menstrual period.
- Follow-up: Within 2 to 3 months to check BP and for side effects and patient's questions.

Oral Contraceptive Pill Problems

Unscheduled Bleeding (Spotting)

Term used for menstrual bleeding that occurs out of usual cycle. The first 3 weeks (21 days) of pills contain active hormones (estrogen/progesterone).

During the fourth week (the last 7 days), the pills are hormone free (when the period occurs).

- Educate patient that she may have spotting/light bleeding during the first few weeks after starting birth control pills.
- Discourage patient from switching to another pill brand during the first 3 months because of spotting. Advise patient that most cases resolve within 3 months.

Menstrual Cramps

Menstrual cramps are treated with non-steroidal anti-inflammatory drugs (NSAIDs), which decrease menstrual cramp pain and bleeding by suppressing prostaglandins. Endometriosis is associated with heavy menstrual periods (menorrhagia) with severe cramping in younger women.

- *Mefenamic acid (Ponstel):* One capsule every 6 hours for pain as needed.
- *Naproxen (Aleve):* One enteric-coated tablet every 6 to 8 hours as needed.
- *Prescription-strength naproxen sodium (Anaprox, Naprosyn):* One tablet BID as needed.

Missing Consecutive Days of Oral Contraceptive Pills

Missed 1 Day

- Take two pills now and continue with same pill pack ("doubling up").

Missed 2 Consecutive Days

- Take two pills the next 2 days to catch up and finish the birth control pill pack (use condoms for the current pill cycle).

Drug Interactions of Oral Contraceptives

These drugs can decrease the efficacy of oral contraceptives. Advise patients to use alternative form of birth control (condoms) when taking these drugs and for one pill cycle afterwards.

- *Anticonvulsants:* Phenobarbital, phenytoin.
- *Antifungals:* Griseofulvin (Fulvicin), itraconazle (Sporanox), ketoconazole (Nizoral).
- *Certain antibiotics:* Ampicillin, tetracyclines, rifampin.
- *St. John's wort:* May cause breakthrough bleeding (BTB).

Emergency Contraception ("Morning-After Pill")

Rule out preexisting pregnancy first. Effective up to 72 hours after unprotected sex. Most effective if taken within the first 24 hours.

Progesterone Only (Plan B, Levonorgestrel 0.75 mg Tabs)

- Effective up to 89%.
- Oral contraceptive pills with levonorgestrel (Ovral, Triphasil, others) in high doses.
- Take first dose as soon as possible (no later than 72 hours after). Take the second dose 12 hours after the first. Using birth control pills for emergency contraception causes more vomiting than Plan B (due to high estrogen content). If vomits tablets within 1 hour, repeat dose.
- Advise patient that if she does not have a period in next 3 weeks, she should return for follow-up to rule out pregnancy.

Pill Danger Signs (Table 17.1)

Thromboembolic events can happen in any organ of the body. These signs indicate a possible thromboembolic event. Advise patient to report these or to call 911 if symptoms of ACHES:

- **A**bdominal pain
- **C**hest pain
- **H**eadaches
- **E**ye problems; change in vision
- **S**evere leg pain.

Oral Contraceptive Pills

- Traditional oral contraceptive pills have 21 days of "active" pills and 7 days of placebo pills.
- The last 7 days are the "hormone-free" days. The menstrual period usually starts within 2 to 3 days after the last active pill was taken (from very low levels of estrogen/progesterone).
- Some brands of birth control pills (e.g., Loestrin FE) contain iron during the last 7 days of the pill cycle (instead of a placebo pill). The last 7 days (hormone-free) of the pill cycle are there to reinforce the habit of daily pill-taking.
- For the *first* pill cycle, advise patient to use "back-up" (an alternative form of birth control).
- All the COCs, the patch, and the NuvaRing contain both estrogen and progesterone (i.e., levonorgestrel, norethindrone, desogestrel, others).
- The preferred birth control pill for breastfeeding women is the progestin-only pills or the "mini pill" (e.g., Microno, Nor-QD). Side effects includes spotting and irregular menses.

Table 17.1 Oral Contraceptive Danger Signs

Complaints	Possible Cause
Chest pain (an acute MI)	Blood clot in a coronary artery
Severe headache	Stroke, TIA
Weakness on one side of the body	Ischemic stroke caused by a blood clot in the brain
Visual changes in one eye	Blood clot in the retinal artery of the affected eye
Abdominal pain	Ischemic pain of the mesenteric area caused by a blood clot
Lower leg pain (DVT)	Blood clot on a deep vein of the leg

- Yaz or Yasmin contains estrogen and drospirenone. Has a higher risk of blood clots, stroke, heart attacks, and hyperkalemia.
- The contraceptive patch (i.e., Ortho Evra) results in higher levels of estrogen exposure compared to COCs (higher risk of blood clots, DVT).
- The estrogen in COCs can elevate blood pressure. Check patient's BP before and 2 to 4 weeks afterward.

OTHER CONTRACEPTIVE METHODS

Intrauterine Device

The second most commonly used method of contraception in the world (female sterilization is the first). Paragard is copper-bearing (effective up to 10 years) and Mirena contains the hormone levonorgestrel, which decreases vaginal bleeding. Mirena intrauterine device (IUD) is effective up to 5 years and is slightly more effective than copper-bearing IUDs.

Contraindications
- Active PID or history of PID within the past year
- Suspected or with STD or pregnant
- Uterine or cervical abnormality (e.g., bicornate uterus)
- Undiagnosed vaginal bleeding or uterine/cervical cancer
- History of ectopic pregnancy

Increased Risk
- Endometrial and pelvic infections (first few months after insertion only)
- Perforation of the uterus
- Heavy or prolonged menstrual periods

Education
- Educate patient to check for missing or shortened string periodically, especially after each menstrual period. If the patient or clinician does not feel the string, order a pelvic ultrasound.

Depo-Provera (6% Typical Failure Rate)

Each dose by injection lasts 3 months. Check for pregnancy before starting dose. Start in first 5 days of cycle (day 1–5) because females are less likely to ovulate at these times. Women on Depo-Provera for at least 1 year (or longer) have amenorrhea because of severe uterine atrophy from lack of estrogen. Do not recommend to women who want to become pregnant in 12 to 18 months. Causes delayed return of fertility. It takes up to 1 year for most women to start ovulating.
- *Black Box Warning:* Avoid long-term use (more than 2 years). Increases risk of osteopenia/osteoporosis that may not be fully reversible. Using Depo-Provera for more than 2 years is discouraged.

History of Anorexia Nervosa
Consider testing for osteopenia/osteoporosis (dual-energy x-ray absorptiometry [DXA] scan). Avoid using Depo-Provera in this population because it will further increase their risk of osteopenia/osteoporosis. Recommend calcium with vitamin D and weight-bearing exercises for patients who are on this medicine.

Diaphragm With Contraceptive Gel and the Cervical Cap (13% Failure Rate)

- The diaphragm must be used with spermicidal gel. After intercourse, leave diaphragm inside vagina for at least 6 to 8 hours (can remain inside vagina up to 24 hours).
- Need additional spermicide before every act of intercourse. Apply the spermicidal foam/gel inside the vagina without removing the diaphragm.
- The cervical cap (Pretif cap) can be worn up to 72 hours. Compared with the diaphragm, the Prentif cap may cause abnormal cervical cellular change (abnormal Pap).

Increased Risk
- UTIs and toxic shock syndrome (rare).

Condoms
Male Condoms (18% Failure Rate)
- More effective than the female condom.

Female Condoms (21% Failure Rate)
- Do not use with any oil-based lubricants, creams, and so on.

Nuvaring (9% Failure Rate)

- Plastic cervical ring that contains etonogestrel and ethinyl lestradiol and is left inside the vagina for 3 weeks, then removed for 1 week (has period). Educate patient on how to apply and remove (the ring should fit snugly around cervix). Absolute and relative contraindications for combined estrogen-progesterone method of contraception are the same as oral contraceptives.

Ortho Evra Contraceptive Patch (9% Failure Rate)

- Higher risk of VTE (releases higher levels of estrogen) compared to oral contraceptive pills. Absolute and relative contraindications for combined estrogen-progesterone method of contraception are the same as oral contraceptives.

Contraceptive Implants (<1% Failure Rate)

- Contains long-acting form of progestin (etonorgestrel). Results in amenorrhea, which is reversible when the implants are removed. May take a few weeks to 12 months to ovulate. Thin plastic rods are inserted on the inner aspect of the upper arm subdermally.
- Norplant II (2 rods) is effective up to 5 years. Implanon (now known as Nexplanon) (1 rod) is effective for up to 3 years.

:☰ DISEASE REVIEW

Fibrocystic Breast

Monthly hormonal cycle induces breast tissue to become engorged and painful. Symptoms occur 2 weeks before the onset of menses (luteal phase) and are at their worst right before the menstrual cycle. Resolves after menses start. Commonly starts in women in their 30s.

Classic Case
Adult to middle-aged woman complains of the cyclic onset of bilateral breast tenderness and breast lumps that start from a few days (up to 2 weeks) before her period for many years. Once menstruation starts, the tenderness disappears and the size of breast lumps decreases. During breast examination, the breast lumps are tender and feel rubbery, and are mobile to touch. Denies dominant mass, skin changes, nipple discharge, or enlarged nodes.

Objective
- Multiple mobile and rubbery cystic masses on both breasts.
- Both breasts have symmetrical findings.

Treatment Plan
- Stop caffeine intake. Vitamin E and evening primrose capsules daily.
- Wear bras with good support.
- *Refer:* Dominant mass, skin changes, fixed mass.

Polycystic Ovary Syndrome (PCOS)
- Hormonal abnormality marked by anovulation, infertility, excessive androgen production, and insulin resistance.

Classic Case
Obese teen or young adult complains of excessive facial and body hair (hirsutism 70%), bad acne, and amenorrhea or infrequent periods (oligomenorrhea). Dark thick hair (terminal hair) is seen on the face, cheek, and beard areas.

Treatment Plan
- Transvaginal ultrasound: Enlarged ovaries with multiple small follicles (sizes vary).
- Serum testosterone, DHEAs, and androstenedione are elevated. FSH levels normal or low.
- Fasting blood glucose and 2-hour oral glucose tolerance test (OGTT) are abnormal.

Medications
- Low-dose oral contraceptives to suppress ovaries.
- Spironolactone to decrease and control hirsutism.
- Provera tablets 10 mg daily for 7 to 10 days (repeat every 2 months to induce menses).
- Metformin (Glucophage) used to induce ovulation (if desires pregnancy). Warn reproductive-aged diabetic females (who do not want to become pregnant) to use birth control.
- Weight loss reduces androgen and insulin levels.

Complications
PCOS patients are at increased risk for:
- Coronary heart disease (CHD)
- Type 2 diabetes mellitus and metabolic syndrome
- Cancer of the breast and endometrium
- Central obesity
- Infertility

VULVOVAGINAL INFECTIONS

Candida Vaginitis

Overgrowth of *Candida albicans* yeast in the vulva/vagina. Considered as normal vaginal flora, but can also be pathogenic. Diabetics, HIV-positive, on antibiotics (i.e., amoxicillin), or any type of immunosuppression are at higher risk. (The male penis can also be infected [balanitis].)

Classic Case

Adult female presents with complaints of white cheese-like ("curdlike") vaginal discharge accompanied by severe vulvovaginal pruritus, swelling, and redness (inflammatory reaction). May complain of external pruritus of the vulva and vagina.

Labs

Wet Smear Microscopy

- Swipe cotton swab with vaginal discharge in the middle of a glass slide.
- Add a few drops of normal saline (to the discharge).
- Cover the sample with a cover slip and examine it under the microscope (set it at high power).
- *Findings:* Pseudohyphae and spores with a large number of white blood cells (WBCs).

Medications

- Miconazole (Monistat), clotrimazole (Gyne-Lotrimin) for 7 days (over the counter).
- *Prescription:* Diflucan 100 mg tab × 1 dose, terconazole (Terazol-3) vaginal cream/ suppository.
- If patient is on an antibiotic such as amoxicillin, recommend daily yogurt or lactobacillus pills.

Bacterial Vaginosis (BV)

Caused by an overgrowth of anaerobic bacteria in the vagina. Risk factors include sexual activity, new or multiple sex partners, and douching. Not an STD. Therefore, sexual partner does not need treatment.

Pregnant women with BV are at higher risk for intrauterine infections and premature labor.

Classic Case

Sexually active female complains of an unpleasant and fishlike vaginal odor that is worse after intercourse (if no condom is used). Vaginal discharge is copious and has milk-like consistency. Speculum examination reveals off-white to light gray discharge coating the vaginal walls. There is no vulvar or vaginal redness or irritation (vaginal anaerobic bacteria does not cause inflammation).

Treatment Plan

Wet Smear Microscopy

- *Findings:* Clue cells and very few WBCs. May see *Mobiluncus* bacteria (mobile bacteria).
- *Clue cells:* Made up of squamous epithelial cells with large amount of bacteria coating the surface that obliterates the edges of the squamous epithelial cells.

Whiff Test
- Apply one drop of KOH to a cotton swab that is soaked with vaginal discharge.
- *Positive:* A strong "fishy" odor is released.

Vaginal pH
- Alkaline vaginal pH >4.5. Normal vaginal pH is between 4.0 and 4.5 (acidic).

Medications
- Metronidazole (Flagyl) BID × 7 days or vaginal gel at HS (bedtime) × 5 days.
- Watch for disulfuram (Antabuse) effect if combined with alcohol (severe nausea, headache, etc.).
- Clindamycin (Cleocin) cream at HS × 7 days.
- Oil-based creams can weaken condoms.
- Sex partners: Treatment not recommended by the CDC because not an STD.
- Abstain from sexual intercourse until treatment is done.

Trichomonas Vaginitis (Trichomoniasis)

Unicellular protozoan parasite with flagella that infects genitourinary tissue (both males and females). Infection causes inflammation (pruritus, burning, and irritation) of vagina/urethra.

Classic Case
Adult female complains of very pruritic, reddened vulvovaginal area. May complain of dysuria. Copious grayish-green and bubbly vaginal discharge. Most males and sex partner may have same symptoms (urethritis) or maybe asymptomatic.

Objective
"Strawberry cervix" from small points of bleeding on cervical surface (punctate hemorrhages). Swollen and reddened vulvar and vaginal area. Vaginal pH >5.0.

Treatment Plan
Microscopy (use low power): Mobile unicellular organisms with flagella (flagellates) and a large amount of WBCs.

Medications
- Metronidazole (Flagyl) 2 g PO × 1 dose (preferred) or metronidazole 500 mg BID × 7 days.
- Treat sexual partner because trichomoniasis is considered an STI. Avoid sex until both partners complete treatment.

Atrophic Vaginitis

Chronic lack of estrogen in estrogen-dependent tissue of the urogenital tract; results in atrophic changes in the vulva and vagina of menopausal women.

Classic Case
Menopausal female complains of vaginal dryness, itching, and pain with sexual intercourse (dyspareunia). Complains of a great deal of discomfort with speculum examinations (i.e., Pap smears).

Pap smear result is "abnormal" secondary to atrophic changes.

Table 17.2 Vaginal Disorders

Type	Signs/Symptoms	Lab Results
Bacterial vaginosis	"Fishlike" vaginal odor; profuse milk-like discharge that coats the vaginal vault Not itchy/vulva not red Overgrowth of anaerobes	Clue cells Whiff test: positive pH >4.5 alkaline
Trichomonas vaginitis	"Strawberry cervix" Bubbly discharge Vulvovagina red/irritated	Mobile protozoa with flagella Numerous WBCs
Candidal vaginitis	Cheesy or curd-like white discharge Vulvovagina red/irritated	*Pseudohyphae*, spores, numerous WBCs
Atrophic vaginitis	Scant to no discharge Less rugae, vaginal color pale. Dyspareunia (painful intercourse). May bleed slightly during speculum examination (if not on hormones)	Atrophic changes on Pap smear test Elevated FSH and LH

Objective
Atrophic labia with decreased rugae; dry, pale pink color to vagina.

Treatment Plan
- If Pap is mildly abnormal (atrophic changes), consider temporary use of topical estrogen vaginal cream for a few weeks and repeat Pap smear.
- Topical estrogens (e.g., Premarin Cream). Need progesterone supplementation (if intact uterus) if using long term to decrease risk of endometrial hyperplasia.

Osteoporosis

A gradual loss of bone density secondary to estrogen deficiency and other metabolic disorders. Most common in older women (White or Asian descent) who are thin and with small body frames, especially if positive family history. Treat postmenopausal women (or men aged 50 years or older) who have osteoporosis (T-score –2.5 or less) or history of hip or vertebral fracture.

Other risk groups include:
- Patients on chronic steroids (severe asthma, autoimmune disorders, etc.) are at high risk for glucocorticoid-induced osteoporosis.
- Rule out osteoporosis in older men on chronic steroids, especially if accompanied by other risk factors (lower testosterone, small frame, thin, White or Asian).
- Androgen deficiency, hypogonadism (low testosterone levels).
- Anorexia nervosa and bulimia.
- Gastric bypass, celiac disease, hyperthyroidism, ankylosing spondylitis, rheumatoid arthritis (RA), and others.

Lifestyle Risk Factors
Low calcium intake, vitamin D deficiency, inadequate physical activity.
- Alcoholic (three or more/day), high caffeine intake.
- Smoking (active or passive).

Bone Density Test Scores

- Use DXA to measure the bone mineral density (BMD) of the hip and spine. Do baseline and repeat in 1 to 2 years (if on treatment regimen) to assess the efficacy of the medicine. If not on treatment, repeat DXA in 2 to 5 years.
- Osteoporosis: T-scores of –2.5 or lower standard deviations (SD) at the lumbar spine, femoral neck, or total hip region.
- Osteopenia: T-scores between –1.5 and –2.4 SD.

Treatment Plan

- Weight-bearing exercises most days of the week.
  - Swimming is not considered a weight-bearing exercise (but good for severe arthritis).
  - Weight-bearing exercises are walking, jogging, biking, aerobic dance classes, most sports.
  - Isometric exercises are not considered as weight-bearing type of exercise.
- Calcium with vitamin D 1,200 mg /day and vitamin D3 (800 mg to 1,000 IU/day).

Bisphosphonates

- First-line drug for treating postmenopausal osteoporosis, osteoporosis in men, and glucocorticoid-induced osteoporosis (men and women).
- Potent esophageal irritant (advise patients to report sore throat, dysphagia, mid-sternal pain). May cause esophagitis, esophageal perforation, gastric ulcers, reactivation/bleeding peptic ulcer disease (PUD).
- Increases BMD and inhibits bone resorption.
- Fosamax (alendronate) 5 mg to 10 mg/day or 70 mg weekly.
- Actonel (risedronate) 5 mg/day or 35 mg weekly (or 150 mg tablet once a month).
  - Take immediately upon awakening in a.m. with full glass (6–8 ounces) of plain water (do not use mineral water).
  - Take tablets sitting or standing and wait at least 30 minutes before laying down.
  - Do not crush, split, or chew tablets. Swallow the tablets whole.
  - Never take these drugs with other medications, juice, coffee, antacids, vitamins.
  - Will cause severe esophagitis or esophageal perforation if lodged in the esophagus.
- *Contraindications:* Inability to sit upright, esophageal motility disorders, history of PUD or history of gastrointestinal (GI) bleeding.
- Osteonecrosis of the jaw (mandible or maxilla) more likely if on chronic high doses of IM bisphosphonates. Complains of jaw heaviness, pain, swelling, and loose teeth.

Selective Estrogen Receptor Modulator (SERM) Class

Evista (raloxifene). Blocks estrogen receptors. A Category X drug.

- Approved for use after menopause.
- Do not use to treat menopausal symptoms (aggravates hot flashes).
- Does not stimulate endometrium or breast tissue.
- Increases risk of venous thrombosis.
- Reduces risk of breast cancer (if taken long term up to 5 years).
- Used as adjunct treatment for estrogen-receptor positive breast cancers.

Other Hormones

Miacalcin (calcitonin salmon, derived from salmon)

- Not a first-line drug.
- Stops bone loss and maintains BMD (but does not rebuild bone).
- May reduce spinal fracture risk.

HRT/ERT (estrogen-replacement therapy)

- Increases bone density and treats menopausal symptoms.
- Increases risk of heart disease, DVT, breast and endometrial cancer.

✍ EXAM TIPS (BIRTH CONTROL)

- Some brands of birth control pills (e.g., Loestrin FE) contain iron during the last 7 days of the pill cycle (instead of a placebo pill).
- Low-dose birth control pills contain 20 mcg to 25 mcg of ethinyl estradiol.
- Desogen, Ortho-Tricyclen, and Yaz/Yasmin are all indicated for treatment of acne.
- Avoid using Depo-Provera in anorexic and/or bulimic patients (very high risk of osteoporosis).
- Women taking Seasonale will have only four periods per year.
- Learn how to use Plan B (contains only progesterone).
- Learn about the two types of IUDs and safety issues.
- Some questions will ask for the best birth control method for a case scenario. Remember the contraindications or adverse effects of each method (e.g., Depo-Provera).
- Problems on absolute versus relative contraindications of birth control pills are designed with answer options that list a true contraindication with a relative contraindication. For example, a question asking for a relative contraindication may have an answer choice such as "history of a blood clot that resolved" (absolute) and "migraine headache" (relative).
- Missing two consecutive days of the pill (take two pills the next 2 days to finish cycle and use condoms until next cycle starts).

✍ EXAM TIPS (OTHER)

- There will be questions on all the types of vaginitis (bacterial vaginosis [BV], trichomonas, candida, atrophic vaginitis). The questions range from diagnosis, workup/lab tests, to treatment.
- Become familiar with BV. "Clue cells" are squamous epithelial cells that have blurred edges due to the large number of bacteria on the cell's surface.
- Menopausal female body changes. If palpable ovary, order an intravaginal ultrasound.
- PE findings (hard irregular mass that is not mobile) and follow-up of breast cancer.
- Learn how to take bisphosphonates (e.g., Fosamax, Actonel) and contraindications.
- Mefenamic acid (Ponstel) is an NSAID that is very effective for menstrual pain.
- Bone density score for osteoporosis (T-score of > −2.5 SD/SD) and for osteopenia (T-score of −1.5 to −2.4 SD/SD).

🗎 CLINICAL TIPS

- Birth control pills can elevate total T4 levels (but not free T4) and triglycerides/lipids.
- Do not recommend Depo-Provera for women who want to become pregnant in 12 to 18 months because it may cause delayed return of fertility. It can take up to 1 year for some women to start ovulating.
- Using a small amount of KY jelly to lubricate the tips of the speculum (with atrophic vaginitis to reduce pain and vaginal bleeding) will not affect the Pap smear results.
- In reproductive-aged teens or women who present with acute pelvic pain or lower abdominal pain, always perform a pregnancy test (use good quality urine hCG tests strips).

Sexually Transmitted Diseases (STDs) or Infections (STIs) Review*

⚠ DANGER SIGNALS

HIV/AIDS

The median time between initial HIV infection and AIDS is 10 years (CDC, 2011). AIDS is defined by an absolute CD4 cell count of less than 200 cells/mm^3 along with certain opportunistic infections and malignancies (e.g., Kaposi's sarcoma, non-Hodgkin's lymphoma). Signs and symptoms that suggest AIDS are oral candidiasis (thrush), fever, weight loss, diarrhea, cough, shortness of breath, purple to bluish-red bumps on the skin, and certain infections. *Pneumocystis (carinii) jirovecii* is the infection that causes the most deaths in patients with HIV.

Acute Retroviral Syndrome (Primary HIV Infection)

An acute and brief illness that occurs in 50% to 80% of persons within a few weeks after initial exposure to the HIV virus. Very infectious during this time period due to extremely high viral load (>100,000 copies/mL) and high concentration of virus in genital secretions. The initial immune response may mimic mononucleosis (low-grade fever, fatigue, generalized red rash, and lymphadenopathy). During this time, the HIV antibody tests may still be negative. If strongly suspect acute HIV infection, order HIV polymerase chain reaction (PCR). Majority (97%) develop antibodies within 3 months after exposure.

Disseminated Gonococcal Disease (Disseminated Gonorrhea)

Sexually active adult from high-risk population complains of petechial or pustular skin lesions of hands/soles (acral lesions); swollen, red, and tender joints in one large joint (migratory asymmetrical arthritis) such as the knee. May be accompanied by signs of STD (i.e., cervicitis, urethritis). If pharyngitis, will have severe sore throat with green purulent throat exudate that does not respond to usual antibiotics used for strep throat. Occasionally complicated by perihepatitis (Fitzhugh syndrome) and rarely endocarditis or meningitis.

---

* Treatment recommendations for this chapter are adapted from the CDC *MMWR* (*Morbidity and Mortality Weekly Report*) Sexually Transmitted Disease Treatment Guidelines (2010).

☑ NORMAL FINDINGS

- Female normal findings covered in Chapter 17: Women's Health.
- Male normal findings covered in Chapter 16: Men's Health genitourinary section.

STD SCREENING

STD Screening Recommended by the CDC

- Routine annual screening for *Chlamydia trachomatis* and gonorrhea of all sexually active females aged 25 years or younger.
- Repeat testing in 3 months is recommended for those who previously tested positive for gonorrhea due to high rates of reinfection (this is not a test-of-cure).
- All 50 states and the District of Columbia explicitly allow minors to consent for their own health services that involve STDs. No state requires parental consent for STD care.
- Minors do not need parental consent if the clinic visit is related to testing, treating, or follow-up of an STD, birth control, or diagnosis of pregnancy.

STD Risk Factors

- Younger ages (from age 15–24 years), initiated sex at a younger age.
- Multiple sexual partners, new sexual partner in past 60 days.
- Inconsistent condom use, unmarried status.
- History of previous STD infection, illicit drug use.
- Genital ulceration (increases risk of HIV transmission).
- Use of alcohol or illicit drugs.
- Adolescents.

CERVICAL ECTROPION

- An immature cervix has a large ectropion (a normal finding). An ectropion looks like a red-colored bumpy surface that emerges out of the cervical os. It is made up of columnar cells, which are easier to infect compared with squamous epithelial cells (the smooth surface of the cervix).
- It can mimic cervicitis, but the mucus is clear (with ectropion). It is purulent with cervicitis.

DISEASE REVIEW

Chlamydia trachomatis

Most chlamydial infections are asymptomatic. The highest prevalence is among persons 25 years of age or younger. *Chlamydia trachomatis* is the most common STD in the United States. It is an obligate intracellular bacteria (an atypical bacteria).

Possible Sites of Infection
- *Females*: Cervicitis, endometritis, salpingitis (fallopian tubes), pelvic inflammatory disease (PID).
- *Males*: Epididymitis, prostatitis.

- *Both genders*: Urethritis, proctitis (from receptive anal intercourse).
- *Complications*: PID, tubal scarring, ectopic pregnancy, infertility, Reiter's syndrome (males).

Laboratory Testing (Both Gonorrhea and Chlamydia)

- Nucleic acid amplification tests (NAAT) are highly sensitive tests for both gonorrhea and chlamydia. Swab samples can be collected from the urine, cervix, urethra, oral, and rectal sites for both males and females.
- *Urine samples:* Collect the first part of the urine stream (15–20 mL).
- *Pharynx and/or rectal samples:* Swab using a NAAT test (do not use the GenProbe).
- *GenProbe:* Use only for the cervix or urethra (not for pharynx or rectum).
- Chlamydial cultures are not used in primary care (use NAAT test).

Other tests (for gonorrhea):

- *Gram-stain:* Polymorphonuclear leukocytes with gram-negative intracellular diplococcic (use for males with gonorrheal urethritis). Not commonly used in primary care.
- Thayer-Martin culture or chocolate agar culture for gonorrhea.

Treatment Plan
Uncomplicated Infections
Chlamydia (Cervicitis, Urethritis, Sex Partners)

- No test of cure is necessary for azithromycin or doxycycline regimen.
- Azithromycin 1 g PO in a single dose (directly observed treatment [DOT] preferred)

OR

- Doxycycline 100 mg BID × 7 days
  - Abdominal pain (take with water). Esophagitis if tablet gets stuck in throat.
  - Nausea, GI upset, photosensitivity (avoid sun or use sunscreen).
  - Category D (stains growing tooth enamel).

Sexual Partners

- Azithromycin 1 g PO in a single dose.
- Expedited partner treatment. The practice of treating the sexual partner(s) of a patient diagnosed with an STD without the sex partner being seen first by the health provider. Expedited partner treatment (EPT) is an alternative, but can have medicolegal consequences (check state regulations).
- Complicated infections.

Pregnant Women

- Test of cure 3 weeks after completion of treatment if pregnant.
- Azithromycin 1 g PO in a single dose

OR

- Amoxicillin 500 mg PO TID × 7 days

Complicated infections
Pelvic Inflammatory Disease

- Ceftriaxone (Rocephin) 250 mg IM × 1 dose plus doxycycline PO BID × 14 days.
- With or without metronidazole (Flagyl) PO BID × 14 days

Neisseria gonorrhoeae

A gram-negative bacterium that infects the urinary and genital tracts, rectum, and pharynx. Unlike chlamydia, gonorrhea can become systemic or disseminated if left untreated.

If positive for *N. gonorrhea*, cotreat for both (even if negative chlamydial tests) because of the high rate of coinfection. Do not use quinolones to treat gonorrhea due to high-level resistance.

Laboratory Tests
Discussed under chlamydia section in this chapter.

Classic Case
Sexually active teenage to young adult female complains of purulent green-colored vaginal discharge. Speculum examination reveals purulent discharge on the cervix, which may be friable (bleeds easily). Males will have penile discharge and dysuria and may report staining of underwear with purulent discharge. History of new partner (less than 3 months) or multiple sexual partners. Inconsistent condom use. Signs and symptoms depend on the organ/site that becomes infected.

Signs and Symptoms (by Site)
- Cervicitis (mucopurulent cervical discharge, pain, mild bleeding after intercourse).
- Urethritis (scant to copious purulent discharge, dysuria, frequency, urgency).
- Proctitis (pruritis, rectal pain, tenesmus, avoidance of defecation due to pain).
- Pharyngitis (severe sore throat unresponsive to typical antibiotics, purulent green-colored discharge on the posterior pharynx).
- Bartholin's gland abscess (cystic lump that is red and warm [or has purulent discharge] that is located on each side of the introitus or vestibule).
- Endometritis (menometrorrhagia [heavy prolonged menstrual bleeding], dysmenorrhea).
- Salpingitis (fallopian tubes) and PID (one-sided pelvic or lower abdominal pain, adnexal pain, dyspareunia or painful intercourse and cervical motion tenderness).
- Epididymitis and prostatitis (discussed in Chapter 16: Men's Health).

CDC-RECOMMENDED STD TREATMENT REGIMENS (TABLE 18.1)

Uncomplicated Infections of the Cervix, Urethra, Rectum, and Pharynx
- If pharyngeal infection, use only the first-line regimen (CDC, 2010).

First Line
- Ceftriaxone (Rocephin) 250 mg IM × 1 dose PLUS cotreat for chlamydia
  PLUS
- Azithromycin 1 g orally × 1 dose
  OR
- Doxycycline 100 mg orally × 7 days
- Test of cure (i.e., repeat testing 3 to 4 weeks after treatment) is not needed if treated with approved CDC regimen. If symptoms persist, obtain specimen for GC culture and sensitivity.

Management of Sex Partners
- Treat male partners of women with PID if sexual contact during the 60 days preceding the patient's symptoms.
- Avoid sex until both finish treatment and no longer have symptoms.

Complicated Gonococcal Infections

Pelvic Inflammatory Disease, Acute Epididymitis, Acute Prostatitis, Acute Proctitis

- Ceftriaxone (Rocephin) 250 mg IM × 1 dose
  Plus (cotreat for chlamydia)
- Doxycycline 100 mg PO BID × 14 days
  With or without
- Metronidazole (Flagyl) 500 mg PO BID × 14 days

Disseminated Gonococcal Infection

Refer to ED or infectious disease specialist. Ceftriaxone (Rocephin) 1 g IM or IV every 24 hours.

Table 18.1 Sexually Transmitted Diseases: Treatment Guidelines

Diseases and Organism	Uncomplicated Infections	Complicated Infections
Chlamydia		
Chlamydia trachomatis Pregnancy*	Azithromycin 1 g × 1 dose OR	Doxycycline 100 mg BID × 14 days
Azithromycin 1 g × 1 dose OR Amoxicillin 500 mg TID × 7 days	Doxycycline 100 mg BID × 7 days	PID, salpingitis
	Mucopurulent cervicitis urethritis	Tubo-ovarian abscess
		Males
	Sexual partner treatment	Epididymitis, prostatitis
Gonorrheae		
Neisseria gonorrhoeae Pregnancy*	Ceftriaxone 250 mg IM × 1 dose PLUS	Ceftriaxone 250 mg IM × 1 dose PLUS
Ceftriaxone 250 mg IM × 1 dose PLUS Azithromycin 1 g × one	Azithromycin 1 g × 1 dose or doxycycline 100 mg BID × 7 days	Doxycycline 100 mg BID × 14 days
		PID, salpingitis
	Mucopurulent cervicitis	Tubo-ovarian abscess
	Urethritis	Males
	Proctitis	Epididymitis, orchitis, prostatitis
	Sexual partner treatment	Disseminated GC
		Above plus asymmetric arthritis and rash
Syphilis		
Treponema pallidum	Benzathine penicillin G 2.4 mU IM × 1 dose	Benzathine penicillin G 2.4 mU IM weekly × 3 weeks
	Primary or secondary syphilis (same dose)	More than 1 year's duration or latent syphilis. Refer.
	Treat sexual partners	Follow-up of cases is mandatory! (any stage of disease)
	Retreat if clinical signs recur or sustained four-fold titers	

* Doxycycline, Cipro, and Floxin are contraindicated in lactation/pregnancy (Category D).

IM, intramuscular; PID, pelvic inflammatory disease.

Source: Adapted from Centers for Disease Control (2010). Sexually Transmitted Disease Treatment Guidelines.

Risk Factors for PID

- History of PID: 25% recurrence
- Multiple partners
- Age 24 or younger
- Oral contraceptives may reduce the risk of PID (because of thickened mucous plug).

Labs

- Reproductive-aged females: Rule out pregnancy first
  - Gen Probe (use only on urethra and cervix)
  - Do not use on the pharynx or rectum
  - NAAT test: Urine tests for chlamydia and gonorrhea (or cervical/urethral sample)
  - Gonorrhea (anaerobic cultures) such as the Thayer-Martin or chocolate agar
  - For pharyngeal and rectal areas but can be used for other sites if indicated
- Mandatory chlamydial (and gonorrheal) cultures with sexual assault (any age)

Gram Stain

- Useful for gonorrhea only. Look for gram-negative diplococci in clusters.

Other STD testing

- HIV, syphilis, hepatitis B, herpes type 2.
- Partners should be tested and treated. No sex until both complete treatment.

UNUSUAL COMPLICATIONS

Fitz-Hugh–Curtis Syndrome (Perihepatitis)

Chlamydial and/or gonococcal infection of the liver capsule (not the liver itself) resulting in extensive scarring between the liver capsule and abdominal contents (i.e., colon). Scars look like "violin strings" (seen on laparoscopy). A complication of disseminated GC and/or PID.

Classic Case

- Sexually active female with symptoms of PID complains of right upper quadrant (RUQ) abdominal pain and tenderness on palpation. The liver function tests are normal.
- Treated as a complicated gonorrheal/chlamydial infection (14-day treatment).

Jarisch–Herxheimer Reaction

Acute febrile reaction that can occur during the first 24 hours after treatment (more likely to occur after treatment for early syphilis). Look for fever, chills, headache, myalgias. An immune-mediated reaction that usually resolves spontaneously. Treatment is supportive.

Reiter's Syndrome

More common in males. An immune-mediated reaction secondary to infection with certain bacteria (e.g., chlamydia) that spontaneously resolves. Treatment is supportive (e.g., NSAIDs).

Classic Case

A male with current history of chlamydia genital infection (i.e., urethritis) complains of dry red and swollen joints that come and go (migratory arthritis in large joints such as knee) and ulcers on the skin of the glans penis.

Mnemonic: "I can't see, pee, or climb up a tree."

✍ EXAM TIPS

- Older and well-known drugs such as doxycycline and ceftriaxone more likely to appear as treatment options.
- Become familiar with the treatment regimens for chlamydia and gonorrhea.
- If GC positive, always cotreat for chlamydia even if the chlamydial test result is negative.
- Inverse not true. If chlamydia, do not prophylax against GC unless indicated.
- Azithromycin used for pregnant patients who have chlamydia. Test of cure after treatment.
- Use GenProbe only for cervix or urethral chlamydial or gonorrheal symptoms.
- HSV-1 infection more common on oral mucosa and HSV-2 more common on the genitals.
- Learn Fitz-Hugh–Curtis or Jarisch–Herxheimer syndrome.
- If STD symptoms with new onset of swollen red knee on side (or another joint), may be caused by disseminated gonorrheal infection (DGI).

📋 CLINICAL TIPS

- PID is a clinical diagnosis (i.e., cervical motion tenderness [CMT]). Even if both GC and chlamydial tests are negative, treat a sexually active patient who has signs and symptoms of PID.
- After treating a patient for PID, follow up within 2 to 3 days and perform vaginal bimanual examination. Symptoms should improve within 2 to 3 days.
- For STDs treated with azithromycin (chlamydia, syphilis), instruct patient and partner not to have sex for at least 7 days afterward.

SYPHILIS

Screen for syphilis if HIV infection, men who have sex with men (MSM), presence of any genital ulcer (especially if painless chancre), previous STD, pregnancy, IV drug use, or high risk.

Treponema pallidum (spirochete) infection. Becomes systemic if untreated.

Classic Case

Signs and symptoms dependent on stage of infection.

Primary

- Painless chancre (heals in 6 to 9 weeks if not treated).
- Chancre has clean base, well demarcated with indurated margins.

Secondary (>2 Years)

- Condyloma lata (infectious white papules in moist areas that look like white warts).
- Maculopapular rash on palms and soles that is not pruritic (may be generalized).

Latent Stage

- Asymptomatic but will have positive titers.

Tertiary (3–10 Years)

- Neurosyphilis, gumma (soft tissue tumors), aneurysms, valvular damage, and so on.

Labs

- Screening test: RPR or VDRL (nontreponemal test).
- Diagnostic test: Fluorescent antibody absorption antibody (FTA-ABS), direct fluorescent antibody testing (DFA-TP), darkfield microscopy (not commonly used anymore).
- First-order screening test (RPR or VDRL). If reactive, next step is to confirm with FTA-ABS.
- Both RPR and FTA-ABS are positive: Diagnostic for syphilis.
- Do not switch tests (if using RPR to diagnose, continue using to monitor response to treatment).

Treatment Plan
Primary Syphilis (Chancre or Chancroid)

- Benzathine penicillin G 2.4 million units IM × 1 dose.

Follow Up

- Recheck RPR or VDRL at 6 and 12 months to monitor treatment response (look for at least a fourfold decrease in the pretreatment and posttreatment titers).
- Treat sexual partner(s) and test them for HIV and other STDs.
- Refer to infectious disease specialist with latent to tertiary syphilis.

✍ EXAM TIPS

- RPR or VDRL are the screening tests for syphilis.
- If positive RPR or VDRL, confirm with FTA-ABS (treponemal test).
- If RPR and FTA-ABS positive, diagnostic for syphilis.
- RPR or VDRL shows fourfold (or higher) decrease in titers if patient is responding to treatment.
- All patients with syphilis or MSM, test for HIV infection (coinfection).
- Signs and symptoms for secondary syphilis (maculopapular rash palms/soles, etc.).
- Do not confuse *Condyloma acuminata* (genital warts) with *Condyloma lata* (secondary syphilis).

📋 CLINICAL TIPS

- False-positive RPR can be caused by autoimmune diseases, chronic, or acute disease.
- Recheck syphilitic chancre in 3 to 7 days after injection (should start healing).
- The most common criterion clinicians use to diagnose PID is cervical motion tenderness.

HIV INFECTION

In the United States, HIV-1 is the most common strain. In Africa, HIV-2 is more common.

Risk Factors

- Sexual intercourse with an HIV-infected person, MSM.
- Received blood products between 1975 to March 1985, history of illicit drug use.

- History of other STDs, multiple partners, homeless, prisoners in jails, and so on.

Viral Load
- Number of HIV RNA copies in 1 mL plasma. Test measures actively replicating HIV virus; progression of disease and response to antiretroviral treatment.
- The best sign of treatment success is an undetectable viral load (<50 copies/mcL).

CD4 T-Cell Counts (by Flow Cytometry)
- Used to stage HIV infection and to determine when to start prophylaxis.
- Full name is "helper T lymphocytes express cluster determinant 4" or CD4.
- Values vary throughout the day. Check at the same time of the day using the same laboratory each time.

CD4:CD8 Ratio
- Used to monitor depletion of CD4 cells (compared with CD8 cells).
- Immunocompetent with ratios of >1.
- HIV-infected usually have ratio <1.

Screening Test: ELISA Test (Enzyme-Linked Immunosorbent Assay)
- Antibody test with high sensitivity for HIV.
- Sensitivity is the ability of a test to identify or to rule out a person *with* a disease.

Confirmatory Test: Western Blot
- Antibody test with high specificity for HIV (99.7% specificity).
- Specificity is the ability of a test to identify or to rule out a person *without* the disease.
- Both the ELISA and Western blot detect only IgG antibodies (not viral RNA).
- If both tests are positive, the next step is to order an HIV PCR/HIV RNA to definitively diagnose HIV infection.
- Window period:
  - 6 weeks to 6 months (<1% up to 36 months).
  - False-negative ELISA/Western blot. If high risk and suspect HIV, order HIV PCR.

Diagnostic Tests (Viral RNA Test)
HIV PCR
- If ELISA and Western blot positive, order HIV PCR.
- Detects HIV-1 RNA (actual viral presence).
- Infants of HIV-positive mothers.
- High-risk patient with negative ELISA or Western Blot test (window period).
- No separate consent form is needed for HIV screening and patients can "opt out" of HIV testing.

Prophylaxis for Opportunistic Infections (Primary Prevention)
- *Pneumocystis jerovecii* pneumonia (previously known as *Pneumocystis carnii* or PCP).
- CD4 lymphocyte count is <200 cells/mm^3.
- *First line:* Trimethoprim-sulfamethoxazole (Bactrim DS) one tab daily. If develops a severe reaction to sulfas, the next step is dapsone 100 mg daily or atovaquone suspension.
- *Alternatives:* Dapsone, atovaquone, or aerosolized pentamindine.

Toxoplasma gondii Infections (Protozoa)
- CD4 count is <100 cells/mm³.
- *First line:* Trimethoprim-sulfamethaxozole (Bactrim DS) one tablet daily.
- Causes brain abscesses (headaches, blurred vision, confusion, imbalance, others).
- Avoid cleaning cat litter boxes and eating undercooked meats.

Monitoring Viral Load: HAART or ART
- Check every 1 to 2 months until viral load is undetectable, then every 3 to 4 months.

Recommended Vaccines
HIV and AIDS patients can receive inactivated vaccines such as: hepatitis A, hepatitis B, annual flu vaccine, pneumooccal vaccine, Td/Tdap, others as needed.

Live Virus Vaccines
HIV patients can receive some live virus vaccines but if CD4 count is <200 cells/ mm³, it is contraindicated. HIV patients have higher mortality rates from measles and chickenpox.
- *MMR Vaccine:* Recommended for asymptomatic HIV-infected children if CD4 >200.
- *Varicella Vaccine:* Recommended for sero-negative children and adults if CD4 >200.

HIV Education
- Do not handle cat litter or eat uncooked lamb, beef, or pork (risk of toxoplasmosis).
- Avoid bird stool since it contains histoplasmosis spores.
- Turtles and other amphibians may be infected with salmonella.
- Use gloves or avoid gardening (soil contains fungal spores, protozoa, bacteria, fecal matter).

Table 18.2 HIV Tests

Types of HIV Tests	Rationale
Enzyme-linked immunosorbent assay (ELISA)	Screening test (antibody test). If positive, next step is Western blot test (done automatically by lab).
Rapid HIV testing kits or point-of-care tests	Also used for screening. Result available in <30 min (antibody test). Can be done at home.
Western blot	Confirmatory test (antibody test). If positive Western blot, next step is HIV PCR.
HIV PCR	Tests for HIV virus directly (antigen test). Used for infants of HIV-positive mothers. Diagnosing acute HIV infection (window stage).
CD4 T-cell counts	Initiation of prophylaxis, staging HIV disease, disease progression, and treatment response. If on HAART or ART, check same time as viral load schedule (below).
Viral load (antigen)	Monitor treatment response. If on HAART or antiretroviral therapy (ART), monitor every 1 to 2 months until nondetectable, then every 3 to 4 months.
CD4:CD8 Ratio	As CD4 cells are depleted, the ratio will decrease. HIV-infected ratio is <1.0. Not checked routinely as often as the CD4.

Preventing HIV Transmission
- Use condom every single time you have sex. Genital ulcers increase risk for HIV.
- Do not share needles or syringes if you inject drugs.
- Do not share any toothbrushes, razors, or other items that may have blood on them.
- For mothers with HIV infection, do not breastfeed your baby.

Occupationally Acquired HIV Infection
- Nurses have the highest rate of all health care occupations of occupationally acquired HIV/AIDS.
- Trauma with large-bore hollow needles that contain contaminated material from patients with high viral loads such as retroviral syndrome, symptomatic patients, or AIDS are highest risk.

Lab Evaluation
Order rapid blood test for HIV ASAP (within 72 hours), ELISA and Western blot test, HBsAg, HCV antibody, and HCV RNA, syphilis, and so on. Recheck at 6 weeks, 3 months, and months.

Postexposure Prophylaxis (PEP)
- Use HAART regimen (within 72 hours of exposure) with zidovudine (ZDV, AZT) + lamivudine (3TC) plus tenofovir (Viread) OR Combivir (ZDV + lamivudine) plus tenofovir (Viread).
  - Drug class: nucleoside reverse transcriptase inhibitors (NRTIs).
  - PEP for exposure to hepatitis B source patient.
  - If unvaccinated, give hepatitis B immune globulin (HBIG) plus vaccinate. If vaccinated responder (check titer—high titer of antibodies), no PEP is recommended.

✍ EXAM TIPS

- PCP prophylaxis when CD4 <200.
- Bactrim DS used first; if allergic to sulfa, use dapsone 100 mg PO daily.
- Bactrim DS is used for both prophylaxis or treatment of PCP.
- Screening test for HIV is the ELISA test (tests for antibodies only).
- Confirmatory test is Western blot (antibody test only).
- HIV RNA or HIV PCR is the diagnostic test (viral RNA).
- HIV-infected pregnant women: start AZT in the second trimester.
- Hairy leukoplakia of tongue, recurrent candidiasis, thrush: Rule out HIV infection.

📋 CLINICAL TIP

- For job-related exposures, contact National Clinician's Postexposure Prophylaxis Hotline (PEPline) at 1-888-448-4911 for advice (open 24/7).

HIV Infection: Pregnant Women
- The HIV drug that is considered the "safest" to use during pregnancy is zidovudine (Retrovir, ZDV, AZT). Avoid breastfeeding.
- *Newborns:* Start treatment with zidovudine (AZT) within first 6 to 12 hours of delivery.

Zidovudine
- Drug of choice for treating pregnant women and infants.
- Reduces rate of perinatal transmission by 70%.

- Ideally, start zidovudine during second trimester of pregnancy until delivery (but can be started earlier if needed for mother's health).

Condyloma Acuminata (Genital Warts)

- Human papilloma virus (HPV) high-risk oncogenic types are 16 and 18.
- HPV vaccine (e.g., Gardasil): age 11 to 12 years (both girls and boys). Between ages 13 and 26, catch-up for patient who did not get the vaccine when younger. HPV vaccine is also recommended for MSM.
- *Genital sites:* Cervix, vagina, external genitals, urethra, anus.
- Other sites that can be infected are the anus, penis, nasal mucosa, oropharynx, conjunctiva.

Cervical HPV

- *HIV-positive women:* Risk for aggressive HPV disease and cervical cancer. HIV-positive women need more frequent Pap testing (every 6 months to monitor).

Pap Smears

- Cervical cancer screening test is the traditional Pap smear or liquid-based Pap testing.
- Koilocytotic changes (large cell nuclei) seen on Pap smear may signify human papilloma virus (HPV) infection. Check for HPV and refer for a colposcopy for high-risk strains.
- Management of abnormal Pap results (i.e., ASCUS) discussed in Chapter 17: Women's Health.

Colposcopy

- A specialized microscope for evaluating and treating cervix. It is used to visualize the cervix and to obtain both endocervical and cervical tissue biopsies.
- Biopsy of cervical tissue: Gold standard for diagnosing cervical cancer.

Acetowhitening

Areas of white-colored skin (leukoplakia-like appearance) on the cervical surface that appear only after acetic acid (distilled vinegar) is swabbed on the cervix. This procedure is done before starting a colposcopic examination and biopsy. HPV-infected skin becomes a bright-white color from the acetic acid exposure and these are the areas on the cervix that are biopsied.

Genital HPV (External Genital Warts)

Majority (90%) are caused by HPV 6 or 11. The cervical surface will look "normal" until it is advanced. External genital warts appear as soft flesh-colored pedunculated, flat, or papular growths. Commonly located on the vaginal introitus or the shaft of the male penis.

Medications
Self-Administered Topical Medications

- Podofilox (Condylox) 0.5% gel or cream (anti-mitotic drug). Contraindicated in pregnancy.
- Imiquimod (Aldara) 5% cream immune-modulating (or immune response modifier) drug that stimulates the production of interferon and other cytokines.
  - Apply a thin layer 3×/week at bedtime for up to 16 weeks. Do not cover with dressing.
  - Leave cream on skin for 6 to 10 hours. Wash off skin with soap and water after.
  - *Side effects:* Irritation, ulceration/erosions, hypopigmentation.
- Cryo, bichloroacetic, or trichloroacetic acid (caustic acids) done in office.

Herpes Simplex: HSV-1 and HSV-2

Asymptomatic shedding (intact skin) also occurs intermittently and patient is still contagious.

- *HSV-1:* Usually oral infection, sometimes genital
- *HSV-2:* Most cases recurrent genital herpes, can be oral

Classic Case

May have prodrome (i.e., itching, burning, and tingling) on site. Sudden onset of groups of small vesicles sitting on an erythematous base. Easily ruptures and is painful. Primary episode more severe and can last from 2 to 4 weeks. Vesicle fluid and crust are contagious.

Treatment Plan

- *Diagnostic test*: Herpes viral culture or RPR assay for HSV-1 and HSV-2 DNA (more sensitive).

Tzanck Smear

An "old test." If herpes virus infection (herpes simplex or varicella), shows multinucleated giant cells.

First Episode

- Acyclovir (Zovirax) 400 mg 3×/day for 7 to 10 days (or 200 mg 5×/day for 7–10 days).
- Famciclovir (Famvir) 1 g BID for 7 to 10 days.
- Valacyclovir (Valtrex) TID for 7 to 10 days.

Episodic Treatment (Flare-Up)

- Best if treatment started within one day of lesion onset
- Famciclovir (Famvir) 125 mg BID for 5 days
- Zovirax BID or TID × 5 days or Valtrex BID × 5 days

Suppressive Treatment

- Acyclovir (Zovirax) 400 mg PO BID or famicyclovir (Famvir) 250 mg PO BID

Evaluation

- For all cases of genital ulcers: Always rule out syphilis and HSV (genital herpes) infection.

🖎 EXAM TIPS

- First episode treatment (Zovirax 5×/day or Valtrex 3×/day or Famvir BID for 7 to 10 days).
- Flare-up treatment (Zovirax or Valtrex or Famvir BID for 5 days).
- Imiquimod for genital warts and how to use.
- HSV-1 and HSV-2 locations.
- HPV strains 16 and 18 are carcinogenic.

19

Adolescents Review

⚠ DANGER SIGNALS

HODGKIN'S LYMPHOMA

Hodgkin's lymphoma presents with enlarged and painless cervical and supraclavicular lymphadenopathy associated with fever (Pel-Epstein sign) and night sweats. May report an episode(s) of severe pain that is located on or over malignant areas a few minutes after drinking alcohol. The most common cancers in teens aged 15 to 19 years are Hodgkin's lymphoma (16%) and germ cell tumors (16%) such as testicular and ovarian cancer.

TESTICULAR CANCER

Teenage to adult male complaints of a testicular or scrotal mass that may be tender to touch or asymptomatic. Some patients may have testicular discomfort, but not pain. The patient reports a sensation of heaviness in the affected testicle. The affected testicle has a firm texture. More common in males from the age of 15 to 35 years. Cryptoorchidism is a strong risk factor.

TESTICULAR TORSION (ACUTE SCROTUM)

Pubertal male awakens with abrupt onset of unilateral testicular pain that increases in severity. Pain may radiate to the lower abdomen and/or groin. Almost all patients (90%) also have nausea and vomiting. Ischemic changes result in severe scrotal edema, redness, induration, and testicular pain. Ipsilateral (same-side) cremasteric reflex is absent. Highest incidence is during puberty.

Urinalysis: Negative for WBCs. Doppler ultrasound is the initial diagnostic test. Testicle not functional after 24 hours if not repaired. Refer to ED. A surgical emergency.

☑ NORMAL FINDINGS

ADOLESCENCE

Defined as the onset of puberty until sexual maturity.

Most Common Cause of Death
- Accidents (i.e., motor vehicle crashes)

PUBERTY

The time period in life when secondary sexual characteristics start to develop because of hormonal stimulation. Girls' ovaries start producing estrogen and progesterone. Boys' testes start producing testosterone. All of these changes result in reproductive capability.

Girls

- Precocious puberty if puberty starts before age 8 years.
- Delayed puberty if no breast development (Tanner Stage II) by age 12 years.

Growth Spurt

Majority of somatic changes occur between the ages of 10 and 13 years.
- Majority of skeletal growth occurs before menses. Afterward, growth slows down.
- Girls start their growth spurts 1 year earlier than boys.

Growth Time Line in Girls

Breast development → peak growth acceleration → menarche. Most of a girl's height is gained before menarche. Skeletal growth in girls is considered complete within 2 years after menarche.

Mittelschmerz

Unilateral mid-cycle pelvic pain that is caused by an enlarged ovarian follicle (or ruptured follicle). Pain may last a few hours to a few days. May occur intermittently.

Menarche

- Average age is about 12 years (12.34 years)
- After Tanner Stage II starts (breast bud stage), girls start menses within 1 to 2 years.
- Delayed puberty if no secondary sexual characteristics at age 12 to 13 years.

Boys

- Precocious puberty if starts before age 9 years.
- Delayed puberty if no testicular/scrotal growth by age 14 years.

Growth Spurt

- Boys' growth spurts are 1 year later than girls' (age 11 to 15 years).

Spermarche

- Average age is 13.3 years.

TANNER STAGES (TABLE 19.1)

Boys

- Stage I: Prepuberty.
- Stage II: Testes begin to enlarge/increased rugation of scrotum.
- Stage III: Penis elongates. Testicular/scrotal growth continues. Scrotal color starts to darken.
- Stage IV: Penis thickens and increases in size. Larger testes and scrotal skin darker.
- Stage V: Adult pattern.

Girls

- Stage I: Prepuberty.
- Stage II: Breast bud (onset of thelarche or breast development).

- Stage III: Breast tissue and areola are in one mound.
- Stage IV: Areola/nipples separate and form a secondary mound.
- Stage V: Adult pattern.

Pubic Hair (Both Genders)

- Stage I: Prepuberty.
- Stage II: Sparse growth of straight hair that is easily counted.
- Stage III: Hair darker and starts to curl.
- Stage IV: Hair curly but not on medial thigh yet as in adult. Hair is coarser.
- Stage V: Adult pattern, hair spreads to medial thigh and lower abdomen.

Table 19.1 Tanner Stages

Stage	Girls	Boys	Pubic Hair
I	Prepuberty	Prepuberty	None
II	Breast bud	Testes enlarges Scrotum rugae	Few straight, fine hairs
III	Breast and areola One mound	Penis lengthens	Darker, coarse Starts to curl
VI	Breast and areola Secondary mound	Penis widens	Thicker, curly Darker, coarse
V	Adult pattern	Adult pattern	Adult pattern Inner thigh

IMMUNIZATION SCHEDULE FOR ADOLESCENTS

The schedule in Table 19.2 is for patients who did not complete immunization or were not immunized as infants.

Table 19.2 Immunization Schedule (Age 7–18 Years)

Vaccine	Immunizations
Tdap (Boostrix, Adacel)	All 11 or 12 year olds: give Tdap as booster, then Td every 10 years for lifetime.
HPV (Gardasil)	All 11 or 12 year olds: give to girls and boys.
OR HPV (Cervarix)	Girls/females only (do not give to males). Minimum age (HPV vaccines): 9 years old. All 11 or 12 year olds: give 1st shot. Booster: 16 years old, give 2nd shot.
Meningococcal/MCV4 (Menactra, Menveo)	College freshmen living in dormitories.
Influenza inactivated	Vaccinate everyone from age 6 months and older.
Influenza live virus (FluMist)	Healthy people 2 to 49 years of age.
Hepatitis B (Recombivax HB)	Catch-up: give the third dose if not completed.
MMR	Catch-up: give the second dose if not completed.
Varicella	If no reliable history of chickenpox (verbal okay). Live virus contraindications.

Note. Adapted from Centers for Disease Control Recommended Immunization Schedule (2012).
This table is a simplified version and is designed for studying for the certification exams only.
Do not use this table as a guideline for clinical practice.

✍ EXAM TIPS

- *All college freshmen living in dormitories:* High risk of meningococcal infection. Meningococcal conjugate vaccine (MCV4) is recommended by the CDC.
- *Live attenuated influenza virus (LAIV) nasal only:* If indicated, use only on healthy persons from ages 2 to 49 years.
- *High risk for flu with vaccination recommended:* HIV, asthma, heart disease, sickle cell, cystic fibrosis, diabetes, others. Household members/health workers caring for or living with any person with the above conditions and infants also need to be vaccinated.
- *Vaccine Adverse Event Reporting System (VAERS):* Governmental program to report clinically adverse events.

LABORATORY TESTS

Elevated Alkaline Phosphatase

Normally elevated from puberty to teenage years, secondary to rapid growth spurts. Enzyme is produced by growing bone or patients healing from major fractures.

LEGAL ISSUES

Right to Consent and Confidentiality

No parental (or guardian) consent is necessary for the following:
- Contraception
- Treatment for sexually transmitted diseases (STDs)
- Diagnosis and management of pregnancy

Emancipated Minor Criteria

These minors may give full consent as an adult without parental involvement:
- Legally married
- Active duty in the armed forces

Confidentiality

Confidentiality can be broken in the following situations:
- Gunshot wounds, stab wounds must be reported to the police (regardless of age).
- Child abuse (actual or suspected abuse) must be reported to the authorities.
- Suicidal ideation and/or attempt (discharge to parents/guardians or hospital).
- Homicidal ideation or intent (especially mental health providers).

"Mature Minor Rule"

A mature minor is an unemancipated minor (from 15 to 17 years of age) with the mental capacity (and intelligence) to understand the consequences of a decision (such as refusing a surgical procedure or medical treatment). The mature minor has the right to refuse or to request treatment (even if the parents disagree with this decision). There are statutory and/or common laws at the state level. Each state has its own laws and statutes.

Example

A 17-year-old male who is scheduled for a procedure calls the NP and tells her that he does not want to have the procedure. After the NP speaks with the patient and listens to his rationale (the patient understands the consequences), she decides to call the hospital's patient liaison/advocate (or ombudsman) to speak with the patient first (instead of calling the parents first).

HEALTH PROMOTION

During a physical examination or wellness visit, assess teenager for high-risk behaviors. Intensive behavior counseling is recommended. The following are high-risk behaviors to screen for:

- *Sexually active:* Use of condoms, birth control, intimate partner violence (i.e., rape), signs/symptoms of STDs.
- *Safety:* Driver safety, seatbelt/helmet use, smoking, alcohol, and drug use.
- *Social history:* Family, peers, school performance, work.
- Signs/symptoms of depression and antisocial behaviors (i.e., gangs).

✍ EXAM TIPS

- Puberty starts at Tanner Stage II in girls (breast bud) or boys (testicular enlargement and scrotal rugation/color starting to become darker). Puberty ends at Tanner Stage V (adult stage).
- Tanner Stage III in boys is elongation of the penis (testes continues to grow). Only Tanner Stages II to IV need to be memorized for the exam.
- There is no need to memorize pubic hair changes for either gender. Memorize only the breast changes (girls) and the genital changes (boys).
- Adolescent health history is obtained from both parent and child initially, then the adolescent is interviewed alone without the parent.
- Memorize the criteria for an emancipated minor. Do not confuse the right to confidentiality with emancipated minor status.

≔ DISEASE REVIEW

Primary and Secondary Amenorrhea

- *Primary amenorrhea:* Absence of menarche by the age of 15 years (with or without development of secondary sexual characteristics). Half are caused by chromosomal disorders (50%).
- *Secondary amenorrhea:* Absence of menses for three cycles or 6 months if previously had menses. Most common cause is pregnancy. Others are ovarian disorders, stress, anorexia, polycystic ovary syndrome (PCOS).

Secondary Amenorrhea Associated With Exercise and Underweight

- Excessive exercise and/or sports participation have a higher incidence of amenorrhea (and infertility) due to relative caloric deficiency.
- "Female athlete triad": Anorexia nervosa/restrictive eating, amenorrhea, and osteoporosis.

Labs

- Pregnancy test (Serum hCG)
- Serum prolactin level (rule out prolactinoma-induced amenorrhea).
- Serum thyroid-stimulating hormone (TSH). Also follicle-stimulating hormone (FSH) and luteinizing hormone (LH) (rule out premature ovarian failure).
- If amenorrhea for more than 6 months, measure bone density.

TREATMENT

- Educate about increasing caloric intake and decreasing exercise.
- Calcium with vitamin D 1,200–1,500 mg daily. Vitamin D 400 IU daily.

Complications

- Osteopenia/osteoporosis (stress fractures). Infertility.
- BMI less than 18.5 associated with excess mortality for smokers and nonsmokers (mechanism unknown).

Anorexia Nervosa

- Onset usually during adolescence. Irrational preoccupation with and intense fear of gaining weight.
- *Two types:* Restriction (dieting, excessive exercise) or binge eating and purging. Some examples of purging are excessive use of laxatives, enemas, diuretics, vomiting.

Clinical Findings

- Marked weight loss (>15% of body weight, BMI <18.5 or less).
- Lanugo (increased lanugo especially in the face, back, and shoulders).
- Stress fractures (osteopenia or osteoporosis from estrogen depletion and low calcium intake).
- Swollen feet (low albumin), dizziness, abdominal bloating.
- ED: Weight <70% of ideal body weight, low pulse (40 or less), vital signs unstable, hypotension.

✎ EXAM TIPS

- Recognize how anorexic patients present (i.e., lanugo, peripheral edema, amenorrhea, weight loss >10% of body weight).
- Increased risk of osteoporosis or osteopenia. For birth control, avoid Depo Provera and other progesterone-only contraceptives since they can cause bone loss.
- Low albumin level.

Gynecomastia (Figure 19.1)

Excessive growth of breast tissue in males. Can involve one or both breasts. Physiologic gynecomastia is benign and is more common during infancy and adolescence. Normal in up to 40% of pubertal boys (peaks at age 14). Most cases resolve spontaneously within 6 months to 2 years.

Classic Case

Pubertal to adolescent male is brought in by a parent who is concerned about gradual onset of enlarged breasts or asymmetrical breast tissue (one may be larger). Child is embarrassed and scared about breast changes. Affected breast may be tender to palpation.

Objective

Round, rubbery, and mobile mound (disc-like) under the areola of both breasts. Skin has no dimpling, redness, or changes. If mass irregular, fixed, hard; rapid growth in breast size; or suspect secondary cause, refer to specialist.

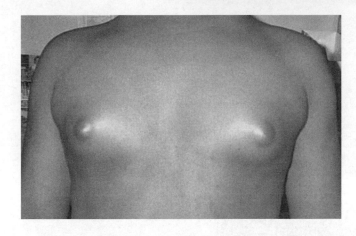

FIGURE 19.1 Gynecomastia (male aged 14 years).

Treatment Plan
- Evaluate for Tanner stage (check testicular size, pubic hair, axillary hair, body odor).
- Check for drug use: both illicit and prescription (i.e., steroids, cimetidine, antipsychotics).
- Rule out serious etiology (testicular or adrenal tumors, brain tumor, hypogonadism, etc.).
- Recheck patient in 6 months to monitor for changes.

Pseudogynecomastia
More common in obese boys. Bilateral enlarged breast is due to fatty tissue (adipose tissue). Both breasts feel soft to touch and are not tender. No breast bud or disc-like breast tissue is palpable.

Labs
None. Diagnosed by clinical presentation.

Adolescent Idiopathic Scoliosis (Figure 19.2)
Screening Test: Adams Forward Bend Test
Lateral curvature of the spine that may be accompanied by spinal rotation. More common in girls (80% of patients). Painless and asymptomatic. Scoliosis will most likely worsen (66% of cases) if it starts in the beginning of the growth spurt. Rapid worsening of curvature is indicative of secondary cause (Marfan or Ehlers–Danlos syndrome, cerebral palsy, myelomeningocele, etc.)

Classic Case
Pubertal to young teen complains that one hip, shoulder, breast, or scapula is higher than the other. No complaints of pain.

Adams Forward Bend Test (or Forward Bend Test)
Bend forward with both arms hanging free. Look for asymmetry of spine, scapula, thoracic, and lumbar curvature. Check height. Measure the Cobb angle (degree of spinal curvature). Full-spine x-rays are used to measure degree of curvature.

Scoliosis Treatment Parameters
- Curves less than 20 degrees:
  - Observe and monitor for changes in spinal curvature.

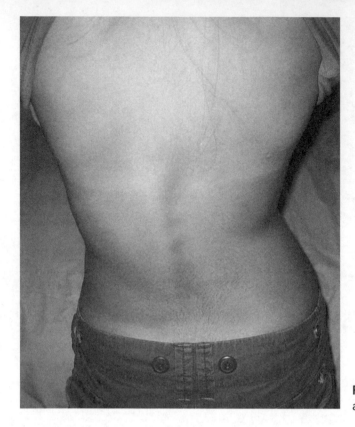

FIGURE 19.2 Scoliosis (female aged 18 years).

- Curves of 20 to 40 degrees:
  - Bracing (i.e., Milwaukee brace).
- Curves greater than 40 degrees:
  - Surgical correction with Harrington rod used on spine and other options.

Management

- Check Tanner stage (Tanner Stage II up to Tanner Stage V).
- Order spinal x-ray (PA view) to measure Cobb angle.

📋 CLINICAL TIP

Refer all patients with scoliosis to a pediatric orthopedic specialist.

Osgood–Schlatter Disease

A common cause of knee pain in young athletes. Caused by overuse of the knee. Repetitive stress on the patellar tendon by the quadriceps muscle causes pain, tenderness, and swelling at the tendon's insertion site (the tibial tuberosity). Usually affects one knee, but can be bilateral. Most common during rapid growth spurts in teenage males who are physically active and/or play sports that stress the patellar tendon (i.e., basketball, soccer, running).

Classic Case

A 14-year-old male athlete undergoing a rapid growth spurt complains of a tender bony mass over the anterior tubercle of one knee. The pain is worsened by some activities (squatting, kneeling, jumping, and climbing up stairs). The knee pain improves with rest and avoidance of aggravating activity. Reports the presence of bony mass on the anterior tibial tubercle that is slightly tender. Almost all cases resolve spontaneously within a few weeks to months. Rule out avulsion fracture (tibial tubercle) if acute onset of pain posttrauma (order lateral x-ray of knee).

Treatment Plan

Follow RICE: Rest affected knee. Use ice pack 3×/day for 10 to 15 minutes. Avoiding aggravating activities or sport will typically reduce/resolve pain. Adolescent may continue to play based on degree of pain after sports participation. Play does not necessarily worsen the condition. Tylenol or nonsteroidal anti-inflammatory drugs (NSAIDs) for pain as needed.

✍ EXAM TIPS

- Scoliosis treatment for a 10-degree curve (observe for worsening).
- Screening test for scoliosis is the "Forward Bend Test."

Delayed Puberty

- Absence of secondary sexual characteristics by the age of 13 years for girls (such as a breast bud) or at the age of 14 years for boys. The child remains in Tanner Stage I (prepubertal).
- *Primary amenorrhea*: Absence of menarche by age of 15 years.

Labs

Serum Pregnancy Test

- Check prolactin level. If prolactin level is elevated, next step is to order a computed tomography (CT) scan of the sella turcica (location of pituitary gland inside the skull).
- For primary amenorrhea (no menses by age 15 years), rule out hypogonadism by checking hormone levels (i.e., estrogen, progesterone, DHEA, FSH, TSH). Rule out chromosomal disorders, absence of uterus/vagina, imperforate hymen. X-ray of the hand is used for estimating "bone age":
  - When the long-bone epiphyses (growth plates) are fused, skeletal growth is finished.
  - Refer to pediatric endocrinologist if no growth spurt, delayed puberty, others.

✍ EXAM TIPS

- Osgood–Schlatter presentation.
- Primary and secondary amenorrhea definitions.
- Gynecomastia vs. pseudogynecomastia (know the difference).
- No parental consent is needed for health services related to sexual activity (STD testing, pregnancy tests, birth control prescriptions).
- If not related to sexual activity, then need parental consent (dysmenorrhea, headache, URI).
- Emancipated minor definition.
- Anorexia nervosa presentation (lanugo, etc.), low albumin (pedal edema).

Professional Issues Review

IV

20

Hospice

HOSPICE

A model of care designed for terminally ill patients who are in the final phase of their disease. Focus is on alleviation of pain and improving quality of life. Emphasis is on palliative care (not curative care).

Palliative Care

Palliative care is what hospice care is all about. The main goal of palliative care is to help improve the patient's quality of life. Pain management is an important aspect of this health model.

Home-Based Residential Care

The majority of hospice care programs are home-based. Patients reside and are cared for in their homes. Some hospice groups have specialized inpatient units that are in local hospitals.

Respite Care

Provides a rest period for the primary caregiver. The patient is cared for by another caregiver for 1 day.

Hospice Admission Criteria

- Physician must write an order for hospice care (also must sign the death certificate).
- Physician certifies that patient has a life expectancy of less than 6 months.
- Patient gives consent to be admitted to a hospice program.
- In addition, the patient agrees not to use life-sustaining equipment if a life-threatening event occurs during the hospice time period. Depending on the insurance benefits, patients who need a physical therapist and speech rehab are allowed to continue in hospice.

Note

If a terminal patient's family wants the patient admitted to hospice, but the patient is not willing, then the patient does not meet hospice admission criteria.

Examples of Terminal Conditions

- Metastatic cancers (e.g., lung cancer, colon cancer).
- End-stage lung disease (e.g., COPD).
- End-stage heart disease (e.g., CHF).
- Amyotrophic lateral sclerosis.
- End-stage dementia (e.g., Alzheimer's disease, Parkinson's disease).

Hospice Team

The hospice team consists of the attending physician, hospice physician, registered nurse, home health aides, social worker/grief counselor, and clergy.

- *Registered nurse* (primary case manager): Coordination of care. Visits patient regularly (from daily to weekly).
- *Home health aides:* Assist patient with personal care, food shopping and preparation, driving patients to go shopping, appointments, others.
- *Hospice physician:* Mainly pain management.
- *Primary attending physician/clinician:* Continuation and follow-up of medications and preexisting health conditions.
- *Social worker:* Grief counseling and emotional issues.
- *Clergy/priest:* Depends on patient's religious affiliation and desire.

Bereavement Care

Both the patient and family members/significant others receive bereavement care. A therapist specializing in hospice counseling will regularly see the patient and the family members/significant others for counseling and support. After a patient's death, bereavement care benefits continue for up to 1 year.

Reimbursement

Hospice care is covered by Medicare Part A, Medicaid, and most private health insurance.

Medicare Hospice Benefits

Medicare Part A covers hospice care for patients aged 65 years and older. Must enroll in a Medicare-approved facility. Both the hospice and the patient's attending physician must certify that the patient has less than 6 months to live. In addition, the patient agrees that he or she cannot be on life-sustaining equipment for a condition that occurs during the hospice period.

Advanced Directives

There are two types, the Living Will and Health Care Proxy.

Living Will

A legal document stating the type of health care that the patient wants if he or she is unable to give legal consent due to a severe mental or neurological condition (coma, dementia). The document must be signed by the patient and a witness (if possible).

Health Care Proxy

Another name for this legal document is the "Durable Power of Attorney." The patient assigns the right to another person to make his or her health decisions in case the patient becomes incapacitated.

21

Medico-Legal, Ethical Guidelines, and Advanced Practice Law

ETHICAL CONCEPTS

Beneficence

The obligation to help the patient. Remove harm, prevent harm, promote good. ("do no harm"). Acting in the patient's best interest. Compassionate patient care.

Example: Health promotion. Educating an obese patient on the harmful effects of obesity and recommending weight loss. Encouraging a patient to stop smoking and enroll in smoking cessation programs. Personal level: Calling the surgeon to get a prescription for stronger pain medications (a narcotic) for a postsurgical patient who complains of severe pain.

Nonmaleficence

The obligation to avoid harm. Protecting a patient from harm.

Examples: A new nurse practitioner (NP) is told to suture a laceration on a patient's face. The NP tells the physician that she has not been trained to suture facial area lacerations and therefore is unable to do it.

    The NP discusses a new anticancer drug that may be more effective in treating a patient's cancer. The NP discusses the known risk versus the benefits of the new drug. The patient declines the treatment.

Utilitarianism

The outcome of the action is what matters with utilitarianism. It also means to use a resource for the benefit of most (e.g., tax money). It may resemble justice, but it is not the same concept (see below).

Example: The Women, Infants, and Children food (WIC) program is only for pregnant women and children. It is not open to adults and elderly males. The reason may be that it would cost society more if women (and their fetuses), infants, and children are harmed by inadequate food intake (affects the brain growth, etc.).

Justice

The lack of bias. The right to fair and equitable treatment. The fair and equitable distribution of societal resources.

Example: Low-income individuals do not pay some types of taxes to the government, but they still have equal access to the postal service and other public services that are supported by taxes.

A homeless alcoholic male without health insurance presents to the ED for abdominal pain. The patient is triaged and treated in the same manner as the other patients who have health insurance.

Dignity

Respect for human dignity is an important aspect of medical ethics. A person's religious, personal, and cultural beliefs can influence greatly what a person considers "dignified" treatmaent.

Example: Hospital gowns should be secured correctly so that when patients get up to walk, their backs are not visible.

Fidelity

Dedication and loyalty to one's patients. Keeping one's promise.

Example: A woman with terminal breast cancer does not want the NP to reveal her poor prognosis to her mother. The patient explains to the NP that her mother is very anxious and she wants to wait until the next week before she tells her mother news. If the NP keeps the prognosis in confidence from the patient's mother, she is exercising the concept of fidelity.

Confidentiality

The obligation to protect the patient's identity, personal information, test results, and medical records.

This "right" is also protected by the Health Insurance Portability and Accountability Act (HIPAA) (release of patient information for electronic billing purposes). Psychiatric and mental health medical records are protected information and require separate consent.

Paternalism

Making decisions for a patient (or for others) because you "believe" that it is for their best interest. The opinion (or desires) of the patient is minimized or ignored. The patient is "powerless."

Example: A 92-year-old male does not want to be on a ventilator if he codes. The son disagrees and quietly tells the NP and physician that he wants this father to be aggressively treated with life support, if it is necessary.

Autonomy

Mentally competent adult patients have the right to make their own health decisions and express treatment preferences. If the patient is mentally incapacitated (dementia, coma), the designated surrogate's choices are respected. A patient can decline or refuse treatment.

Examples: An alert elderly female with periods of forgetfulness and who has breast cancer decides to have a mastectomy after discussing the treatment options with her oncologist. The woman's daughter tells the NP that she does not want her mother to have a mastectomy because she thinks her mother is too old and confused. The NP has the duty to respect the patient's decision. This case is also a good example of the NP acting as the patient advocate.

Accountability

Health care providers are responsible for their own choices and actions and do not blame others for their mistakes.

Veracity

The duty to present information honestly and truthfully.

Example: An elderly woman is recently diagnosed with advanced pancreatic cancer. The patient thinks that she has a very good chance of being cured. The oncologist explains to the patient her poor prognosis. The oncologist is being truthful and honest to the patient about her prognosis.

✎ EXAM TIP

- Become familiar with some of the ethical concepts (e.g., beneficence, veracity, autonomy, utilitarianism) and how they are applied (look at the examples).

The American Nurses Association (ANA) Code of Ethics for Nurses

The ANA Code of Ethics for Nurses with Interpretive Statements (2001) contains "the goals, values and ethical precepts that direct the profession of nursing." According to the ANA, the Code "is nonnegotiable." Each nurse "has an obligation to uphold and adhere to the code of ethics."

LEGAL ISSUES

Ombudsman

A person who acts as an intermediary (or as a liaison) between the patient and an organization (long-term care or nursing homes, hospitals, governmental agencies, courts). The ombudsman represents the patient and works in the best interests of the patient.

Guardian Ad Litem

A court-appointed guardian who is assigned by a court (and has the legal authority) to act in the best interest of the "ward." The ward is usually a person who is a child, frail, or vulnerable.

Advanced Health Care Directive

Living Will

A document that contains the patient's instructions and preferences regarding health care if the patient becomes seriously ill or is dying. It contains the patient's preferences (or not) for aggressive life-support measures. Health care providers should have a copy of the document in the patient's chart.

Health Care Power of Attorney

Also known as the "Durable Power of Attorney for Health Care." The patient designates a person (family member or a close friend) who has the legal authority to make future health care decisions for the patient in the event that the patient becomes mentally incompetent or incapacitated (i.e., comatose).

Power of Attorney

A person who is designated by the patient, and who has the legal authority to make decisions for the patient.

This role is broader and encompasses not only health care decisions but also other areas of the patient's life, such as financial affairs.

Health Insurance Portability and Accountability Act (HIPAA)*

Also known as the "HIPAA Privacy Rule" (or Public Law 104–191). The law was passed by the U.S. Congress and enacted in August, 1996. The law provides protections for:

"the use and disclosure of individuals' health information"—called "protected health information" by organizations subject to the Privacy Rule— called "covered entities."

Covered Entities

Any health care provider, health insurance company, health care plans, and third-party administrators (TPAs) who "electronically transmit health information" must follow the HIPAA regulations.

What Is a TPA?

A third-party administrator is the organization that does the processing of claims and administrative work for another company (health insurer, health plans, retirement plans).

HIPAA Requirements (Not Inclusive)

- Health providers are required to provide each patient with a copy of their office's HIPAA policy (patient to sign the form).
- The HIPAA form must be reviewed and signed annually by the patient.
- Patients have the right to review their medical files.
- A mental health provider has the right to refuse patients' requests to view their psychiatric and mental health records.
- When patients request to review their medical records, the health provider has up to 30 days to comply.
- Patients are allowed (under HIPAA) to correct errors in their medical records.
- Must keep identifying information (name, DOB, address, Social Security number) and any diagnosis/disease or health concerns private except with allowed exceptions (see list below).

Patient Consent Is Not Required in the Following Cases

- The health plan/insurance company that is paying for the medical care.
- A third party or business associate (e.g., accounting, legal, administrative) that the insurance company or doctor's office hires to assist in payment of their services (e.g., medical billing services).
- Health care operations (medical services review, sale of health care plan, audits).
- Collection agency for unpaid bills.
- Victims of abuse/neglect or domestic violence.
- No separate consent is needed to consult with other health care providers.

HIPAA Case Scenarios

Health providers cannot disclose sensitive patient information, including laboratory and test results (e.g., laboratory results, mammogram results) to persons whom the patient has not given consent to view his or her records.

Examples

- If a family member or spouse requests for a patient's lab result, but the patient has not given authorization for that family member, the record cannot be released to that person.

---

* U.S. Department of Health and Human Services. Health Information Privacy. www.HHS.gov/ocr/privacy/hipaa/

- If a staff member (who is not involved in the patient's care) calls the attending NP and wants to discuss a patient's progress, the NP cannot release information to the staff member.
- Laboratory, tests, and procedure results (even if normal) cannot be left on an answering machine. Instead, the staff member who is calling the patient can leave the NP's or office's contact information (with a message for the patient to call back).

Outpatient Clinics

Examples: When a patient is inside an examining room, the medical chart should be turned backward so that the patient's name is not exposed.

The sign-in list on the front desk must be covered so that the previous patient's names are not visible to other patients.

Psychiatric and Mental Health Records

A psychiatric diagnosis and/or mental health records may not be released without a specific signed authorization by the patient. Patients can be denied access to their psychotherapy records.

Minors

The health records of a minor (less than 18 years old) can be released to parents or legal guardians without the minor's consent. If authorization is needed to release a minor's medical record, the parent or legal guardian must sign for it (except for emancipated minors). Emancipated minors can sign their own legal documents.

✍ EXAM TIPS

- Become familiar with how HIPAA is applied in real life. Study the HIPAA case scenarios.
- Learn the definitions of beneficence, justice, and veracity (and the other ethical concepts).
- No consent is required for entities that pay the patient's health bills, such as health insurance companies, health maintenance organizations (HMOs), medical billers, collection agencies (or third-party contractors hired by the company to pay or to process claims).

MALPRACTICE INSURANCE

The two types of malpractice insurance are occurrence-based and claims-based.

Claims-Based Policy

This type of malpractice insurance will cover claims only if the NP is still enrolled with the same insurance company at the time the claim is filed in court.

Example: A claim is filed in court against an NP in January 2011 for an incident that occurred in January 2009. The NP remains enrolled with the same malpractice insurance company. Therefore, the claim will be covered. But if the NP has changed jobs or is retired (and does not carry tail coverage), the claim will not be covered even if the NP was insured at that time.

What is "tail" insurance or "tail coverage"? When an NP with claims-based malpractice insurance retires or changes to a new job, it is advisable to buy "tail" coverage insurance. The tail coverage insurance will cover the NP for malpractice claims that may be filed against him or her in the future.

Occurrence-Based Policy

This type of malpractice policy is not affected by job changes or retirement. When a claim is filed against the NP in the future, it is covered if he or she had an occurrence-based policy at the time the incident occurred.

Example: An NP who has been retired for 2 years has a claim filed against her for an incident that occurred while she was employed. Since she carried an occurrence-based policy, the claim will be covered.

MALPRACTICE LAWSUITS

Plaintiff (the patient or whoever is acting on behalf of the patient).
Defendant (the health care provider).

Elements of a Case

The plaintiff must prove that all of the following occurred:
- A duty is owed (a legal duty exists).
- The duty was breached (e.g., not following standard of care, etc.).
- The breach caused an injury (proximate cause).
- Damage occurred.

Phases of a Medical Malpractice Trial

- A lawsuit is filed in the appropriate court.
- The "discovery" phase (requesting of medical records, depositions, expert opinions, etc.).
- Plaintiff (the patient or patient's representative who files the lawsuit claiming injury and/or damage by another party) has the "burden of proof." The defendant is the party that responds to the lawsuit filed by another party that claims an injury and/or damage (e.g., NP, hospital).
- Court trial phase (or settle out of court or arbitration).
- The judgment is given.
- Either the case is dismissed or damages awarded (physical harm, emotional/mental harm, etc.).

Expert Witnesses

Ideally, the NP who will testify as an expert witness should be someone who practices in the same specialty and geographic area as the NP defendant. For example, an NP who practices in Los Angeles, CA, may not be the best choice as an expert witness for an NP who is being sued and who is practicing in Miami, FL.

Reimbursement

The Balanced Budget Act (1997) broadened Medicare coverage of nurse practitioner services.

NPs can be reimbursed directly by Medicare Part B, Medicaid, Tricare, and some health insurance plans. Medicare will reimburse NPs 85% of the usual and customary fee (paid to a physician). The NP must file the charges under his or her name and provider number to get reimbursed for services. Previously, only NPs who practiced in certain rural/designated areas in the United States were allowed to bill Medicare for reimbursement.

NPI (National Provider Identifier) Number

The NPI is a unique identification number for covered health care providers and health plans. The NPI is a 10-position numeric identifier (10-digit number). Covered health care providers must use the NPIs in the administrative and financial transactions adopted under HIPAA.

Medical Coding

What Is the ICD-10 (International Classification of Diseases, 10th Edition)?

The ICD-10 is the code that is used in the United States to indicate the diagnosis, including family history disorders. Each disease is assigned an ICD-10 code.

What Is an ICD-10 "V-Code" (or Modifiers)?

V-codes indicate the reason for the visit. V-codes are not to be used for procedures. There are many situations in which a V code can be used. It can be used as the primary or secondary diagnosis.

What Is the Current Procedural Terminology (CPT)?

The CPT is a list of descriptive identifying codes that are used to identify procedures (e.g., suturing, incision, and drainage or I&D) and other medical services. It is owned by the American Medical Association (AMA).

HEALTH INSURANCE

The Affordable Care Act (ACA, 2010)*

Signed by President Obama in March 2010. Parts of the ACA are already in effect (e.g., children under age 26 can be insured under the parents' health care insurance); the ACA will take full effect starting 2014. It is a comprehensive bill that reforms health care insurance law in this country. According to the website (www.healthcare.gov/law/index.html), it will provide for "comprehensive reforms that improve access to affordable health coverage for everyone." It will improve "access to care for our most vulnerable," expand coverage, and lower health care costs. Starting in the year 2014, it will be illegal for insurance companies to deny coverage to individuals with preexisting conditions.

The Consolidated Omnibus Budget Reconciliation Act (COBRA)

Also known as "COBRA coverage." Provides for the continuation of preexisting group health insurance (from the employer) for individuals who lose their coverage (between jobs, quit job, or are fired) for a fixed period of time.

Health Maintenance Organizations

Patients are assigned a primary care provider (PCP). The PCP is the "gatekeeper." The patient has a set "co-pay" per visit, and the participating physician/health provider is paid a set fee (per patient) monthly. The physician receives a monthly check from the HMO.

- Specialist/consultant: The PCP must first approve the referral. The patient is limited to seeing the physicians/specialists who are enrolled in the HMO's network.
- "Out of network physicians" or not referred by the PCP: The visit may not be covered or it will be reimbursed at a lower rate.

---

* Upheld by the U.S. Supreme Court (May 2012).

Preferred Provider Organization (PPO)

The patient can visit any provider in the network without a referral. Not assigned a primary care provider (as in HMOs). The patient can choose his or her own PCP. No referral is needed to see a specialist. Specialists are part of the PPO panel. PPOs are usually more expensive than HMOs.

MEDICARE AND MEDICAID

Both the Medicare and Medicaid programs are under the Centers for Medicare and Medicaid Services (CMS). The CMS is one of the agencies of the U.S. Department of Health and Human Services (DHHS).

Medicare Part A (Inpatient Hospitalization)

"Automatic" at age 65 if the person paid the premiums (automatically deducted from paycheck by the employer). If the person never paid the premiums (e.g., full-time house-wife), the person is not eligible for Medicare coverage. Also covers persons with end-stage renal diseases at any age.

Certain religious groups (e.g., Amish Mennonites) do not participate in Medicare.

Medicare Part A will pay for the following "medically necessary" services:

- Inpatient hospitalization (including inpatient psychiatric hospitalization).
- Hospice care.
- Home health care.
- Skilled nursing facility.

Medicare Part A will not pay for custodial care (nursing homes, retirement homes).

Medicare Part B (Outpatient Insurance)

Medicare Part B is a voluntary program with monthly premiums. Must enroll during the "general enrollment period" (happens once a year).

- Medicare Part B will pay for the following "medically necessary" services:
  - Outpatient visits (including walk-in clinics, urgent care clinics, emergency room visits).
  - Laboratory and other types of tests (electrocardiogram, x-rays, computed tomography scans).
  - Durable medical equipment.
  - "Second opinions" with another physician (surgery).
  - Kidney dialysis, organ transplants, and many others.
- Medicare Part B does not pay for:
  - Most eyeglasses and eye exams (except following cataract surgery that implants an intraocular lens).
  - Hearing aids.
  - Most dentures and dental care.
  - Cosmetic plastic surgery (unless it is medically necessary).
  - Over-the-counter drugs and most prescription drugs.
- Part B also pays health prevention services:
  - Flu shots once a year. Pneumovax (once in a lifetime).
  - Screening mammogram (once every 12 months for women age 40+).
  - Screening colonoscopy or flexible sigmoidoscopy (aged 50 years or older) every 10 years if low risk.

- Routine Pap smears (once every 2 years, or once every 12 months for women at high risk).
- Prostate cancer screening (once a year after age 50).
- Lipid profile (cardiovascular screening every 5 years).
- Bone density testing.
- HIV screening.
- Physical exams (once a year).
- Smoking cessation.

Medicare Part D

- Also known as the Medicare prescription drug benefit. Only individuals who are enrolled (or eligible) for Medicare Part A and/or Part B are eligible. One type of Part D coverage is called the Medicare Advantage plan (MA).
- All prescription drug plans have a list of preferred drugs (the formulary). If a non-formulary drug is used, it may not be covered and the patient has to pay for it "out–of–pocket."

Medicaid

Authorized by Title XIX of the Social Security Act. A federal and state matching program.

Provides health insurance coverage for low-income individuals and their families who meet the federal poverty level criteria. Provides health insurance for children, pregnant women, parents, seniors, and individuals with disabilities (i.e., blindness). Pays for health care and prescription drugs.

THE NURSE PRACTITIONER ROLE

History

Loretta C. Ford, PhD, RN, and Henry K. Silver, MD, introduced the NP role. The University of Colorado started the first NP program in 1978 and was pivotal in helping to develop the NP role. The first NPs were pediatric NPs who practiced in poor rural areas where there were no physicians (due to a severe shortage of primary care physicians).

Regulation of Nurse Practitioners

Educational Requirements

A nurse practitioner must meet the minimal educational requirements that are mandated by the Nurse Practice Act of the state (where she/he plans to practice).

State Nurse Practice Act*

The nurse practitioner's legal right to practice is derived from the state Nurse Practice Act. The Nurse Practice Act contains the regulations that mandate the educational requirements, responsibilities, and the scope of practice for nurse practitioners and for other nurses (i.e., RNs, licensed practical nurses, midwives, etc.) who practice in the state.

NP practice is not regulated by either the federal government, the AMA, or the Department of Health & Human Services.

---

* ANA web site. Professional Standards. Accessed on 5/28/2012 from www.nursingworld.org. http://ana.nursingworld.org/MainMenuCategories/EthicsStandards/CodeofEthicsforNurses/AboutTheCode.aspx

State Board of Nursing

The state board of nursing (BON) is responsible for enforcing the state's Nurse Practice Act. The BON is a formal governmental agency that has the statutory authority to regulate nursing practice. The BON has the legal authority to license, monitor, and to discipline nurses. The BON is also authorized to revoke a nurse's license (after formal hearings).

Title Protection

Professional designations such as registered nurse (RN) or nurse practitioner (NP, advanced registered nurse practitioner [ARNP], advanced practice registered nurse [APRN]) are protected by law. It is illegal for any person to use these titles without a valid license. Title protection is under the Nurse Practice Act. Title protection protects the public from unlicensed "nurses."

Licensure and Certification

Licensure is a legal requirement to practice as an NP. It is done through a governmental entity, the state Board of Nursing. The NP must meet the minimal educational and clinical requirements in order to become licensed.

Certification is generally a "voluntary" process and is done through a nongovernmental entity such as a professional nursing association or specialty organization. The majority of states in the United States now mandate board certification (or certification) as a condition to obtain licensure.

Scope and Standards of Practice

A document that contains "authoritative statements" that are used to evaluate and measure the nursing "quality of practice, service, or education" (ANA, 1996). They are developed by professional societies (e.g., ANA) as well as specialty organizations. For example, the American Academy of Nurse Practitioners publishes "Standards of Practice for Nurse Practitioners."

Collaborative Agreements

A written agreement between a supervising physician and nurse practitioner outlining the nurse practitioner's role and responsibility to the clinical practice. Also known as "protocols."

Physicians and Dentists

Nurse practitioners can sign collaborative agreements with physicians (MD), osteopaths (DO), and dentists/dental surgeons (DDS or DMD). Physcians are the only ones that can legally sign the death certificate. Chiropractors are not consedered physicians under the Nurse Practice Act.

Prescriptive Privileges

The majority of states requires nurse practitioners to have a written protocol with a supervising physician(s) in order to prescribe drugs. The protocol usually contains the list of drugs (by name, by class, or by condition) that the nurse practitioner is allowed to prescribe. Many states now allow nurse practitioners to prescribe certain controlled drugs, but with limitations.

Prescription Pads

The NP's prescription pad should contain the following:
- NP's name, designation, and license number.
- Clinic's name, address, and phone number. If the practice has several clinics, the other clinics where the NP practices should also be listed on the pad.

Budget Reconciliation Act of 1989 (HR 3299)

The first law allowing NPs to be reimbursed directly by Medicare. Only certified pediatric and family nurse practitioners were allowed as primary providers as long as they practiced in designated "rural" areas.

RESEARCH-BASED CLINICAL CARE

Evidence-Based Medicine (EBM)

Also known as "evidence-based practice." EBM is the result of the use and integration of solid clinical evidence (finding the best evidence) into clinical care. Research evidence (results from experiments and studies) is critically evaluated for the validity, impact (size of effect), and applicability.

Treatment Guidelines

Guideline contents are based on the systematic review of available clinical evidence. Guidelines are written by national expert panels (e.g., JNC 7) and/or specialty organizations (e.g., Infectious Disease Society of America, American Academy of Pediatrics). The "National Guideline Clearinghouse" contains a huge database of treatment guidelines (www.guideline.gov).

CASE AND RISK MANAGEMENT

Case Managers

Health care case managers are usually experienced RNs who act as coordinators for the outpatient management of patients with certain diagnoses (usually chronic diseases). The process is called "case management." Case management is mainly done by telephone.

Examples: COPD, chronic heart failure, diabetes.

Quality Improvement Programs

Patient outcomes are important indicators of a health system's quality. The goal of these programs is to improve the quality of care, decrease complications, decrease hospitalizations, lower patient mortality, decrease system errors, and increase patient satisfaction.

Example: A "problem" is identified (diabetic complications such as peripheral neuropathy, retinopathy, etc.). Then outcome measures are identified (such as an A1c of less than 6.5 %, etc.). Be familiar about what a good outcome is for a disease (for diabetics, a good outcome is A1c less than 6.5%) and what a poor outcome is (A1c greater than 8%).

Health Risk Management

A systematic organizational process to identify risky practices to minimize adverse patient outcomes and corporate liability. For example, high-risk areas that are usually checked by risk managers are medication errors, hospital-acquired infections, patient identification problems, and falls.

Accreditation

Accreditation is a voluntary process in which a nongovernmental association evaluates and certifies that an organization (e.g., hospital, clinic, nursing program) has met the requirements and excels in its class. For example, the American Nurses Credentialing

Center and the National League for Nursing Accrediting Commission, Inc., are accreditation organizations.

Culture and Nursing

Respect a patient's cultural beliefs/practices—if the cultural belief or the traditional healer's advice does not cause harm to the patient, then the NP should support the practice. If a cultural practice has an adverse effect on a patient's health, then the NP needs to explain to the patient in a sensitive manner the reason for not following the practice.

Example: A patient tells the NP that her shaman/curandero "told me not to take my medicine, but to drink herbal tea instead" or "he told me not to drink water for 2 days"—the NP respectfully communicates/explains to the patient why the practice is harmful to her health.

Madeleine Leininger's Theory of Cultural Care Diversity and Universality

Defined culture as "the specific pattern of behavior that distinguishes any society from others and gives meaning to human expressions of care." Founder of transcultural nursing and credited with the construct of "culturally congruent care." Nursing care should be in agreement with a person's or group's cultural beliefs, values, and practices.

CULTURAL AWARENESS*

It is defined as "being knowledgeable about one's own thoughts, feelings, and sensations, as well as the ability to reflect on how these can affect one's interactions with other" (Giger et al., 2007).

Muslims

In traditional Muslim families, women must cover their head and hair. Some wear a body cloak called the "burka" or "burqa." Females are not allowed to be alone with males who are not family members. Male children are preferred. The male is in charge of the household.

If a woman is seen by a male health provider, her husband or another male family member must be present in the room. The female patient may refuse to undress (examine with the gown on).

The Qur'an (Koran) forbids eating pork or blood or meat not slaughtered in the "halal" manner.

Example: A 22-year-old Muslim woman is seen for a complaint of recurrent abdominal pain. The NP gives the patient a paper gown with instructions and leaves the room. When the NP returns, the patient is still clothed and refuses to undress. The nurse practitioner's best action is to:
A) Ask the patient if she prefers to be seen by a male physician.
B) Tell the patient what to expect and perform a modified physical exam.
C) Instruct the patient to go to the closest ED for an abdominal sonogram.
D) Lecture the patient about the importance of performing an abdominal exam without clothing on the skin.
   The correct answer is Option B.

---

*Adapted from the AACN's Tool Kit of Resources for Culturally Competent Education for Baccalaureate Nurses, August 2008.

Latinos/ Hispanics

"Susto" is a cultural illness (*susto* means "fright"). "Mal ojo" or the "evil eye" is a folk illness (usually of a baby/child). It is caused by an adult who stares with envy at the child. The evil eye is also practiced in some Muslim and Mediterranean cultures.

Family ties are important and several generations may live in the same household.

Asians (China, Vietnam, Cambodia, Korea, Japan, etc.)

Listening quietly without questioning is considered as a sign of respect. Asians highly value college education and have high regard (respect) for doctors. Some think that asking questions (or disagreeing) with the treatment plan is a sign of disrespect. Elderly are held in high esteem. Their opinion is highly respected. Kinship ties are very important. Several generations may live in the same household. Some Asian cultures have some form of "ancestor veneration" practices.

Vietnamese

May stop taking prescription medicine when symptoms resolve. It is common to save large quantities of left-over or half-used prescription drugs. Blood tests and surgery are feared because they think that blood loss worsens illness. Believe that Western medicine will put the body out of balance.

Traditional Chinese Medicine (TCM)

Life energy (chi or qi) imbalance or blockage is believed to be the cause of disease.
- Yin is the female and yang is the male. Acupuncture and cupping correct energy imbalance.
- Cupping will create large round reddened marks or bruises on back.
- Coining is when a coin is rubbed vigorously on skin to create welts. Both of these practices may produce lesions that may be misinterpreted as signs of abuse. The NP should question how a child received the lesions before reporting as abuse.

Jehovah's Witness

They do not believe in blood transfusions, but will accept plasma expanders.

Amish/Mennonites

They do not participate in Medicare or Social Security. The community pays for health care. Traditional roles for women. Prefer large families with several children. Prefer giving birth (using midwives) and dying at home.

THEORETICAL CONCEPTS

Health Belief Model (HBM)

A model that attempts to explain why people engage in health behavior(s). According to the HBM, a person is more likely to engage in healthier behavior if he or she feels threatened by the condition (perceived susceptibility), and believes that he or she can overcome the barriers (perceived barriers), will benefit, and can successfully perform the action (self-efficacy) (Rosenstock, Stretcher, & Becker, 1988).

Example: Who is more likely to perform healthier behavior—a 50-year-old smoker who recently had a myocardial infarction (MI), or 16-year-old girl who is obese?

In this case, it is probably the 50-year-old smoker who is more likely to quit smoking due to the seriousness of a MI and his older age, rather than the teenager who has to lose weight.

Family Systems Theory

All parts of a system are interrelated and dependent on each other. If one part of the system is damaged or dysfunctional, the rest of the system is also affected.

Families develop at different rates. If one family member becomes dysfunctional, it will affect the whole family. Another family member may compensate and take over some of the duties or the role of the dysfunctional family member.

Example: A family member is an alcoholic (the mother). She is married with three children. The oldest child is a 12-year-old girl. The daughter will most likely take over some of her mother's tasks such as cooking for the family or helping her father take care of the younger siblings.

Human Genetic Symbols

A new development in the exam is questions about genetic symbols. The symbol for a healthy male is an empty square; for a diseased/affected male, it is a filled square. The symbol for a healthy female is an empty circle; for a diseased/affected female, it is a filled circle. A diagonal dash across a symbol means that the person is dead.

Gender	Symbol	Description
Healthy male	□	Empty square
Diseased male	■	Filled square
Healthy female	○	Empty circle
Diseased female	●	Filled circle
Death	☒	Diagonal dash across a symbol

✎ EXAM TIP

- Learn the symbol for a diseased (or affected) male and female.

22

Nursing Research Review

DEFINITION

Nursing research is the "systematic inquiry that uses disciplined methods to answer questions or solve problems" (Polit & Hungler, 2004).

SOURCES OF DATA

Primary Sources (Preferred)

In research, primary sources are preferred. It is the original research where the data came from.

Secondary Sources

Secondary sources are created when the original data (primary data) are interpreted or analyzed by another person (not the original researcher).

Institutional Review Boards (IRBs)

An important duty of the IRB is to ensure the rights of human subjects who are participating in research studies in their hospital or clinic. IRBs have the right and responsibility to approve or reject research proposals that are submitted to their institution or hospital.

IRB Committee Members

The members of the IRB committee are the staff members and others who are affiliated with the institution. The members usually consists of staff members (registered nurses, nurse practitioners, physician assistants, physicians), staff pharmacist and/or affiliated consultants, and research faculty members. The size of the IRB and its members depend on the type of institution. Therefore physicians, clinicians, providers, or retail pharmacists who are not affiliated with the institution are generally not included in an IRB committee.

Vulnerable Populations

Almost all types of biomedical and behavioral research in the United States require informed consent. Groups considered "vulnerable populations" have additional paperwork and consent requirements. The following groups have special protections and have additional informed consent requirements:

- Infants and children under the age of 18 years.
- Pregnant women.

- Prisoners.
- Persons at risk for suicide.
- Persons with impaired decision capacity (e.g., mental retardation, Down's syndrome, etc.).

Belmont Report

A paper that outlines the important ethical principles that should be followed when doing research involving human subjects. It was issued by a national commission of experts in the United States in 1978.

Tuskegee Syphilis Experiment

An infamous study of 600 African American sharecroppers (1932 to 1972) from Alabama. The men were all tested for syphilis infection and those with positive results were never informed or treated. Due to this study, laws were passed that protect human subjects' rights and mandate informed consent.

Informed Consent of Human Subjects

Research subjects must be informed that they have the right to withdraw from the research study at any time without adverse consequences or penalty. There are additional requirements for minors and vulnerable subjects.

- Description of the study. Inform the subject of what he/she is expected to do (e.g., questionnaires, labs).
- Describe the risk or the discomforts of participating in the study in the present and the future (if applicable).
- Describe the benefits of participating in the study in the present and the future (if applicable).
- Discuss the alternatives to the study.
- Discuss if there is any compensation or reward for participation.
- Discuss how confidentiality and data will be secured to protect the subject's identity.
- Give the number and/or email address of the contact for the study so that the subject can contact that person if there are any concerns or problems with the study.

Minors

Any person who is under 18 years of age.

Emancipated Minor Criteria

- Legal court document declaring that the minor is an "emancipated minor."
- Active duty in the U.S. military.
- Legally binding marriage (or divorced from a legally binding marriage).

Consent Versus Assent

A minor (who is not emancipated) as young as the age of 7 years up to age 17 years can give assent to participate in a research study, but cannot give consent legally. The parent or legal guardian must first consent to the minor's participation in the study. In addition, the researcher needs parental permission to speak with the minor in order to obtain assent (the child signs a separate assent form).

Statistical Terms

- α: Also known as the significance level or the "*p*-value." It is usually set as either *p* <.05 or *p* <.01. A significance level of *p* <.05 means that there is a 5% probability that the data from the study are due to chance.

  A significance level of *p* <.01 means that there is only a 1% probability that the data from the study are due to chance. Therefore, an α of *p* <.01 is "better" than an α of *p* <.05.
- *Control group:* The subjects in an experiment who do not receive treatment.
- *Hypothesis:* The proposed explanation for (or prediction of) a phenomenon.
- *Median:* The numerical value separating the higher half from the lower half. The middle value in a list of numbers. The numbers are sorted from the lowest to the highest value.
- *Mode:* The most common value in a list of numbers.
- N: The symbol to indicate the total size of the sample.
- n: The symbol to indicate the number of subjects in the group.
- *Significance level:* Also known as the "α" or a "*p*-value." It is the probability that the study results are due to chance. The *p*-value is usually set at either *p* <.05 or *p* <.01.
- *Null hypothesis:* There is no significant relation between the variables of the study. If the null hypothesis is rejected, it means that the results of the study are not due to chance.

TYPES OF RESEARCH

Prospective Versus Retrospective Studies

Prospective

Studies that are done in the present (to the future) time frame.

Retrospective

Studies done on events that have already occurred (e.g., chart reviews, recall of events). Another name for this study design is "Ex post facto."

Longitudinal Studies

A long-term study follows the same group of subjects (or a subpopulation) over many years to observe and measure the same variables over time. It is an observational study (there is no manipulation or intervention). For example, the Framingham Heart Study has tracked the same research subjects (N = 5,029) from the town of Framingham, MA. The goal is to study the development and identify the factors that are associated with the development of cerebrovascular disease.

Variable

A characteristic, an object, or an event that is being measured.

Independent Variable

The variable that is not affected by the other variables. It is the variable that is manipulated. The result from the manipulation is called the dependent variable.

Dependent Variable

The variable(s) that is the result of the manipulation of the independent variable.

TYPES OF STUDIES

Qualitative Versus Quantitative Studies

Quantitative

Systematic gathering of data. The study's data are measurable and numerical. Data are evaluated by using statistical methods. Quantitative research is deductive.

Qualitative

The researcher uses observation and detailed interviews to gather data. Qualitative research is inductive. Identifies phenomena and concepts. Asks broad questions. The study's data are gathered as "words" and not numerical data.

Inductive Versus Deductive Reasoning

Inductive reasoning is the process of developing a generalization after studying specific information.

Deductive reasoning is figuring out a problem after evaluating some broad generalization(s).

RESEARCH DESIGNS

Experimental Versus Quasiexperimental Studies

Experimental Design

Considered the "gold standard" in research design. An important criterion is the use of random sampling to recruit research subjects. There is an intervention (or treatment) group and a control group. For example, a simple two-group experimental design will contain a control group and an intervention group that are "matched." Pretest (before intervention) and posttest data are measured. Data are numerical and evaluated using rigorous statistical testing.

Quasiexperimental Design

The design is similar to an experimental study except there is no randomization of the research subjects. Instead, recruitment of subjects is by convenience sample.

Case Study

An intensive and in-depth study of one person.

Cohort Study

A study of a group of individuals with one or more common characteristics. For example, the Framingham study has a subpopulation of nurses (a cohort of nurses) whose health habits have been tracked for many years.

Descriptive Versus Correlational Studies

Descriptive

Describes and measures the characteristics of a group or a phenomenon. Data are measurable, numerical, and are evaluated by statistical testing. No correlations are measured between the variables. Also known as surveys.
Example: "HIV knowledge of college students."

Correlational

Describes and measures relationships between two or more variables (or interrelationships). Data are measurable and are numerical. Data are subjected to statistical testing.
Example: "Is there a relationship between HIV knowledge and safe sex behaviors of college students?"

Cross-Sectional

A correlational study that evaluates for interrelationships between two or more groups.

✍ EXAM TIPS

- Primary data are the preferred source in research (original study that produced the data).
- Experimental studies use randomization.
- A correlational study describes and measures the interrelationships among the study's variables.
- A cross-correlational study describes and measures the interrelationships among the study's variables between two groups (or more).
- Definition of a cohort study, case study.
- What is a dependent or independent variable?
- Which groups are considered vulnerable populations?
- Definition of an IRB's role.
- Any staff or consultant of the hospital can become a member of the IRB. Community-based health professionals (e.g., retail pharmacist) cannot be part of an IRB (unless they are hired as consultants).
- Define a longitudinal study, descriptive study.
- The IRB's most important role is to protect the rights of the human subjects enrolled in the study.
- Definition of assent. Assent refers to minors because they legally cannot give consent (unless an emancipated minor).
- Definition of an emancipated minor.
- What is the significance level (the α or the p-value)? It is usually set at either $p < .05$ or $p < .01$. A significance level of $p < .05$ means that there is a 5% probability that the data from the study are due to chance.
- Learn definition of "median."

Gerontology Review

23

Professional, Medico-Legal, Support Services, and Reimbursement Considerations

CERTIFICATION EXAMS

Nurses who specialize in working with the aged prefer the broad term of "gerontology" to geriatrics.

ANCC Adult-Gerontology Primary Care Nurse Practitioner
Age Groups
- Adolescents (12–17 years)
- Adults (18–64 years)
- Older adults (age 65 years and older)

AANPCP Adult-Gerontology Nurse Practitioner (A-GNP)
Age Groups
- Late adolescents (16–20 years)
- Adults (21–64 years)
- Elderly (age 65 years and older)
- Older adults: Age classification:
  - Young–old (65–74 years)
  - Middle–old (75–84 years)
  - Oldest–old (85 years and older)

U.S. Census Bureau (2010): United States
Persons Greater Than 65 Years
Health care for elders is responsible for 1/3 of physician resources and 1/4 of medication use in the United States.

Population
- Age 65 years or older: 40.3 million people in the United States.
- Average American lifespan (both genders): 78.5 years.
- By the year 2030: 71.5 million (20% of population).
- Age 85 years or older (the "old–old"): by 2030, this will increase to 9.6 million (up to 19 million by 2050).

Leading Causes of Death*

- Heart disease
- Cancer
- Chronic obstructive pulmonary disease (COPD)

Life Expectancy*

- Average lifespan: 78.5 years.
- At age 65 years, the average American can expect to live another 19 years.
- Death rate (age 65 years or older): 794 deaths per 100,000 population.
- Average life expectancy:
  - Women: 80 years.
  - Men: 75 years.

Females

Generally, women live about 5 years longer than men (2010). Average life expectancy for women is 80 years (for men, it is 75 years). By the age of 85 (or older), there are 49 men for every 100 women.

By the age of 65, women are expected to live another 20 years (males will live another 17 years).

Ageism

"Ageism" is the belief in negative societal stereotypes about aging. Avoid the following actions when speaking with an older/elderly adult:

Example:

- Speaking in a loud voice (assumption of hearing loss).
- Speaking slowly (assumption of decreased mental capacity).
- Using terms such as "sweetie" or "granny" or "old guy."

Gerontological Nursing

Timeline Highlights

- 1981: American Nurses Association (ANA) Division of Gerontological Nursing first published the scope of practice for the specialty (revised in 1987).
- 1987: Scope of Practice of Gerontological Nursing revised.
- 1998: ANA offers certification for geriatric nurse practitioners and gerontologic clinical nurse specialists.
- 2008: The new specialty called the "Adult-Gerontologic" nurse will replace the "gerontologic" nursing programs by 2015 per the Consensus** expert panel (40 organizations). First group to take the new certification exam was the December 2012 graduates from Adult-Gerontology NP programs.
- A graduate of an ANP-only program or a GNP-only program cannot take the new exam.
- According to the ANCC (2012), the model is designed "to align the inter-relationships among licensure, accreditation, certification, and education to create a more uniform practice across the country."

---

*U.S. Census Bureau Data (2012).

**Consensus Model for advanced practice nursing registered (APRN). Regulation: Licensure, Accreditation, Certification, and Education (2008).

Gerontology Nurse Practitioner

A specialty area in advanced practice nursing that focuses on the aged (healthy and ill). May function in a variety of settings such as in skilled nursing facilities (SNFs), long-term care facilities (LTCF), hospice care, home care, academia, or the community setting.

The Gerontological NP and Adult NP roles were combined into "adult-gerontology" by the "National Consensus Model for APRN Regulation" on 2008. Educational programs for the ANP and the GNP will be completely phased out by 2015. NPs who are already certified in these two separate specialties will continue with their certifications (ANP or GNP). Certification can be renewed every 5 years by continuing education and clinical practice hours.

National Consensus Model for APRN Regulation: Licensure, Accreditation, Certification, and Education

The "consensus" group consisted of an Expert Panel (in adult and gerontologic nursing) in collaboration with organizations such as the American Association of Colleges of Nursing (AACN), National Organization of Nurse Practitioner Faculty (NONPF), Hartford Institute of Nursing, ANCC, AANPCP, and many others. The regulatory model has been endorsed by 45 national nursing organizations. The consensus group was jointly facilitated by Drs. Joan Stanley, AACN, and Katherine Crabtree, NONPF.

Adult-Gerontology Primary Care Nurse Practitioner

A new specialty of APRN. The population age group starts with adolescents until death. Practice settings includes those mentioned above plus private clinics, public health, urgent care, internal medicine clinics, college health clinics, home health, and others. The roles of the adult-gerontology nurses are many (nurse, health care provider, patient advocate, teacher, consultant, case manager).

The new advanced practice nursing specialty is the result of the national *Consensus Model for APRN Regulation: Licensure, Accreditation, Certification, and Education*, which was finalized in 2008. Full implementation is expected by 2015. The AACN published the *Adult-Gerontology Primary Care Nurse Practitioner Competencies* in March 2010.

New Regulatory Model

Advanced practice nurses have six population foci:
- Entire lifespan (FNP)
- Adult-gerontology
- Neonatal
- Pediatrics
- Women's health
- Psychiatric/mental health

The Consensus Model assigned four roles for the advanced practice nurse:
- Nurse practitioner (NP)
- Clinical nurse specialist
- Nurse-midwife
- Nurse anesthetist

Educational Requirements

A minimum of a master's degree level of education is mandatory. The AACN endorsed the "Position Statement on the Practice Doctorate in Nursing," which called for moving the current level of preparation necessary for advanced nursing practice from the master's degree to the doctorate level (Doctor of Nurse Practice) by the year 2015.

Professional Specialties in Gerontology/Geriatrics

- *Geriatrics*: Broad term associated with the "medical care" of the aged.
- *Gerontology*: Broad term relating to health care of the aged. The preferred term for nurses.
- *Geropsychology*: Branch of psychology that focuses on the psychology and mental health of the aged. Psychologists have a PhD degree.
- *Social gerontology*: focus is on the social aspects of aging. Degree in social work, sociology, or other fields.
- *Adult-Gerontology Primary Care Nurse Practitioner* (AGPCNP).
- *Gerontologic Nurse Practitioner*.

Organizations for Older Adults*

American Bar Association Commission on Law and Aging

A 15-member interdisciplinary organization that operates under the American Bar Association (ABA). Its members are experts (social services, law, academics, advocates, health professionals, advocates) whose mission is "to strengthen and secure the legal rights, dignity, autonomy, quality of life, and quality care of elders" (AoA.gov, 2011).

Administration on Aging (AoA)

A federal agency under the U.S. Department of Health and Human Services (DHHS). Its mission is "to develop a comprehensive, coordinated, and cost-effective system of home and community-based services that helps elderly individuals maintain their health and independence in their homes and communities" (AoA.gov, 2011).

Alzheimer's Association

A voluntary health organization whose mission is to "eliminate Alzheimer's disease through the advancement of research" and to help enhance the lives of individuals with Alzheimer's disease.

American Association of Homes and Services for the Aging (AAHSA)

A nongovernmental group that represents not-for-profit nursing homes, continuing care retirement communities, assisted-living facilities (ALFs), and other health care facilities for the aged.

American Association of Retired Persons (AARP)

A nongovernmental organization of retired persons aged 50 years or older in the United States. Based in Washington, DC. One of the most powerful lobbying and advocacy groups. Offers services and discounts for members such as Medicare supplemental and Medigap health insurance, prescription drug discounts, travel/car discounts, life insurance discounts. Founder is Ethel Percy Andrus, PhD (1958).

American Geriatrics Society (AGS)

A nonprofit organization for health professionals (multidisciplinary) who are involved in the field of geriatrics. Its goal is to improve elderly people's quality of life, health, and independence.

---

* For a full list of organizations for the elderly, go to www.aoa.gov.

Centers for Medicare and Medicaid Services (CMS)
A federal agency that is responsible for the Medicare and Medicaid programs.

John A. Hartford Foundation Institute for Geriatric Nursing
A not-for-profit charitable foundation that funds educational programs and research grants that address older adult/elderly health care and health care delivery issues.

National Council on the Aging (NCoA)
A membership organization of professionals whose goal is to help promote the "dignity, self-determination, well-being, and contributions of older persons" (ncoa.org, 2011).

Elder Abuse

National Center on Elder Abuse
An organization under the AoA. It administers a telephone "hotline" for reporting elder abuse. A locator (by state) is on their website. The Eldercare Locator phone number is 1-800-677-1116.

The National Center on Elder Abuse (NCEA) defines a "vulnerable" adult as "a person who is being mistreated or is in danger of mistreatment and who, due to age and/or disability, is unable to protect himself or herself."

Adult Protective Services (APS) or Protective Services
Administered by each state. Provides services to "insure the safety and well-being of elders and adults with disabilities who are in danger of being mistreated or neglected" (AoA, 2011). APS caseworkers are usually the "first responders" in many states on reports of elder abuse, exploitation, and/or neglect.

Adult Protective Services Interventions
Receive and investigate reports of elder abuse. Casework services includes obtaining emergency housing, medical care, legal assistance, housing, law enforcement, and other supportive services.

Mandatory Reporting
There are differences between states regarding mandatory reporting of elder abuse. Each state has its own statute or law about the types of professions that must report abuse. In most states, certain professions are mandated reporters (e.g., social workers, mental health providers, professional nurses, school personnel, nursing home employees).

Gunshot wounds must be reported to the local police. Sexual assault cases are referred to the emergency department for evaluation, treatment, and for gathering of evidence of the assault.

Avoid contaminating possible evidence (avoid washing clothing, sheets). Document on the resident's chart the facts regarding the incident, scene, and possible evidence.

Types of Elder Abuse
There are several types of elder abuse: financial abuse neglect, emotional abuse, physical abuse, sexual abuse, and excessive physical restraints. Caregivers who are under high stress are more likely to abuse elders in their care. Respite care is recommended for providers who are stressed.

Financial Abuse
Clues include withdrawals from an ATM, large withdrawals from a bank account, excessive credit card use, identity theft, checks/documents with signatures that do

not match the elder's signature (or if the elder is unable to write or is confused), a stranger who is a "close friend" and is managing the patient's finances and assets. Other types of perpetrators are family members, the person who is designated as the durable power of attorney, a financial conservator, or a construction contractor (home improvement scams).

Neglect

Neglect is also considered abuse. Signs of neglect include poor hygiene (uncombed/matted hair, dirty, foul smelling), dehydration, or malnutrition.

Emotional Abuse

Frequent screaming or "verbal assault," threats, intimidation.

Physical Abuse/Assault

Unexplained bruises/welts (or with as an outline such as a belt), patches of hair missing from scalp, bites, injuries with incompatible explanations.

Sexual Abuse/Assault

Bloody or torn undergarments, purulent and/or blood-tinged vaginal discharge, onset of new sexually transmitted disease.

Physical Constraints

Locking elderly persons inside their bedrooms, preventing them from seeing friends, isolating patients, using restraints to limit mobility, and excessive "drugging" with psychotropic medications.

Patient Rights

The Ominibus Budget Reconciliation Act of 1987 (OBRA, 1987) included major reforms and regulations to address abuses in nursing homes. A "Patient Bill of Rights" poster must be posted on the wall in a visible area in health care facilities (e.g., LTCFs, hospitals). The telephone number of the local ombudsman's office is also included in the poster.

Patients have the right to:

- Review their care plan.
- Be informed when their treatment changes.
- Voice grievances and to communicate freely without fear of reprisal.
- Dignity and privacy.
- Self-determination.
- Participate in resident groups and family groups.
- Freedom from mistreatment and abuse.

Physical Restraints

A "resident has the right to be free from any physical or chemical restraints imposed for purposes of discipline or convenience and not required to treat a resident's medical symptoms" (Medicare Long-Term Care User Manual). A resident who is of sound mind can legally refuse the use of physical restraints (or any type of medical treatment).

Types of Physical Restraints

Vests, belts, wrist restraints, and ankle restraints. State laws and federal law (for Medicare or Medicaid-certified LTCFs) prohibit the use of physical restraints unless medically necessary.

Illegal use of a physical restraint is considered a type of physical assault.

Adverse Effects

Functional decline, contractures, pressure ulcers, urinary incontinence, increased agitation, decreased mobility, decreased self-image, strangulation, and death.

Chemical restraint is the excessive and unnecessary use of psychotropic meds (e.g., haloperidol).

Prescribing Physical Restraints

1) Staff should document the interventions done to ensure patient's safety and the results. If it is determined that physical restraints are medically necessary, a prescription is written.
2) The type of physical restraint device, indication, and directions are written on the prescription.
3) Document the patient's response and condition (vital signs, behaviors) while on restraints.
4) Check the patient's extremities for pulse and the skin for cyanosis regularly if on wrist and/or ankle restraints. Check the restraints for proper placement.
5) Resident must be released at least every 2 hours (or repositioned if bedridden). Check if patient needs to use the toilet. If incontinent, check incontinence briefs for soiling at least every 2 hours.

Residences and Facilities for Older Adults

All health care facilities must be licensed and regulated by the state (e.g., Department of Health) where the facility is located. Since most accept Medicare and Medicaid, they must also be certified by the Centers for Medicare and Medicaid Services (CMS) and follow federal rules and regulations.

Long-Term Care Facility

Also known as "nursing homes." Emphasis is on 24-hour custodial care. Custodial care is non-medical care of people with chronic illnesses or disability (e.g., helping people with bathing, grooming, or other activities of daily living [ADL], or shopping, finances, or other instrumental activities of daily living [IADL]). The majority of patients with moderate to severe dementia are taken care of in nursing homes. The typical nursing home resident is a female with multiple impairments in ADLs (greater than 3 ADLs) who is 80 years of age or older.

Skilled-Nursing Facilities (SNFs)

Provides transitional care (after hospital discharge), rehabilitation (physical and/or occupational therapy), and skilled nursing and medical care. Age group is not limited to older adults. Examples of patient groups are those who need chronic skilled nursing care such as those in a coma, with spinal cord injuries, or on chronic respiratory ventilators.

Assisted-Living Facilities

A facility for older adults who may need minimal assistance with ADLs and/or IADLs. Usually provides nursing home aides to assist residents. Residents are alert (not for dementia patients).

Group Homes

Residents live with others in a residential type of setting. Usually privately owned. Age groups may vary.

Green House
Consists of home-like dwellings that accommodate from 8 to 10 older adult residents. The Green House model was created by geriatric specialist Dr. William Thomas (2004) and is an "alternative to traditional long-term care facilities" (Mauk, 2009).

Adult Day Care
Community-dwelling older adults who need constant supervision can be enrolled in adult day care.

Home Health Care
Care is delivered in a home setting. Higher-skilled care given by registered nurses (RNs) or LPNs. ADL and IADL assistance is given by certified nursing assistants (CNAs). May be temporary or permanent ("medical home").

Respite Care (For Health Caregivers Only)
Provides short-term "relief" or a break for the long-term primary health caregiver (usually a family member). Ranges from a few hours to a day. An alternate caregiver (nurse or aide) is hired to care for the patient temporarily.

Independent Living Retirement Communities
Also known as "independent living" or "retirement communities." The residents are from age 55 years (and older) who require minimal to no help with daily activities. Housing ranges from free-standing homes to apartments and condominiums. The campus usually has health clubs, golf courses, planned activities, restaurants, and transportation. Requires a large entry fee ($40,000–$400,000) plus monthly fees.

Continuing Care Retirement Communities
Continuing care retirement communities (CCRCs) offer a spectrum of care in one setting. Resident packages range from completely independent (independent living) ALFs to skilled nursing care facilities (SNFs), which are all, located in one community. For example, if an independent resident falls and fractures a hip, the resident can be moved (temporarily) to the SNF for skilled nursing care and rehab. When the resident recovers, he/she can move back into the independent living campus. An advantage is that only one entrance fee is required (plus the monthly fees).

Retirement Communities
Only those aged 55 years or older are allowed to live in this type of community. The resident must buy a housing unit (apartment, condo, house) and pay a monthly fee (yard maintenance, recreation centers). A retirement community may also be part of a CCRC.

Subsidized Senior Housing
The U.S. Department of Housing and Urban Development (HUD) subsidizes senior housing complexes for low-income seniors. There is a high demand for this program and waiting lists can extend for several years. Therefore, early planning is important.

PAYMENT METHODS

Reimbursement Glossary
- *Accelerated Death Benefit*: a type of life insurance policy benefit that allows an insured person to use some of the policy's death benefit prior to death. For example, it can be used to pay for long-term care.
- *Assignment of Benefits*: a person with a long-term care insurance policy can assign his or her benefits to be paid directly to the providers of care (e.g., nursing home) instead of receiving the payment directly.

- *Authorized Representative or Representative Payee*: A person (usually a lawyer) who is chosen by an older adult who has Social Security benefits to represent him/her in any business with the Social Security Administration.
- *Benefit Maximum*: A limit on a covered benefit. A service or supply may be limited by dollar amount, duration, or number of visits. An example of a benefit maximum is that well-woman exams are typically limited to one per calendar year. Another example, the insurance company may only allow a set amount of reimbursement for a surgery such as a hysterectomy.
- *Benefit Period*: Medicare's hospitalization insurance has a limit (time period) of 60 consecutive days after discharge from a hospital or SNF before a new benefit period starts. There is a set number of benefit periods that a person can have.
- *Certificate of Need (CON)*: A hospital (or "builder") must prove that there is a need for more hospital beds (or a new hospital, SNF) in the local area before it can receive a certificate of need.
- *Conservatorship*: A legal term. If a person is deemed by the court to be incapable of managing his or her property (due to dementia, in jail, chronic drug abuse, under-aged), the property can be managed by others (e.g., bank, lawyer). The conservator manages the finances and pays for the person's support and allowance.
- *Deductible*: A yearly amount that is required by an insurance carrier (Medicare, health insurance) that is the patient's responsibility. After the deductible is met, the insurer pays for future costs.

Reimbursement: Government Programs

Although most of these terms are covered in the Non-Professional Issues in Section IV under the Medico-Legal, Ethical Guidelines, and AP Law, they are important topics to become familiar with in the field of gerontological nursing.

Medicare does not pay, for "custodial care" (e.g., nursing homes). Custodial care is nonskilled care that most people perform for themselves such as grooming, dressing, or using the bathroom. Medicaid does pay for nursing home care of eligible low-income persons.

Medicare Part B

Will pay for skilled care for nursing home residents that is medically necessary.

Other Forms of Payment (For Nursing Home Care)
- Veterans benefits (armed services).
- Long-term care insurance/policy (cheaper if bought at younger ages).
- Life insurance settlement (life insurance value is converted into cash).
- Reverse mortgages (value of home is converted into cash/mortgage).

Medicaid
A federal and state program that pays for health care services for individuals/children with low incomes and limited assets. The largest group supported by Medicaid is dependent children of low-income persons. Will pay for nursing home care of low-income people. Eligibility and coverage vary by state.

Medicare Review
Medicare is a federal health insurance program that is administered by the CMS. Medicare is a fee-for-service program. Payment is collected through monthly payroll deductions (Social Security taxes). There are now four parts to Medicare.

Medicare Part A

Pays for inpatient health services. Automatic at age of 65 years, but if a person never paid Medicare taxes (e.g., housewife), then he or she is not eligible for Medicare. Best to enroll a few months before the 65th birthday.

Medicare Part B

Pays for outpatient care. Must pay a monthly premium. Must enroll during the "open enrollment period." Pays for outpatient care such as doctor visits, laboratory tests, outpatient procedures, and medically necessary durable medical equipment (DME) such as wheelchairs and oxygen. DME must be "prescribed" (written prescription).

Medicare Part C

Also known as "Medicare Advantage." Voluntary. Person must enroll. Allows person to receive health care services through a provider organization such as an HMO. These type of coverage will pay for both inpatient and outpatient health services and prescription drugs (has formulary or list of drugs that are covered). Formerly called "Medicare + Choice."

Medicare Part D

Prescription drug coverage. Voluntary. Must enroll and pay monthly premiums. Person must enroll in an approved plan.

Medicare Supplemental Insurance ("Medigap")

Covers "gaps" in coverage (e.g., prescription drugs) of original Medicare Part B plan. Sold by private insurance companies or may be partially funded by employers or unions as a benefit. Must enroll and pay a monthly premium.

Personal Resources and Assets

Another method of payment and frequently combined with other methods such as private insurance, co-pay, and deductible amounts.

Glossary of Joint Commission (JC) Terms

The Joint Commission

An independent, not-for-profit organization that accredits health care organizations (hospitals, nursing homes, home care, laboratories) via inspection and evaluation of their facilities (charged a fee). Achieving JC certification means that a facility has met or surpassed their strict requirements.

Root Cause Analysis (RCA)

A JC requirement for investigating problems/adverse events in a health care system (e.g., clinic, hospitals). The hospital/clinic looks for the factors that may have contributed to the problem (root cause). The possible contributing factors are then identified. The gathered data are analyzed for the root causes (usually a combination of human factors, environmental and system factors) and a plan to remedy the problem is carried out to correct the problem (and to prevent it in the future).

Example: Adverse event occurs (e.g., injuries). The "root cause" that contributed must be identified (worker stress, time limitations, patient load, low staff morale, lacking certain skills, others). These factors are analyzed and a plan is proposed to remedy/prevent the problem (e.g., more staff, staff education, etc.).

Sentinel Event (SE) Reporting

The JC requires reporting of a SE, which is an unexpected occurrence that resulted in a death or serious injury (such as loss of a limb). The type, setting, sources, outcomes, the reporting, and response to the event are evaluated.

Examples:

Presence of these events adversely affects reimbursement for LTCFs by Medicare and Medicaid. Sentinel events are monitored by JACHO, Quality Assurance and Risk Management teams.

- Incidence of retained foreign objects (sponges) after surgery
- Health care worker fatigue and patient safety.
- Patient injury/deaths from using certain medications (anticoagulants, opioids, etc.).
- Patient injuries/deaths from anticoagulants.
- Pressure ulcers (type III and type VI).

Legal Terms

- *Ombudsmen*: assigned to protect the rights of an individual versus the health care system (e.g., LTCF, hospitals, etc.). If contacted, will investigate complaints and negotiate for the individual.
- *Power of Attorney (or Durable Power of Attorney) for Health Care*: a legal document that designates a person (picked by the resident/patient) to act on the patient's behalf to make health decisions in the event that the patient is incapacitated (physical and/or mental). Power is only for health care decisions (no power with financial assets).
- *Power of Attorney (Broad)*: a legal document that designates a person (picked by the resident/patient) to act on the patient's behalf to make all decisions in the event that the patient is incapacitated (physical and/or mental). Involves all aspects of the resident's/patient's life (health care, finances, assets).

Long-Term Care Facilities

As of 2012, it is estimated that about 9 million Americans over the age of 65 years will need long-term care in nursing homes. By the year 2020, the number will climb up to 12 million Americans due to the large number of aging "baby boomers." Most older adults (70%) are taken care of in private homes (not in nursing homes) by family members. There is usually one primary caregiver (family member or friend).

The most common cause of death in nursing home residents is pneumonia. The other common causes of death are heart disease, pulmonary embolism, cachexia/malnutrition, and dehydration.

INTERDISCIPLINARY TEAMS: GERIATRIC SETTINGS

Types of Clinical Teams

Multidisciplinary

A group composed of members from different disciplines/specialties. Each team member develops a treatment plan independently from each other. For example, the physical therapist writes a treatment plan that addresses the patient's exercise goals, and the dietician writes a goal of helping the patient to gain weight. Each member (depending on the specialty) conducts an individual assessment. Primary care provider typically writes prescriptions, makes referrals to specialists, seeks consultations, and oversees care.

A case manager whose role is to coordinate the patient's care and avoid duplication of services may be involved.

Intradisciplinary Team

An intradisciplinary team is composed of team members who are from the same specialty or discipline area, but are at different levels of educational training. For example, a team composed of an NP, RN, and an LPN. The term may be confused with a multidisciplinary team.

Geriatric Assessment Interdisciplinary Teams

Composed of several individuals from different disciplines/specialties who work together as a team. The team's goal is to maximize the resident's/patient's health care, continuity of care, and quality of life. A team can be made up of three or more members. Members of the team a.. those who are involved with the patient's care.

Geriatric Team Members and Roles

Geriatrician

A physician (MD or DO) who has a specialty in geriatrics. Specializes in the medical care of the aged.

Physician, Nurse Practitioner (NP), Physician Assistant (PA)

Physicians, NPs, and PAs are responsible for the medical or health care of residents/patients.

In addition, a physician can function as the medical director of the facility. PAs are under the supervision of a physician.

Contact physician, NP, or PA for the following:

- Admitting new patients (for admission orders).
- Prescription (or refills) of medication, including OTCs.
- Prescription for laboratory or imaging testing.
- Prescriptions (e.g., meds, physical restraint devices, oxygen, medical equipment).
- Prescriptions and referral for rehabilitation (physical therapist [PT], occupational therapist [OT], speech therapy).
- Referrals and consults with physician specialists (e.g., endocrinologist for diabetic patient), hospice.
- Hospitalization/discharge or transfer of the resident/patient.

Registered Nurse

May function as the director of nursing, a supervisor, or as a staff nurse. RNs can supervise and delegate to other RNs, LPNs, and medical assistants.

Contact RN for the following:

- Patient admissions, transfers, and discharge; telephone orders; documentation.
- Medication issues, patient assessment, signs/symptoms of health problems, to contact physician.
- Behavioral issues; incidents (patient falls, etc.).
- Must file incident report. Assesses patient's injury. Notify nursing supervisor.

Director of Nursing

Responsible for entire nursing staff (including medical assistants and nurses aides). Can hire and fire nursing staff. Contact Director of Nursing (DON) or Assistant DON, and/or nurse supervisor if problems with understaffing, nursing personnel conflicts, or conflict with medical staff.

LPNs
Educated through vocational education schools or in community colleges. LPNs are directed and supervised by RNs. LPNs with special training may administer IV solutions with RN supervision (states may differ).

Medical Assistant or Nurse's Aide
Most are certified and have the designation of CMA (Certified Medical Assistant) or CNA (Certified Nurse's Aide). Educated through vocational education programs. CNAs in LTCFs typically care for many patients. Responsible for basic patient care such as assisting patient with oral intake and walking, toileting, bathing, brushing teeth, and assisting patient with transfers (e.g., from bed to chair). Medical assistants usually are charged with repositioning or turning bedridden patients every 2 hours. Common activities include recording vital signs, oral and food intake, and intake and output.

Registered Dietician
Contact to evaluate new patients, for consultations, dietary assessment.

Physical Therapist or PT Assistant
PT will evaluate person's ability to walk and other gross motor skills. PT will make recommendations on type of rehabilitation, frequency, and duration.

Occupational Therapist
Focus is more on hands/fine motor-related disabilities. OT will evaluate patient and make recommendations. For example, stroke patients can be trained to feed themselves. OT may make recommendations on type of assistive equipment (nonslip pad for dishes, forks/spoons with special handles).

Speech Therapist
Focus is on teaching and training patients with speech problems.

Priest
Contact local priest if Catholic patient requests the "last rites" (Prayer of the Sick).

Minister/Pastor
Other Christians may request a minister for prayers.

Social Worker
Master's in Social Work (MSW). Social workers function as mental health therapists or as caseworkers. Casework involves knowledge of local and federal assistance, social programs, local community resources, legal resources, financial resources such as Medicaid/Medicare, and others.

Social workers assist low-income patients by helping them find local social agencies.

Psychologist
May specialize in gerontology (geropsychology). Psychologist cannot prescribe medications. May function as a consultant or a mental health therapist.

Psychiatrist or Gerontologic NP or Adult-Gerontology NP or Psychiatric NP
May specialize in gerontology or mental health. They typically write prescriptions and refill psychotropic medications.

Neurologist
Refer patient for dementia evaluation and testing, seizures, and other neurological disease.

Pharmacist

Responsible for filling prescriptions and refills; may be consulted about potential drug interactions. The pharmacist may notify the prescriber of potential problems with the prescribed medications.

Geriatric Interdisciplinary Team Training Program*

The Geriatric Interdisciplinary Team Training (GITT) program was developed with the John A. Hartford Foundation. Its goal is to provide training and educational materials for geriatric interdisciplinary team training.

Phases of Team Formation (GITT program)

- *Forming*: creation of a group. Conflict is not discussed at this stage.
- *Norming*: appoint a leader. Establish common goals and ground rules. Conflicts may become evident, but are not addressed yet.
- *Confronting or Storming*: conflicts can no longer be avoided. Increased conflicts over leadership.
- *Performing*: productivity and problem solving are emphasized. Meeting attendance is regular/consistent.
- *Leaving*: team may break up. Individuals or some members may withdraw.

Ineffective Behaviors

- Interrupting another team member while speaking.
- Starting a meeting late, lack of an agenda.
- Sarcasm and lack of respect.
- Lack of effective leadership, unresolved team conflict.
- Members are not sure of their role in the team.
- Beepers, cell phones, snacking during the meeting.
- Avoid long breaks for "coffee and donuts" since it will delay and extend meeting times.

Recommendations

To minimze ineffective behavior:

- Practice good leadership skills: leader facilitates meeting, refocuses group (as necessary), uses collaborative language.
- Team members are clear about their roles and responsibilities.
- Conflicts between members are addressed directly.
- Team members respect each other.
- Members avoid interrupting while others are speaking.
- Schedule follow-up meeting.

---

* Adapted from the John A. Hartford Foundations GITT website. What is team training? Accessed December 20, 2012, at www.gittprogram.org.

24

Theory and Conceptual Models Applied to Gerontology

STAGES OF CHANGE (PROCHASKA AND DICLEMENTE)

Also known as the "Transtheoretical" model (TTM). A five-stage model to help assess a person's readiness to change. Originally used in alcoholism addiction research, but now used in other areas such as in smoking cessation, weight loss, drug addiction, and the like.

Stage	Description	Application: Weight Loss
Precontemplation	In denial, rationalization Rebels and not ready to change	May report "I'm big-boned" or "just overweight" or "I love to eat." Does not feel that she has a problem
Contemplation	Fully or partially aware of problem. Ambivalent about changing "Sitting on the fence"	Not sure of wanting to change yet, investigates options but does not commit
Preparation	Admits the problem. Ready to change behavior. Planning stage	Writes down goals, looks for recipes, plans exercise schedule
Action	Takes action in changing lifestyle, adopting healthier behaviors. Looks for social support (tells friends about plans, what to avoid)	Grocery shopping for healthier foods, exercises, attends weight loss meetings (Weight Watchers)
Maintenance	Successful, takes measures to avoid relapse, social supports	Continues with healthier eating plan, exercises consistently

SELF-EFFICACY AND SOCIAL COGNITIVE THEORY (ALFRED BANDURA)

Alfred Bandura created the concept of "self-efficacy." He defined self-efficacy as the belief about one's ability to successfully perform a behavior(s) in certain situations.

He is also the creator of Social Cognitive Theory. This model posits that people learn new behaviors by modeling and observation. It contains four primary variables (explained below).

Application: Cigarette Advertisements

A good-looking model (attracts attention) is smoking in a party of young beautiful adults. The unspoken message is that people who smoke are more attractive to the opposite sex (the motivation). The person viewing the advertisement remembers (retention) and mimics the smoking behavior (reproduction).

HEALTH BELIEF MODEL

A model that attempts to explain why people adopt healthier behaviors. The Health Belief Model (HBM) has many constructs and variables. The most popular constructs are listed here in tabular form.

Construct	Definition
Perceived susceptibility	A person's belief about the severity of a condition
Perceived barriers	A person's belief about the barriers to changing a behavior
Perceived severity	A person's belief that the disease/addiction is severe and life threatening
Perceived benefits	A person's belief that the benefits of adapting the new behavior outweigh negative risk
Perceived efficacy	A person's belief that he or she will be successful

Application

Which of the following individuals is more likely to change his or her behavior?
A) Overweight teenager who has dropped out of high school.
B) A middle-aged male who was discharged after recovering from an acute myocardial infarction (MI).
C) An adult who has been smoking since the age of 10.
D) An older adult who drinks one glass of wine with the evening meal.

The correct answer is option B. The middle-aged adult recovering from an acute MI is most likely to change behavior. Task is to engage in productive activity, including such activities as a job or raising a family. Rule out option D since the person is not considered an alcoholic. The adult smoker is not ill (rule out option C).

Developmental Theories

Regarding developmental theories, only the stages that occur in older adults are discussed in this chapter. The younger age groups are discussed under the Pediatrics and Adolescent sections.

ERIK ERIKSON'S STAGES OF PSYCHOSOCIAL DEVELOPMENT

The first five stages occur from birth to age 18 years. After 18 years of age, there are three stages.

Intimacy Versus Isolation

Early adulthood. Task is to develop intimate relationships. May be married. Enjoys friendships and relationships.

Failure: social isolation and lack of emotional commitment.

Generativity Versus Stagnation

Middle age. Task is to hold a productive job; may have a family. May become involved with social causes.

Failure: unable to hold down a job or refuses to work, self-centered, not contributing to society.

Table 24.1 Maslow's Hierarchy of Needs

Stage	Examples
Self-actualization (highest level)	Pursues hobbies, creativity, and spiritual needs. Attends church groups, spiritual retreats
	Volunteers. Involved with social issues. Personal growth activities
Self-esteem	Doing well in one's job, feeling competent, confidence, feeling respected by others, fame
Love and belonging	Relationships, friends and family. Marriage/significant other. Sexual intimacy
Safety needs	Shelter, clothing, public laws to protect citizens from crime, military, police
Physiologic/biologic needs (lowest level)	Eating, breathing, elimination, sleep, physical activity, and sexual activity

Ego Integrity Versus Despair

Older adult to frail elderly. Satisfaction with life accomplishments (i.e., career, family, children). Wants to leave a "legacy" to the future generation. For example, grandmother may sew a quilt for each of her grandchildren and give them as gifts.

Failure: many regrets about life and at high risk for depression (despair).

ABRAHAM MASLOW'S HIERARCHY OF NEEDS

There are five stages in the original model. Basic physiologic needs must first be met before one can progress to the highest stage (self-actualization). A pyramid/triangle is often used to show this model. The basic needs are listed on the bottom (base), and the highest stage is at the apex of the triangle (Table 24.1).

✎ EXAM TIP

One of the best clues for identifying a stage is to look at the age group. Older adult stage appears often (generativity vs. despair). Learn to recognize "real-life" examples.

STAGES OF COGNITIVE DEVELOPMENT (JEAN PIAGET)

This stage attempts to identify cognitive development. The last stage of the theory is the "formal operational stage." This stage usually starts at about the age of 11 (or older). People with intellectual impairment remain in the "concrete" phase and never reach this stage.

Formal operational stage: starts at age 11 years. At this stage, the older child can understand abstract ideas (abstract thinking). Logical thinking is more developed. More aware of the future. Can think in "gray" instead of "black or white" or "all or nothing" terms. Some adults never reach this stage and remain "concrete" thinkers.

STAGES OF PSYCHOSEXUAL DEVELOPMENT (SIGMUND FREUD)

The last stage of this model is the "Genital Stage," which starts in puberty. At this stage, the genitals are seen as an important source of pleasure.

Sexuality and Aging

Some older adults (up to their mid-80s) remain sexually active. Some of the factors that affect sexuality as we age are gender, physiologic changes (e.g., atrophic vaginitis), disease, medications, cognition, and mobility. STDs (including HIV) should be considered in sexually active older adults who present with signs and symptoms and have risk factors (i.e., new partner in the past 60 days; Table 24.2).

Table 24.2 Nursing Theory

Name	Concepts	Theorist
Theory of Cultural Care Diversity Nursing care should be culture-specific and culturally sensitive	Transcultural nursing, culturally congruent care, culturally competent care, cultural awareness	Madeleine Leininger
Self-Care Deficit Theory Nurses help patients to maintain or assist them with self-care activities	Self-care deficit occurs when one is unable or has difficulty performing "self-care" activities or "self-care agency" Self-care are activities that a person performs independently to maintain his or her health (e.g., eating, grooming, elimination, walking)	Dorothea Orem
Roy's Adaptation Model Promote adaptation of individuals/ group by assessing behaviors/factors that affect adaptive capabilities	Stimuli of three types (focal, contextual, residual) Model identified six steps to nursing process: Adaptive/ineffective responses, cognator or regulator adaptive systems, others	Sister Calista Roy
Theory of Caring Caring is an important component of nursing (focus is on the person, not technology)	"Carative" factors include humanistic-altruistic values, faith–hope, sensitivity to self/others, establishing helping–trusting relationships	Jean Watson
Neuman Systems Model Each person is a complete system and any changes in the "subparts" will affect the entire system; nurses help maintain stability of the system	Person is an open system, concentric circles used to represent the energy resources, "central core," lines of defense, lines of resistance, stressors, nursing actions (primary, secondary, tertiary)	Betty Neuman

25

Body and Metabolic Changes in the Older Adult

Skin Findings

Skin atrophy. Thinner epidermis, dermis, and subdermal fat. Less collagen (less elasticity). Fragile skin and slower healing. Slower nail growth. Lower oil production and drier skin (xerosis) due to decrease in sebaceous and sweat gland activity. Fewer melanocytes leading to graying of hair and vitamin D synthesis. Decrease in the skin's sensory ability.

Seborrheic Keratoses

Soft wart-like skin lesions that appear "pasted on." Mostly seen on the back/trunk. Benign.

Senile Purpura

Bright purple-colored patches with well-demarcated edges. Located on the dorsum of the forearms and hands. Lesions eventually resolved over several weeks. Benign.

Lentigines

Also known as "liver spots." Tan- to brown-colored macules on the dorsum of the hands and forearms. Due to sun damage. More common in light skinned individuals. Benign.

Stasis Dermatitis

Affects primarily lower legs and ankles secondary to chronic edema (from PVD).

Senile Actinic Keratosis

Secondary to sun exposure; potential for malignancy.

Nails

Growth slows and become brittle, yellow, and thicker. Longitudinal ridges develop.

Eyes

Presbyopia is caused by loss of elasticity of the lenses, which makes it difficult to focus on close objects. Close vision is markedly affected. Onset is during early to mid-40s.

Can be remedied with "reading glasses" or bifocal lenses. Cornea less sensitive to touch. Arcus senilis, cataracts, and glaucoma are more common.

Arcus Senilis (Corneal Arcus)

Opaque grayish to white ring at the periphery of the cornea. Develops gradually and not associated with visual changes. Caused by deposition of cholesterol and fat. In younger patients (<40 years), can be a sign of elevated cholesterol. Check fasting lipid profile.

Cataracts

Cloudiness and opacity of the lens of the eye(s) or its envelope (posterior capsular cataract). Three types (nuclear, cortical, and posterior capsular). Color is white to gray. Gradual onset of decreased night vision, sensitivity to glare of car lights (driving at night), and hazy vision. The red reflex disappears.

Test: Red reflex (reflection is opaque gray versus orange-red glow).

Macular Degeneration

Loss of central visual fields results in loss of visual acuity and contrast sensitivity. May find Drusen bodies. Use Amsler grid to evaluate central vision changes.

Ears

Presbycusis (Sensorineural Hearing Loss)

High-frequency hearing lost first (e.g., speaking voice is high-frequency). Degenerative changes of the ossicles, fewer auditory neurons, and atrophy of the hair cells resulting in sensorineural hearing loss.

Cardiac

Elongation and tortuosity (twisting) of the arteries. Thickened intimal layer of arteries and arteriosclerosis resulting in increased systolic blood pressure (BP) due to increased vascular resistance (isolated systolic hypertension). Thicker mitral and aortic valves, which may contain calcium deposits.

Baroreceptors less sensitive to changes in position. Decreased sensitivity of the autonomic nervous system. Blunted BP response. Decrease in maximum heart rate. Higher risk of orthostatic hypotension.

S4 heart sound a "normal finding" in the elderly if not associated with heart disease. The left ventricle hypertrophies with aging (up to 10% of thickness).

Lungs

Total lung capacity remains relatively the same as we age. Both the residual volume and the forced expiratory volume in 1 second (FEV1) increase due to the decrease in lung and chest wall compliance. The chest wall becomes stiffer and the diaphragm is flatter and less efficient.

Mucociliary clearance (less cilia) and coughing are less efficient. The airways collapse sooner during expiration. Responses to hypoxia and hypercapnia decreases. Decreased breath sounds and crackles are commonly found in the lung bases of elderly patients without presence of disease. Instruct the patient to "cough" several times to inflate the lung bases (the benign crackles will disappear). Increased anterior–posterior (AP) diameter related to normal body changes.

Liver

Liver size and mass decreases due to atrophy (20%–40%). Liver blood flow and perfusion decreases (up to 50% in some elders). Fat (lipofuscin) deposition in the liver is more common. The liver function test (aspartate aminotransferase [ALT], alanine aminotransferase [AST], alkaline phosphatase) result is not significantly changed. Metabolic clearance of drugs is slowed by 20% to 40% because the cytochrome P450 (CYP 450) enzyme system is less efficient. The low-density lipoprotein (LDL) and cholesterol levels increase with aging.

Renal Function

Renal size and mass decreased by 25% to 30%. The steepest decline in renal mass occurs after the age of 50. Starting at the age of 40 years, the glomerular filtration rate (GFR) starts to decrease. By age 70, up to 30% of renal function is lost. Renal clearance of drugs is less efficient. The serum creatinine is a less reliable indicator of renal function in the elderly due to the decrease in muscle mass, creatine production, and creatinine clearance. Serum creatinine can be in the normal range even if renal function is markedly reduced. The risk of kidney damage from nonsteroidal anti-inflammatory drugs (NSAIDs) is much higher. The renin-angiotensin levels are lower in the elderly.

Musculoskeletal System

Kyphosis: Compression fractures of vertebrae (a sign of osteoporosis). Deterioration of articular cartilages common after age of 40. Stiffness in the morning. Osteoarthritis (degenerative joint disease [DJD]) very common. Muscle mass and muscle strength markedly decrease, with more muscle loss on the legs compared with the arms. Osteoporosis and osteopenia common. Slower healing of fractures due to decrease in the number of osteoblasts. Bone resorption is more rapid than bone deposition in women compared with men (4:1).

Gastrointestinal System

Receding gums and dry mouth common. Decreased sensitivity of taste buds results in decrease in appetite. Decreased efficiency in absorbing some vitamins (i.e., folic acid, B12) and minerals (e.g., calcium) by the small intestines. Delayed gastric emptying. Higher risk of gastritis and GI damage from decreased production of prostaglandins. Diverticuli common. Large bowel (colon) transit time is slower. Constipation more common. Increased risk of colon cancer (age greater than 50 years is strongest risk factor). Fecal incontinence common due to drug side effects, underlying disease, and/or neurogenic disorders. Fecal impaction may lead to small amount of runny soft stool. Laxative abuse more common.

Endocrine

Minor atrophy of the pancreas. Increased levels of insulin along with mild peripheral insulin resistance. Changes or disorders of the circadian rhythm hormonal secretion (growth hormone, melatonin, and other hormones) can cause changes in sleep patterns.

Sex Hormones

Testes active for the entire life cycle of males. Produce less dehydroepiandrosterone (DHEA) and testosterone.

Females: estrogen and progesterone production decrease significantly due to ovarian failure (menopause).

Adipose tissue is able to synthesize very small amounts of estrogen.

Immune System

Less likely to present with fever during infections. Typical body temperature is slightly lower. Decreased antibody response to vaccines. Immune system is less active. Higher risk of infection. Cellular immunity is affected more by aging than humoral immunity. Humoral immunity is associated with B-lymphocytes and antibody (immunoglobulins or IgG) production. Cell-mediated or cellular immunity involves the activity of T-lymphocytes, macrophages, and the cytokines.

Hematologic System

There are no changes in the red blood cell (RBC) lifespan, the blood volume, or the total number of circulating leukocytes. Higher risk of thrombi and emboli due to increased platelet responsiveness. Increased risk of iron and folate-deficiency anemia due to decreased efficiency of the GI tract to absorb Vitamin B12 and folate.

Neurologic System

Cranial nerve testing may show differences in ability to differentiate color, papillary response, and decreased corneal reflex. Decreased gag reflex. Deep tendon reflexes may be brisk or absent. Neurological testing may be impaired by medications causing slower reaction times. Benign essential tremor more common.

Pharmacologic Issues

Drug clearance is affected by: renal impairment, less efficient liver CYP 450 system, malabsorption, and relatively higher fat:muscle tissue (extends fat-soluble drugs). Older adults have an increased sensitivity to benzodiazepines, hypnotics, tricyclic antidepressants (TCAs), and antipsychotics. The American Geriatric Society's has made a list of inappropriate medications for the elderly (Updated Beers Criteria, 2012).

✍ EXAM TIPS

- Total lung volume remains the same, but the FEV1 decreases resulting in an increase in the residual volume of the lungs (decreased lung elasticity).
- Kidney size decreases as we get older (up to 30% atrophy). Creatinine clearance decreases with age.
- Actinic keratosis: precursor of squamous cell cancer. Memory tip: the letter "C" in ACTINIC is a reminder for CANCER.
- Do not confuse this with seborrheic keratosis, which is benign (common mistake).
- Most common cause of blindness in the United States is macular degeneration. In developing countries, cataracts are the most common cause of blindness.
- Become familiar with skin changes in the elderly.

26

Health Screening and Health and Safety Promotion*

MINIMUM DATA SET 3.0

1) The Minimum Data Set (MDS) is a mandatory state and federal requirement for all Medicare/Medicaid certified long-term care facilities (LTCFs).
2) The MDS is "a standardized primary screening and assessment tool of health status that forms the foundation of the comprehensive assessment for all residents in a Medicare and/or Medicaid-certified long-term facility."
3) The MDS provides a "multidimensional view of the patient's functional capacities and helps staff to identify health problems" (Centers for Medicare and Medicaid Services, 2012).
4) The MDS contains information about a nursing-home patient's physical, mental, psychosocial, and functional status.
5) The MDS was developed as a response to the U.S. Ominibus Budget Reconciliation Act of 1987 (OBRA). The latest version is the MDS 3.0, which was released in October 2010.
6) The MDS manual defines a "physician" as an MD, doctor of osteopathy (DO), nurse practitioner (NP), physician assistant (PA), or clinical nurse specialist (CNS).
7) The MDS forms must be started within 48 hours after a new resident's admission. If a person is discharged early (within 24 hours after admission), completion of the MDS is not required.
8) The MDS data set results must be submitted electronically to Medicare or Medicaid through a secure broadband connection.
9) All Medicare and Medicaid bills must be submitted electronically through a secure broadband connection.

MINIMUM DATA SET: RESIDENT ASSESSMENT

- *Diagnosis and health/medical history* (registered nurses [RNs]): perform intake and comprehensive history.
- *Medications* (including over-the-counter [OTCs] drugs): obtain record/history of current prescriptions. RN will obtain admitting orders and the necessary prescriptions (patient's medications) from the attending "physician."

---

* Adapted from Hartford Institute for Geriatric Nursing. Shelkey M, Wallace M. Katz Index of Independence in Activities of Daily Living (ADL). ConsultGeriRN.org

- *Polypharmacy* (including herbs, alternative therapy): ask patient or family to bring all of the resident's medications, vitamins, and other alternative medicines in a "brown bag."
- *Cognition:* use Mini-Cog, Mini-Mental Status Examination (MMSE), clock-drawing test. Look for signs of dementia, history of depression, bipolar disorder, stroke.
- *Behaviors:* use behavioral assessment tool. Assess if combative, confused, dementia, sundown phenomenon.
- *Communication:* unable to communicate, confused, aphasia, history of stroke.
- *Sensory deficits:* check hearing, vision, prescription glasses, use of hearing aid, peripheral neuropathy. Perform neurologic exam.
- *Oral/nutritional evaluation* (dietician and nurse): missing teeth, dentures, oral ulcers from poor-fitting dentures, anorexia, dysphagia, weight loss, body mass index (BMI). Can the patient swallow solids or does food need to be pureed? Ability to feed self, specialized equipment.
- *Activities:* interview patient and/or family about routine and favorite activities.
- *Treatments:* pressure ulcers, others.
- *Advanced directives:* obtain a copy. If resident has dementia, ask patient's family if one is on file.
- *Elimination:* ask for history of fecal or urinary incontinence, constipation.
- *Skin:* assess skin for pressure ulcers, bruises, condition of skin.

RESIDENT ASSESSMENT INSTRUMENTS (RAI)

MDS-CHESS Scale (Changes in Health, End-Stage Disease, Symptoms and Signs or CHESS)

A tool to predict survival and mortality risk. Detects frailty and health instability. Originally designed for nursing-home residents.

The CHESS scale contains nine items. Scores range from 0 (no instability) to 5 (health highly unstable). Higher scores are correlated with a reduction in survival time and adverse outcomes (i.e., hospitalization).

Fulmer SPICES Tool

SPICES is an acronym for the common syndromes of the elderly requiring nursing intervention. Developed by Terry Fulmer, PhD, FAAN (New York University College of Nursing). An overall assessment tool of older adults.

S: Sleep disorders
P: Problems with eating or feeding
I: Incontinence
C: Confusion
E: Evidence of falls
S: Skin breakdown

COGNITIVE PERFORMANCE SCALES

- Mini-Mental Exam
- Mini-Cog Exam

- Geriatric Depression Rating Scale
- ADL Self-Performance Hierarchy Scale
- Pain Scale and Pain-Behavioral Assessment Scale
- Index of Social Engagement Scale

FUNCTIONAL ASSESSMENT

Activities of Daily Living (ADLs):
ADLs are self-care activities that are necessary for "independent" living depending on the person's environment (i.e., home, retirement community, ALF, nursing home).

Examples
- Eating (self-feeding, preparing meals, grocery shopping).
- Personal hygiene (brushing teeth, bathing, dressing, grooming).
- Ambulation (walking, canes, wheelchairs).
- Bowel and bladder management.

Instrumental Activities of Daily Living (IADL):
ADLs are associated with the use of "instruments" or finance.

Examples
- Shopping (groceries, clothing).
- Housework (vacuuming, sweeping).
- Using electronics (stoves, microwaves, telephones, television).
- Driving a car.

Assessment Tools

Katz Index of Independence in Activities of Daily Living
- A measure to assess an older adult's independence. Contains 6 items. Each item is scored a "1" or "0." The highest score is 6 points (independent) and the lowest is 0 points (patient very dependent).
- Independence (1 point): ability to perform with no supervision, direction, or personal assistance.
- Dependence (0 point): need of supervision, direction, personal assistance, or total care.

Activities
Independence is defined as:
- *Bathing*: able to bathe self completely or needs help in bathing with only one body part (e.g., back, genitals).
- *Dressing*: can get clothes from closet/drawer and puts on clothes without help (except tying shoelaces).
- *Toileting*: able to get on/off toilet including pants/underwear, cleans genital area without help.
- *Transferring*: able to move in/out of bed or chair unassisted. Mechanical transfer aids acceptable.
- *Continence*: has complete control (urination and defecation).
- *Feeding*: can get food from plate into mouth, able to feed self (okay if another person prepares food).

Falls

Fall injuries include head injuries, pelvic injuries, lacerations, and others. About 90% of hip fractures are due to falls. White women are at highest risk for hip fractures compared with African Americans. Elderly are at higher risk of death from a fall. The majority of deaths (82%) from falls were among people aged 65 years or older.

High-risk of fall: history of two or more falls prior to 12 months, difficulty walking or balance.

Risk Factors

1) Frailness and older age (more common after age 75 years). Postural hypotension.
2) Adverse or side effects from certain medications. Polypharmacy (four or more drugs).
3) Dementia and cognitive impairment. Neurologic deficits. Chronic illness.
4) Poor eyesight, decreased hearing, decrease in night vision. Balance problems.
5) Use of area rugs, poor fit of shoes/slippers. Poor lighting.
6) Lives alone. History of previous falls.
7) Urinary tract infections (UTIs).

Fall Assessment

1) Assess for risk of falls (history of falls, gait and balance problems, vision problems, hypotension, postural hypotension, arrhythmias, osteoporosis, type of shoes, assistive devices).
2) Medications: polypharmacy, sedating meds, anticholinergic burden, beta-blockers.
3) Gait, balance, and mobility assessment (refer to physical therapy [PT] if necessary for in-depth assessment).
4) Muscle strength (check hand grip strength, ability to support weight, transfer from chair to bed).
5) Visual acuity: check whether patient has glasses, cataracts, history of glaucoma.
6) Heart rate and rhythm: 12-lead ECG, history of CAD, MIs, arrhythmias.
7) Postural hypotension: check if on meds that cause hypotension (antihypertensives).
8) Feet and footwear: shoes too loose or tight, shoes have thick rubber soles.
9) Environment: area rugs, uneven floors, low light.

Factors That Decrease Fall Risk

1) Proper lighting especially in bathrooms and hallways.
2) Grab bars by the toilet and by the tub/shower, higher level of toilet seat.
3) Regular weight-bearing exercises. Leg strength exercise. Gait training PRN.
4) Tai Chi programs have been found to promote balance and muscle strength.
5) Adequate calcium and vitamin D intake. Annual eye exams.
6) Take all meds and vitamins in a "brown bag" to health provider to check.
7) Physical therapy (PT) or occupational therapy (OT) for gait training.
8) May need adaptive devices—refer to PT or OT for further evaluation.
9) Ensure that patient's food and fluid intake is adequate. Malnutrition markedly affects strength.

Adaptive Equipment

Bathing and Toilet Safety

- Elevated toilet seats, especially after hip fracture and hip replacement.
- Grab bars: place on the bathroom wall(s) and on the side of the tub.

- Shower chairs: for patients who cannot stand/walk, too weak.
- Avoid area rugs. If patient wants a rug, avoid thick rugs. Choose a thin rug with rubber backing (nonslip).

Walking

Refer patient to PT for evaluation of gait and recommendations for adaptive equipment. PT will teach patients how to use a cane, walker, or other equipment.

Other Equipment

Medicare, Medicaid, Tricare (health insurance of U.S. Armed Forces), and most insurance health plans will pay up to 80% for some medically necessary durable medical equipment.

Canes: check weight limits of the cane if the patient is obese. Several types: regular, foldable, quad foot, etc. Instruct patient or medical assistant to periodically check the bottom of the cane (if rubber foot is thinning or is missing). Replace as needed.

Walkers: several types. Foldable or nonfoldable. With or without casters. Some patients like to have bags/baskets attached to the front of the walker. Refer patient to PT if gait is unsteady or falling for evaluation and recommendations.

Wheelchairs: many styles and uses. Adult and child sizes. There are now wheelchairs designed for the obese.

Scooters (electric wheelchairs): expensive (price $1,000 and up). Contains a motor in specialized chair with handlebars and brakes. Most can take up to 300 lb of weight. Popular with very obese patients, patients with spinal cord injuries.

Vision and Hearing

Blindness

Legal blindness is defined as the best corrected visual field of 20/200 (or less) in the better eye. The ophthalmic nerve (retina) is cranial nerve II (CN II). The most common cause of legal blindness in persons aged 65 years or older in the United States is age-related macular degeneration (AMD). Other eye conditions that are more common in the elderly are giant cell arteritis, acute-closure glaucoma, and several types of hemianopsia associated with certain types of CVAs or stroke.

Vision Loss: Signs

- Prefers to use one eye ("dominant" eye) or squinting.
- Tilts head slightly or moves head to side when reading street signs.
- Problems reading (near vision).
- After a stroke, may not eat/touch foods on the blind side (i.e., homonymous hemianopsia).

Assess Medications: Adverse Effects on Vision

- Digoxin: yellow to greenish color to vision.
- Sildenafil (Viagra): bluish tinge to vision, ischemic optic neuropathy (permanent).
- Anticholinergics (decongestants, antihistamines, etc.): can precipitate acute angle glaucoma.

Visual Aids

- Magnifying glass/binoculars and electronic magnifiers.
- Computer magnifiers: digital magnification of text and objects (special software or apps).
- Talking watches or alarm clocks.

- Large-print watches, books, or telephones with large keys.
- Vision training such as scanning training (compensate for missing visual field).

Hearing

Involves the brain, cranial nerve 8 (CN VIII), inner ear, middle ear, and external ear canal.

Sensorineural

Involves the inner ear (cochlear hair cells and vestibulocochlear nerve). Presbycusis (or age-related hearing loss) is a type of sensorineural hearing loss. It is the most common cause of hearing loss in the world. Look for gradual onset of progressive loss that is symmetric (both ears). If hearing loss is only in one hear, it is not due to presbycusis. High-frequency hearing lost first (e.g., human speech).

Symptoms of Hearing Loss

- Family or friends complain that patient sets the TV volume or radio "too loud."
- Problems hearing or understanding speech in noisy areas (e.g., restaurant).
- Complains of problems understanding or hearing conversation.
- May look puzzled or will ask person to repeat a question several times.
- Difficulty hearing speech/voice during telephone calls.
- Complains of tinnitus.

Assess Medications: Ototoxic Meds

- Aminoglycosides (gentamycin, vancomycin).
- Aspirin/salicylic acid.
- High chronic doses of furosemide.
- Chemotherapeutic drugs.

Hearing Evaluation

Examine external ear and tympanic member. Remove cerumen if unable to view TM. Look at TM landmarks such as the "cone of light," retraction, or bulging of TM, erythema.

Higher Risk of Hearing Loss

- History of chronic tinnitus
- Older age
- Ototoxic meds
- Chronic exposure to loud noises
- Comorbid conditions such as diabetes

Gold Standard

Diagnostic test is audiometry using soundproof booth performed by a professional audiologist.

Screening Tests

Weber Test

Normal: sound is heard in both ears. If sound heard only in one ear, abnormal (lateralization).
Example: With cerumenosis, the sound will be lateralized on the "good" ear (will not hear sound with the plugged ear).

Rinne Test

Normal: air conduction (AC) greater than bone conduction (BC).
Example: If bone conduction greater than air conduction, rule out conductive hearing loss. Weber test will also show lateralization.

Whisper Test

Stand about 2 feet behind patient. Occlude one ear (press tragus toward ear). Whisper the alphabet or count numbers. Another option is to rub the patient's hair together in front of each ear.

Tympanogram

If fluid/pus inside middle ear (otitis media) or cerumen is present, the TM will have little to no mobility.
    The result will be abnormal (flat line, small peak, to no peak on printout result).

NUTRITIONAL ASSESSMENT

USDA MyPlate System

The USDA Food Pyramid has been replaced with the "MyPlate" system (www.choose MyPlate.gov).

Recommendations:

1) Educate patients about the MyPlate system (free handouts at website).
2) Drink 8 glasses of water per day (if not contraindicated or in heart failure).
3) Exercise at least 150 minutes per week (30 minutes/5× per week) if it is not contraindicated.
4) For protein, consider eating seafood twice a week. Cold-water fish (salmon, sardines) are preferred since they contain omega-3 oils (vegan source is flax seed oil).
5) Reduce intake of solid fats and added sugars (SoFAS) since studies show that they make up to 35% calories of daily total caloric intake.
6) Solid fats come from animal fats and lard (some fried foods, baked goods).
7) Added sugars include corn syrup, sucrose (table sugar), fructose, brown sugar.
8) Calorie-free forms of sugar are: sugar alcohols (xylitol, mannlitol), saccharin, aspartame, sucralose (Splenda), stevia, and others. Eating high amounts of sugar alcohols may cause bloating and flatulence.
9) Eat a variety of fruits and vegetables that are of different colors (red, yellow, orange, green).
10) Reduce sodium intake (table salt, prepared and pickled foods, chips, pickles).
11) Limit sodium intake to less than 3 g/day (Figure 26.1, Table 26.1).

Assessment

Perform a comprehensive dietary history, health history, and anthropomorphic measurements.

History

- Check past medical and health history such as celiac disease, colitis, diarrhea, GERD, others.
- Check patient's preferred foods, appetite patterns, snacking, and fluid intake.
- Check for unintentional weight loss.

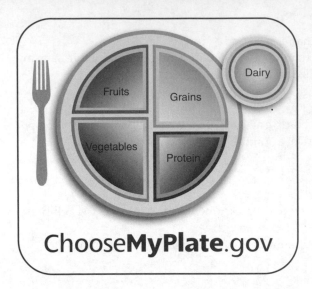

FIGURE 26.1 USDA MyPlate System.

Table 26.1 Dietary Guidelines for Americans 2010 (Adapted for Age 50 or Older)

Type of Food	Servings Per Day	Foods
Vegetables	2 to 3½ cups 1 cup cut-up vegetables = 2 cups of uncooked leafy vegetables	Leafy greens, cabbages, carrots, red peppers, etc.
Fruits	1½ to 2½ cups	Apples, prunes, plums, oranges, bananas, berries, dried fruits
Grains	5 to 10 ounces	Whole grains preferred. If celiac, use rice—avoid wheat, rye, barley. Kamut is a type of wheat (avoid if celiac)
Proteins	5 to 7 ounces	Chicken, fish, beef, lamb, others Vegetarian: 1 egg, ¼ cup cooked beans or tofu, 1 tbsp. peanut butter, ½ ounce nuts/seeds
Dairy	3 cups of fat-free or low-fat milk	1 cup milk = 1 cup yogurt 1 cup = 2 ounces cheese
Oils	5 to 8 teaspoons	Olive oil, canola oil, flax seed oil, nuts, avocado
SoFAS	Limit intake	Lard, animal fats

Adapted from the National Institute of Aging. AgePage. Healthy Eating After 50.

Unintentional Weight Loss

- Defined as unintentional weight loss of greater than 5% in the past 30 days or if greater than 10% over the past 180 days (6 months).
- Assess dental health, gum disease, missing teeth, use of dentures, and oral ulcers.
- Rule out mental health issues such as major depression, anemia, hypothyroidism.

Assess for Risk Factors of Malnutrition

- Decreased taste sensation.
- Poor dentition (check for poor-fitting dentures, oral ulcers).
- Adverse effects of medications.
- Depression and feelings of loneliness and isolation.
- Dementia.

Elderly and BMI*:

- Overweight: BMI 25.0 to 29.9. Obese: BMI 30 to 39. Extremely obese: BMI 40 or higher.
- BMI of between 25 and 27 has been found to result in less mortality in elderly than a BMI less than 25.

Laboratory testing:

- *Pre-albumin*: a hepatic protein that is a sensitive test for malnutrition (not the same as albumin). High-risk patients can have the test done as often as once to twice a week.
- *Albumin*: decreased levels are associated with higher mortality.
- *CBC*: check for anemia (iron-deficiency anemia is most common anemia).
- *Folate and B12 levels*: assess for deficiency and macrocytic anemia.
- *Vitamin D levels*: many elderly are low in Vitamin D and may need supplementation.

Check anthropomorphic measurements:

- *Weight and height*.
- *Waist-to-hip ratio (WHR)*: women whose WHR is greater than 0.8 are at increased risk and men with WHR greater than 1.0 are at increased risk (abdominal obesity) for heart disease, metabolic syndrome, and type 2 diabetes.

Handgrip strength:

- An indicator of functional status. Weak hand grip is present with malnutrition. Residents with severe malnutrition have very weak hand grips.

Management Plan

- Correct the factors that are adversely affecting oral food intake if possible.
- Dietician referral: can calculate basal energy and caloric requirements and dietary requirements.
- Consider multivitamin supplementation, calcium with vitamin D 1200 mg/day.
- Encourage resident to eat in the dining room with others (avoids isolation).
- Assess for depression and grieving. If depressed, consider prescribing SSRI that increases appetite such as mirtazapine (Remeron). Remeron causes the most weight gain compared with other SSRIs.
- Check if wearing dentures during meal times.
- Give the patient food choices and snacks.

Community-Dwelling Older Adult

- Assess if assistance is needed with grocery shopping, food preparation, and/or feeding self.
- The patient can enroll for food assistance ("food stamps") and Medicaid if eligible.
- Meals on Wheels programs deliver meals to eligible persons two to three times per day (daily).
- Will be charged a low price of $2.00 to $4.00 per meal.

---

* MedlinePlus. U.S. National Library of Medicine and National Institutes of Health, Dec. 2012.

Appetite Stimulants

- Not a first-line approach due to side effects. Some malnourished and underweight patients with anorexia who do not respond to usual measures can be given a trial of appetite stimulant.
- *Megestrol acetate (Megace)*: a progesterone-type of drug that causes weight gain in patients with anorexia (elderly, cancer-related). Covered by Medicare Part D.
- *Side effects*: water retention may exacerbate or cause heart failure. Monitor patients for edema and signs of heart failure (dyspnea, edema, bibasilar rales).
- *Mirtazapine (Remeron)*: an SSRI that causes more weight gain compared with other SSRIs.

Types of Diets

Clear Liquids or Full Liquid Diets

- Use for only 2 to 3 days (if without supplementation).

Mechanical Soft (Pureed Diet)

- Indicated for patients who have problems chewing or swallowing.

Soft Diet

- Indicated for residents who have problems with chewing and swallowing, GI irritation.
- Foods: milk (all types), instant breakfast, cream cheese, soft lean meats.
- Avoid seeds, nuts, dried fruits, fried fish, hot dogs, crunchy foods.

Low Residue (Low-Fiber Diet)

- Indicated for certain patients with GI disorders, after bowel surgery, or if GI tract irritated (diverticulitis).
- Foods: white rice, white pasta, soups, fruits and vegetables with low pulp or canned, eggs.
- Avoid whole wheat bread, whole grain foods, dried fruits, popcorn, seeds, and nuts.

Renal Diet

- Indicated for chronic kidney disease, acute renal failure. Fluids are limited. Low-protein diet may be recommended.
- Restrict salt, potassium (avoid salt substitutes, citrus, apricots, sports drinks). Limit calcium and phosphorus (minimize dairy since high levels of both).

Hepatic Diet

- Indicated for liver disease, cirrhosis. Restricts protein intake (reduces ammonia blood levels). Liver unable to make enough glycogen. Diet is very high in carbohydrates (carbs are the major source of calories).
- Foods: high carbohydrates (breads, grains, starchy foods), moderate fat intake. Low protein.
- Vitamin supplementation (B-complex vitamins).
- Avoid too much meats, seafoods. Avoid organ meats.

Enteral Feeding

Patients with terminal dementia who refuse to eat or are unable to chew and swallow adequately may become malnourished. If the patient has an intact and functioning GI tract, then tube feedings are an alternative. Initial options are either the orogastric tube or the nasogastric tube. Check for placement after first insertion by ordering a plain chest radiograph (chest x-ray). Should be checked for placement before each feeding by aspirating for stomach contents.

NG tube placement complications: pneumothorax, perforations, empyema, bronchopleural fistula, aspiration pneumonia.

Nutrition Glossary

- *Anorexia*: loss of appetite that has many causes such as dementia, drug side effect, changes in taste and smell, and major depression.
- *Cachexia*: a multifactorial metabolic disorder that is associated with an illness or disease. Associated with increased risk of falls and morbidity. Check serum albumin (low).
- *Sarcopenia*: loss of muscle mass, strength, and performance. Multiple causes such as low hormone levels (testosterone and estrogen), immobility, low levels of physical activity, low protein intake, and others. Higher risk of falls, hip fracture, functional decline, and morbidity.
- *Satiety*: the subjective feeling of "fullness" that follows a meal. If a patient complains of early satiety or dysphagia (especially if accompanied with weight loss), it is a worrisome finding. Rule out cancers of the colon or esophagus. Refer to GI specialist for colonoscopy.

Screening for Dementia

The most common cause of dementia is Alzheimer disease (60%–80%). The second most common cause is vascular dementia (previously known as multi-infarct or post-stroke dementia). The most helpful method of diagnosing dementia is by eliciting a thorough history of the changes in the patient's memory, behaviors, functional changes, and personality changes from family members and close contacts of the patient.

Best imaging test is the MRI scan (brain biopsy rarely done, but is the "gold standard"; Table 26.2).

Table 26.2 Types of Dementia

Disease	Brain Findings	Presentation
Alzheimer's disease (AD)	Deposits of beta amyloid protein (plaques) and neurofibrillary tangles affecting the frontal and temporal lobes	Early signs are short-term memory loss such as difficulty remembering names and recent events; depression
		Progression to impaired judgment, executive skills, confusion, behavioral changes. Terminal stage with difficulty speaking, swallowing, and walking
Dementia with Lewy-bodies (DLB)	Alpha-synuclein protein (Lewy bodies)	Initially, has sleep disturbance, vivid visual hallucinations, muscle rigidity and movement disorders like Parkinson's disease plus symptoms of dementia (AD-like symptoms)

(continued)

Table 26.2 *Continued*

Disease	Brain Findings	Presentation
Vascular dementia	Ischemic damage due to atherosclerotic plaques, bleeding, and/or blood clots	Risk factors are hypertension, diabetes, etc. Signs and symptoms of stroke with memory loss, confusion, etc.
Parkinson's disease	Loss of dopamine receptors in the basal ganglia of the substantia nigra	Movement disorders: rigidity, bradykinesia, difficulty initiating voluntary movements, pill-rolling tremor, masked face plus features of DLB (sleep disturbance, visual hallucinations)
Frontotemporal dementia (Pick's disease)	Orbital and frontal areas of brain (orbitofrontal)	Lack of insight into personality change (social withdrawal, loss of spontaneity, loss of motivation/desire to do task (abulia), impulsive, disinhibition. Utilization behavior (i.e., uses and reuses same object as in using a spoon to eat, comb hair, waving it, etc.)
Mixed dementia	Mixture of two or more types (e.g., Alzheimer's and Lewy-body dementia)	Signs and symptoms are mixture of the dementia type
Wernicke–Korsakoff dementia (or Wernicke's encephalopathy)	Chronic thiamine (vitamin B1) deficiency due to chronic alcohol abuse causes brain damage	Confusion, disorientation, indifference, horizontal movement nystagmus (both eyes). Thiamine IV in high doses can help, but late diagnosis, permanent brain damage

NEUROLOGICAL FINDINGS

- *Abulia*: loss of motivation or desire to do tasks, indifference to social norms (e.g., urinates in public).
- *Akinesia*: reduced voluntary muscle movement (e.g., Parkinson's disease).
- *Amnesia*: memory loss. Anterograde amnesia is memory loss of recent events (occurs during disease) and retrograde amnesia is memory loss of events in the past (before the onset of disease).
- *Anomia*: problems recalling words or names.
- *Aphasia*: difficulty of using (speech) and/or understanding language; can include difficulty with speaking, comprehension, and written language.
- *Apraxia*: difficulty with or inability to remember learned motor skill.
- *Astereognosis*: inability to recognize familiar objects placed in the palm (place a coin on palm with eyes closed and ask patient to identify object).
- *Ataxia*: difficulty coordinating voluntary movement.
- *Broca's aphasia*: speech ability is intact but ability to comprehend language is lost.
- *Confabulation*: "lying" or fabrication of events due to inability to remember the event.
- *Dyskinesia*: abnormal involuntary muscle rigidity.

FOLSTEIN MINI-MENTAL STATUS EXAMINATION

A brief screening exam to assess for cognitive impairment. Sensitivity of 87% and specificity of 82%. Maximum score is 30 points (range 0–30). A score of less than 24 points is suggestive of dementia or delirium. Low scores are seen in dementia, delirium, and schizophrenia. Five subject areas are tested.

1) *Orientation*:
   - Date, day of the week, state, country, home address, and so forth.
2) *Attention and calculation*:
   - Serial 7s (ask patient to subtract 7 from 100 and so on). Stop after 5 correct answers.
   - Spell "world" (or another word) backward.
3) *Recall*:
   - Name three objects. Ask patient to repeat names after 5 minutes (short-term memory).
4) *Write a sentence*:
   - Instruct the patient to write a sentence. Do not give hints. The sentence must be a full sentence.
5) *Three-stage command*:
   - Tell patient to "take a paper in your right hand," then "fold it in half and put it down on the floor."
6) *Copy a design*:
   - Examiner uses a handout that is designed for the MMSE. It is pre-drawn with intersecting lines, such as two pentagons.
   - Examiner draws a square or a triangle and tells the patient to copy the design.

"MINI-COG" TEST

- Quick method for assessing dementia. If abnormal, screen further with MMSE.
- Use these two methods: the clock drawing test with word recall test (three unrelated words).
  - Instruct patient to draw a clock and mark it with the hands showing a certain time.
    - *Example*: Instruct patient to "Draw a clock that shows twenty minutes past four."
  - Scoring clock test: hands point to correct time and numbers on clock are in correct sequence.

✎ EXAM TIPS

1) A question will ask you to identify the MMSE "activity" that is being performed.
2) When a person is asked to interpret a proverb (given by the NP), it is a test of abstract thinking.
3) Abstract thinking starts at about age 11 years (early abstract thinking stage).
4) Korsakoff–Wernicke dementia brain damage caused by Vitamin B1 (thiamine).

SAMPLE QUESTION

A nurse practitioner instructs a patient to copy a square (or spell "world" backward, subtract 7 from 100, etc.). Which of the following tests is being performed:

A) MMPI (or Minnesota Multiphasic Personality Inventory; for personality testing).
B) CAGE (for alcohol abuse screening in primary care).
C) MMSE (correct answer).
D) Beck's Inventory (a depression screening tool).

The correct answer is option C, the MMSE.

PHARMACOLOGIC CONCEPTS: OLDER ADULTS

Drugs: Higher risk of adverse effects (avoid with frail/elderly)

- *Antihistamines*: diphenhydramine (Benadryl) is the most sedating antihistamine. Avoid antihistamines, if possible. Claritin less likely to cause sedation.
- *Tricyclic antidepressants*: amitriptyline (Elavil) is the most sedating. Also causes confusion, delirium, hallucinations. All tricyclic antidepressants (TCAs) cause sedation. Given at bedtime.
- *Benzodiazepines*: confusion, dizziness, ataxia resulting in falls, other accidents.
- *Hypnotics*: avoid long-acting (e.g., Halcion). Prefer shorter duration (e.g., Ambien).
- *Narcotics*: start at lower doses; lasts longer in the elderly.
- *Propranolol, others* (beta blockers): depression, fatigue, slowing, hypotension.
- *Digoxin, warfarin sodium*: high doses cause visual changes, fatigue, depression.
- *Muscle relaxants* (Soma, Skelaxin, Norflex): drowsiness, confusion, delirium.
- *High anticholinergic effects* (antihistamines, antipsychotics, atropine, Ditropan, etc.).
- *Atypical antipsychotics*: Black Box Warning of the high risk of mortality in elderly (from long-term care facilities) with dementia who are treated with atypical antipsychotics (Seroquel, etc.; Table 26.3).

Table 26.3 American Geriatric Society Beer's Criteria (2012)

Drug Class	Drugs to Avoid
Antihistamines	Diphenhydramine/Benadryl and others. Newer generation has lower incidence (Claritin). Sedation, confusion, poor balance, risk of falls, paradoxical reactions (stimulation)
Benzodiazepines	Alprazolam (Xanax), lorazepam (Ativan), triazolam (Halcion)
Short—intermediate acting	Diazepam (Valium), clonazepam (Klonopin)
Long-acting	Risk of confusion, slowing, sedation and confusion increases risk of falls
Antipsychotics	Thioridazine (Mellaril), mexoridazine (Serentil)
Atypical antipsychotics	Quetiapine (Seroquel), olanzapine (Zyprexa)
	Black Box Warning: higher risk of death in nursing-home patients. Excessive sedation increases risk of falls
TCAs	Amitriptyline (Elavil), imipramine (Tofranil)
	Anticholinergic effects, excessive sedation. Give at HS. TCAs used for post-herpetic neuralgia, chronic pain. Use SSRIs for depression instead of TCAs

(continued)

Table 26.3 Continued

Drug Class	Drugs to Avoid
Cardiac drugs	Orthostatic hypotension
Alpha blockers (terazosin, prazosin)	Bradycardia
Central alpha agonist (clonidine)	Dizziness
	Not recommended for routine treatment of hypertension
Nifedipine (immediate release)	Hypotension with risk of syncope and falls
Sulfonylureas (long-acting first generation)	Glyburide (Diabeta), chlorpropamide (Diabenase: higher risk of hypoglycemia and falls due to prolonged half-life of 24 hours
NSAIDs (except COX-inhibiting)	Indomethacin (Indocin), diclofenac (Voltaren), others
	Ketorolac and indomethacin (Indocin)
	Risk GI bleed, kidney damage, exacerbate hypertension
Mineral oil (oral)	Aspiration into lungs. Aspiration pneumonia
Antispasmodics	Dicyclomine (Bentyl), scopolamine, belladonna
	Anticholinergic effects risk, dry eyes, blurred vision
Other medications	Metoclopramide (Reglan, except for gastroparesis)
	Sliding-scale insulin dosing
	Causes sedation and confusion in some elderly

* List is not all-inclusive.

DISEASE PREVENTION AND HEALTH MAINTENANCE

1) Designs health maintenance and disease prevention interventions that are age, gender, and health status appropriate.
2) Develops, implements, and evaluates age-appropriate health screening and health promotion programs (Table 26.4).

HEALTHY PEOPLE 2020

Leading health indicators for older adults:

- Enhance Fitness Program (1-hour classes 3×/week in 5-week sessions).
- Strength training (wrist/ankle weights), aerobics, stretching, and balance exercises.
- Arthritis Foundation Exercise Program, National Institute on Aging Exercise Guide.
- Eating more than five servings of fruits and vegetables daily.
- Obesity.
- Current smoking.
- Hip fracture hospitalizations.
- Disability.
- Flu vaccine in past year.
- Mammogram within past 2 years.
- Cholesterol check within past 5 years.

Table 26.4 USPSTF Clinical Preventive Services for Older Adults

Topic	USPSTF Recommendation
Abdominal aorta aneurysm screening (men only)	Men age 65 to 75 years who have ever smoked with ultrasound (one-time screen only)
Aspirin to prevent CVD	
Men	Men age 45 to 79 years if potential benefit (reduction of MIs) outweighs the risk to GI bleeding
Women	Women age 55 to 79 years if potential benefits (reduction of ischemic strokes) outweighs the risk of GI bleeding
Breast cancer screening	Baseline at age 50 years, then every 2 years (biennial) until age 74. Family history of *BRCA1* or *BRCA2*, refer for genetic testing/counseling
Cholesterol screening	
Men	Men aged 35 and older should be screened for lipid disorders
Women	Women aged 45 years or older with risk factors for heart disease
Colorectal cancer screening	Start at age 50 years with baseline colonoscopy, sigmoidoscopy, or high-sensitivity fecal occult blood test (FOBT)
Osteoporosis	Women aged 65 years or older routine screening. Consider starting at age 60 years if at high risk for osteoporosis
Alcohol use	Behavioral counseling interventions (Alcoholics Anonymous,
Cigarette smoking	therapy). Discuss tobacco use and educate about smoking cessation (every office visit).
Falls prevention	Exercise or physical therapy and/or attend a falls prevention course

Adapted from the U.S. Preventive Services Task Force "USPSTF A and B Recommendations"; www.uspreventiveservicestaskforce.org/uspstf/uspsabrecs.htm.

IMMUNIZATIONS

Influenza vaccine (trivalent inactivated vaccine or TIV):

- Start giving the flu injection in November of each year (fall to winter season). Health care personnel (HCP) who work with patients greater than 50 years should be vaccinated with the TIV injection (not the intranasal LAIV) flu vaccine.

FluMist intranasal vaccine (live attenuated influenza virus or LAIV):

- Age limit is 49 years. Do not use with elderly. FluMist intranasal vaccine only for healthy persons from ages 2 to 49 years.

Pneumococcal polysaccharide vaccine (PPSV23):

- Give one dose of "Pneumovax" at age of 65 years or older (IM or SQ).

Tetanus-diphtheria-acellular pertussis (Tdap) vaccine:

- Replace one tetanus (tetanus-diphtheria [Td]) vaccine booster with one Tdap (once/lifetime). Then, use Td form every 10 years.

Zoster vaccine:

- Give one dose at age 65 years or older (regardless if history of prior episode of shingles). Contraindication: pregnancy, immunocompromised (e.g., HIV/AIDS), drugs affecting the immune system (e.g., steroids, biologics), cancer of the bone marrow/lymphatic system (lymphoma)

MMR (measles, mumps, and rubella vaccine):

- Adults born before 1957 are generally considered immune to measles and mumps (Table 26.5).

Table 26.5 Recommended Immunizations for Older Adults

Vaccine	Generic Name	Recommendation
Influenza vaccine	Trivalent inactivated vaccine (TIV)	Start giving in November annually
Influenza vaccine (intranasal)	Live attenuated influenza virus (LAIV)	Contraindicated after age 49 years
Tetanus vaccine	Tetanus-diphtheria-acellular pertussis (Tdap) or Td (tetanus-diphtheria)	Substitute Tdap for one Td booster (once in a lifetime)
Shingles vaccine	Herpes zoster vaccine (Zostavax)	Age 65 years or older
Pneumococcal vaccine	Pneumococcal vaccine	Age 65 years or older

Source: CDC, 2012.

27

Common Disorders in Geriatrics

⚠ DANGER SIGNALS

Severe Bacterial Infections

Atypical presentation is common. Older adults/elderly with bacteremia or sepsis may be afebrile. About one-third to one-half of people with severe bacterial infections do not develop fever and/or chills. Some present with slightly lower than normal body temperature (less than 37°C or 98.6°F). The white blood count (WBC) can be normal. Atypical presentations also include a sudden decline in mental status (confusion, dementia), the new onset of urine/bowel incontinence, falling, worsening inability to perform activities of daily living (ADLs), and/or loss of appetite. Serious infections include pneumonia, pyelonephritis, bacterial endocarditis, sepsis, and others. The most common infection in older adults (greater than 65 years) is urinary tract infection (UTI).

Temporal Arteritis (Giant Cell Arteritis)

Temporal headache (one sided) with tenderness or induration over temporal artery; may be accompanied by sudden visual loss in one eye (amaurasis fugax). Scalp tenderness of affected side. Screening test is the sedimentation rate, which will be elevated. Considered a medical emergency (can cause blindness).

Acute Closure Glaucoma

Older adult with acute onset of severe eye pain, severe headache, and nausea and vomiting. The eye(s) is reddened with profuse tearing. Complains of blurred vision and halos around lights. Call 911. Do not delay treatment. Tonometry is done in the emergency room to quickly measure the intra-ocular pressure.

Cerebrovascular Accident (CVA)

Sudden onset of neurological dysfunction that worsens within hours. Also called a "brain attack." Deficits can include changes such as blurred vision, slurred speech, one-sided upper and/or lower extremity weakness, confusion. Signs and symptoms dependent on location of infarct. In comparison, a transient ischemic attack (TIA) is a temporary episodes that generally lasts less than 24 hours.

Actinic Keratosis (Precursor of Squamous Cell Carcinoma)

Small rough pink to reddish lesions that do not heal. Located in sun-exposed areas such as the cheeks, nose, back of neck, arms, chest, and so on. More common in light-skinned individuals. Squamous cell precancer skin lesions. Diagnostic method of choice is biopsy. Small number of lesions can be treated with cryo. Larger numbers with wider distribution treated with 5-fluorouracil cream.

Fractures of the Hip

Acute onset of limping, guarding, and/or inability/difficulty with bearing weight on the affected side. New onset of hip pain; may be referred to the knee or groin. Unequal leg length. Affected leg is abducted (turned away from the body). History of osteoporosis or osteopenia. Fractures of the hip are a major cause of morbidity and mortality in the elderly. Up to 20% of elderly with hip fractures die from complications (e.g., pneumonia).

Elder Abuse

- Presence of bruising, skin tears, lacerations, and fractures that are poorly explained.
- Presence of sexually transmitted disease, vaginal, and/or rectal bleeding, bruises on breasts are indicators of possible sexual abuse.
- Malnutrition, poor hygiene, and pressure ulcers. Screen for abuse and financial exploitation.

Interview Elder Alone With These Three Questions
Do you feel safe where you live?
Who handles your checkbook and finances?
Who prepares your meals?

Top Three Leading Causes of Death (Greater Than Age 65 Years)
1. Heart disease (myocardial infarction [MI], heart failure, arrythymias).
2. Cancers (lung and colorectal).
3. Chronic lower respiratory diseases (COPD).

Cancer in Older Adults

Cancer with highest mortality: lung cancer (both genders). Cancer with second highest mortality: colon cancer.

Aging and advancing age are the most common risk factors of cancer. Up to 60% of newly diagnosed malignancies occur in older adults (age 65 years or older). Cancers among older adults may be caused by gene-related DNA damage, familial genetics, decrease in immunity, decreased healing rates, and hormonal influences.

Lung Cancer*

The cancer with the highest mortality for older adults (both genders). Lung cancer is also the most common cancer in the world. Most patients with lung cancer are older adults. The 5-year survival rate for lung cancer is low (16%) compared with colon cancer (65%).
- *Most common risk factor:* Smoking (causes 90% of cases), history of radiation therapy.
- *Most common type of lung cancer:* Small cell (80%) and non-small cell (90%) carcinoma.
- *Screening:* There is no screening test for lung cancer.

Classic Case
An older male smoker (or ex-smoker) presents with a new onset of cough that is productive of large amounts of thin mucoid phlegm (bronchorrhea). Some patients have blood-tinged phlegm. The patient complains of worsening shortness of breath or dyspnea. Some will report persistent and dull achy chest pain that does not go

---

* American Lung Association. Lung Cancer Fact Sheet (2012).

away. If the tumor is obstructing a bronchus, it can result in recurrent pneumonia of the same lobe. Some may have weight loss.

Management
- Order chest radiograph (nodules, lesions with irregular borders).
- The next imaging exam is a computed tomography (CT) scan. Gold standard is a positive lung biopsy.
- Baseline labs include the CBC, FBOT, chemistry panel, and urinalysis.
- Refer patient to a pulmonologist for bronchoscopy and tumor biopsy.

Colon Cancer

Also known as colorectal cancer. It is the second most common cause of cancer deaths in the United States. It is staged using the TNM staging system (Stage I to Stage IIIC).
- *Risk factor:* Advancing age (most common), inflammatory bowel disease, or a family history of colorectal cancer, colonic polyps.
- *Lifestyle risk factors:* Lack of regular physical activity, high-fat diet, low-fiber diet, obesity, and so on.
- *Screening:* Start at age 50 years with baseline colonoscopy (every 10 years), sigmoidoscopy (every 5 years), or a high-sensitivity fecal occult blood test (annually).

Classic Case
Most patients with colorectal cancer present with abdominal pain and a change in bowel habits with hematochezia or melena. The patient may report anorexia and unintentional weight loss. Iron-deficiency anemia is present in a few cases (11%).

Management
- Baseline labs includes the CBC, FBOT, chemistry panel, and urine.
- Check occult fecal blood in stool (guaiac-based, stool DNA, others).

Multiple Myeloma

Myeloma is a cancer of the bone marrow that affects the plasma cells of the immune system (production of monoclonal immunoglobulins). The racial background with the highest incidence are people of African descent (doubled or tripled compared with Whites). Multiple myeloma is a cancer found mostly in older adults.

Classic Case
Typical patient is an older to elderly adult who complains of bone pain with generalized weakness. The bone pain is usually located on the chest and/or the back and usually does not occur at night. The majority have anemia (73%).

Management
- Baseline labs include CBC, FBOT, chemistry panel, and urinalysis.
- Refer patient to a hematologist.

📋 CLINICAL TIPS

- Any patient with unexplained iron-deficiency anemia who is older, male, or postmenopausal should be referred for a colposcopy.
- If the chemistry profile shows marked elevations in the serum calcium and/or alkaline phosphatase, it is usually indicative of cancerous metastasis of the bone.

GERIATRIC ASSESSMENT

- *Assessment team:* Physician/nurse practitioner, nurse, social worker, dietician, physical therapist, others.
- *ADLs:* Dressing, feeding self, grooming, bathing.
- *Instrumental ADLs*: Driving, grocery shopping, laundry, cooking.
- *Cognition and mood disorders:* Depression, geriatric bipolar disorder.
- *Risk of falls:* History of falls, gait and balance, vision, hypotension, postural hypotension, arrythymias, osteoporosis, type of shoes, assistive devices.
- *Polypharmacy* (including herbs, alternative therapy): Advise patient to bring all meds, vitamins, and other alternative medicines in a "brown bag."

RISK FACTORS IN THE ELDERLY

Falls

- Injuries from falls include head injuries, pelvic injuries, lacerations, and others.
- About 90% of hip fractures are due to falls. White women are at higher risk for hip fractures than Black women.
- During 2008, the majority of deaths (82%) from falls were among people aged 65 years or older.

Factors That Increase Fall Risk

- Frailness and older age (more common after age 75 years). Postural hypotension.
- Adverse or side effects from certain medications. Polypharmacy (4 or more drugs).
- Dementia and cognitive impairment. Neurologic deficits. Chronic illness.
- Poor eyesight, decreased hearing, decrease in night vision. Balance problems.
- Use of area rugs, poor fit to shoes/slippers. Poor lighting.
- Lives alone. History of previous falls.
- UTIs.

Factors That Decrease Fall Risk

- Proper lighting, especially in bathrooms and hallways.
- Grab bars by the toilet and by the tub/shower, higher level of toilet seat.
- Regular weight-bearing exercises. Leg strength exercises. Gait training PRN.
- Tai Chi programs. Exercises to improve balance.
- Adequate calcium and vitamin D intake. Annual eye exams.
- Take all meds and vitamins in a "brown bag" to health provider to check.

Drugs: Higher Risk of Adverse Effects (Avoid With Frail/Elderly)

- *Antihistamines:* Diphenhydramine (Benadryl) is the most sedating antihistamine. Avoid antihistamines, if possible. Claritin less likely to cause sedation.
- *Tricyclic antidepressants:* Amitriptyline (Elavil) is the most sedating. Also causes confusion, delirium, hallucinations. All tricyclic antidepressants (TCAs) cause sedation. Given at bedtime.
- *Benzodiazepines:* Confusion, dizziness, ataxia resulting in falls, other accidents.
- *Hypnotics:* Avoid long-acting (e.g., Halcion). Prefer shorter duration (e.g., Ambien).
- *Narcotics:* Start at lower doses; lasts longer in the elderly.
- *Propranolol, others* (beta-blockers): Depression, fatigue, slowing, hypotension.

- *Digoxin (warfarin sodium):* High doses cause visual changes, fatigue, depression.
- *Muscle relaxants* (Soma, Skelaxin, Norflex): Drowsiness, confusion, delirium.
- *High anticholinergic effects* (antihistamines, antipsychotics, atropine, Ditropan, etc.).
- *Atypical antipsychotics:* Black Box Warning of the high risk of mortality in elderly (from long-term care facilities) with dementia who are treated with atypical antipsychotics (Seroquel, etc.).

✎ EXAM TIPS

- S4 heart sound is seen with left ventricular hypertrophy and with many elderly.
- Residual volume increases with age. Total lung volume same. Decrease in forced expiratory volume in 1 second and forced vital capacity.
- Senile arcus. Red reflex; know how to perform and what it is for (screening for cataracts).
- Red reflex is missing with cataracts. Cataracts do not allow light through to reflect off optic vessels. It looks dull white.
- Delirium is reversible; dementia is irreversible.
- Reversible causes of delirium: high fever, infections, metabolic derangements, certain drugs, dehydration, others.
- Irreversible causes of dementia: Alzheimer's disease, CVAs, severe chronic B12 deficiency, Parkinson's disease, others.
- Do not confuse reversible versus irreversible causes of dementia/ delirium on the exam.
- The most common side effects from digoxin overdose are gastrointestinal (GI) effects such as nausea and abdominal discomfort. Halos around lights are not an early symptom of overdose.
- Fall risk factors.

📋 CLINICAL TIPS

- Try to prescribe shorter-acting drugs. For example, for benzodiazepines, Xanax has a shorter effect (half-life of 4 hours) versus that of Valium (can last 12 hours).
- Avoid using diphenhydramine (Benadryl) in elderly, especially those with dementia.

SCREENING FOR DEMENTIA

Folstein Mini-Mental Status Examination (MMSE)

A brief screening exam to assess for cognitive impairment. Sensitivity of 87% and specificity of 82%. Maximum score is 30 points (range 0–30). A score of less than 24 points suggestive of dementia or delirium. Low scores are seen in dementia, delirium, and schizophrenia. Six subject areas are tested:

- Orientation
  - Date, day of the week, state, country, home address, and so on.
- Attention and calculation
  - Serial 7s (ask patient to subtract 7 from 100 and so on). Stop after 5 correct answers.
  - Spell "world" (or another word) backward.
- Recall
  - Name three objects. Ask patient to repeat names after 5 minutes (short-term memory).

- Write a sentence
  - Instruct the patient to write a sentence. Do not give hints. The sentence must be a full sentence.
- Three-stage command
  - Tell patient to "take a paper in your right hand," then "fold it in half and put it down on the floor."
- Copy a design
  - Examiner uses a handout that is designed for the Mini-Mental State Examination (MME). It is pre-drawn with intersecting lines, such as two pentagons.
  - Examiner draws a square or a triangle and tells the patient to copy the design.

"Mini-Cog" Test

- Quick method for assessing dementia. If abnormal, screen further with MMSE.
- Use these two methods: the clock drawing test with word recall test (three unrelated words).
- Instruct patient to draw a clock and mark it with the hands showing a certain time.
- *Example:* Instruct patient to "Draw a clock that shows 20 minutes past 4."
  - *Scoring clock test:* Hands point to the correct time and numbers on clock are in correct sequence.

✍ EXAM TIPS

- A question will ask you to identify the MMSE "activity" that is being performed.
- When a person is asked to interpret a proverb (given by the NP), it is a test of abstract thinking.
- Abstract thinking starts at about age 11 years (early abstract thinking stage).

Sample Question
A nurse practitioner instructs a patient to copy a square (or spell *world* backwards, subtract 7 from 100, etc.). Which of the following tests is being performed?
A) Minnesota Multiphasic Personality Inventory for personality testing
B) CAGE (for alcohol abuse screening in primary care)
C) MMSE (correct answer)
D) Beck's Inventory (a depression screening tool)
The correct answer is Option C, the MMSE

IMMUNIZATIONS

Pneumovax Vaccine (Pneumococcal Polysaccharide Vaccine)
Start vaccinating healthy older adults at the age of 65 years. The patient needs only one dose per lifetime if healthy. If patient received first vaccine before age 65 years, another dose of the vaccine may be given.

Influenza Vaccine
Given annually starting in November of each year. Vaccine strains changes every year due to the viral mutations. Immunity from the flu vaccine lasts only a few months.

Tetanus Vaccine (Td and Tdap)

Booster every 10 years. Adults 50 years or older should receive one dose of Tdap regardless of time since last immunization. This is particularly important for adults caring for infants and young children. Tdap can replace one of the regular Td boosters. For contaminated wounds, give a booster if the last one was given 5 years or more before the incident.

Zoster Vaccine (Zostavax)

Indicated for adults aged 60 years or older (regardless if they report a prior episode of shingles).

Person must have a history of chickenpox or varicella titer before giving vaccine.

HEARING AND VISION

Hearing

The process of hearing is complex. It involves the brain, cranial nerve VIII (vestibulocochlear nerve), the cochlea, the ossicles, the tympanic membrane, and a patent external ear canal.

The area of the brain that is responsible for hearing, memory, and language comprehension is located in the temporal lobes.

Conductive Hearing Loss

Involves the external ear (external canal, pinna, tragus) and/or the middle ear (eustachian tube, tympanic membrane [TM], and the ossicles).
- *Example*: Cerumenosis (earwax impaction).

Otitis Externa

Perforation of the tympanic membrane.

Sensorineural Hearing Loss

Involves the inner ear (cochlear hair cells and vestibulocochlear nerve).

Examples
- Presbycusis (or age-related hearing loss) is a type of sensorineural hearing loss.
- Most common cause of hearing loss in the world.
- Progressive and symmetric (both ears) hearing loss.
- High-frequency hearing lost first (e.g., human speech).

Signs and Symptoms of Hearing Loss
- Family or friends complain that patient sets the TV volume or radio "too loud."
- Problems hearing or understanding speech in noisy areas (e.g., restaurant).
- May look puzzled or will ask person to repeat at question several times.
- Complains of difficulty hearing phone conversations.
- Complaints of tinnitus.

Ototoxic Medications
- Aminoglycosides (e.g., gentamycin, vancomycin)
- Aspirin/salicylic acid
- Furosemide
- Some chemotherapeutic drugs

Evaluation

- Examine external ear and TM. Remove cerumen if unable to view TM. Look at TM landmarks such as the "cone of light," retraction or bulging of TM, erythema.
- Check history of tinnitus, ototoxic meds, signs/symptoms of otitis media, ear infections, chronic exposure to loud noises, diabetes, and so on.
- Perform screening testing (Weber, Rinne). Tympanogram testing.

Screening Tests

Weber Test

- *Normal*: Sound is heard in both ears. If sound is heard only in one ear, abnormal (lateralization).
- Place handle of tuning fork between the brows on the forehead. Ask patient if sound is heard on both sides or if the sound is heard in one ear (called lateralization).

Example:

With cerumenosis, the sound will be lateralized on the "bad" ear (will hear sound better in plugged ear).

Rinne Test

- *Normal*: AC (air conduction) > than BC (bone conduction).
- Place handle of tuning fork over the mastoid bone behind the ear, then move the tuning fork to the front of the ear. Instruct patient to indicate when the sound stops on each side.

Example:

- If BC > AC, it is highly suggestive of conductive hearing loss (e.g., cerumenosis, otitis media). Rule out conductive hearing loss. Weber test will also show lateralization (hears better in the affected/bad ear if it is conductive hearing loss).

Whisper Test

- Stand about 2 feet behind. Occlude one ear (press tragus toward ear). Whisper the alphabet or count numbers. Another option is to rub patient's hair together in front of each ear.

Tympanogram

- If fluid/pus inside middle ear (e.g., otitis media) or cerumen is present, the TM will have little to no mobility.
- The result will be abnormal (flat line, small peak to no peak on printout result).
- Diagnostic test: audiometry using soundproof booth (refer to audiologist for testing and hearing aid fitting).

VISION

Visual processing involves the brain, the optic nerve (CN II), and the structures of the eyes.

The retina is the neural tissue that first encounters the light.

Vision is fully developed (to 20/20) by the age of 6 years. Sudden visual loss is always an emergency. Refer to the ED.

Visual Problems

Normal

Difficulty reading or unable to see small print, holds magazine at arm's length in order to read print. This is normal at this age, and it starts during the early 40s (refer to optometrist for prescription glasses).

Abnormal

- Tilts head slightly to the side and scans when reading street signs (visual field defect).
- Reports that light poles and wall edges appear bent or crooked (hemianopsia, retinal pathology).
- Complains of excessive glare of lights that interferes with driving (glaucoma).
- Complains of running into objects, falling, knocking over drinks (hemianopsia).
- Consistently leaves foods/drinks untouched on one area of the food tray (hemianopsia).
- Complains of a yellowish to green tint to everything (adverse effect digoxin).
- Male complains of bluish tinge to vision (check if taking sildenafil/Viagra).
- Complains of acute onset of floaters with blurred vision (retinal detachment; refer to ED).
- Acute onset of severe eye pain, tearing, redness, blurred vision, nausea, and vomiting (acute glaucoma is emergent; refer to the ED).
- Presbyopia is caused by stiffening of the lens of the eye (not as flexible). It makes it harder to focus on close objects (such as reading). Reading glasses or prescription glasses are used to "correct" vision.

Plan

- Perform visual exam. Check distance vision using the Snellen chart.
- Check near vision by asking patient to read a paragraph from a book or magazine.
- Eye problems are more common in older adults (glaucoma, diabetic or hypertensive retinopathy, macular degeneration).
- Older adults should have an eye exam at least once a year. Older diabetics usually get eye exams twice a year.

Drugs With Adverse Effects on Vision

- *Sildenafil (Viagra)*: Causes bluish tinge to vision and ischemic optic neuropathy, which causes blindness (permanent). Avoid prescribing if eye problems. If older diabetic, refer for eye examination with ophthalmologist first to find out severity of retinopathy. Consider referring to physician.
- *Anticholinergics* (decongestants, antihistamines, etc.): Can precipitate acute-angle glaucoma.

Visual Aids

- Prescription eye glasses. Adequate light?
- Magnifying glass and electronic magnifiers.
- Large-print watches, books, or telephones with large keys.
- Computer magnifiers: digital magnification of text and objects (special software).
- Talking watches or alarm clocks.

Homonymous Hemianopsia

Visual field loss involving either the two left halves (or the two right halves) of the visual field. Most common cause is stroke. There are many types of hemianopsia.

- *Screening test*: Visual field by confrontation.

Left-Sided Homonymous Hemianopsia

The diagram at right shows the intact and missing visual fields of a person who has left-sided homonymous hemianopsia. The "X" signifies the missing visual fields and the equal sign "==" is the intact visual field.

Left Eye	*Right Eye*
xxxxx====	xxxx====
xxxxx====	xxxx====
xxxxx====	xxxx====

Plan

- Refer to ophthalmologist for evaluation.
- When placing food or drinks in front of the patient, position on the right side of the tray. Tell patient what is on the tray.
- Vision training, such as scanning training, compensates for missing visual field.

☰ DISEASE REVIEW

Atypical Presentation in Elderly

Atypical disease presentations are more common in this age group. The immune system is less robust as we age and is less likely to become stimulated by bacterial and viral infections. Vaccines in the elderly may not be as effective compared with the young because of decreased immune response (result is lower antibody production).

Older adults and the elderly are more likely to be asymptomatic or to present with subtle symptoms. The elderly are less likely to have high fever during an infection. Instead, they are more likely to suffer acute cognitive dysfunction such as confusion, agitation, and delirium. One of the reasons for cognitive dysfunction may be that many have multiple comorbid conditions, resulting in many prescriptions. Polypharmacy increases the chances of adverse drugs reactions and drug–drug interactions.

Examples

The management of these diseases is covered in the respective organ system. For example, the management and treatment of pneumonia is in the "pulmonary" chapter.

Bacterial Pneumonia

Fever and chills may be missing or mild. Coughing may not be a prominent symptom. The cough may be mild and produce little to no sputum (especially if the patient is dehydrated). May stop eating and drinking water and start losing weight. More likely to become confused and weak with loss of appetite. May become incontinent of bladder and bowel. Tachycardia usually present. Increases the risk of falls. The WBC count may be normal or mildly elevated. Streptococcccal pneumonia causes the most deaths from pneumonia in the elderly.

Urinary Tract Infections

The most common infection in elderly nursing home residents. Patients usually have no fever or can be asymptomatic. May become acutely confused or agitated. May become septic with mild symptoms. At higher risk of falls.

Acute Abdomen

Elderly patients may have more subtle symptoms such as the absence of abdominal guarding and other signs of acute abdomen. The abdominal pain may be milder.

The WBC count may be only slightly elevated. Patient will have anorexia and weakness.

Acute Myocardial Infarction

May be asymptomatic. Symptoms may consist of back pain or mild chest pain.

Hypothyroidism

Subtle and insidious symptoms such as slowing and depression. Problems with memory. If severe, may mimic dementia. Slower movements. Appears apathetic.

Pressure Ulcers

Prolonged pressure and shearing forces over areas of tissue located over bony prominences cause ischemic damage to the skin and underlying tissue. Treatment depends on the stage.

Common locations: hips (trochanter), the back (sacrum, ischium), shoulders, elbows, knees, ankles (malleolus), heels, back of the head (occiput).

Risk factors: immobility, disabilities, spinal cord injuries, older age (especially greater than 75 years), malnutrition, incontinence, and so on.

Staging

- *Stage I*: Reddened area on intact skin that does not go away. Non-blanchable. The affected area may feel warm and firm (induration). Darker color of skin, affected area appears darker than surrounding skin.
- *Stage II*: Damage to epidermis. Blisters form, which erupt into red shiny skin or shallow superficial ulcers. The wound bed is pink to red in color.
- *Stage III*: Damage to epidermis and dermis. Ulcers are deeper and involve subcutaneous tissue. Base may be red, pink, or yellowish. Ulcer borders are obvious and firm. Fat may be visible. Tendon, bone, or muscle is not visible.
- *Stage IV*: Deep ulcers with visible muscle, tendon, fascia, and/or bone. Undermining on wound edges or tunneling is common. Higher risk of osteomyelitis.
- *Unstageable/Unclassified*: Damaged skin with eschar or sloughing that cannot be staged (until the base is visible).

Chronic Constipation

There are two types of constipation: idiopathic and functional constipation.

Constipation is the most common GI complaint. Self-treatment is common with OTC fiber and laxatives. Constipation has many secondary causes such as prescription and OTC drugs, neurological disease (Parkinson's disease, dementia), IBS, diabetes, hypothyroidism, others. There are lifestyle factors that contribute to constipation: Immobility, low-fiber diet, dehydration, milk intake, ignoring the urge to have bowel movement.

Drugs that cause constipation: Iron supplements, beta-blockers, calcium channel blockers, antihistamines, anticholinergics, antipsychotics, opiates, calcium-containing antacids.

Classic Case

Older adult complains of history of long-term constipation (years). Describes stool as dry and hard "ball-like" pieces or as large-volume stools that are difficult to pass. Reports of straining often to pass the stool. Accompanied by feelings of fullness and bloating. Some patients take laxatives daily (laxative abuse). Usually accompanied by hemorrhoids, which may become exacerbated (reports bright red blood on toilet paper and blood streaks on stool surface).

Treatment Plan

- Education and behavior modification. Teach "toilet" hygiene such as going to the bathroom at the same time each day; advise not to ignore the urge to defecate.
- Dietary changes such as eating dried prunes and/or drinking prune juice.
- Bulk-forming fibers (25–35 g/day) once to twice a day. Take with full glass of water (can cause intestinal obstruction).
- Increase physical activity.
- Increase fluid intake from 8 to 10 glasses/day (if no contraindication).
- Consider laxative treatment (Table 27.1). Avoid using laxatives daily (except for fiber supplements) and chronic treatment with laxatives.

Dementia

An irreversible disorder with gradual and insidious onset. Global intellectual decline. Terminal stage is about 10 years in Alzheimer's disease (most common cause). Patient is usually incoherent to nonverbal; unable to ambulate, eat, or perform self-care as disease progresses.

Duration: lifetime.

Etiology

- Alzheimer's disease (most common cause of dementia in the United States). Caused by neurofibrillary plaques and tangles, which can be detected if the brain is biopsied.

Table 27.1 List of Laxatives

Type of Laxative	Name	Notes
Bulk-forming	Psyllium (Metamucil) Wheat dextrin (Benefiber) Methylcellulose (Citrucel) Polycarbophil (Fibercon)	Two types: soluble or insoluble fiber (bran). Absorbs water adding bulk to stool. Constipation, IBS, diverticulitis.
Stimulants (irritants)	Bisacodyl (Dulcolax) PO and supp. Senna extract (Senokot) PO Aloe vera juice	Stimulates colon directly causing contractions. Drug class: anthraquinone.
Osmotics (hyperosmotic agents)	Sorbitol Polyethylene glycol or PEG (Miralax) Lactulose (Cephulac)	Draws fluid by osmosis to increase fluid retention in the colon.
Saline laxatives	Magnesium citrate Magnesium hydroxide (Milk of Magnesia) Magnesium sulfate (Epsom salts)	Saline attracts water into the intestinal lumen (small and large intestines). Side effects: Fluid and electrolyte imbalance.
Chloride channel activators	Lubiprostone (Amitza)	Idiopathic chronic constipation, IBS. Contraindications: history of mechanical obstruction.
Lubricants	Mineral oil	Lubricants are not absorbed.
Stool softeners	Docusate sodium (Colace)	Softens stool (does not stimulate colon). Stool becomes soft and slippery.

IBS, irritable bowel syndrome; PEG, polyethylene glycol.

- "Dementia with Lewy bodies" is the second most common cause of dementia in the United States. It is caused by brain deposits of Lewy bodies. Patient symptoms of this type of dementia are visual hallucinations, cognitive fluctuations, and parkinsonism.
- Stroke or CVA or vascular dementia.
- Parkinson's disease (up to 40% develop dementia).

Management
- Important to obtain a thorough health/medical/drug history.
- Patient should be accompanied by family during the interview. Family members (and friends) will report patient's signs and symptoms. Refer to neurologist for further assessment.

Differential Diagnosis
- Rule out correctable causes: B12 deficiency, hypothyroidism, major depression, infection, adverse/drug interactions, heavy metal poisoning, others.
- Drugs commonly used to slow down cognitive decline in Alzheimer's disease are Aricept, Namenda, Exelon, and Cerefolin (folate, B12, and acetylcysteine). There is no cure.

Delirium (Acute Confusional State)
A reversible process that is temporary. Acute and dramatic onset. Duration is usually brief (hours to days). May be excitable, irritable, and combative. Short attention span, memory loss, and disorientation. Secondary to medical condition, drug, intoxication, adverse reaction to medicine.

Etiology
- Polypharmacy (drug–drug interactions, adverse reaction).
- Abrupt drug withdrawal (alcohol, benzodiazepines, drugs).
- Preexisting medical conditions, intensive care unit patients.
- Infections (UTIs and pneumonia most common infections), sepsis.
- GI distress (constipation, diarrhea).

Treatment Plan
- Remove and/or treat illness, infection, or metabolic derangement and delirium will resolve.

"Sundowning"
- Seen in both delirium and dementia.
- Starting at dusk/sundown, the patient becomes very agitated, confused, and combative. Symptoms resolve in the morning. Seen more with dementia. Recurs commonly.

Treatment Plan
- Avoid quiet and dark rooms.
- Well-lighted room with a radio, TV, or clock.
- Familiar surroundings important. Do not move furniture or change decor.
- Avoid drugs that affect cognition (antihistamines, sedatives, hypnotics, narcotics).

Alzheimer's Disease
- Accumulation of neurofibrillary plaques/tangles cause permanent damage to brain.

- The median survival time after diagnosis is 10 years.
- Three As: aphasia, apraxia, agnosia.
  - Aphasia (difficulty verbalizing).
  - Apraxia (difficulty with gross motor movements such as walking).
  - Agnosia (inability to recognize familiar people or objects).

Classic Case

- *Mild (from 2 to 4 years)*: Getting lost on familiar routes. Problems managing personal finances and money. Forgets important dates. Repeats same questions. Poor judgment. Becomes withdrawn, anxious, and/or depressed. Easily upset.
- *Moderate (from 2 to 10 years)*: Wanders and gets lost. Problems with speech and following instructions. Stops paying bills. May start a conversation and forget to complete sentences. Loses ability to read and write. Problems recognizing familiar people (agnosia).
- *Severe/Stage 3 (from 1 to 3 years)*: Needs total care. Unable to feed self. Incontinent of bowel and bladder. Stops walking. Uses wheelchair or bedridden. Incoherent or mute. Apathetic.

Medications

- Cholinesterase inhibitor (increases acetylcholine synthesis): moderate to severe cases.
- Memantine (Namenda) by mouth (po) daily to twice a day (BID), donepezil (Aricept) po once a day.
- Improvement within 3 to 6 months. Stop if not effective anymore.

Adjunct Treatment

- Physical activity and exercise have been shown to decrease the risk of dementia.
- *Gingko biloba*: May help with memory (do not mix with aspirin or warfarin).
- Omega-3 fatty acids, vitamin B supplementation.

Treatment Plan

Most patients with dementia are taken care of at home by a family member or caregiver during the early stages of the disease. As disease progresses, many patients are placed in skilled nursing facilities, or assisted-living dementia units. In later stages of the disease, families may consider hospice care.

Complications

- Death usually due to an overwhelming infection such as pneumonia and sepsis.
- Hip fractures are also a common cause of death (from complications).

Essential Tremor

- Essential tremor is classified as an action or an intentional tremor (postural tremor). It is not curable, but the symptoms can be controlled by treatment with beta-blockers.

Treatment Plan

- Propranolol 60 to 320 mg per day. Long-acting propranolol (Inderal LA) is also effective but it provides the same response as "regular" propranolol.
- Alternative treatment is primidone 50 to 1,000 mg per day.

Parkinson's Disease

Progressive neurodegenerative disease (marked decrease of dopamine receptors). More common after 60 years of age. Depression common (up to two-thirds of all patients). The classic three symptoms are tremor (worse at rest), rigidity, and bradykinesia. Parkinson's dementia is common (up to 41%).

Classic Signs

An elderly patient complains of a gradual onset of motor symptoms such as pill-rolling tremors of the hands, cogwheel rigidity with difficulty initiating voluntary movement. Walks with slow shuffling gait. Poor balance and falls often. Generalized muscular rigidity with masked facies. Difficulty with executive function (making decisions, planning, tasks). May have signs and symptoms of dementia. Worsening of seborrheic dermatitis (white scales, erythema).

Treatment Plan

Consider treatment: moderate to severe hand tremors or gait disturbance, patient preference, and so on.

Medications

- *First Line*: Levodopa-carbidopa (Sinemet) TID (dopamine precursor). Start at low doses (half tablet) and titrate up slowly to control symptoms.
  - Adverse effects (Sinemet): dizziness, somnolence, nausea, headache.
  - After 5 to 10 years on medication: motor fluctuations (wearing off phenomenon), tardive dyskinesia (treat with amantadine, others).
- Selegiline (Eldepryl) once a day (MAO B inhibitor). Do not combine with MAOIs or serotonin antagonist (SSRIs, triptans).
- Amantadine (Symmetrel) once a day to TID for tardive dyskinesia.
- Benztropine (Cogentin) BID (anticholinergic), and others.
- Nonpharmacologic: exercise, physical therapy, speech therapy.

Complications

- *Acute Akinesia*: Loss of voluntary movement. Sudden exacerbation of Parkinson's disease.
- Dementia.
- Frequent falls may result in fractures of the face, hips, and so on.

✍ EXAM TIPS

- Essential tremor is an "action" tremor (not a resting tremor).
- First-line treatment for essential tremor are beta-blockers (propranolol).
- Recognize classic presentation of Parkinson's and Alzheimer's diseases.
- If a case scenario presents a patient aged 65 years who is being seen for a wellness visit during November or the fall, the patient needs to be vaccinated with both the Pneumovax and flu vaccines.
- If the patient is older than 65 years of age, then only needs the flu vaccine. FluMist indicated for healthy adults up to age of 50 years.
- Recognize sundowning phenomenon.

📋 CLINICAL TIP

- Eldepryl is a specialized MAO inhibitor. Do not combine with meds that affect serotonin in the brain (SSRIs, triptans, TCAs). Increases risk of serotonin syndrome (see Chapter 15).

Transient Ischemic Attack (TIA)

A TIA is a transient episode of neurologic dysfunction caused by focal ischemia (brain, spinal cord, or retinal ischemia) without acute infarction of the brain as seen in stroke (2009). The timing of 24 hours has been removed (previous definition). It is now known that permanent neurologic damage can happen with TIAs (as seen in CVAs). TIA is also known as a "mini-stroke" or "minor stroke." These patients are at very high risk for stroke. Rule out conditions that can mimic TIAs such as complex migraine, seizures, hypoglycemia.

Classic Case

Older adult with history of hypertension reports new onset of one-sided weakness that started on the face and is descending downward. Accompanied by sudden onset of headache, blurred vision, and slurred speech. Complains that one side of the face is drooping. Speech is slurred. Patient may appear confused or have problems with comprehension. Depending on severity of the TIA, the signs and symptoms can be subtle to severe. The longer the episode of the TIA, the higher the risk of ischemic brain damage or weakness. The TIA can progress into a full-blown stroke. Signs and symptoms of CVA or stroke can be insidious and start a few days before the major episode occurs.

"ABCD" Stroke Scoring System

A clinical tool used to predict patient's risk of stroke.
- A is age.
- B is blood pressure (systolic > 140 mm Hg or diastolic > 90 mm Hg).
- C is clinical features (unilateral weakness, isolated speech disturbance, other).
- D is diabetes.

Hospitalization Criteria

- Consider hospitalization within first 24 to 48 hours.
- It is the patient's first TIA or the duration of the TIA is 1 hour or longer.
- High risk for cardiac emboli (e.g., atrial fibrillation).
- Symptomatic internal carotid stenosis greater than 50%.
- Hypercoagulable state.
- High risk of early stroke.

Treatment Plan

- Refer patient to ED for further evaluation. Workup to find the extent of brain damage and the cause of the TIA (or stroke).
- CT and/or MRI scan as soon as possible (within first 24 hours of the episode). The diffusion-weighted MRI is the preferred imaging method.

Cerebrovascular Accident or Stroke

A stroke can be caused either by emboli or bleeding. Both result in permanent neurologic damage that results in ischemia to the affected brain tissues. The most common cause of stroke is hypertension. Other causes are aneurysms, trauma, bleeding abnormality, cocaine/illicit drugs, diabetes, warfarin/anticoagulants.

The sources of bleeding can be from intracerebral hemorrhage and a subarachnoid hemorrhage (SAH). A thrombotic stroke is due to emboli that broke off from thrombus formation in the body. Common locations are the lower extremities and the heart (atrial fibrillation).

Bleeding

- SAH or ICH: Sudden onset of severe headache that is described as "the worst headache of my life." Vomiting is more common in hemorrhagic strokes (compared with embolic strokes). Usually caused by a ruptured aneurysm.

Physical Exam

- Complains of severe headache with slurred speech, double vision (diplopia), poor balance, and difficulty walking. Problems expressing self or with speaking. Speech may be incoherent.
- Focal abnormalities such as one-sided weakness (drooping on one side of the face and weakness of the extremity on the same side).

Management

Call 911. Assess the "ABCs" as soon as possible. Check for airway patency, chest movement, breath sounds from both lungs, and circulation. Check vital signs next.

Emergency Department Management

Assess ABCs. Stabilize patient. Initial imaging study in the ED is CT scan (without contrast), then an MRI study. Decide if patient is a candidate for antithrombolytic therapy, and so on.

Labs

- Prothrombin time, partial thromboplastin time, international normalized ratio.
- CBC with differential and platelet count. Serum blood glucose.
- Total lipid profile (cholesterol, low-density lipoprotein, high-density lipoprotein, triglycertides).

Examples of Brain Damage

Temporal Lobe Damage

- *Apraxia*: Difficulty with performing purposeful movements.
- *Broca's aphasia*: Also known as "non-fluent aphasia." Patient comprehends speech relatively well (and can read), but has extreme difficulty with the motor aspects of speech. Speech length is usually less than four words.
- *Wernicke's aphasia*: Also known as "fluent aphasia." Patient has difficulty with comprehension, but has no problem with producing speech. Reading and writing can be markedly impaired.
- *Frontal lobe damage*: The frontal lobes are the areas where intelligence, executive skills, logic, and personality reside. Damage will cause dementia, memory loss/difficulties, inability to learn, etc.

OTHER COMMON GERIATRIC CONDITIONS

These diseases are covered under their respective organ systems.

Acute diverticulitis (Chap. 10)
Anemia (Chap. 13)
Bacterial pneumonia (Chap. 8)
COPD (Chap. 8)
Congestive heart failure (Chap. 7)
Diabetes type 2 (Chap. 9)
Glaucoma (Chap. 5)
Heart disease/murmurs (Chap. 7)
Hyperlipidemia (Chap. 7)

Hypertension (Chap. 7)
Macular degeneration (Chap. 5)
Menopause/atrophic vaginitis (Chap. 17)
Temporal arteritis (Chap. 12)

PHARMACOLOGIC ISSUES: OLDER ADULTS (TABLE 27.2)

Drug clearance is affected by: renal impairment, a less efficient liver CYP 450 system, malabsorption, and relatively higher fat:muscle tissue (extends half-life, fat-soluble drugs). Older adults have an increased sensitivity to benzodiazepines, hypnotics, TCAs, and antipsychotics. The American Geriatric Society has made a list of inappropriate medications for the elderly (Updated Beers Criteria, 2012; Table 27.2).

NUTRITIONAL ISSUES

Nutrition issues are common in older adults, especially in the frail elderly or the "old-old."

Clinically significant weight loss is defined by the minimum data set criteria as weight loss of 5% of usual body weight (in 30 days) or weight loss equal to at least 10% of the usual body weight (in 6 months). Weight loss involve loss of muscle mass and body fat. A patient with edema and fluid retention may have "normal weight" even if she is malnourished.

Table 27.2 Potentially Inappropriate Medications for Older Adults (Beer's Criteria List)

Drug Class	Drugs to Avoid
Antihistamines	Diphenhydramine/Benadryl and others. Newer generation has lower incidence (Claritin)
Benzodiazepines	
Short–intermediate acting	Alprazolam (Xanax), lorazepam (Ativan), triazolam (Halcion)
Long-acting	Diazepam (Valium), clonazepam (Klonopin)
Antipsychotics	Thioridazine (Mellaril), mexoridazine (Serentil)
Atypical antipsychotics	Quetapine (Seroquel), olanzapine (Zyprexa)
TCA	Amitriptylin (Elavil), imipramine (Tofranil)
Cardiac drugs	Orthostatic hypotension.
Alpha-blockers	Terazosin (Hytrin), prazosin (Minipress)
Central alpha agonist	Clonidine (Catapres)
Nifedipine (immediate release)	Not recommended for routine treatment of hypertension
Sulfonylureas (long-acting first generation)	Glyburide (Diabeta), chlorpropamide (Diabenase)
NSAIDs (except COX-inhibiting)	Indomethacin (Indocin), diclofenac (Voltaren), others
	Ketorolac and indomethacin (Indocin); high risk of GI bleeding
Mineral oil (oral)	Aspiration into lungs
Antispasmodics	Dicyclomine (Bentyl), scopolamine, belladonna
Other	Metoclopramide (Reglan except for gastroparesis)
	Sliding-scale insulin dosing

* List is not all-inclusive.

Terms

- *Anorexia*: Loss of appetite that has many causes such as dementia, drug side effect, changes in taste and smell, and major depression.
- *Cachexia*: Defined as a complex multifactorial metabolic disorder that is associated with an illness or disease. Associated with increased risk of falls and morbidity.
- *Sarcopenia*: Loss of muscle mass, strength, and performance. Multiple causes such as low hormone levels (testosterone and estrogen), immobility, low levels of physical activity, low protein intake, and others. Higher risk of falls, hip fracture, functional decline, and morbidity.
- *Satiety*: The subjective feeling of "fullness" that follows a meal. If a patient complains of early satiety or dysphagia (especially if accompanied with weight loss), it is a worrisome finding. Rule out cancers of the colon or esophagus. Refer to GI specialist for colonoscopy.

Nutritional Screening Tools

- Body fat and lean muscle mass estimation using bioelectrical impedance.
- Measurement of upper arm circumference.
- Dietary diary or estimated dietary intake (dementia), types of foods preferred, snacking.
- There are several screening tools for malnutrition.

Questionnaires
Mini Nutrition Assessment-Short-Form

- Contains six questions. A global assessment that includes anthropomorphic measurements.

Simplified Nutrition Assessment Questionnaire

- Contains four items. Has a sensitivity of 88% and a specificity of 84%.

Interventions

- Encourage resident to eat in the dining room with others (avoid isolation).
- Give the patient a choice of the type of food and drink preferred.
- Nutritional supplements and drinks. Encourage patient to eat high-caloric foods.
- If community-dwelling, assess if assistance is needed for grocery shopping and food preparation.
- The patient can enroll for food assistance ("food stamps").

Treatment Plan

- Perform thorough health, medical, and medicines assessment (including OTC, herbs).
- Find out the factors that are affecting food intake and correct (if possible).
- Assess dental health, gum disease, missing teeth, use of dentures, and oral ulcers.
- Rule out major depression, anemia, hypothyroidism.
- *Labs*: CBC, biochemical profile, thyroid-stimulating hormone, folate and B12 level, vitamin D level.
- Refer to the dietician for evaluation and dietary recommendations.
- Handgrip strength: one of the indications of functional status. Weak hand grip abnormal and is present in malnutrition (severe malnutrition associated with very weak hand grip).
- Give multivitamin supplement.
- Consider short-term trial of prescription appetite stimulants.

Appetite Stimulants

- Megestrol acetate (Megace): A progesterone-type of drug that causes weight gain in patients with anorexia (e.g., elderly, cancer-related).
  - Side effects: water retention may exacerbate or cause heart failure. Monitor patients for edema and signs of heart failure (dyspnea, edema, bibasilar rales).
- Mirtazapine (Remeron): An SSRI that causes more weight gain compared with the other SSRIs.
  - Has same Black Box Warning as the other SSRIs.

28

Pressure Ulcers, Wounds, Wound Treatment, and Advanced Practice Procedures

The last few pages of this chapter cover clinical procedures that can be performed (with training) by adult nurse practitioners, gerontological nurse practitioners (GNPs), and adult-gerontology nurse practitioners such as wound debridement, wound care, local anesthesia (digital block and infiltration), suturing, and skin biopsy.

PRESSURE ULCERS

A pressure ulcer (pressure sore, bed sore, decubitus ulcers) is formed when there is prolonged pressure over localized area of skin and underlying tissue (usually over a bony prominence) or when there is prolonged pressure combined with shearing forces and friction. Do not confuse pressure ulcers with ulcers that are caused by arterial or venous insufficiency or by diabetes.

Risk factors: immobility, older age, skin too wet or too dry, smoking, urine or bowel incontinence, maceration, diabetic, PVD (lower extremity ulcers), malnutrition, spinal cord injuries, etc.

Nutritional indicators: low serum albumin, anemia, poor appetite/anorexia, underweight.

Prevention of Pressure Ulcers (Decubiti)

Nutrition

Assess nutritional status by checking albumin (low), CBC (anemia), hydration status, food and fluid intake, weight/BMI, and diet. Supplement diet with high-protein mixed with oral nutritional supplements or tube feedings, in addition to person's normal diet. May need to refer to dietician for consult about increasing dietary calories and snacks.

Positioning
- Avoid 90° side-lying position (increases pressure).
- Avoid semi-recumbent position (increases pressure).
- Turn patient every 2 hours in bed. Clean urine/feces as soon as possible and change clothes if soiled or wet. Keep skin clean and dry.
- Positioning: right side, back, left side (30° tilt on each side) every 2 hours.
- When supine, use heel protectors and position legs with slight flexion of the knee.
- Use transfer aids to reduce shearing and friction. Do not drag patient on the bed— lift using folded sheet while repositioning patient to avoid shearing and rubbing.

Skin

- Skin that is frequently moist or is very dry places a person at higher risk for pressure ulcers. For dry skin, use skin emollients (e.g., Eucerin cream, cocoa butter).
- Protect from excessive moisture by using heavy creams as a waterproof barrier (zinc creams, Desitin cream).
- If incontinent, change adult diaper when soiled.
- Do not use "massage" for pressure ulcer prevention. If the skin is inflamed, massage is contraindicated (may damage skin further).
- If patient is a smoker, give smoking cessation education. Wounds take longer to heal in smokers.

Pressure-Relieving Devices

- Avoid using doughnut-, cutout-, or ring-shaped chair cushions/devices, synthetic sheepskin (real sheepskin works), shaped cushions.
- Use rolled towels, pillows, sheepskin, or wedge to help bedridden patient with position changes.
- Pressure-reducing mattress: higher specification foam mattresses (not standard type), alternating-pressure mattress, but do not use small-cell size (less than 10 cm) types.
- Pressure-reducing beds, air-loss beds, air-fluidized beds.
- Chair cushions: pressure-redistributing seat cushions, chair cushions (gel, foams), natural sheepskin.
- Teach wheelchair patients to shift body weight every 15 to 20 minutes.

TOOL FOR PREDICTING RISK OF PRESSURE SORES

Braden Scale for Predicting Pressure Sore Risk

Used to predict pressure ulcer risk. Helpful in identifying risk factors so that interventions can be started early to help prevent or delay ulcer development.

The Braden Scale contains six categories. It measures the following factors: sensory perception, moisture (skin), activity, mobility, nutrition, and friction and shear. A Braden score of 12 or less is considered "high risk" for development of bed sores, and a Braden score of 9 or below is considered "very high risk."

Staging Pressure Ulcers

See Table 28.1.

Management

Important to monitor and document condition of the pressure ulcer daily. Use the PUSH tool to document the surface area, exudate, and the type of wound tissue of the ulcer.

Pressure Ulcer Healing Chart (PUSH Tool version 3.0)

The PUSH tool is an observational rating scale from the National Pressure Ulcer Advisory Panel. It is used to document the healing progress of the ulcer. The PUSH score ranges from 1 to 17 points (healed = 0). When using the tool, always use the same type/brand of centimeter ruler and always measure it the same way each time.

Table 28.1 Pressure Ulcer Stages

Ulcer Stage or Category	Description
Stage/Category I	Intact skin. Red, nonblanchable local area of skin that may feel tender. If darker colored skin, difficult to assess blanching. Look for signs of ischemic damage such a localized area with that feels firm and warm (or cool skin). Affected area usually located on a bony prominence
Stage/Category II (partial thickness)	Shiny or dry shallow ulcer without slough or bruising. Wound bed is pink to red. May have blisters (serous or blood-tinged serous) that erupt resulting in a red, shiny, shallow ulcer
Stage/Category III (full thickness)	Full-thickness loss (epidermis and dermis). Deeper ulcers. Ulcer borders are obvious and firm. Thickness depends on location. Ulcers located on ear, occiput, malleolus are shallower
Stage/Category VI	Full-thickness tissue loss with exposed bone, tendon, or muscle. Sometimes undermining and tunneling is present. Slough or eschar may be present. Ulcers located on ear, occiput, malleolus are shallower
Unstageable	Presence of eschar or sloughing interferes with staging. Slough covers wound (yellow, tan, gray, green or brown). Wound needs to be cleaned and debrided
Suspected deep tissue injury	Purple or maroon colored skin that feels very firm. Some with blood-filled blister. Can be preceded by tissue that feels painful, firm, boggy, warmer or cooler. Some may have blistering

Source: National Pressure Ulcer Advisory Panel (NPUAP, 2007).

Length × Width

Measure at greatest length and greatest width (side to side). How: Multiply (length × width) to obtain the surface area in square centimeters (cm^2). Use disposable measuring tapes.

Exudate Amount

- Estimate amount from none to light, moderate, or heavy.
- *Tissue type*: describe the type of tissue that is on the wound bed. Use the below terms:
  - *Eschar (necrotic tissue)*: "black, brown, or tan colored tissue that adheres firmly to the wound bed or ulcer edges." Texture is "either firmer or softer than surrounding skin."
  - *Slough*: "yellow or white tissue that adheres to the ulcer bed." Slough is tissue that is attached to the ulcer bed and looks like "strings or thick clumps or is mucinous."
  - *Granulation tissue*: look for "pink or beefy red tissue with shiny, moist, granular appearance."
  - *Epithelial tissue*: "for superficial ulcers, appears like "new pink or shiny tissue (skin) that grows in from the edges or as islands on the ulcer surface."
  - *Closed/resurfaced*: "the wound is completely covered with epithelium (new skin)."

Wound Treatment

Debridement Stage

- *Hydrogels or hydrocolloid dressings*: can be used to protect stoma skin from maceration. Avoid using with high-exudate wounds. Can be used for many wound types.

- *Wound types*: pressure ulcers, burns, macerated skin, fistula, stoma, others.
- *Examples*: DuoDerm, Derma-Gel Hydrogel, Elasto-Gel Occlusive Dressing, Aquagel.

Granulation Stage

- Foam dressing works well for most wound types. Works well with high-exudate wounds. Low adherence of foam dressing decreases wound trauma (dressing changes). Several types of foam (e.g., true foam, polyurethane, silicone foam). Some types have an adhesive border and some do not. Can be left in place for 3 to 4 days.
- *Examples*: 3M Tegaderm, Opsite, others.
- *Wounds*: leg ulcers, pressure ulcers, skin graft donor sites, minor burns, diabetic ulcers, etc.

Epithelialization Stage

- Hydrocolloid and low-adherence dressings are used during the epithelialization stage.

Wound Dressings

Most wounds heal faster in a moist environment (40% faster). Moisture facilitates migration of epidermal cells, which helps with the healing process (granulation; Table 28.2).

Table 28.2 Types of Wound Dressings for Pressure Ulcers

Dressing Type	Action	Wound Types
Hydrogels Aquasorb PolyDerm	Cleans and debrides wounds by liquefying necrotic tissue. Keeps wounds moist. Breathable films prevent bacteria from entering wound	Wounds with little to no exudate. Avoid with high-exudate wounds.
Foam, Silicone foam	Soaks up excess exudate. Low adherence	Works well with most wound types. Can be used as the secondary dressing
Alginates Silver alginate	Forms gel on contact. Derived from brown seaweed. Silver alginate has antimicrobial properties	Soaks up exudate Moderate to heavy exudate wounds. Cover with absorbent gauze and secure in place with secondary dressing
Enzymes Collagenase, fibrolysin	Cleans and debrides wounds by liquefying tissue	Necrotic wounds
Semi-permeable or semi-occlusive films Tegaderm (3M)	Waterproof semi-transparent film made from polyurethane. High-moisture vapor transmission rate (MVTR)	Protects wounds and keeps it moist. Use with non-draining wounds as primary or secondary dressing
Packing gauze	Some types are impregnated with antimicrobials	Wounds with cavities Tunneling wounds Deep wounds Needs secondary dressing such as silicone foam dressing

DEBRIDEMENT

Pressure Ulcers

Necrotic tissue impairs wound healing and increases the risk of infection. Debridement of wounds is the process of removing necrotic tissue. There are several methods.

Procedure

Sharp Debridement

Tools: scalpel or scissors and forceps.

Gently lift up necrotic tissue with forceps, then cut it gently with either scalpel or sharp scissors. Do not perform sharp debridement on thick heel eschars because of the risk of bone trauma (risk of osteomyelitis). Clean wound and apply dressing.

Enzymatic Debridement

Topical proteolytic enzymes: collagenase, fibrinolysin, deoxyribonuclease.

Apply proteolytic enzyme to the pressure ulcer. Be careful with the amount; avoid placing too much because it can leak to the normal skin surrounding the ulcer. Produces large amount of exudate.

Autolytic Debridement

Cover pressure ulcer with hydrogel or semi-occlusive transparent film. Works better in wounds with minimal to no discharge. Retains the enzymes produced by the wound. Enzymes break down the necrotic tissue.

Jet Lavage Wound Debridement

Water is used under pressure to clean and debride wound. A large syringe is connected to a short tube with a silicone needle tip. A "jet" of water is produced that is used to clean and debride the wound.

COMPLICATIONS: PRESSURE ULCERS

The most common complication of pressure ulcers is local infection. Chronic pressure ulcers or wounds are always colonized by bacteria. But if the bacterial load is too high, the patient's wound will become infected. Common organisms are *Proteus mirabilis*, group D streptococci, *Escherichia coli*, *Staphylococcus* species, *Pseudomonas* species, and *Corynebacterium* organisms. Infection can be localized or it can spread to surrounding skin (cellulitis), to the bone (osteomyelitis), and the body (sepsis). Treat if there is clinical evidence of an infection.

Possible infection: Look for purulent or darkening color of discharge, necrotic tissue, foul odor, systemic symptoms.

Management of Complications of Pressure Ulcers

Superficial Pressure Ulcer Infections

- Initial actions are better wound care and debridement of necrotic tissue and slough.
- Avoid using povidone-iodine (Betadine), hydrogen peroxide, or chlorhexidine on the ulcer wound because they impede healing (toxic to fibroblasts).
- Trial of topical antibiotics for 2-week duration (combination antibiotic ointment or silver sulfadiazine 1% cream).

- Do not use a superficial swab specimen to obtain specimen for a wound culture. Deep tissue specimen is needed. It can be obtained by a wound biopsy or by needle aspiration (if applicable). Collect specimen from the area of the wound that appears infected.
- Refer: osteomyelitis, bacteremia/sepsis, septic arthritis (infected joint), endocarditis. Hospitalize for high-dosed IV antibiotics.

Osteomyelitis

- Deeper ulcers (stage III and VI) are at higher risk for osteomyelitis. May complain of bone pain or may be asymptomatic.
- If suspect osteomyelitis, order a plain x-ray (radiograph). If abnormal (i.e., inflammation), refer to physician or order MRI (preferred) or CT scan. Other tests are blood cultures, erythrocyte sedimentation rate (ESR), C-reactive protein (CRP), WBC, bone biopsy for C&S.
- Hospitalization (IV antibiotics, bone debridement). Mild case, oral antibiotics (e.g., Cipro × 6 weeks.).

Marjolin Ulcer

Malignant transformation of a chronic wound or scar (rare). An aggressive form of squamous cell carcinoma. Obtain a tissue biopsy from the ulcer and refer to a dermatologist.

Other complications are osteomyelitis, cellulitis, sepsis, fistula formation, tunneling, malignant transformation (Marjolin ulcer), severe scarring.

WOUNDS

A wound is a disruption or damage to the skin. There are four phases involved in wound healing. Some of the factors that impair the wound healing process are older/mature age, poor nutrition, impaired immune system, impaired mobility, stress (affects immune system), diabetes, certain medicines (impair clot formation, steroids), cigarette smoking, and secondary bacterial infection (Table 28.3).

Categories of Wound Healing

- *Primary healing (primary closure)*: Wound is closed within 24 hours by suturing or by application of tissue glue or butterfly strips (so that edges of wounds are well approximated). Causes the least amount of scarring.
- *Secondary intention*: Wound is left open with formation of granulation tissue and scarring. Wound heals from the bottom of the wound up. Wound edges are not well approximated. Causes more scarring than primary closure.

Table 28.3 Phases of Wound Healing

Phase	Healing Event
Hemostasis	Constriction of local blood vessels, platelet aggregation, fibrin (clot) formation
Inflammation	Macrophages and lymphocytes proliferate, presence of inflammatory mediators such as cytokines and leukotrienes
Proliferation	Proliferation of basal and epithelial cells
	Angiogenesis
Remodeling	Remodeling of collagen, scar formation (cicatrix)

- *Tertiary intention (delayed primary closure)*: wounds with heavy contamination or poor vascularity (crush injuries) are best left open to heal by secondary intention (granulation) and wound contraction. Then the wound edges are approximated in 3 to 4 days. Produces more scar tissue.

High-Risk Wounds: Consider Referral

1) Infected wounds (pus, wound is not healing; devitalized tissue, wound becomes hot and swollen).
2) Closed-fist injuries.
3) Facial wounds with risk of cosmetic damage (e.g., large wound, bites, cartilage injury).
4) Suspected foreign body or embedded object in wound that cannot be removed.
5) Injury of a joint capsule. If joint capsule penetrated, joint can become infected.
6) Electrical injuries.
7) Paint-gun or high-pressure wounds.
8) Chemical wounds (especially alkali-related damage) of the eyes or skin.
9) Suspected physical or child abuse.
10) Wounds with cosmetic concerns (cartilage wounds in the ears, nose). Cartilage does not heal. Refer to plastic surgeon or ED.

Infected Wounds

1) Do not suture infected wounds (open greater than 24 hours). Wound will heal by secondary intention.
2) Treat infection with antibiotics such as cephalexin (Keflex) QID or dicloxacillin for 10 days.
3) Infection can spread (cellulitis); may need to hospitalize for systemic antibiotics.

Closed-Fist Injuries and Bite Wounds

1) Refer close-fist injuries to the ED or urgent care center. X-ray of the hand to rule out foreign body (i.e., teeth) and fracture. Sometimes, ultrasound is used to view foreign bodies that do not show up on x-rays.
2) Test distal pulses, skin color, range of motion (ROM), tendon damage, nerve damage, fracture.
3) Do not suture bite wounds or puncture wounds due to high risk of infection.
4) Antibiotic prophylaxis needed for animal and human bite wounds. First line is amoxicillin-clavulanic acid (Augmentin po BID × 10 days).
5) Tetanus vaccine if last dose was greater than 5 years. Use Tdap vaccine (tetanus, diptheria, and acellular pertussis) (if never had Tdap) in patients of age greater than 7 years.

Retained Foreign Bodies

1) Higher risk of infection. If unable to remove, refer to ER. Plain x-ray is first-line imaging test. Ultrasound is used if suspected object or object does not show on x-rays (radiolucent).
2) May not be visible on x-rays:
   - Small glass splinters or particles.
   - Splinters, thorns, fish bones.
   - Plastics.

Minor Burns

Wash area with water and mild soap. Using sterile tongue blade, apply thin layer of 1% silver sulfadiazine (Silvadene) to burned area. Cover burned area with non-stick gauze (e.g., Telfa). Secure with stretch-conforming gauze (e.g., Kerlix).

Apply Silvadene once to twice a day until the burn is healed. After skin is healed, consider using Desitin daily for 1 to 2 weeks to protect area from sunlight. Do not expose recently healed burned skin to sunlight (causes hyperpigmentation).

Wound Care

During history, ask about mechanism of injury and other details about the incident. Check for allergy to iodine, rubber, latex, lidocaine. If patient has rubber or latex allergy, do not use latex gloves. Use silicone-based disposable gloves. Do not forget tetanus prophylaxis. If last dose was greater than 5 years, give Tdap booster.

Procedure

1) Irrigate wound with normal saline (do not mix with Betadine, hydrogen peroxide, Hibiclens) and/or wash area with mild soap and water. Remove dirt.
2) Assess wound for neurovascular and tendon damage. Check distal pulses. Depending on injury, rule out foreign body.
3) Treatment depends on the type of wound and patient characteristics.

PRIMARY CARE PRACTICE: PROCEDURES

Procedures

Local Anesthesia

There are two types of lidocaine 1% (plain or mixed with epinephrine). Do not use lidocaine with epinephrine on areas of body at high risk of ischemia (tip of nose, ears, fingertips, toes, penis).

Contraindications to local anesthesia: infected injection site, allergy to anesthetic, or devascularized/ischemic tissue damage.

Adverse complications: allergic reaction, infection, injecting solution directly into blood vessel, injury to nerves and tendons in the area.

Example of anesthesia use: wounds that need suturing, incisions (e.g., embedded splinter or paronychia), biopsy, and others.

Drug: lidocaine 1% (plain) onset of action is from 2 to 5 minutes. Duration of action is from 30 minutes to 2 hours. Advise patient he/she will feel a burning sensation at the start of the injection, which will go away.

Procedure

Digital Nerve Block (Fingers)

1) Clean web space on each side of the involved finger with Betadine swab and allow to dry.
2) Draw up about 3 mL of plain lidocaine 1% from vial using a 5 to 10 cc syringe with an #18 gauge needle. Then change needle to smaller gauge (#25 to #30 gauge, 1½ inches).
3) Place needle in perpendicular position above web space and insert into subcutaneous tissue space.

4) Before injecting, aspirate first to check for placement. If there is no blood, slowly inject the lidocaine into the web space (volar aspect). Inject slowly and use small amounts.

5) If blood is aspirated, withdraw needle slightly and reposition slightly (without removing the needle from the skin).

6) Reposition needle slightly and continue to infiltrate drug into the web space on each side of the injured finger.

7) Instruct patient that it may take 15 minutes for the anesthesia to become effective. Ask patient if area is numb (test by using tip of needle to test sensation) before suturing.

Infiltration Technique

Apply Betadine on intact skin around wound. Slowly insert syringe (as directed above). Aspirate for blood. Slowly infiltrate the edges of the wound, then withdraw slightly to move it to another area. Slowly infiltrate wound edges. Needle is inserted into the subcutaneous layer only. The amount of lidocaine that is used varies based on the size of the wound and the location.

Suturing

General rules about suturing:
1) Do not suture puncture wounds or human or animal bites.
2) Do not suture heavily contaminated wounds.
3) Lacerations that are greater than 12 hours old are at higher risk of infection. Do not suture infected wounds.
4) Do not suture wounds that have been open longer than 24 hours (high bacterial load).

Types of Sutures and Needles

- *Example*: Skin laceration.
- Use nonabsorbable synthetic suture (i.e., nylon, Prolene).
- Preferred suture size is from 3-0 to 5-0 (middle range).
- Preferred needle type to suture skin is a curved cutting needle.
- *Suture size*: the higher the number, the smaller the diameter (the same concept is used for needle size). (Size range is 00 to 10-0.) The smallest diameter suture is 00 (about the size of human hair). It is used to repair small blood vessels.

Suture Technique

1) Evert the edges of the wound by inserting needle at 90° angle (ensures that wound edges are well approximated).
2) Use needle holder to hold needle. Use forceps to grab wound edges.
3) Usually, simple sutures are used on skin lacerations. Each suture is individually tied, then cut (simple interrupted sutures).
4) When cutting suture thread, do not cut too short. Leave a short tail (easier to remove).
5) Non-absorbable synthetic sutures are preferred for lacerations/wounds of the skin.
6) If suturing scalp of a person with black hair, blue-colored suture thread is easier to visualize (for removal).

Suture Removal

Most sutures are removed within 7 to 10 days. Sutures on the face are removed within 5 days to minimize scarring. Stitches that are left beyond 10 days may develop scars that resemble a "railroad track."

- Face: from 5 to 7 days.
- Scalp: from 10 to 12 days.
- Arms/legs/hands/feet: from 7 to 10 days.

Procedure

Use forceps and lift suture from the skin. Cut it with scissors. Use forceps to grasp the knot and pull the suture gently out of the wound.

Skin Biopsy

Punch Biopsy

Check for history of bleeding disorder and use of drugs that affect bleeding time (aspirin, warfarin). Patients with INR greater than 2.5 should not be biopsied. Check scar history (history of keloids or hypertrophic scarring?).

Refer to dermatologist: facial biopsies, biopsy of areas with cartilage, suspected melanoma, history of keloid/hypertrophic scarring, bleeding disorder, etc.

Ask if allergic to lidocaine or rubber/latex (use silicone gloves).

Procedure

1) Prep skin site with alcohol wipes and allow to dry.
2) Using a tuberculin syringe, draw lidocaine 1% and epinephrine 1:100,100 (do not use with epinephrine if area is on the nose, ears, fingertips, toes, penis).
3) Inject slowly under the epidermis until a small bleb is formed. The color of the skin over the bleb area becomes paler due to the vasoconstricting effect of epinephrine.
4) Check site for numbness by using the point of the syringe and testing sensation on the bleb area. The skin will become numb within 5 to 10 minutes (lasts about 45–60 minutes).
5) Using a 3-mm skin punch, position instrument at 90° (perpendicular to the skin).
6) Twist the punch instrument gently in a "drilling" motion until it has pierced the epidermis (there should be about ½ inch of the blade visible on top of the skin).
7) Remove from skin and lift plug gently with forceps (do not crush). Use a scalpel to cut the plug at the base. Immediately place it on the biopsy specimen container. Do not forget to label the specimen cup with the patient's name, location of the biopsy site, and the type of tissue obtained.
8) Cover area with sterile 2 × 2 gauze with tape (if bleeding) or with Band-Aid if minimal bleeding. Instruct patient to change Band-Aid once a day.
9) Instruct patient to keep the site dry. Instruct to avoid submerging site in water (avoid tub bath, swimming, hot tubs) until it is healed. Site will scab within a few days.

Note

This book is written for review purposes only. It is not designed for clinical practice.

Practice Questions
and Answers

VI

29

Practice Questions

1. During a physical examination, the nurse practitioner instructs the patient to make a fist by folding his thumb and then covering the thumb with the other fingers. The patient complains of pain (positive Finkelstein's sign). Which of the following conditions is this test indicative of?

    A) Depuytren's contracture
    B) DeQuervain's tenosynovitis
    C) A "trigger" finger
    D) A severe case of carpal tunnel syndrome

2. Which of the following statements is true regarding claims-based professional malpractice insurance?

    A) All malpractice claims made are paid as long as the nurse practitioner is in active practice
    B) Claims made during the insured periods are covered provided the nurse practitioner is currently enrolled in the malpractice insurance program with the company
    C) Although the nurse practitioner is no longer insured by the same insurance company, any claims made against her on the dates that her malpractice insurance was active are still eligible for coverage
    D) Malpractice insurance will pay claims that are eligible if the nurse practitioner is found to be not at fault

3. Which of the following is a true statement regarding the serum glycosylated hemoglobin test?

    A) It is the average blood glucose level during the previous 3 months
    B) It detects the fasting blood glucose level in the previous 3 months
    C) It is a test to detect the amount of glucose and lactose in the blood
    D) The test is more sensitive in type 2 diabetes than in type 1 diabetes

4. A 21-year-old female, complaining of random palpitations along with dizziness, is diagnosed with mitral valve prolapse (MVP) by the nurse practitioner. Her echocardiogram reveals redundant and thickened leaflets. On physical examination, a grade III/VI systolic murmur with an ejection click is noted. Which of the following is a true statement regarding this condition?

   A) Endocarditis prophylaxis is indicated for some dental, urologic, and gastrointestinal invasive procedures
   B) No endocarditis prophylaxis is indicated for any procedures
   C) Warfarin sodium (Coumadin) is always indicated for older patients
   D) Endocarditis prophylaxis is necessary for dental procedures only

5. All of the following services are covered under Medicare Part A except:

   A) Inpatient hospitalizations
   B) Medicines administered to a patient while hospitalized
   C) Nursing home care
   D) Radiology tests done in a hospital

6. The nurse practitioner would test the obturator and iliopsoas muscles to evaluate a possible case of which of the following conditions?

   A) Acute cholecystitis
   B) Acute appendicitis
   C) Inguinal hernia
   D) Gastric ulcer

7. The Dawn phenomenon is best described as which of the following?

   A) It is due to abnormally low levels of serum glucose very early in the morning that stimulate the liver to secrete glucagon
   B) It is an increase in the blood glucose level early in the morning due to the physiologic spike of growth hormone
   C) It is an autoimmune disorder resulting in a very high fasting blood glucose level
   D) It is a rare phenomenon that occurs only in diabetics

8. An 18-year-old male is brought in by his mother to an urgent care center. She tells the nurse practitioner that he returned from a camping trip 3 days ago and now has a high fever, severe headache, myalgias, and neck discomfort. She reports that her son started to break out with rashes; some of which are turning into dark-red to purple lesions. On physical examination, the temperature is 103.0°F, the pulse is 110 beats per minute, and the respiratory rate is 22/minute. The blood pressure is 90/50 mmHg. Which of the following conditions is it most likely to be?

   A) Stevens-Johnson syndrome
   B) Meningococcemia
   C) Rocky Mountain spotted fever
   D) Erythema multiforme

9. A 22-year-old student is seen in the college health clinic with complaints of fatigue, rhinitis, and a cough for 2 weeks. The cough is productive of small amounts of sputum. The patient has a negative health history, is not on any prescription medications, and denies a history of allergies. Physical examination reveals a temperature of 99.9°F, respirations of 18/minute, and a pulse of 100 beats per minute. Lung examination reveals fine crackles on the left lower lobe of the lung. A chest radiograph (x-ray) shows diffuse infiltrates on the same lobe. What is the diagnosis most likely to be?

A) *Streptococcus* pneumonia
B) *Mycoplasma* pneumonia
C) Allergic rhinitis
D) Legionnaire's disease

10. Which of the following antihypertensive medications should the nurse practitioner avoid when treating patients with emphysema?

A) Calcium channel blockers
B) ACE inhibitors
C) Beta-blockers
D) Diuretics

11. Linda B., a 30-year-old chef, complains of a sudden onset of hives that started to break out all over her body after she returned from lunch. It is accompanied by chest tightness and a dry cough. She tells a coworker that she has a history of eczema and had mild asthma during childhood. She appears anxious and is not sure of what is to be done next. Which of the following is the best intervention to follow for this patient?

A) Immediately administer a treatment of nebulized albuterol mixed with saline and repeat in 10 minutes if the patient's symptoms are not better
B) Administer an injection of cimetidine (Tagamet) and an antihistamine as soon as possible
C) Administer an injection of epinephrine 1:1,000 intramuscularly immediately
D) Immediately administer an injection of prednisone and epinephrine 1:1,000 intramuscularly and call for emergency assistance

12. In which of the following conditions would the cremasteric reflex be absent?

A) Acute epididymitis
B) Testicular torsion
C) Acute prostatitis
D) It is always present

13. Which of the following is not associated with B12-deficiency anemia?

A) Spoon-shaped nails and pica
B) A red and swollen tongue (glossitis) and a vegan diet
C) Macrocytes and multisegmented neutrophils
D) Tingling and numbness in both feet

14. A diabetic patient has a urinalysis ordered. The results are: 4+ ketones, trace leukocytes, negative nitrites, and negative red blood cells. Which of the following would the nurse practitioner do next?

    A) Order an ultrasound of the kidneys to rule out subacute renal failure
    B) Check the patient's blood glucose
    C) Order a 24-hour urine for microalbumin
    D) Assess for a history of illicit drug or alcohol use

15. All of the following are true statements about diverticula except:

    A) Diverticula are located in the colon
    B) A low-fiber diet is associated with the condition
    C) Diverticula in the colon are colonized with bacteria
    D) Supplementing with fiber such as psyllium (Metamucil) is never recommended

16. Patients who are diagnosed with gonorrhea are also treated for the following because of high rates of coinfection:

    A) *Mycoplasma pneumoniae*
    B) *Chlamydia trachomatis*
    C) Syphilis
    D) Pelvic inflammatory disease

17. An older woman complains to the nurse practitioner that she has leakage of urine when she sneezes or is laughing. The patient thinks that it is getting worse. Which of the following would be appropriate initial intervention?

    A) Educate the patient about Kegel exercises
    B) Recommend that she limit her fluid intake to less than 1 L per day
    C) Refer the patient to a urologist for a cystoscopy
    D) Advise the patient that she will be given medicine to help her with bladder control

18. A 15-year-old high school student who is going through a growth spurt has a baseline laboratory test done during a routine physical examination. The serum alkaline phosphatase level is expected to be:

    A) Normal
    B) Higher than normal
    C) Lower than normal
    D) None of the above

19. Which of the following antihypertensive medications has beneficial effects for an elderly White female with osteoporosis?

    A) Calcium channel blockers
    B) ACE inhibitors
    C) Beta-blockers
    D) Diuretics

20. The Lachman maneuver is used to detect which of the following?

    A) Instability of the knee due to anterior cruciate ligament damage
    B) Nerve damage of the knee due to past injury
    C) The integrity of the patellar tendon
    D) Tears on the meniscus of the knee

21. When an adolescent male's penis grows in length more than in width, in which of the following Tanner stages is he classified?

    A) Tanner Stage II
    B) Tanner Stage III
    C) Tanner Stage IV
    D) Tanner Stage V

22. An obese patient who is being discharged on anticoagulants from the local hospital for deep vein thrombosis (DVT) wants to know if there is anything he can do to minimize the recurrence of the disorder. Which of the following is a false statement?

    A) Use thromboembolic stockings as much as possible
    B) Avoid prolonged inactivity
    C) Continue your anticoagulants as prescribed and report any bleeding in the gums and excessive bruising
    D) Start exercising vigorously as soon as possible so that the circulation in the affected lower extremity improves

23. Human papilloma virus (HPV) infection of the larynx has been associated with:

    A) Laryngeal cancer
    B) Esophageal stricture
    C) Cervical cancer
    D) Metaplasia of the squamous cells

24. Mr. Brown is a 65-year-old carpenter complaining of morning stiffness and pain in both his hands and right knee on awakening. He feels some relief after warming up. On examination, the nurse notices the presence of Heberden's nodes. Which of the following is most likely?

    A) Osteoporosis
    B) Rheumatoid arthritis
    C) Osteoarthritis
    D) Reiter's syndrome

25. A positive posterior drawer sign in a soccer player signifies:

    A) An abnormal knee
    B) Instability of the knee
    C) A large amount of swelling on the knee
    D) An injury of the meniscus

26. Valgus stress means:

    A) The force is being directed toward the midline of the body
    B) The force is being directed away from the body
    C) The patient is emotionally distressed
    D) The vagal nerve is inflamed

27. Healthy People 2020 has several focus areas. All of the following are focus areas except:

    A) Mental health disorders
    B) Injury prevention
    C) Diabetes and HIV (human immunodeficiency virus)
    D) Sexual abstinence

28. What is the most common laboratory test used in primary care to evaluate for the glomerular filtration rate (GFR) in a patient with diabetes mellitus?

    A) Electrolyte panel
    B) Creatinine
    C) Alkaline phosphatase
    D) BUN-to-creatinine ratio

29. All of the following are false statements regarding acute gastritis except:

    A) Chronic intake of nonsteroidal analgesics (NSAIDs) can cause the disorder
    B) Chronic lack of dietary fiber is the main cause of the disorder
    C) The screening test for the disorder is the barium swallow test
    D) The gold standard to evaluate the disorder is a colonoscopy

30. Signs and symptoms of depression include all of the following except:

    A) Anhedonia
    B) Low self-esteem
    C) Apathy
    D) Apraxia

31. Which of the following is an accurate description of eliciting for Murphy's sign?

    A) On deep inspiration by the patient, palpate firmly in the right upper quadrant of the abdomen below the costovertebral angle
    B) Bend patient's hips and knees at 90 degrees, then passively rotate hip externally, then internally
    C) Ask the patient to squat, then place the stethoscope on apical area
    D) Press into the abdomen deeply, then release it suddenly

32. A pregnant woman complains of a painful right knee after playing with her 3-year-old son. She wants to be treated for the pain because it is keeping her awake at night. Which of the following is the most appropriate drug to give this patient?

    A) Low-dose ibuprofen (Advil)
    B) Acetaminophen (Tylenol)
    C) Naproxen sodium (Aleve)
    D) Baby aspirin (Bayer)

33. Epidemiologic studies show that Hashimoto's disease occurs most commonly in:

    A) Middle-aged to older women
    B) Smokers
    C) Obese individuals
    D) Older men

34. A 48-year-old woman is told by her physician that she is starting menopause. All of the following are possible findings in premenopausal women except:

    A) Hot flashes that may interfere with sleep
    B) Irregular menstrual periods
    C) Severe vaginal atrophic changes
    D) Cyclic mood swings

35. A 63-year-old patient with a 10-year history of poorly controlled hypertension presents with a cluster of physical examination findings. Which of the following indicate target organ damage commonly seen in hypertensive patients?

    A) Pedal edema, hepatomegaly, and enlarged kidneys
    B) Hepatomegaly, arteriovenous (AV) nicking, bibasilar crackles
    C) Renal infection, S3, neuromuscular abnormalities
    D) Glaucoma, jugular vein atrophy, heart failure

36. The following skin lesions are found more commonly in the elderly except:

    A) Actinic keratosis
    B) Solar lentigines
    C) Tinea cruris
    D) Seborrheic keratosis

37. A 30-year-old female who is sexually active complains of a large amount of milk-like vaginal discharge. A microscopy slide reveals squamous epithelial cells with blurred margins. The vaginal pH is at 6.0. Which of the following is most likely?

    A) Trichomonas infection
    B) Bacterial vaginosis
    C) Candidal infection
    D) A normal finding

38. The Pap smear result on a 20-year-old sexually active student who uses condoms inconsistently shows a large amount of inflammation. Which of the following is the best follow up?

    A) The NP needs to do cervical cultures to verify the presence of gonorrhea
    B) Treat the patient with metronidazole vaginal cream over the phone
    C) Call the patient and tell her she needs a repeat Pap smear in 6 months
    D) Advise her to use a Betadine douche at H (half strength) × 3 days

39. During a routine Pap smear done on a 53-year-old, several areas of flat white skin lesions are found on the patient's vulva. The skin lesions look thin and atrophic. The patient reports that the area is sometimes itchy and has been present for several years. Which condition is best described?

    A) Chronic scabies infection
    B) Lichen sclerosus
    C) Chronic candidal vaginitis
    D) A physiologic variant

40. The heart sound S2 is caused by:

    A) Closure of the atrioventricular valves
    B) Closure of the semilunar valves
    C) Opening of the atrioventricular valves
    D) Opening of the semilunar valves

41. Diabetes mellitus is the leading cause of:

    A) Lower limb amputations
    B) Decubitus ulcers
    C) Dementia
    D) Heart attacks

42. All of the following are covered under Medicare Part B except:

    A) Persons aged 65 years or older
    B) Durable medical equipment
    C) Mammograms annually starting at age 50
    D) Anesthesiologists' services

43. All of the following patients are at higher risk for suicide except:

    A) A 66-year-old White male whose wife of 40 years recently died
    B) A high school student who binges on alcoholic drinks but only on weekends
    C) A depressed 45-year-old female with family history of suicide
    D) A grandmother who has recently been diagnosed with both hypertension and hypothyroidism

44. A 70-year-old male patient complains of a bright red-colored spot in his left eye for 2 days. He denies eye pain, visual changes, or headaches. He has a new onset of cough from a recent viral upper respiratory infection. The only medicine he is on is Bayer aspirin, 1 tablet a day. Which of the following is most likely?

    A) Corneal abrasion
    B) Acute bacterial conjunctivitis
    C) Acute uveitis
    D) Subconjunctival hemorrhage

45. Which of the following is appropriate follow-up for this 70-year-old patient?

A) Referral to an optometrist

B) Referral to an ophthalmologist

C) Advise the patient that it is a benign condition and will resolve spontaneously

D) Prescribe an ophthalmic antibiotic solution

46. Jason, a type 1 diabetic, is being seen for a 3-day history of frequency and nocturia. He denies flank pain and is afebrile. The urinalysis result shows negative ketones, trace amounts of blood, negative nitrites, and 3+leukocytes. He has a trace amount of protein. Which of the following is the best test to order initially?

A) Urine for culture and sensitivity

B) 24-hour urine for protein and creatinine clearance

C) 24-hour urine for microalbumin

D) An intravenous pyelogram (IVP)

47. During an episodic visit, a blood pressure reading of 172/90 is found in a woman with a 10-year history of controlled stage I hypertension and osteoarthritis. Her knees are slightly deformed and she is currently complaining of severe pain in her left knee. She has been self-treating with over-the-counter naproxen sodium (Aleve) 2 tablets twice a day (BID) for the past 2 months. How do nonsteroidal anti-inflammatory drugs (NSAIDs) affect hypertension?

A) They increase the drug level of diuretics in the body

B) They affect the kidneys and can elevate blood pressure

C) A drug–drug interaction is a common finding in these patients

D) They are not associated with adverse effects for patients with hypertension

48. Which of the following pharmacologic agents is used to treat nicotine dependence (smoking cessation)?

A) Sertraline (Zoloft)

B) Bupropion (Zyban)

C) Multivitamins

D) Diazepam (Valium)

49. Rocky Mountain spotted fever is caused by the bite of which of the following?

A) Mosquito

B) Tick

C) Flying insect

D) Flea

50. All of the following are false statements about atopic dermatitis except:

A) Contact with cold objects may exacerbate the condition

B) It does not have a linear distribution

C) It is associated with bullae

D) It is not pruritic

51. A 65-year-old grandmother tells the nurse practitioner that on waking up in the morning, she noticed that her left eye was very painful and tearing profusely. She had noticed crusty small round rashes on the side of her left forehead along with a few on the tip of her nose. Which of the following conditions is most likely?

A) Varicella zoster virus infection of the cornea
B) Corneal ulcer
C) Viral conjunctivitis
D) Bacterial conjunctivitis

52. A 22-year-old sexually active woman is complaining of amenorrhea and vaginal spotting. On examination, her left adnexa is tender and cervical motion tenderness is positive. Which test should the nurse practitioner initially order?

A) Flat plate of the abdomen
B) Complete blood count (CBC) with white cell differentials
C) Pregnancy test
D) Pelvic ultrasound

53. Which of the following heart sounds is associated with heart failure?

A) S3
B) S1, S2, and S3
C) S1, S2, and S4
D) Still's murmur and S4

54. A crossing guard complains of twisting his right knee while walking that morning. The knee is swollen and tender to palpation. The nurse practitioner suspects a grade II sprain. The initial treatment plan includes which of the following?

A) Intermittent application of cold packs during the first 24 hours followed by applications of low heat at bedtime
B) Elevation of the affected limb with episodic applications of cold packs for the next 48 hours
C) Rechecking the knee in 24 hours and isometric exercises
D) The application of an Ace bandage to the affected knee and a warm shower

55. Trimethoprim-sulfamethoxazole (Bactrim) is contraindicated in which of the following conditions?

A) G6PD-deficiency anemia
B) Lead poisoning
C) Beta thalassemia minor
D) B12-deficiency anemia

56. An 18-year-old male with a history of sickle cell anemia calls the nurse practitioner on the phone complaining that he woke up with a painful penile erection 4 hours ago. The nurse practitioner would follow which of the following treatment plans?

   A) Insert a Foley catheter and measure the patient's intake and output for the next 24 hours
   B) Insert a small Foley catheter to obtain a specimen for a urinalysis and for culture and sensitivity
   C) Recommend an increase in the fluid intake up to 2 L per day and application of warm packs
   D) Recommend immediate referral to the emergency department

57. A patient is being given a physical examination for an elective surgical procedure. The patient reports taking an herbal substance. The nurse practitioner is well aware that the patient should be educated to stop taking the substance a few days before surgery. Which of the following herbs should be stopped a few days before surgery to minimize the risk of an adverse drug interaction between the herb and anesthetics?

   A) St. John's wort
   B) Echinachea
   C) Saw palmetto
   D) Mint tea

58. Folic acid supplementation is recommended for women who are planning pregnancy, in order to:

   A) Prevent renal agenesis
   B) Prevent anencephaly
   C) Prevent kidney defects
   D) Prevent heart defects

59. All of the following are possible etiologies for secondary hypertension except:

   A) Acute pyelonephritis
   B) Pheochromocytoma
   C) Renovascular stenosis
   D) Coarctation of the aorta

60. Fitz-Hugh–Curtis syndrome is associated with which of the following infections?

   A) Syphilis
   B) *Chlamydia trachomatis*
   C) Herpes genitalis
   D) Lymphogranuloma venereum

61. A nursing home resident's previous roommate is started on treatment for tuberculosis. They shared a room for 3 months. What is the minimum size of induration considered positive for this patient?

   A) 3 mm
   B) 5 mm
   C) 10 mm
   D) 15 mm

62. A patient with AIDS (acquired immunodeficiency syndrome) wants to be vaccinated. Which of the following vaccines is contraindicated for this patient?

A) Diphtheria and tetanus
B) Hepatitis A and hepatitis B
C) Varicella and nasal flu vaccine (FluMist)
D) Influenza and mumps

63. A 40-year-old woman who is undergoing treatment for infertility complains of not having a menstrual period for several weeks. The night before, she started spotting and is now having pain in her lower abdomen. Her blood pressure is 160/80, the pulse rate is 110 beats per minute, and her temperature is 99.0°F. All of the following are differential diagnoses to consider in this patient except:

A) Irritable bowel syndrome (IBS)
B) Threatened abortion
C) Ectopic pregnancy
D) Acute pelvic inflammatory disease (PID)

64. A 13-year-old adolescent who is not sexually active is brought in by her mother for an immunization update and physical examination. According to the mother, her daughter had two doses of hepatitis B vaccine 1 year ago. All of the following are indicated for this visit except:

A) Hepatitis B vaccine
B) Tetanus vaccine
C) Screen for depression
D) HIV test

65. Rh-negative pregnant women with negative rubella titers should be vaccinated at what time period in pregnancy?

A) At any time in her pregnancy
B) During the second trimester
C) During the third trimester
D) During the postpartum period

66. Medicare Part B will pay for all of the following services except:

A) Outpatient physician visits
B) Durable medical equipment
C) Outpatient laboratory tests
D) Eyeglasses and routine dental care

67. A 38-year-old woman with a history of rheumatoid arthritis and systemic lupus erythematosus (SLE) is being seen for a routine follow-up visit. The results of the complete blood count (CBC) are the following: hemoglobin of 11.0 mg/dL, hematocrit of 34%, and a mean corpuscular volume (MCV) of 85 fL. The serum ferritin level is mildly elevated, and the transferring and total iron-binding capacity (TIBC) are within normal range. Which of the following is most likely?

A) Microcytic anemia
B) Normocytic anemia
C) Macrocytic anemia
D) Hemolytic anemia

68. A 67-year-old retired clerk presents with complaints of shortness of breath and weight gain during a 2-week period. A nonproductive cough accompanies her symptoms. The lung examination is positive for fine crackles and egophony on both bases. Which of the following conditions is most likely?

A) Acute exacerbation of asthma
B) Left heart failure
C) Right heart failure
D) Chronic obstructive pulmonary disease (COPD)

69. Which of the following drugs is most likely to relieve the cause of this patient's symptoms?

A) Captopril (Capoten)
B) Trimethoprim/sulfamethoxazole (Bactrim DS)
C) Furosemide (Lasix)
D) Hydrocodone/guaifenesin syrup (Hycotuss)

70. A 20-year-old patient has recently been diagnosed with migraine headache. The nurse practitioner is educating the patient about factors that are known to trigger migraine headaches. Which of the following is incorrect advice?

A) Avoid foods with high tyramine content
B) Avoid foods with high potassium content
C) Get enough sleep
D) Avoid fermented foods

71. A 21-year-old female with a history of mitral valve prolapse (MVP) is requesting prophylaxis before her dental surgery. Which of the following would you prescribe this patient?

A) Amoxicillin 2.5 g 30 minutes before and repeat 2 hours after the procedure
B) Amoxicillin 2 g 60 minutes before the procedure
C) Amoxicillin 3 g 1 hour before and 3 hours after the procedure
D) Prophylaxis is not recommended for this patient

72. Small red spots with bluish-white centers located in the buccal mucosa by the upper molars are called:

    A) Buccal cysts
    B) Koplik's spots
    C) Lentigenes
    D) Fordyce spots

73. Stella, a 21-year-old mother, complains that she has been feeling irritable and jittery almost daily for the past few months. She complains of frequent palpitations and more frequent bowel movements along with weight loss. Her blood pressure is 160/70, her pulse is 110, and she is afebrile. All of the following conditions should be considered in the differential diagnosis except:

    A) Hashimoto's disease
    B) Graves' disease
    C) Generalized anxiety disorder
    D) Illicit drug use

74. An elderly patient with a productive cough and fever is diagnosed with pneumonia. All of the following organisms are capable of causing community-acquired pneumonia except:

    A) *Haemophilus influenzae*
    B) *Mycoplasma pneumoniae*
    C) *Treponema pallidum*
    D) *Moxarella catarrhalis*

75. The "blue dot" sign, which is not considered a true surgical emergency, is usually located on the upper pole of the testicle. It is caused by:

    A) A testicular torsion
    B) Blood underneath the scrotal skin
    C) An acute infection with either chlamydia or gonorrhea
    D) Torsion of a testicular appendage

76. A triglyceride level of 800 mg/dL is noted in the laboratory report. Which of the following conditions is a serious complication from high triglyceride levels?

    A) Acute renal failure
    B) Acute appendicitis
    C) Acute pancreatitis
    D) Familial hypertriglyceremia

77. An emergency department nurse presents to the employee health clinic 10 hours after a needle stick incident while starting an intravenous line on a patient. She tells the nurse practitioner in the clinic that she had forgotten to write up the incident because she was too busy the night before. All of the following are appropriate interventions except:

    A) Tetanus vaccine
    B) Western blot test
    C) Hepatitis B testing
    D) An ELISA test

78. An elderly woman has been on digoxin (Lanoxin) for 10 years. Her EKG is showing a new onset of atrial fibrillation. Her pulse is 60 beats per minute. She complains of gastrointestinal upset. Which of the following interventions is most appropriate?

    A) Order an electrolyte panel and a digoxin level
    B) Order a serum TSH, a digoxin level, and an electrolyte panel
    C) Order a serum digoxin level and cut her digoxin dose in half while you wait for results
    D) Discontinue the digoxin and order another 12-lead EKG

79. Which of the following maneuvers may be positive in a patient who is complaining of an acute onset of high fever, chills, severe headache, photophobia, and nausea that is accompanied by limited range of motion of the neck?

    A) Anterior drawer sign
    B) Kernig's sign
    C) Cullen's sign
    D) Lachman's sign

80. Which is a true statement regarding occurrence-based malpractice insurance policies?

    A) If the insurance company's lawyer finds the nurse practitioner negligent, it is the nurse's responsibility to pay for the claim
    B) Claims against the nurse practitioner are covered as long as she had an active malpractice policy at the time of the incident
    C) Claims against the nurse practitioner are usually paid if she is found not to be negligent
    D) Claims against the nurse practitioner are covered even if she had not paid her premiums at the time of the incident

81. The most common pathogen found in acute epididymitis in younger males is:

    A) *Escherichia coli*
    B) *Chlamydia trachomatis*
    C) *Staphylococcus aureus*
    D) Ureaplasma

82. An asthmatic patient who was seen for a viral upper respiratory infection presents to the nurse practitioner's office complaining of a recent onset of shortness of breath, inspiratory and expiratory wheezing, and chest tightness. He has been using his inhaler from four to six times a day. When the nurse practitioner quickly evaluates the patient, he notices that the patient is diaphoretic and tachypneic. Which of the following interventions is not indicated?

    A) Administer oxygen by nasal cannula at 7 L per minute
    B) Give the patient an injection of epinephrine subcutaneously immediately
    C) Quickly assess the patient's blood pressure and pulse
    D) Initiate cardiopulmonary resuscitation (CPR) immediately

83. A 35-year-old male walks into an urgent care clinic complaining of extremely painful headaches that started during the past week. The headaches occur several times a day in brief attacks of severe, lacerating-type pain. The patient has noticed that the headache pain causes ipsilateral ptosis (drooping eyelid) and lacrimation accompanied by clear rhinorrhea. The patient is pacing and appears distressed. Which of the following conditions is being described?

    A) Cluster headache
    B) Migraine headache with aura
    C) Trigeminal neuralgia
    D) Basilar migraine

84. A 21-year-old male college student has recently been informed that he has a human papilloma virus (HPV) infection on the shaft of his penis. Which of the following methods can be used to visualize subclinical HPV lesions on the penile skin?

    A) Perform a KOH (potassium hydroxide) examination
    B) Scrape off some of the affected skin and send it for a culture and sensitivity
    C) Apply acetic acid to the penile shaft and look for acetowhite changes and confirm by biopsy
    D) Order a serum herpes virus titer

85. Carol M. is a 40-year-old bank teller who has recently been diagnosed with obsessive-compulsive disorder by her therapist. Her symptoms would include:

    A) Ritualistic behaviors that the patient feels compelled to repeat
    B) Attempts to ignore or suppress the repetitive behaviors increasing her anxiety
    C) Frequent intrusive and repetitive thoughts and impulses
    D) All of the above

86. Which of the following medications is indicated for the treatment of obsessive-compulsive disorder?

    A) paroxetine (Paxil CR)
    B) haloperidol (Haldol)
    C) alprazolam (Xanax)
    D) imipramine (Elavil)

87. You would advise an 18-year-old female student who has been given a booster dose of MMR at the college health clinic that:

    A) She might have a low-grade fever during the first 24 to 48 hours
    B) She should not get pregnant within the next 4 weeks
    C) Her arm will be very sore on the injection site in 24 to 48 hours
    D) Her arm will have some induration on the injection site in 24 to 48 hours

88. Jean, a 68-year-old female, is suspected of having Alzheimer's disease. Which of the following is the best initial method for assessing the condition?

    A) CT scan of the brain
    B) Mini-Mental Exam
    C) Obtain the history from the patient, friends, and family members
    D) EEG

89. A 55-year-old woman who has type 2 diabetes is concerned about her kidneys. She has a history of three urinary tract infections within the past 8 months but is currently asymptomatic. Which of the following is the best course to follow?

    A) Recheck the patient's urine during the visit and then refer her to the nephrologist
    B) Order a monthly urinalysis test
    C) Order a nuclear scan of the kidney
    D) Refer the patient to a urologist

90. A nurse practitioner is giving dietary counseling to a 30-year-old male alcoholic who has recently been diagnosed with folic acid deficiency anemia. Which of the following foods should the nurse practitioner recommend to this patient?

    A) Tomatoes, oranges, and bananas
    B) Cheese, yogurt, and milk
    C) Lettuce, beef, and dairy products
    D) Spinach, liver, and whole wheat bread

91. The ELISA and Western blot tests are both used to test for the HIV virus. Which of the following statements is correct?

    A) They are both tests to detect viral RNA
    B) A positive ELISA screening does not mean the person has HIV infection
    C) They are both tests used to detect for antibodies against HIV
    D) They are both the best diagnostic tests for HIV

92. All of the following conditions are contraindications for metformin (Glucophage) except:

    A) Renal disease
    B) Gross obesity
    C) Alcoholism
    D) Liver disease

93. Terazosin (Hytrin) is classified under which of the following drug classes?

    A) Alpha-blockers
    B) Beta-blockers
    C) Calcium channel blockers
    D) Tricyclic blockers

94. A 67-year-old female with a 50-pack-per-year history of smoking presents for a routine annual physical examination. She complains of becoming easily short of breath and of fatigue. Physical examination reveals diminished breath sounds, hyperresonance, and hypertrophied respiratory accessory muscles. Her complete blood count (CBC) results reveal that her hematocrit level is slightly elevated. Her pulmonary function test (PFT) results show increased total lung capacity. What is the most likely diagnosis for this patient?

    A) Bronchogenic carcinoma
    B) Chronic obstructive pulmonary disease
    C) Chronic bronchitis
    D) Congestive heart failure

95. Your patient of 10 years, Mrs. Leman, is concerned about her most recent diagnosis. She was told by her dermatologist that she has an advanced case of actinic keratosis. Which of the following is the best explanation for this patient?

    A) It is a benign condition
    B) It is a precancerous lesion and needs to be followed up with her dermatologist
    C) Apply hydrocortisone cream 1% BID for 2 weeks and most of it will go away
    D) It is important for her to follow up with an oncologist

96. The Nursing Code of Ethics contains how many provisions?

    A) 7 provisions
    B) 8 provisions
    C) 9 provisions
    D) 10 provisions

97. Which of the following laboratory examinations is most commonly used to measure the size of red blood cells in a sample of blood?

    A) TIBC (total iron-binding capacity)
    B) MHC (mean hemoglobin concentration)
    C) MCV (mean corpuscular volume)
    D) Hemoglobin electrophoresis

98. A 55-year-old male patient describes an episode of chest tightness in his substernal area that radiated to his back while he was jogging. It was relieved immediately when he stopped. Which of the following conditions does this best describe?

    A) Angina pectoris
    B) Acute myocardial infarction
    C) Gastroesophageal reflux disease
    D) Acute costochondritis

99. Which of the following would you recommend to this 55-year-old patient?

    A) Start an exercise program with walking instead of jogging
    B) Consult with a cardiologist for further evaluation
    C) Consult with a gastroenterologist to rule out acute cholecystitis
    D) Take ibuprofen (Advil) 600 mg for pain every 4 to 6 hours as needed

100. An 83-year-old male with a history of hypertension complains to the nurse practitioner of some weakness in his left arm that slowly progressed to his left leg. It is accompanied by dizziness and slightly blurred vision. He has had the symptoms for the past 24 hours. Which of the following conditions is most likely?

    A) Cerebrovascular accident (CVA)
    B) Acute vertigo
    C) Multiple sclerosis (MS)
    D) Transient ischemic attack (TIA)

101. All of the following measures have been found to help lower the risk of osteoporosis except:

A) Drinking organic juice
B) Eating low-fat dairy foods
C) Performing weight-bearing exercises
D) Vitamin D supplementation

102. A 28-year-old male nurse of Hispanic descent with hypertension complains of a sore throat and nasal congestion that started 1 week ago. He tells the nurse practitioner at the employee health office that his other symptoms have resolved except for a dry cough that started a few days afterward. The patient denies allergies. His vital signs are stable and he is afebrile. Which of the following medications is best initiated at this visit?

A) Clarithromycin (Biaxin) 500 mg po BID (twice a day) for 10 days
B) Dextromethorphan and guaifenesin (Robitussin DM) 1 to 2 teaspoons every 4 hours
C) Pseudoephedrine (Sudafed) 30 mg QID (4 times a day)
D) Diphenhydramine (Benadryl) 25 mg at bedtime

103. Which of the following has orchitis as a possible complication?

A) Rubella
B) Mumps
C) Varicella
D) Hepatitis B

104. The Jarisch-Herxheimer reaction is best described as:

A) An immune-mediated reaction precipitated by the destruction of a large number of spirochetes due to an antibiotic injection
B) Severe chills and elevated blood pressures
C) Caused either by infection with *Chlamydia trachomatis* or gonorrheal infection of the liver capsule
D) Associated with certain viral illnesses

105. During breast examination of a 30-year-old nulliparous female, the nurse practitioner palpates several rubbery mobile areas of breast tissue. They are slightly tender to palpation and are present in both breasts. There are no skin changes and no nipple discharge. The patient is expecting her menstrual period in 5 days. Which of the following interventions is the best choice?

A) Referral to a gynecologist for further evaluation
B) Tell her to return 1 week after her period so her breasts can be rechecked
C) Advise the patient to return in 6 months so that you can recheck her breasts
D) Schedule the patient for a mammogram

106. Pulsus paradoxus is more likely to be seen in all of the following conditions except:

A) Status asthmaticus
B) Pleural effusion
C) Abdominal aortic aneurysm
D) Cardiac tamponade

107. Which of the following should you expect to find on a wet-mount slide of a patient diagnosed with bacterial vaginosis?

A) Tzanck cells
B) A large number of leukocytes and epithelial cells
C) A large number of squamous epithelial cells whose surfaces and edges are coated with large numbers of bacteria along with a few leukocytes
D) Epithelial cells and a small amount of blood

108. A 30-year-old female is in the office complaining of palpitations and some light headedness for the past 6 months. These are random episodes. The nurse practitioner notices a midsystolic click with a late systolic murmur that is best heard in the apical area during auscultation of the chest. You would suspect:

A) Atrial fibrillation
B) Sinus arrhythmia
C) Mitral stenosis
D) Mitral valve prolapse (MVP)

109. Your 35-year-old patient is being worked up for microscopic hematuria. The following are differential diagnosis of microscopic hematuria except:

A) Kidney stones
B) Bladder cancer
C) Acute pyelonephritis
D) Renal artery stenosis

110. During a routine physical examination of a 60-year-old Black woman, the nurse practitioner notices a triangular thickening of the bulbar conjunctiva on the temporal side of the patient's face. It is encroaching on the cornea. The patient denies pain and visual changes. Which of the following is most likely?

A) Corneal arcus
B) Pterygium
C) Pinguecula
D) Chalazion

111. Mr. J. has been on pravastatin (Pravachol) 20 mg HS (half strength) for the past 3 months. He complains of feeling very fatigued lately and denies lack of sleep. He has noticed that his urine has been a darker color for the past 2 weeks. You would:

A) Discontinue his pravastatin and order a liver-function profile
B) Continue the pravastatin but on half the dose
C) Schedule him for a complete physical examination
D) Schedule him for a liver-function profile

112. Which of the following conditions is a contraindication for pioglitazone (Actos)?

A) Severe congestive heart failure
B) Chronic infections
C) Underweight patients
D) Patients with severe depression

113. A teenage girl complains that she has never had a period. On examination, the nurse practitioner notes that she is at Tanner Stage II. What are the physical examination findings during this stage?

A) Breast buds and some straight pubic hair
B) Fully developed breasts and curly pubic hair
C) Breast tissue with the areola on a separate mound with curly pubic hair
D) No breast tissue and no pubic hair

114. The Phalen test is used to evaluate for:

A) Inflammation of the median nerve
B) Rheumatoid arthritis
C) Degenerative joint changes
D) Chronic tenosynovitis

115. Which of the following treatment regimens is recommended to treat a *Helicobacter pylori* infection?

A) Metronidazole (Flagyl) BID, doxycycline BID, and omeprazole (Prilosec) daily
B) Bismuth subsalicylate (Pepto-Bismol) tablets QID, metronidazole (Flagyl) QID, azithromycin (Zithromax), and cimetidine (Tagamet) daily
C) Amoxicillin BID, sulfamethoxazole trimethoprim (Bactrim DS) BID, and ranitidine (Zantac) daily
D) Clarithromycin (Biaxin) BID, amoxicillin BID, and omeprazole (Prilosec) QD daily

116. All of the following are known to cause chronic cough except:

A) Chronic bronchitis
B) Allergic rhinitis
C) Acute viral upper respiratory infection (URI)
D) Gastroesophageal reflux disease (GERD)

117. The following are true statements about aspirin and its action on platelets except:

A) Its effects on platelets are irreversible
B) Its effects on platelets may last up to 3 weeks
C) It is used for prophylaxis against strokes and acute myocardial infarctions
D) Its effects only last 2 weeks and are reversible

118. All of the following agents are used to control the inflammatory changes seen in the lungs of asthmatics except:

A) Albuterol inhaler (Proventil)
B) Triamcinolone (Azmacort)
C) Montelukast (Singulair)
D) Cromolyn sodium inhaler (Intal)

119. All of the following antibiotics are contraindicated for children younger than 18 years of age except:

    A) Minocycline (Minocin)
    B) Ciprofloxacin (Cipro)
    C) Ceftriaxone (Rocephin)
    D) Levofloxacin (Levaquin)

120. All of the following are useful in treating allergic rhinitis except:

    A) Allergy injections
    B) Oral antihistamines
    C) Systemic steroids
    D) Oral decongestants

121. Erysipelas is caused by which of the following organisms?

    A) *Escherichia*
    B) *Haemophilus influenzae*
    C) Group A beta-hemolytic *Streptococcus*
    D) *Staphylococcus aureus*

122. A 62-year-old female with a 10-year history of severe low back pain reports to the nurse practitioner a new onset of difficulty controlling her urine that is associated with numbness on her perineal area. She denies trauma. You would suspect which of the following?

    A) Fracture of the lower spine
    B) A herniated disc
    C) Cauda equina syndrome
    D) Ankylosing spondylitis

123. A 38-year-old White female with a BMI of 32 complains of colicky pain in the right upper quadrant of her abdomen that gets worse if she eats fried food. During physical examination, the nurse practitioner presses deeply on the left lower quadrant of the abdomen. After the NP releases her hand, the patient complains of pain on the right side of the lower abdomen. What is the name of this examination?

    A) Rebound tenderness
    B) Rovsing's sign
    C) Murphy's sign
    D) Psoas test

124. Which of the following viral infections is associated with possible abnormal lymphocytes that resolve a few weeks after the acute infection?

    A) CMV (cytomegalovirus)
    B) EBV (Epstein-Barr virus)
    C) HPV (human papilloma virus)
    D) Coxsackie virus

125. The following is a screening test for scoliosis:

A) Straight leg raising test
B) Adam's forward bend test
C) Growth hormone titers
D) Serum alkaline phosphatase

126. Jenny, who is a type 1 diabetic, complains of a 1-week episode of dysuria, frequency, and a strong odor to her urine. She denies fever and .chills. This is her second episode during the year. What is the best treatment option for this patient during this visit?

A) Treat the patient with a 7-day course of antibiotics and order a urine test for culture and sensitivity (C&S) before and after treatment
B) Order a urine C&S and hold treatment until you get the results of the test from the laboratory
C) Treat the patient with antibiotics and encourage her to drink more fluids, especially cranberry juice
D) Treat the patient with a 3-day course of antibiotics and order a urine test for C&S after treatment to document the complete resolution of the infection

127. All of the following are infections affecting the labia and vagina except:

A) Bacterial vaginosis
B) Candidiasis
C) Trichomoniasis
D) *Chlamydia trachomatis*

128. During eye examination of a 50-year-old hypertensive patient complaining of a severe headache, the nurse practitioner finds that the borders of the disc margins of both eyes are slightly blurred. The veins are larger than the arteries and there is no arteriovenous (AV) nicking. What is the significance of this clinical finding?

A) They are all normal findings
B) The patient has hypertensive retinopathy
C) The intracranial pressure (ICP) of the brain is increased
D) The patient has acute closed-angle glaucoma

129. A 30-year-old overweight high school teacher complains of a dry cough that has been present for 3 months. The cough worsens when he is supine. He complains of a few episodes of a sour taste in the back of his throat. The patient's cough may be caused by:

A) Asthma
B) Gastroesophageal reflux disease (GERD)
C) Pneumonia
D) Chronic postnasal drip

130. The red reflex is elicited by shining a light on the eyes at an angle with the light about 15 inches away. The nurse practitioner is screening for:

    A) Cataracts
    B) Strabismus
    C) Blindness
    D) The blinking response

131. A 44-year-old patient with Down syndrome develops impaired memory and difficulty with his usual daily life routines. He is having problems functioning at his job, which he has been doing for 10 years. The physical examination and routine labs are all negative. The vital signs are normal. His appetite is normal. The most likely diagnosis is:

    A) Tic douloureux
    B) A stroke
    C) Alzheimer's disease
    D) Delirium

132. Which of the following findings is associated with the chronic use of chewing tobacco?

    A) Cheilosis
    B) Glossitis
    C) A geographic tongue
    D) Leukoplakia of the tongue

133. Which of the following is a recommended treatment for erythema migrans (or early Lyme's disease)?

    A) Doxycycline (Vibramycin) 100 mg PO BID × 21 days
    B) Ciprofloxacin (Cipro) 250 mg PO BID × 14 days
    C) Erythromycin (E-Mycin) 333 mg PO TID × 10 days
    D) Dicloxacillin 500 mg PO BID × 10 days

134. Nurse practitioners and clinical nurse specialists derive their legal right to practice from:

    A) The Nurse Practice Act of the state where they practice
    B) The laws of the state where they practice
    C) The Medicare bill
    D) The Board of Nursing from the state where they practice

135. You are checking a 67-year-old female's breast during an annual gynecological examination. The left nipple and surrounding areolar skin are scaly and reddened. The patient denies pain and pruritis. She has noticed this scaliness on her left nipple for many months. Her dermatologist gave her a topical steroid that she used on the rash twice a day for 1 month. The patient never went back for the follow-up. She still has the rash and wants an evaluation. The nurse practitioner suspects Paget's disease of the breast. Which of the following is the best treatment plan for this patient?

    A) Prescribe another potent topical steroid and tell the patient to use it twice a day for 4 weeks
    B) Order a mammogram and refer the patient to a breast surgeon

C) Advise her to stop using soap on both breasts when she bathes to avoid drying up the skin on her areola and nipples

D) Order a sonogram of the breast and fine needle biopsy of the breast

136. The following are considered at higher risk for tuberculosis except:

A) A teenager recently diagnosed with leukemia

B) A nurse who works in a community clinic in the inner city

C) A 60-year-old male working in a homeless shelter

D) A 22-year-old female recently diagnosed with asthma

137. During a sports physical examination of a 20-year-old athlete, the nurse practitioner notices a split of the S2 component of the heart sound during deep inspiration. She notes that it disappears on expiration. The heart rate is regular and no murmurs are auscultated. Which of the following is correct?

A) This is an abnormal finding and should be evaluated further by a cardiologist

B) A stress test should be ordered

C) This is a normal finding in some young athletes

D) An echocardiogram should be ordered

138. Mrs. J.L. is a 55-year-old female with a BMI of 30 and a history of asthma. She has hypertension that has been under control with hydrochlorothiazide 12.5 mg PO daily. Her total cholesterol is 230 g/dL. How many risk factors for coronary heart disease (CAD) does she have?

A) 1 risk factor

B) 2 risk factors

C) 3 risk factors

D) 4 risk factors

139. A common side effect of metformin (Glucophage) therapy is:

A) Weight gain

B) Lactic acidosis

C) Hypoglycemic episodes

D) Gastrointestinal upset

140. While doing a cardiac examination on a 75-year-old male, the nurse practitioner notices an irregularly irregular rhythm with a pulse rate of 110 beats per minute. The patient is alert and is not in distress. Which of the following is most likely?

A) Atrial fibrillation

B) Ventricular fibrillation

C) Cardiac arrhythmia

D) First-degree right bundle branch block

141. The following are patients who are at high risk for complications due to urinary tract infections. Who of the following does not belong in this category?

A) A 38-year-old diabetic patient with a HgbA1c of 6.0%
B) A woman with a history of rheumatoid arthritis who is currently being treated with a regimen of methotrexate and low-dose steroids
C) A 21-year-old woman who is under treatment for a sexually transmitted infection
D) Pregnant women

142. A 68-year-old woman with hypertension and diabetes is seen by the nurse practitioner for a dry cough that worsens at night when she lies in bed. She has shortness of breath that worsens when she exerts herself. The patient's pulse rate is 90/min and regular. The patient has gained 6 pounds during the past 2 months. She is on a nitroglycerine patch and furosemide daily. The best explanation for her symptoms is:

A) Kidney failure
B) Congestive heart failure
C) ACE-inhibitor-induced coughing
D) Thyroid disease

143. A nurse practitioner is doing a funduscopic examination on a 35-year-old female during a routine physical examination. He notices that she has sharp disc margins and a yellowish-orange color to her optic disc. The ratio of veins to arteries is 3:2. What is the next most appropriate action?

A) Advise the patient that she had a normal examination
B) Advise the patient that she had an abnormal examination
C) Refer the patient to the emergency department
D) Refer the patient to an ophthalmologist

144. During a sports physical, the nurse practitioner records a vision of 20/30. Which of the following statements is true?

A) The patient can see at 20 feet what a person with normal vision can see at 30 feet
B) The patient can see at 30 feet what a person with normal vision can see at 20 feet
C) The patient cannot engage in contact sports
D) The patient needs to be referred to an ophthalmologist

145. Carol, a 30-year-old type 1 diabetic, is on regular and NPH (neutral protein Hagedorn) insulin in the morning and evening. She recently started attending aerobic classes in the afternoon. Because of her workouts, her blood sugars have dipped below 50 mg/dL very early in the morning. The hypoglycemia is stimulating her liver into secreting glucagon. As a result, the patient's fasting blood sugar levels in the morning have been elevated above normal. Which of the following is being described correctly?

A) Somogyi phenomenon
B) Dawn phenomenon
C) Raynaud's phenomenon
D) Insulin resistance

146. A 40-year-old female is positive for anti-HCV. Which test is appropriate for follow-up?

A) HCV RNA
B) HCV antibodies
C) HCV core antigen
D) Hepatitis C surface antigen

147. To evaluate a 55-year-old male patient who is a smoker and has peripheral vascular disease (PVD), the nurse practitioner would initially start with the following intervention:

A) Order a venogram
B) Order TED hose
C) Check the apical pulse
D) Check the pedal and posterior tibial pulses

148. All of the following drugs can interact with theophylline (Theo-24) except:

A) Erythromycin
B) Montelukast (Singulair)
C) Phenytoin sodium (Dilantin)
D) Cimetidine (Tagamet)

149. You note a high-pitched and blowing pansystolic murmur on a 50-year-old male. It is grade II/VI and is best heard at the apical area. Which of the following is most likely?

A) Ventricular septal defect (VSD)
B) Tricuspid regurgitation
C) Mitral regurgitation
D) Mitral stenosis

150. Which of the following drugs is the preferred treatment for a skin infection with the organism called *Bacillus anthracis* (anthrax)?

A) Amoxicillin/clavulanic acid (Augmentin)
B) Ciprofloxacin (Cipro)
C) Ceftriaxone (Rocephin) injections
D) Erythromycin

151. An 18-year-old female with a history of hypothyroidism presents to an urgent care clinic complaining of numbness and tingling in the fingertips on both her hands for several hours. On examination, both radial pulses are at +2 and equal bilaterally. The patient reports a history during the past several months of identical episodes that last several hours. The skin color changes range from blue to white, and then a dark red. Eventually, the skin returns to normal and the tingling and numbness disappear. Which of the following conditions is best described?

A) Hashimoto's disease
B) Raynaud's disease
C) Peripheral neuropathy
D) Vitamin B12 deficiency anemia

152. Which of the following clinical findings is associated with a measles (rubeola) infection?

    A) Multiple crops of papules that evolve into vesicles and pustules
    B) Small red spots with bluish centers located by the posterior molaris
    C) Fever
    D) Myalgia

153. You are reviewing a Pap smear report on a 25-year-old female. Which of the following cells should be on a Pap smear to be classified as a satisfactory specimen?

    A) Clue cells and endometrial cells
    B) Vaginal cells and cervical cells
    C) Squamous epithelial cells and endocervical cells
    D) Leukocytes and red blood cells

154. Which of the following T-scores derived during the dual-energy x-ray absorptiometry (DEXA) test of an 80-year-old woman's bones is indicative of osteoporosis?

    A) T score of less than –2.50
    B) T score of less than –2.00
    C) T score of above –1.00
    D) T score of above 1.50

155. A 56-year-old man complains of several episodes of severe lacerating pain that shoots up to his right cheek and is precipitated by drinking cold drinks or chewing. These episodes start suddenly and end spontaneously after a few seconds with several episodes per day. He denies any trauma, facial weakness, or difficulty swallowing. He has stopped drinking cold drinks because of the pain. Which of the following is most likely?

    A) Trigeminal neuralgia
    B) Cluster headache
    C) Acute sinusitis
    D) Sinus headache

156. The KOH (potassium hydroxide) prep is helping with the diagnosis of all of the following conditions except:

    A) Tinea infections
    B) *Candida albicans* infections on the skin
    C) Bacterial vaginosis
    D) Atypical bacterial infections

157. Which of the following is classified as an atypical antidepressant?

    A) Amitriptyline (Elavil)
    B) Lorazepam (Ativan)
    C) Sertraline (Zoloft)
    D) Bupropion hydrochloride (Wellbutrin)

158. All of the following pulmonary tests require the patient's voice to perform correctly except:

A) Egophony
B) Tactile fremitus
C) Whispered pectoriloquy
D) Auscultation

159. Which of the following interventions is not indicated for an acute case of deep vein thrombosis (DVT) in a 35-year-old female who was on oral contraceptive pills?

A) Special support stockings
B) Have the woman continue oral contraceptives
C) Elevation of the affected limb
D) Anticoagulation therapy

160. All of the following infections are reportable diseases except:

A) Lyme disease
B) Gonorrhea
C) Nongonococcal urethritis
D) Syphilis

161. A menopausal woman with osteopenia is attending a dietary education class. Which of the following foods are recommended?

A) Yogurt and sardines
B) Spinach and red meat
C) Cheese and red meat
D) Low-fat cheese and whole grain

162. All of the following dietary factors should be avoided by patients on oral anticoagulation therapy with warfarin sodium (Coumadin) because:

A) Green leafy vegetables have high levels of vitamin K that can bind with the blood-clotting cascade and increase bleeding time
B) Yellow and green-colored vegetables have high amounts of beta carotene that can inactivate the active metabolite of the drug
C) Food with high potassium content increases risk for cardiac arrhythmias
D) Currently, no food restrictions are indicated because research has shown that food has minimal effect on the bleeding time

163. You are following up a 65-year-old male who has been on a new prescription of fluvastatin (Lescol) for 6 weeks. During a follow-up visit, he reports feeling extremely fatigued and having dark-colored urine. He denies any generalized muscle soreness. Which of the following is the most appropriate treatment plan?

A) Order a CBC with differential
B) Order a liver function profile
C) Recommend an increase in fluid intake and rest
D) Order a urine culture and sensitivity test

164. What would you advise him regarding his fluvastatin (Lescol) prescription?

    A) Continue taking the medicine until the laboratory results are available
    B) Take half the usual daily dose until the laboratory results are available
    C) Take the medicine every other day instead of daily until the laboratory results are available
    D) Stop taking the medicine until the laboratory results are available

165. A 56-year-old male presents to the nurse practitioner complaining of a history of back pain for the past 4 months. On examination, the range of motion of the patient's spine is mildly limited while bending forward. The other joints in the patient's body are normal. Only the spine seems to be affected. The patient reports that a laboratory test from a previous doctor showed increased ESR (sedimentation rate), a negative antinuclear antigen (ANA), and a negative rheumatoid factor. Which of the following is best described?

    A) Rheumatoid arthritis
    B) Lupus erythematosus
    C) Degenerative joint disease of the spine
    D) Ankylosing spondylitis

166. A postmenopausal woman who has been on low-dose estrogen and progesterone replacement hormone therapy for her severe vasomotor symptoms complains to the nurse practitioner that she has had a few episodes of small amounts of vaginal bleeding that seem to occur at random over the past 4 months. She denies uterine cramping and dyspareunia. Which of the following is the best treatment plan for this patient?

    A) Recommend a D&C (dilatation and curettage) procedure, which is very helpful in cases of postmenopausal bleeding
    B) Schedule the patient for a uterine ultrasound and uterine biopsy
    C) Prescribe a 13-day course of progesterone pills to induce uterine shedding of the thickened endometrial lining at the end of the month
    D) Refer the patient to a gynecologist for further evaluation

167. Which of the following drug classes is useful in the management of chronic obstructive pulmonary disease (COPD) symptoms?

    A) Anticholinergics
    B) Antibiotics
    C) Systemic corticosteroids
    D) Antimalarial drugs

168. All of the following statements are correct regarding the Td vaccine except:

    A) Fever occurs in up to 80% of the patients
    B) A possible side effect is induration on the injection site
    C) The Td is given every 10 years
    D) The DPT and DT should not be given beyond the seventh birthday

169. Which of the following is recommended by the Joint National Committee on Prevention, Detection, Evaluation, and Treatment of High Blood Pressure (JNC 7) as first-line treatment for hypertension for patients with microalbuminuria?

    A) Angiotensin-converting enzyme (ACE) inhibitors
    B) Diuretics
    C) Calcium channel blockers
    D) Beta-blockers

170. A 20-year-old woman who is sexually active complains of copious milk-like vaginal discharge. On microscopy, the slide reveals a large number of mature squamous epithelial cells. The vaginal pH is 5.0. There are very few leukocytes and no red blood cells seen on the wet smear. Which of the following is most likely?

    A) Atrophic vaginitis
    B) Bacterial vaginosis
    C) Trichomoniasis
    D) This is a normal finding

171. A test called the visual fields by confrontation is used to evaluate for:

    A) Peripheral vision
    B) Central vision
    C) Visual acuity
    D) Accommodation

172. The following skin findings are considered macules except:

    A) Freckles
    B) Petechiae
    C) Acne
    D) A flat 0.5-cm brown-colored birthmark

173. Clara is a 20-year-old college student who reports to the student health clinic with a laceration of her left hand. She tells the nurse practitioner that she cut her hand while working in her garden. Her last tetanus booster was 5½ years ago. Which of the following is the best treatment plan?

    A) Administer a booster dose of the Td vaccine
    B) Administer the Td vaccine and the tetanus immune globulin (HyperTet)
    C) Administer tetanus immune globulin (HyperTet) only
    D) She does not need any tetanus immune globulin (HyperTet) or a Td booster

174. The apex of the heart is located at:

    A) Second ICS to the right of the sternal border
    B) Second ICS to the left of the sternal border
    C) The left lower sternal border
    D) The left side of the sternum at the fifth ICS by the midclavicular line

175. A middle-age female with blonde hair and blue eyes complains of small acne-like papules on the sides of her mouth and on her chin that do not seem to respond to topical acne medicine. It is not pruritic. She complains of flushing easily, especially when she drinks beer and wine. Her mother has a history of the same lesions. Which of the following is most likely?

A) Adult-onset acne
B) Rosacea
C) Atopic dermatitis
D) Perioral folliculitis

176. Koilonychia is associated with which of the following conditions?

A) Lead poisoning
B) Beta thalassemia trait
C) B12-deficiency anemia
D) Iron-deficiency anemia

177. What type of cancer causes the highest mortality among White, Black, Asian/Pacific Islander, and American Indian/Alaska Native women?

A) Breast cancer
B) Lung cancer
C) Colon cancer
D) Uterine cancer

178. All of the following are correct statements regarding the S3 component of the heart sound except:

A) It occurs very early in diastole and is sometimes called an opening snap
B) It is a normal finding in some children, healthy young adults, and athletes
C) It can be a normal variant if heard in a person aged 40 or older
D) It signifies congestive heart failure

179. A positive straight leg-raising test is indicative of which of the following conditions?

A) Myasthenia gravis
B) Inflammation of the sciatic nerve/herniated disc
C) Multiple sclerosis
D) Parkinson's disease

180. Which of the following would you recommend on an annual basis for an elderly patient with type 2 diabetes?

A) An eye examination with an ophthalmologist
B) Follow-up visit with a urologist
C) Periodic visits to an optometrist
D) Colonoscopy

181. A 72-year-old White female complains of a crusty and nonhealing small ulcer on her upper lip that she has had for several months. She also has light red-colored lesions with a roughened texture on both her upper cheeks. Which of the following would be the most appropriate intervention for this patient?

A) Triamcinolone acetonide (Kenalog) cream BID for 2 weeks
B) Triple antibiotic ointment BID × 2 weeks
C) Hydrocortisone 1% cream BID for 2 weeks
D) She needs to be evaluated by a dermatologist

182. Which of the following drugs is considered a "rescue" drug for asthmatics?

A) Formoterol (Foradil) inhalers
B) Albuterol (Ventolin) inhalers
C) Montelukast (Singulair) tablets
D) Triamcinolone (AeroBid) inhalers

183. Bouchard's nodule is found in which of the following?

A) Rheumatoid arthritis
B) Degenerative joint disease
C) Psoriatic arthritis
D) Septic arthritis

184. The red blood cell (RBC) peripheral smear in pernicious anemia will show:

A) Microcytic and hypochromic cells
B) Microcytic and normochromic cells
C) Macrocytic and normochromic cells
D) Macrocytic and hypochromic cells

185. You notice a medium-pitched harsh systolic murmur during an episodic examination of a 37-year-old woman. It is best heard at the right upper border of the sternum. Which of the following is most likely?

A) Mitral stenosis
B) Aortic stenosis
C) Pulmonic stenosis
D) Tricuspid regurgitation

186. A small abscess on a hair follicle of the eyelid is called:

A) Hordeolum
B) Pterygium
C) Pinguecula
D) Ptosis

187. Which of the following is indicated for the prophylactic treatment of migraine headache?

A) Ibuprofen (Motrin)
B) Naproxen sodium (Anaprox)
C) Propranolol (Inderal)
D) Sumatriptan (Imitrex)

188. A 40-year-old male complains to the nurse practitioner of severe episodic lanci-nating pains behind his left eye for the past 2 weeks. The pain does not seem to affect his vision. It is always accompanied by some nasal congestion and rhinitis. He complains that it is so painful that sometimes he feels like he wants to die. The patient's temperature is 98.8°F, the pulse is 92 beats per minute, and the respiratory rate is 14 per minute. Neurological examination is within normal limits. Which of the following conditions is most likely?

A) Migraine headache with aura
B) Cluster headache
C) Tic douloureux
D) Cranial neuralgia

189. Which of the following drugs is most likely to cause abdominal side effects?

A) Sucralfate (Carafate)
B) Acetaminophen (Tylenol)
C) Clarithromycin (Biaxin)
D) Penicillin

190. All of the following statements are true regarding domestic abuse except:

A) There is no delay in seeking medical treatment
B) The pattern of injuries is inconsistent with the history reported
C) Injuries are usually in the "central" area of the body instead of the extremities
D) Pregnant women have a higher risk of domestic abuse

191. Which of the following patients is least likely to become an alcohol abuser?

A) A 50-year-old construction worker who drinks 1 beer nightly while watching sports programs on television
B) A 30-year-old nurse who complains to her coworker that her mother's com-ments about her recreational drinking are starting to annoy her and her spouse
C) A 19-year-old college student who binges on alcoholic drinks but only on the weekends
D) A 70-year-old male who feels better after drinking rum in the morning

192. Alpha thalassemia minor (Cooley's anemia) and sickle cell anemia testing are eval-uated by using what diagnostic test?

A) Ferritin
B) Hemoglobin electrophoresis
C) Total iron-binding capacity (TIBC)
D) Folate level

193. Potential complications of mitral valve prolapse (MVP) include all of the following except:

A) Severe mitral regurgitation
B) Endocarditis
C) Increased risk of stroke and TIA
D) Mitral stenosis

194. A new patient is complaining of severe pruritis that is worse at night. Several family members also have the same symptoms. On examination, areas of excoriated papules are noted on some of the interdigital webs of both hands and on the axillae. This finding is most consistent with:

A) Contact dermatitis
B) Impetigo
C) Larva migrans
D) Scabies

195. An elderly woman with a history of rheumatoid arthritis reports to the nurse practitioner that she has been taking ibuprofen BID for many years. Which of the following organ systems has the highest risk of damage from chronic nonsteroidal anti-inflammatory drug (NSAID) use?

A) Cardiovascular system
B) Neurological system
C) Gastrointestinal system
D) Renal system

196. Ted, who is 15 years old, has just moved into the community and is staying in a foster home temporarily. There is no record of his immunizations. His foster mother wants him to be checked before he enters the local high school. Which of the following does this patient need?

A) Meningococcal
B) Measles–Mumps–Rubella (MMR)
C) Tdap
D) All of the above

197. Which cranial nerve is being evaluated when a patient is instructed to shrug his shoulders?

A) CN IX
B) CN X
C) CN XI
D) CN XII

198. A laboratory technician has a 10.5-millimeter area of redness and induration in his left forearm after getting a Mantoux test 48 hours before from the employee health nurse. The Mantoux test done by the same nurse 12 months ago was at 5 millimeters of induration. The technician denies cough, night sweats, and weight loss. Which of the following is a true statement?

A) The patient is at higher risk for active tuberculosis disease within the next 2 years
B) A chest radiograph and sputum culture are indicated.
C) A sputum for culture and sensitivity and referral to an infectious disease specialist are indicated
D) The laboratory technician should not be allowed to draw blood from immunosuppressed patients

199. Learning how to drive with a therapist after a stroke is considered:

   A) Primary prevention
   B) Secondary prevention
   C) Tertiary prevention
   D) Health prevention

200. Which of the following individuals is at higher risk for osteoporosis?

   A) 70-year-old female of African ancestry who walks daily for exercise
   B) 42-year-old obese woman taking prednisone 10 mg daily for severe asthma for 2 years
   C) 55-year-old White female who is an aerobics instructor
   D) 45-year-old Asian female who has been on high-dose steroids for 1 week

201. Patients with celiac sprue should avoid which of the following in their diets?

   A) Organ meats
   B) Lactose
   C) Phenylalanine
   D) Gluten

202. Which of the following eye findings are seen in patients with diabetic neuropathy?

   A) AV nicking
   B) Copper wire arterioles
   C) Flame hemorrhages
   D) Microaneurysms

203. The following conditions are absolute contraindications for the use of oral contraceptives except:

   A) A benign hepatoma
   B) History of emboli that resolved with heparin therapy 15 years ago
   C) A family history of migraines with aura
   D) A history of gallbladder disease during pregnancy

204. The most common cause of cancer mortality in this country is:

   A) Lung cancer
   B) Prostate cancer
   C) Colon cancer
   D) Skin cancer

205. Which of the following findings are seen in a patient with folate-deficiency anemia?

   A) Microcytic and hypochromic red blood cells
   B) Microcytic and normochromic red blood cells
   C) Normal size and color of the red blood cells
   D) Macrocytic and normocytic red blood cells

206. When confirming a case of temporal arteritis, the sedimentation rate (ESR) is expected to be:

A) Normal
B) Lower than normal
C) Elevated
D) Indeterminate result

207. Mrs. Green, age 45, is complaining of generalized morning stiffness, especially in both her wrists and hands. It is much worse in the morning after she wakes up and lasts for a few hours. She also complains of fatigue and generalized body aches that have been present for the past few months. Which of the following is most likely?

A) Osteoporosis
B) Rheumatoid arthritis
C) Osteoarthritis
D) Gout

208. All of the following may cause delirium in susceptible individuals except:

A) Severe infection
B) Metabolic derangement
C) Intoxication with certain substances
D) Creutzfeldt-Jakob disease

209. Which of the following drugs is effective therapy in a middle-aged African American male who is having an acute exacerbation of gout on his right great toe?

A) Acetaminophen (Tylenol)
B) Systemic steroids
C) Indomethacin (Indocin)
D) Allopurinol (Zyloprim)

210. The complications of untreated gout include:

A) Loss of joint mobility and renal failure
B) Loss of joint mobility and liver failure
C) An increased risk of urinary tract infections
D) Bladder cancer

211. According to Healthy People 2002, all of the following are considered leading health indicators except:

A) Weight and obesity
B) Immunizations
C) Access to health care
D) International health-promotion programs

212. You note bony nodules located at the proximal interphalangeal joints on both hands of your 65-year-old female patient. Which of the following is most likely?

A) Bouchard's node
B) Heberden's node
C) Osteoarthritic nodules
D) Deposits of uric acid crystals

213. Which chronic illness disproportionately affects the Hispanic population?

    A) Diabetes mellitus
    B) Hypertension
    C) Alcohol abuse
    D) Skin cancer

214. A lipid profile done on a newly diagnosed hypertensive patient shows a triglyceride level of 950 mg/dL, total cholesterol 240 mg/dL, LDL (low-density lipoprotein) 145 mg/dL, and HDL (high-density lipoprotein) of 35 mg/dL. What is the next best intervention for this patient?

    A) Educate the patient about lifestyle changes that will help lower the cholesterol levels.
    B) Initiate a prescription of pravastatin (Pravachol) as soon as possible.
    C) Recommend that the patient avoid eating fatty or fried foods.
    D) Initiate a prescription of nicotinic acid (niacin, Niaspan).

215. The McMurray test is useful for evaluating the stability of an injured knee. Which of the following is being evaluated?

    A) Anterior cruciate ligament of the knee
    B) Posterior cruciate ligament of the knee
    C) The patellar tendon
    D) The meniscus of the knee

216. The "gold standard" for the diagnosis of active *Helicobacter pylori* infection of the stomach or duodenum is:

    A) An *H. pylori* titer
    B) An endoscopy with tissue biopsy
    C) An upper GI (gastrointestinal) series
    D) A urea breath test

217. On which of the following dates did the American Nurses Association (ANA) House of Delegates and the board vote to accept all of the major provisions of the revised *Code of Ethics*?

    A) April 1999
    B) May 2000
    C) June 2001
    D) July 2002

218. A Hispanic middle-aged woman with a BMI (body mass index) of 29 complains of chronic tiredness and feeling thirsty despite drinking up to 10 glasses of water a day. The nurse practitioner wants to rule out type 2 diabetes mellitus. All of the following tests are acceptable methods for diagnosing diabetes, according to the American Diabetes Association (ADA), except:

    A) HgbA1c
    B) Fasting blood glucose
    C) Postprandial serum blood glucose
    D) All of the above

219. A bulla is defined as:

A) A solid nodule less than 1 cm in size
B) A superficial vesicle filled with serous fluid greater than 1 cm in size
C) A maculopapular lesion
D) A shallow ulcer

220. A 30-year-old nurse from the emergency department is shown to have a positive result in the Mantoux test. According to the nurse, she has always had negative results. Which of the following is not true?

A) The highest risk of having tuberculosis disease is within the next 2 years after seroconversion
B) Isoniazid (INH) prophylaxis is not recommended for persons aged 30 years or older because of higher risk of hepatic injury
C) A chest x-ray is recommended
D) The nurse should be asked about the signs and symptoms of active tuberculosis disease

221. Which of the following is the confirmatory test for HIV (human immunodeficiency virus)?

A) ELISA test for HIV
B) Western blot
C) HIV polymerase chain reaction (PCR) test
D) HIV antibody

222. All of the following clinical findings are associated with syphilis except:

A) Condyloma lata
B) Condyloma acuminata
C) Painless chancre
D) Rashes on the palms of the hands and the soles of the feet

223. All of the following are mechanical barrier methods of contraception except:

A) Diaphragm with spermicidal gel
B) The sponge
C) Condoms
D) Depo-Provera injections

224. Women with a history of pelvic inflammatory disease (PID) have an increased risk for all of the following complication(s) except:

A) Ectopic pregnancy
B) Scarring of the fallopian tube(s)
C) Infertility
D) Ovarian cysts

225. The differential diagnosis for genital ulceration includes all of the following except:

    A) Syphilis
    B) Genital herpes
    C) Chancroid
    D) Molluscum contagiosum

226. Lead poisoning can cause which type of anemia?

    A) Macrocytic anemia
    B) Normocytic anemia
    C) Microcytic anemia
    D) Hemolytic anemia

227. Hypovolemic shock would most likely occur with fractures of the:

    A) Spine
    B) Pelvis
    C) Femur
    D) Humerus

228. Podagra is associated with which of the following?

    A) Rheumatoid arthritis
    B) Gout
    C) Osteoarthritis
    D) Septic arthritis

229. While assessing for a cardiac murmur, the first time that a thrill can be palpated is at:

    A) Grade II
    B) Grade III
    C) Grade IV
    D) Grade V

230. A medium-pitched harsh midsystolic murmur is best heard at the right second intercostal space (ICS) of the chest. It radiates into the neck. Which of the following is best described?

    A) Aortic stenosis
    B) Pulmonic stenosis
    C) Aortic regurgitation
    D) Mitral stenosis

231. Which type of hepatitis virus infection is more likely to result in cirrhosis of the liver and an increased risk of developing hepatocellular carcinoma?

    A) Hepatitis A virus
    B) Hepatitis B virus
    C) Hepatitis C virus
    D) Both hepatitis B and hepatitis C

232. Which of the following cranial nerves is involved in Bell's palsy?

   A) CN IX and X
   B) CN VIII
   C) CN VII
   D) CN V

233. A 19-year-old male has recently been diagnosed with acute hepatitis B. He is sexually active and is monogamous and reports using condoms inconsistently. Which of the following is recommended for his male sexual partner, who was also tested for hepatitis with the following results: HBsAg (–), anti-HBs (–), anti-HCV (–), anti-HAV (+)?

   A) Hepatitis B vaccination
   B) Hepatitis B immune globulin
   C) Hepatitis B vaccination and hepatitis B immune globulin
   D) No vaccination is needed at this time

234. All of the following conditions are associated with an increased risk for normocytic anemia except:

   A) Rheumatoid arthritis
   B) Discoid lupus
   C) Chronic autoimmune disorders
   D) Pregnancy

235. You can determine a pulse deficit by counting the:

   A) Apical and radial pulses at the same time, then subtracting the difference between the two
   B) Apical pulse first, then the radial pulse, and subtracting the difference between the two
   C) Apical pulse and the femoral pulse at the same time and subtracting the difference between the two
   D) Radial pulse first, then counting the femoral pulse, and subtracting the difference between the two

236. Which of the following is recommended treatment for a woman with a bacterial vaginosis?

   A) Azithromycin (Zithromax)
   B) Doxycycline (Dynapen)
   C) Ceftriaxone (Rocephin)
   D) Metronidazole (Flagyl)

237. Patients who are being screened for tuberculosis (TB) and are immunocompromised should be evaluated for anergy. Which of the following is the best description of anergy testing?

   A) Apply Candida or mumps antigen to the right forearm and the PPD (purified protein derivative) on the left forearm and read results in 48 to 72 hours
   B) Apply Candida or mumps antigen and PPD on left forearm only and check for a reaction in 24 hours

C) Mix the Candida or mumps antigen with the PPD and apply it to both forearms

D) Apply the Candida or mumps antigen 24 hours before the PPD on the left forearm

238. A nurse practitioner is evaluating an 85-year-old male from a nursing home. He instructs the patient to remember the words *orange*, *street*, and *tiger*. The patient is instructed to recite back these words to the nurse practitioner in 10 minutes. Which of the tests is being described?

A) Becker Inventory
B) Mini-Mental Status Exam
C) Minnesota Multiphasic Personality Inventory (MMPI)
D) The CAGE test

239. Patients younger than the age of 18 years may give consent to a health care provider without the prior knowledge of a parent or legal guardian in all of the following cases except:

A) Treatment of chlamydia cervicitis
B) Treatment for mild acne
C) Pregnancy testing
D) Sexually transmitted disease (STD) testing

240. A hypertensive middle-aged man who is Native American has recently been diagnosed with mild renal insufficiency. He has been on lisinopril (Accupril) for many years. Which of the following laboratory values should be carefully monitored?

A) Hemoglobin, hematocrit, and MCV (mean corpuscular volume)
B) Serum creatinine and potassium level
C) AST and ALT
D) Serum sodium, potassium, and magnesium

241. All of the following are correct statements regarding the role of the person named in a durable power of attorney except:

A) Their decisions are considered legally binding
B) They can take control in other areas of the patient's life, such as financial issues
C) They can decide for the patient who is on life support when it can be terminated
D) The patient's spouse has a right to override the attorney's decisions

242. What is the most common cause of left ventricular hypertrophy in the United States?

A) Chronic atrial fibrillation
B) Chronic hypertension
C) Mitral valve prolapse
D) Pulmonary hypertension

243. Asthmatics may have all of the following symptoms during an acute exacerbation except:

A) Tachycardia
B) Severe wheezing
C) Chronic coughing
D) Tachypnea

244. A nurse practitioner's right to practice is regulated under:

A) Medicare regulations
B) The Board of Medicine
C) The federal government
D) The Board of Nursing

245. An athlete with a history of exercise-induced asthma wants to know when he should use his albuterol inhaler. The nurse practitioner should advise the patient to:

A) Premedicate himself 20 to 30 minutes before starting exercise
B) Wait until he starts to exercise before using the inhaler
C) Premedicate 60 minutes before starting exercise
D) Wait until he finishes his exercises before using his inhaler

246. Atrophic macular degeneration (AMD) of the aged is the leading cause of blindness in the elderly in the United States. Which of the following statements is correct?

A) It is a slow or sudden painless loss of central vision
B) It is a slow or sudden painless loss of peripheral vision
C) It is an occlusion of the central retinal vein causing degeneration of the macular area
D) It is commonly caused by diabetic retinopathy

247. A 20-year-old woman is complaining of a 2-week history of facial pressure that worsens when she bends over. She complains of tooth pain on her upper molars. She notices that over-the-counter decongestants are not giving her relief. On physical examination, her lungs and heart sounds are normal. Which of the following is most likely?

A) An acute dental abscess
B) Chronic sinusitis
C) Acute sinusitis
D) Severe allergic rhinitis

248. Which of the following conditions is potentially a life-threatening disorder?

A) Hashimoto's disease
B) Higher than normal levels of TSH (thyroid-stimulating hormone)
C) A thyroid storm
D) Myxedema

249. What is the best procedure for evaluating a corneal abrasion?

    A) Tonometry
    B) Fluorescein stain
    C) Visual field test
    D) Funduscopy

250. You are examining a patient who has just been diagnosed with Bell's palsy. Bell's palsy is characterized by all of the following except:

    A) Drooling
    B) Inability to swallow
    C) Inability to close the eye on the affected side
    D) Drooping of the corner of the mouth on the affected side

251. Which of the following agents is preferred treatment for a diabetic with stage II hypertension?

    A) Angiotensin-converting enzyme (ACE) inhibitor
    B) Calcium channel blockers
    C) Loop diuretics
    D) Alpha-blockers

252. A peak expiratory flow (PEF) result of 60% to 80% of predicted range with 30% variability of symptoms is classified as which of the following?

    A) Mild intermittent asthma
    B) Mild persistent asthma
    C) Moderate persistent asthma
    D) Severe asthma

253. Which of the following conditions is associated with Auspitz's sign?

    A) Contact dermatitis
    B) Seborrheic dermatitis
    C) Systemic lupus erythematosus
    D) Psoriasis

254. Which of the following is used to confirm a diagnosis of Hashimoto's thyroiditis?

    A) Serum TSH
    B) Free T4 test
    C) Antimicrosomal antibody test
    D) Any of the above

255. Which of the following conditions is most likely to cause cupping of the optic disc?

    A) Brain tumor
    B) Brain abscess
    C) Acute glaucoma
    D) Acute intracranial bleeding

256. A patient is suing a local physician for malpractice. Which of the following is a false statement?

A) The nurse practitioner, hospital, and other personnel who have taken care of the patient can be included in the lawsuit by the plaintiff's lawyer

B) The nurse practitioner may be exempted from the lawsuit if documentation is thorough and can be verified

C) An expert witness should be from the same area of practice

D) The nurse practitioner's documentation can be subpoenaed by the plaintiff's lawyer

257. The best screening test for detecting hyperthyroidism and hypothyroidism is:

A) The total T3

B) Thyroid-stimulating hormone (TSH)

C) Thyroid profile

D) Palpation of the thyroid gland

258. A patient who recently returned from a vacation in Latin America complains of a severe headache and stiff neck that have been accompanied by a high fever for the past 12 hours. While examining the patient, the nurse practitioner flexes the patient's neck while observing the patient's hips and legs for a reaction. The name of this test is:

A) Kernig's maneuver

B) Brudzinski's maneuver

C) Murphy's sign

D) Homan's sign

259. Which of the following groups has been recommended to be screened for thyroid disease?

A) Women aged 50 years or older

B) Adolescent females

C) Elderly males

D) School-aged children

260. A 65-year-old Hispanic woman has a history of type 2 diabetes. A routine urinalysis reveals a few epithelial cells and is negative for leukocytes, nitrites, and protein. Which of the following would you recommend next?

A) Order a urine test for culture and sensitivity

B) Order a 24-hour urine for microalbumin

C) Since it is negative, no further tests are necessary

D) Recommend a screening intravenous pyelogram (IVP)

261. RhoGAM's mechanism of action is:

A) The destruction of Rh-positive fetal red blood cells that are present in the mother's circulatory system

B) The destruction of maternal antibodies against Rh-positive fetal red blood cells

C) The stimulation of maternal antibodies so that there is a decreased risk of hemolysis

D) The destruction of maternal antibodies against fetal red blood cells

262. A chest radiograph shows an area of consolidation on the left lower lobe. Which of the following conditions is most likely?

    A) Bacterial pneumonia
    B) Acute bronchitis
    C) Chronic obstructive pulmonary disease (COPD)
    D) Atypical pneumonia

263. What type of breath sounds are best heard over the base of the lungs?

    A) Fine breath sounds
    B) Vesicular breath sounds
    C) Bronchial sounds
    D) Tracheal breath sounds

264. The Joint National Committee on Prevention, Detection, Evaluation, and Treatment of High Blood Pressure's (JNC 7) most current recommendation for blood pressure goals in diabetics and for patients with coronary heart disease is:

    A) <140/90
    B) <130/85
    C) <130/80
    D) <125/75

265. Which of the following is considered a mast cell stabilizer?

    A) Nedocromil sodium (Tilade)
    B) Albuterol (Ventolin) inhalers
    C) A long-acting oral theophylline (Theo-Dur)
    D) Fluticasone inhaler (Flovent)

266. All of the following clinical findings are considered benign oral findings except:

    A) A patch of leukoplakia
    B) Fordyce spots
    C) Torus palatinus
    D) Fishtail uvula

267. Which of the following interventions is most appropriate if a professional nurse is suspected of being impaired due to a possible addiction to narcotics?

    A) Document the nurse coworker's behavior and file an incident report
    B) Refer the nurse to a special rehabilitation program for impaired health professionals
    C) Report the nurse directly to the state's Board of Nursing
    D) Refer the nurse to a psychiatrist for further evaluation

268. During a routine physical examination of a 90-year-old woman, a low-pitched diastolic murmur grade II/VI is auscultated. It is located on the fifth intercostal space (ICS) on the left side of the midclavicular line. Which of the following identifications is correct?

    A) Aortic regurgitation
    B) Mitral stenosis
    C) Mitral regurgitation
    D) Tricuspid regurgitation

269. Which of the following situations is considered emergent?

A) A laceration on the lower leg of a patient on aspirin (Bayer) 81 mg every other day
B) Rapid breathing and tachycardia in a patient with a fever
C) An elderly man with abdominal pain whose vital signs appear stable
D) A 37-year-old male biker with a concussion due to a fall who appears agitated and does not appear to understand instructions given by the medical assistant checking his vital signs

270. Which of the following is considered an objective finding in patients who have a case of suppurative otitis media?

A) Erythema of the tympanic membrane
B) Decreased mobility of the tympanic membrane as measured by tympanogram
C) Displacement of the light reflex
D) Bulging of the tympanic membrane

271. Pulsus paradoxus is more likely to be associated with:

A) Sarcoidosis
B) Acute bronchitis
C) Status asthmaticus
D) Bacterial pneumonia

272. An older adult male complains of feeling something in his left scrotum. On palpation, soft and moveable blood vessels that feel like a "bag of worms" are noted underneath the scrotal skin. The testicle is not swollen or reddened. The most likely diagnosis is:

A) Chronic orchitis
B) Chronic epididymitis
C) Testicular torsion
D) Varicocele

273. All of the following are true statements regarding elder abuse except:

A) The elderly aged 80 years or older are at the highest risk for abuse
B) A delay in medical care is a common finding
C) A new onset of a sexually transmitted disease (STD) in an elderly patient may signal sexual abuse
D) Decreased anxiety and depression are common symptoms of abuse in the elderly

274. The S1 heart sound is caused by:

A) Closure of the atrioventricular valves
B) Closure of the semilunar valves
C) Opening of the atrioventricular valves
D) Opening of the semilunar valves

275. Patients with Down's syndrome are at higher risk for all of the following except:

    A) Atlantoaxial instability
    B) Congenital heart disease
    C) Early onset of Alzheimer's disease
    D) Melanoma

276. Duvall and Miller used developmental theory to describe the family. Which of the following statements is true?

    A) Each family is developmentally unique in comparison to another family
    B) Families demonstrate common forms of membership across developmental stages
    C) Families complete each developmental task separately
    D) Families change over time because of the influence of environmental factors

277. The following abnormal laboratory results may be seen in patients with acute mononucleosis except:

    A) Lymphocytosis and/or atypical lymphocytes
    B) Positive EBV (Epstein–Barr virus) titers for IgM (immunoglobulin M) and IgG (immunoglobulin G)
    C) Elevated liver function tests
    D) Elevated creatinine and BUN (blood–urea–nitrogen)

278. Which of the following is considered an abnormal result on a Weber test?

    A) Lateralization to one ear
    B) No lateralization in either ear
    C) Air conduction lasts longer than bone conduction
    D) Bone conduction lasts longer than air conduction

279. All of the following are considered benign physiologic variants except:

    A) Xerosis (dry skin)
    B) Supernumerary nipples
    C) Split uvula
    D) Cheilosis

280. A 65-year-old woman's bone density result shows severe demineralization of cortical bone. All of the following pharmacologic agents are useful in treating this condition except:

    A) Raloxifene (Evista)
    B) Calcitonin (Miacalcin)
    C) Medroxyprogesterone (Depo-Provera)
    D) Conjugated estrogen (Premarin)

281. A fracture on the navicular area of the wrist is usually caused by falling forward and landing on the hands. The affected wrist is hyperextended to break the fall. The NP is well aware that all of the following statements are true regarding a fracture of the scaphoid bone of the wrist except:

A) It has higher rate of nonunion compared with the other bones on the wrist when it is fractured

B) The fracture frequently does not show up on an x-ray film when it is taken after the injury

C) The x-ray film will become positive if it is repeated in a few weeks

D) These fractures always require surgical intervention to stabilize the joint

282. John, a 21-year-old, has type 1 diabetes. His late afternoon blood sugars over the past 2 weeks are averaging about 220 mg/dL. He is on 10 units of regular and 15 units of neutral protamine Hagedorn (NPH) insulin in the morning and the same dose in the afternoon. Which of the following is the best course to follow?

A) Increase both doses of insulin

B) Increase only the NPH insulin in the morning

C) Decrease the afternoon dose of NPH insulin

D) Decrease both NPH and regular insulin doses in the morning

283. The mother of an adult male with Down syndrome is in the nurse practitioner's office and wants a sports physical done for her son. She reports that he wants to join the football team at his school. Which of the following is the best advice for this patient's mother?

A) Her son can play a regular football game as long as he wears maximum protective football gear

B) Her son cannot participate in any contact sports because of an increased risk of cervical spine injury

C) Her son can participate in some sports after he has been checked for cervical instability

D) None of the above

284. The nurse practitioner is performing a physical examination on a 20-year-old male. The patient complains of a single nonpruritic and red maculopapular rash that is round in shape. The rash has been slowly enlarging over time and some areas in the center of the rash have already cleared. It is starting to resemble a target. The patient reports that he went hunting 4 weeks ago. Which of the following is most likely?

A) Erythema migrans

B) Rocky Mountain spotted fever

C) Stevens–Johnson syndrome

D) Larva migrans

285. Some pharmacologic agents may cause confusion in the elderly. Which of the following pharmacologic agents is most likely to cause confusion in this population?

A) Cimetidine (Tagamet), digoxin (Lanoxin), diphenhydramine (Benadryl)
B) Acetaminophen (Tylenol), aspirin (Bayer), indomethacin (Indocin)
C) Sucralfate (Carafate), docusate sodium (Surfak), psyllium (Metamucil)
D) Cephalexin (Keflex), amoxicillin (Amoxil), clarithromycin (Biaxin)

286. A 55-year-old female with a history of migraine headaches has recently been diagnosed with stage II hypertension. Her EKG strips reveal second-degree heart block. The chest x-ray is normal. All of the following drug classes are contraindicated in this patient with the exception of:

A) ARBs (angiotensin receptor blockers)
B) Beta-blockers
C) Alpha-blockers
D) Calcium channel blockers

287. Which of the following cranial nerves is evaluated when a wisp of cotton is lightly brushed against the corner of the eye?

A) CN II
B) CN III
C) CN IV
D) CN V

288. A nurse practitioner suspects that a new patient who is an alcoholic may have an acute case of pancreatitis. All of the following laboratory tests are more likely to demonstrate pancreatic injury except:

A) Lipase
B) Amylase
C) Serum blood glucose
D) Gamma glutamyl transpeptidase (GGT)

289. Which of the following is a possible side effect from ACE (angiotensin-converting enzyme) inhibitor therapy?

A) Dry cough
B) Mild wheezing
C) Hypokalemia
D) Increased serum uric acid level

290. All of the following statements are false regarding the rehabilitation of alcoholics except:

A) Al-Anon is designed for family members of alcoholics
B) Disulfiram (Antabuse) is always effective
C) Alcoholics Anonymous is not an effective method for treating this condition
D) Avoid foods or drinks that contain alcohol, such as cough syrups

291. A 35-year-old soccer player presents at an urgent care clinic with a complaint of swelling and pain on the medial aspect of the right knee. The patient reports that the soccer ball hit him on the other side of the same knee. On examination, the knee is swollen with tenderness on the joint line of the medial side of the knee. To assess for possible injury to the meniscus, which maneuver will yield the best information to the nurse practitioner?

A) Anterior drawer test
B) Posterior drawer test
C) Lachman test
D) McMurray's test

292. All of the following are incorrect statements regarding the Healthy People 2010 objectives except:

A) The document's objectives are applicable not only nationally, but also internationally
B) One of the objectives of the document is to help people achieve not only physical health, but social and emotional health as well
C) The document's objectives are applicable only to people of the United States of America
D) The document is formulated by a special committee formed by an alliance of all the state health departments

293. The Pap smear result on a 20-year-old sexually active student who uses condoms inconsistently shows a large amount of white blood cells on the wet smear. During the speculum examination, the patient's cervix bled easily (friable) and a small amount of purulent discharge was found on the surface of the cervix. What is the next appropriate action?

A) The NP needs to do cervical cultures to verify gonorrhea
B) Call the patient and instruct her to use metronidazole vaginal cream
C) Call the patient and tell her she needs a repeat Pap smear in 6 months
D) Advise her to use a Betadine douche at bedtime × 3 days

294. All of the following are covered under the provisions of the ANA's Code of Ethics except:

A) Advocacy for civil rights
B) Acceptance of accountability and responsibility
C) Preservation of patients' dignity
D) Social reform

295. Which of the following is not an absolute contraindication for oral contraceptive pills?

A) Smoking under age 35 years of age and history of deep venous thrombosis (DVT)
B) A family history of migraines with aura
C) Depression and a history of gallbladder disease during pregnancy
D) Controlled hypertension and diabetes mellitus with vascular changes

296. Which of the following is the most common cause of cancer deaths for males in the United States?

    A) Prostate cancer
    B) Lung cancer
    C) Colon cancer
    D) Heart disease

297. Human papilloma virus infection in women has been associated with the development of:

    A) Ectopic pregnancy
    B) Infertility
    C) Cervical cancer
    D) Pelvic inflammatory disease

298. All of the following criteria are included in the diagnosis of patients with AIDS (acquired immunodeficiency syndrome) except:

    A) Reactivation of an Epstein-Barr virus (EBV) infection
    B) Oral thrush
    C) Kaposi's sarcoma
    D) Hairy leukoplakia of the tongue

299. Which of the following conditions is the most common cause of sudden death among athletes?

    A) Brain aneurysm
    B) Hypertrophic cardiomyopathy
    C) Left ventricular hypertrophy
    D) Aortic stenosis

300. The span of the normal adult liver is:

    A) 15 to 18 cm in the midclavicular line
    B) 12 to 16 cm in the right midclavicular line
    C) 2 to 6 cm in the midsternal line
    D) 4 to 8 cm in the midsternal line

301. The tandem gait is used to test which of the following?

    A) Cerebellum
    B) Sacral nerves
    C) Motor movements
    D) Sensory input

302. A neighbor's 18-year-old son, who is active in basketball, complains of pain and swelling on both knees. On physical examination, tenderness is detected over the anterior tubercle of both knees. Which of the following is most likely?

    A) Chondromalacia patella
    B) Left knee sprain
    C) Osgood–Schlatter disease
    D) Tear of the medial ligament

303. A 27-year-old kindergarten teacher presents with a severe sore throat accompanied by a pink generalized rash with sandpaper-like texture. She is currently treated with amoxicillin 500 mg three times a day for 10 days. Which of the following conditions is best described?

A) Scarlatina
B) Rash due to an allergic reaction to amoxicillin
C) Reactivated mononucleosis
D) *Pityriasis rosea*

304. During a physical examination, a 40-year-old patient who has hypertension is noted to have a few beats of horizontal nystagmus on extreme lateral gaze that disappeared when the patient's eyes returned toward midline. Which of the following statements best describes this clinical finding?

A) It is caused by occult bleeding of the retinal artery
B) This is a normal finding
C) It is a sign of a possible brain mass
D) This is a borderline result and requires further evaluation

305. An urgent care nurse practitioner is assessing a 45-year-old White woman with a BMI of 32 for complaints of intermittent right upper quadrant pain that is precipitated by fatty meals over the past few weeks. On examination, the patient's heart and lungs are normal. There is no pain over the costovertebral angle (CVA). During abdominal examination, the bowel sounds are hyperactive. Murphy's sign is positive. Which of the following is best described?

A) Acute cholecystitis
B) Acute appendicitis
C) Acute gastroenteritis
D) Acute diverticulitis

306. Which of the following drugs is recommended by the Centers for Disease Control and Prevention (CDC) as first-line treatment for infections caused by *Bacillus anthracis* (anthrax)?

A) Clindamycin (Cleocin)
B) Doxycycline (Vibramycin)
C) Penicillin G injection
D) Ciprofloxacin (Cipro)

307. Cullen's sign is associated with:

A) Severe appendicitis
B) Acute pancreatitis
C) Hemorrhage
D) Acute hepatitis

308. Which of the following activities is considered a weight-bearing exercise?

A) Swimming
B) Dancing
C) Passive range of motion
D) Bicycling

309. Mary, who is 65 years of age, comes into the clinic on the first week of November for her annual visit. Her last Td booster was 9 years ago. Which immunization(s) would you recommend?

A) Influenza vaccine only
B) Td and influenza vaccine
C) Pneumococcal (Pneumovax) and influenza vaccines
D) No vaccination need be administered during this visit

310. Acute bronchitis is characterized by:

A) High fever
B) Purulent sputum
C) Paroxysms of coughing that is dry or productive of mucoid sputum
D) Slow onset

311. The nurse practitioner notices a gray ring on the edge of both irises of an 80-year-old male. The patient denies visual changes or pain and reports that he has had the "ring" for many years. Which of the following is most likely?

A) Arcus senilis (senile arcus)
B) Pinguecula
C) Peripheral cataracts
D) Macular degeneration

312. Which of the following is not indicated for the treatment of psoriasis?

A) Psoralens
B) Goeckerman's regimen (coal tar followed by UVB phototherapy)
C) Oral and topical steroids
D) Gold salt injections

313. The cones in the retina of the eye are responsible for:

A) Central vision
B) Peripheral vision
C) Night vision
D) Double vision

314. The nurse practitioner would refer all of the following below to a physician except:

A) Severe facial burns
B) Electrical burns
C) Burns that involve the cartilage of the ear
D) Second-degree burns on the lower arm

315. On auscultation of the chest, a split S2 is best heard at:

A) Second intercostal space, right sternal border
B) Second intercostal space, left sternal border
C) Fifth intercostal space, midclavicular line
D) Fourth intercostal space, left sternal border

316. According to the guidelines outlined in the Joint National Committee on Prevention, Detection, Evaluation, and Treatment of High Blood Pressure (JNC 7), the normal blood pressure is defined as:

    A) <140/90
    B) <130/85
    C) <120/80
    D) <110/75

317. Which of the following would be classified as a second-degree burn?

    A) A severe sunburn with blistering
    B) Burns that involve the subcutaneous layer of skin
    C) A reddened finger after touching a hot iron
    D) Burns that involved eschar

318. The mother of a 17-year-old boy is concerned that her son is not developing normally. On physical examination, the patient is noted to have small testes with no pubic or facial hair. You would advise the mother:

    A) Her son is developing normally
    B) Her son's physical development is delayed and should be evaluated by a pediatric endocrinologist
    C) Her son should be rechecked in 3 months; if he still does not have secondary sexual characteristics, a thorough hormonal workup would be initiated
    D) Her son's physiological development is slower than normal but is within the lower limits for his age group

319. Robert, who is 65 years of age, complains of a new onset of a headache on the right temple accompanied by skin sensitivity in the scalp and blurred vision of the right eye. The patient denies nausea or vomiting. The patient, who is a smoker with a history of glaucoma, also complains of a flare-up of his allergies. During physical examination, there is an indurated area that is tender to touch on the right temple. The pupils are equal in size. The patient's nasal turbinates are swollen and have a bluish tinge. Which one of the following conditions is the top priority for the nurse practitioner to treat?

    A) Temporal arteritis (giant cell arteritis)
    B) Glaucoma
    C) Allergic rhinitis
    D) Nicotine dependence

320. All of the following sexually transmitted infections can become disseminated if not treated, with the exception of:

    A) *Neisseria gonorrhoeae*
    B) *Treponema pallidum*
    C) HIV (human immunodeficiency virus)
    D) *Chlamydia trachomatis*

321. Which of the following cranial nerves is evaluated by the Rinne test?

A) CN VII
B) CN VIII
C) CN IX and X
D) CN XI

322. Robert, a homeless man with an extensive history of alcohol abuse, is confused and combative when he arrives at the clinic. Friends report that Robert hasn't consumed alcohol in 2 days and has progressively become uncontrollable. Likely causes for Robert's behavior would include all except:

A) Subdural hematoma
B) Acute delirium related to alcohol withdrawal
C) Thiamine intoxication
D) Gastrointestinal hemorrhage

323. Laura, who has adult-onset acne, is being followed up for acne by the nurse practitioner. During the facial examination, papules and pustules are seen mostly on the forehead, cheeks, and chin areas. The patient has been using medicated soap and other over-the-counter acne medications without much improvement. The nurse practitioner advises the patient that she has moderate acne. Which of the following would you recommend next?

A) Isotretinoin (Accutane)
B) Oral tetracycline
C) Erythromycin topical solution
D) Retin-A 0.25% gel

324. The following statements are all true regarding herpes zoster except:

A) It is due to reactivation of latent varicella virus
B) The typical lesions are bullae
C) It is usually more severe in immunocompromised individuals
D) Infection of the trigeminal nerve ophthalmic branch can cause corneal blindness

325. A 45-year-old construction worker complains of recurrent episodes of painful, large, dark-red nodules, pustules, and abscesses on both his axillae that resolve with antibiotic treatment. The nodules are tender to palpation. Several pustules and abscesses have started to drain purulent green discharge. In addition, severe scarring and sinus tracts are noted on the axillary area. The nurse practitioner explains to the patient that it is caused by bacterial infection of the sweat glands in his axillae. Which of the following conditions is best described?

A) Hidradenitis suppurativa
B) Severe nodular cystic acne
C) Granuloma inguinale
D) Cat scratch fever

326. A possible side effect from the use of nifedipine (Procardia XL) is:

    A) Hypokalemia
    B) Hyperkalemia and tetany
    C) Edema of the ankles and headaches
    D) Dry hacking cough and hyperuricemia

327. Which of the following is contraindicated in patients with acute prostatitis?

    A) Vigorous massage of the prostate
    B) Serial urine samples
    C) Rectal exams
    D) Gentle palpation of the epididymis

328. All of the following conditions are recommended screening for 25-year-old males except:

    A) Prostate-specific antigen (PSA)
    B) Substance abuse
    C) Seatbelt use
    D) Safe-sex practice

329. What is the first-line antibiotic recommended by the American Thoracic Society (ATS) for patients younger than 60 years of age who are diagnosed with uncomplicated community-acquired pneumonia?

    A) First-generation cephalosporins
    B) Second-generation cephalosporins
    C) Macrolides
    D) Beta-lactam antibiotics

330. All of the following are eye findings found in patients with chronic uncontrolled hypertension. Which of the following eye findings is not associated with the disorder?

    A) AV nicking and silver wire arterioles
    B) Copper wire arterioles
    C) Flame-shaped hemorrhages and cotton wool spots
    D) Neovascularization and microaneurysms

331. While reviewing some laboratory reports, the nurse practitioner notices that one of her teenage male patients' laboratory results are abnormal. The alkaline phosphatase level is elevated. The liver function tests are all within normal limits. The patient is a member of a soccer team with no history of recent injury. Which of the following statements is true?

    A) It is an indication of possible liver damage from alcohol; order a liver ultrasound to rule out fatty liver
    B) This is a normal finding due to the skeletal growth spurt in this age group
    C) The patient needs to be evaluated further for pancreatic disease
    D) The patient needs an ultrasound of the liver to rule out fatty liver and referral to a pediatric rheumatologist

332. Which of the following would be appropriate initial management of a second-degree burn?

A) Irrigate with hydrogen peroxide and apply Silvadene cream BID
B) Irrigate with normal saline and apply Silvadene cream BID
C) Irrigate with tap water and apply Neosporin ointment BID
D) Unroof all intact blisters and apply antibiotic ointment BID

333. A male patient is positive for the anti-HCV (hepatitis C antibody) test. All of the following are included in the patient's treatment plan except:

A) Advise the patient that he is immune to hepatitis C and no further testing is indicated
B) Order an alanine aminotransferase (ALT) test
C) Obtain a subjective history to find factors for the disease
D) Order an HCV RNA (hepatitis C ribonucleic acid test) test

334. An 80-year-old woman complains about her "thin" skin. You explain that it is caused by all of the following except:

A) Lower collagen content
B) Loss of subcutaneous fat
C) Atrophy of the sebaceous glands
D) Damage from chronic sun exposure

335. All of the following statements are correct regarding licensure for nurse practitioners except:

A) It ensures a minimum level of professional competency
B) It grants permission for an individual to practice in a profession
C) It requires verification of educational training from an accredited graduate program
D) It reviews information via a nongovernmental agency

336. Which of the following is the correct statement regarding the size of the arterioles and veins on the fundi of the eye?

A) The veins are larger than the arterioles
B) The arterioles are larger than the veins
C) The arterioles are half the size of the veins
D) The veins and the arterioles are equal in size

337. All of the following factors have been found to increase the risk of atrial fibrillation in predisposed individuals except:

A) Hypertension and hyperthyroidism
B) Too much alcohol intake in predisposed patients
C) Theophylline and stimulants
D) Ovarian hormonal imbalance

338. A homeless middle-aged male complains of a migratory arthritis and dysuria. Currently, his right knee is swollen and painful. On examination, green-colored purulent penile discharge is noted. Which of the following is most likely?

A) Gonorrhea
B) Chlamydia
C) Nongonococcal urethritis
D) Acute epididymitis

339. You would associate a positive iliopsoas muscle test result with the following condition:

A) Cerebral vascular accident (CVA)
B) Urinary tract infection (UTI)
C) Autoimmune diseases
D) Acute abdomen

340. Which cranial nerves innervate the extraocular muscles (EOMs) of the eyes?

A) CN II, CN III, and CN VI
B) CN III, CN IV, and CN VI
C) CN IV, CN V, and CN VII
D) CN V, CN VI, and CN VIII

341. The most sensitive and specific diagnostic test for both sickle cell anemia and thalassemia is:

A) Hemoglobin electrophoresis
B) A bone marrow biopsy
C) A blood peripheral smear
D) Reticulocyte count

342. All of the following patients have an increased risk of developing adverse effects from metformin (Glucophage) except:

A) Patients with renal disease
B) Patients who are dehydrated
C) Overweight patients
D) Patients who are alcoholics

343. A 65-year-old homeless male presents to a public health clinic with complaints of an acute onset of chills and cough that started 2 days ago. The cough is productive of rust-colored sputum. The patient complains of sharp chest pain whenever he coughs. He denies pressure or radiation of the pain to his arms, neck, and jaw. His vital signs are the following: temperature: 102°F, pulse of 100 per minute, and a blood pressure of 130/80. The urinalysis shows a few epithelial cells and no leukocytes. Which of the following is most likely?

A) Atypical pneumonia
B) Viral pneumonia
C) Bacterial pneumonia
D) Acute bronchitis

344. Which of the following drugs would you recommend for this patient?

   A) Doxycycline (Dynapen) BID × 10 days
   B) Azithromycin ER (Zmax)
   C) Trimethoprim sulfamethoxazole (Bactrim DS) BID × 10 days
   D) Erythromycin BID × 10 days

345. Which of the following antihypertensive agents should be weaned off in patients who have taken the drug for many years before the drug is discontinued?

   A) Diuretics
   B) Beta-blockers
   C) ACE inhibitors
   D) Calcium channel blockers

346. A 70-year-old male with open-angle glaucoma is prescribed Betimol (timolol) ophthalmic drops. All of the following are contraindications to Betimol ophthalmic drops except:

   A) Overt heart failure or sinus bradycardia
   B) Asthmatic patients
   C) Second- or third-degree AV block
   D) Migraine headaches

347. The side effects of antihistamines are mostly due to their:

   A) Anticholinergic effects
   B) Sedating effects
   C) Anti-inflammatory effects
   D) Immune system effects

348. "Sundowning" is sometimes seen in elderly patients with dementia. Which of the following is the best description of this phenomenon?

   A) The patient becomes very agitated, confused, and aggressive after sunset and throughout the night with resolution of symptoms in the morning
   B) The patient becomes less disoriented and less fearful after sunset
   C) The patient starts hallucinating before sundown with resolution of symptoms in the morning
   D) The patient becomes more forgetful and anxious during the night

349. A 30-year-old male patient with a history of bipolar I disorder refuses to take his afternoon dose of pills. The nurse tells him of the possible consequences of his action, but the patient still refuses to cooperate. Which of the following is the best course for the nurse to follow?

   A) Document in the patient's record his behaviors and the action taken by the nurse
   B) Reassure the patient that he will be fine after taking the medicine
   C) Document only the patient's behavior
   D) Document only the nurse's action

350. While performing a sports physical on a young adult, the nurse practitioner notes a split S2 during inspiration that disappears during expiration. The patient denies chest pain and dyspnea. The mother is with the patient and is concerned. What is the best advice for this patient's mother?

A) The patient needs to be referred to a cardiologist
B) Educate the mother that it is a benign finding
C) Advise the mother that because the patient is an athlete, he should have a stress EKG as soon as possible
D) The patient should avoid strenuous physical exertion until further evaluation

351. Patients who are considered mentally competent need to be advised about their recommended treatment or procedure. This is called:

A) Informed consent
B) Durable power of attorney
C) Competence
D) Advance directives

352. The following lifestyle modifications are an important aspect in the treatment of hypertension. Which of the following is incorrect?

A) Reduce intake of potassium because of its cardiac effects
B) Reduce intake of sodium and saturated fats
C) Exercise at least 3 to 4 times per week
D) Maintain an adequate intake of potassium, magnesium, and calcium

353. At what level of prevention is art therapy considered for patients who have history of a stroke?

A) Primary prevention
B) Secondary prevention
C) Tertiary prevention
D) Health prevention

354. Kyphosis is a late sign of:

A) Old age
B) Osteopenia
C) Osteoporosis
D) Osteoarthritis

355. Which of the following methods is used to diagnose gonorrheal proctitis?

A) Serum chlamydia titer
B) Gen-Probe
C) Thayer-Martin culture
D) RPR (rapid plasma reagent) and VDRL (Venereal Disease Research Laboratory) test

356. The first nurse practitioner program was started by:

   A) Alfred Bandura
   B) President John F. Kennedy
   C) The federal government
   D) Loretta Ford, PhD

357. Terazosin (Hytrin) is used to treat which of the following conditions?

   A) Benign prostatic hypertrophy (BPH) and hypertension
   B) Chronic prostatitis and atrial fibrillation
   C) Urinary tract infections and arrhythmias
   D) Benign prostatic hypertrophy (BPH) and chronic prostatitis

358. All of the following are possible etiology for papilledema except:

   A) Intracranial abscess
   B) Ruptured aneurysm
   C) Basilar migraine headaches
   D) Cerebral edema

359. Which of the following clinical findings can mimic a case of testicular torsion?

   A) The blue dot sign
   B) Cullen's sign
   C) Prehn's sign
   D) Murphy's sign

360. Paroxysmal nocturnal dyspnea is found predominantly in patients with which type of heart failure?

   A) Left heart failure
   B) Right heart failure
   C) Both left and right heart failure
   D) Partial heart failure

361. All of the following factors increase the risk of mortality for patients diagnosed with bacterial pneumonia except:

   A) Alcoholism
   B) Very young age or the elderly
   C) Multiple lobar involvement
   D) Hypertension

362. The bacteria responsible for the highest mortality in patients with community-acquired pneumonia is:

   A) *Streptococcus pneumoniae*
   B) *Mycoplasma pneumoniae*
   C) *Moxarella catarrhalis*
   D) *Haemophilus influenzae*

363. Mr. R. J. is a 40-year-old asthmatic male with hypertension. For the past 6 months, he has been following a low-fat, low-sodium diet and walking three times a week. His blood pressure readings from the past two visits were 160/95 and 170/100. On this visit, it is 160/90. What is the most appropriate action for the nurse practitioner to follow at this visit?

A) Continue the lifestyle modifications and recheck his blood pressure again in 4 weeks
B) Initiate a prescription of hydrochlorothiazide 12.5 mg PO daily
C) Initiate a prescription of atenolol (Tenormin) 25 mg PO daily
D) Refer the patient to a cardiologist for a stress EKG

364. When initially treating an adult for acute bronchitis, which of the following should the nurse practitioner be least likely to order?

A) Expectorants
B) Antibiotics
C) Bronchodilators
D) Antitussives

365. According to JNC 7 criteria, which of the following are considered cardiac risk equivalents?

A) Microalbuminuria and diabetes
B) Congestive heart failure
C) Acute renal failure and chronic bronchitis
D) Patients on anticoagulation therapy

366. Which of the following is one of the best screening tools to rule out alcohol abuse?

A) Alcoholics Anonymous
B) The Becker Depression Inventory
C) Mini-Mental Status Exam
D) CAGE test

367. Mrs. Nottam, who has a body mass index (BMI) of 29, has a 20-year history of essential hypertension. She has been on hydrochlorothiazide 25 mg PO daily with excellent results. On this visit, she is complaining of feeling thirsty all the time even though she drinks more than 10 glasses of water per day. She reports to the nurse practitioner that she been having this problem for about 6 months. On reading the chart, the nurse practitioner notes that the last two fasting blood glucose levels have been 140 mg/dL and 168 mg/dL. A random blood glucose is at 210 mg/dL. Which of the following is the best treatment plan to follow at this visit?

A) Order another random blood sugar test in 2 weeks
B) Initiate a prescription of metformin (Glucophage) 500 mg PO BID
C) Order a 3-hour glucose tolerance test (GTT)
D) Order an HgbA1c level

368. A newly diagnosed middle-aged type 2 diabetic wants to start an exercise program. All of the following statements are true except:

A) If the patient is unable to eat due to illness, antidiabetic agents should not be taken until the patient is able to eat again

B) Strenuous exercise is contraindicated for most type 1 diabetics because of a higher risk of hypoglycemic episodes

C) Exercise increases the body's ability to metabolize glucose

D) Patients who exercise vigorously in the afternoon may have hypoglycemic episodes in the evening or at night if they do not eat

369. What is the least common pathogen found in community-acquired atypical pneumonia?

A) *Moxarella catarrhalis*

B) *Streptococcus pneumoniae*

C) *Pseudomonas aeruginosa*

D) *Mycoplasma pneumonia*

370. All of the following are considered target organs that are more likely to become damaged due to chronic hypertension except:

A) Eyes

B) Heart

C) Adrenal glands

D) Kidneys

371. A 56-year-old mechanic is brought to your office complaining of heavy pressure in the substernal area of his chest that is radiating to his jaw. The pain began while he was lifting up a tire. He now appears pale and is diaphoretic. His blood pressure is 100/60 mm Hg, and his pulse rate 50. What is the most appropriate action?

A) Perform a 12-lead electrocardiogram (EKG)

B) Dial 911

C) Administer a morphine injection for pain

D) Observe the patient in the office

372. Which of the following is indicated for initial treatment of an uncomplicated case of *H. pylori* negative peptic ulcer disease (PUD)?

A) Omeprazole (Prilosec)

B) Metoclopramide (Reglan)

C) Ranitidine (Zantac)

D) Misoprostol (Cytotec)

373. Erythromycin inhibits the cytochrome P-450 system. The following drugs should be avoided because of a potential for a drug interaction except:

A) Theophylline (Theo-Dur)

B) Warfarin (Coumadin)

C) Diazepam (Valium)

D) Furosemide (Lasix)

374. If left untreated, Zollinger-Ellison syndrome can cause which of the following?

A) Severe ulcers in the stomach or duodenum
B) Toxic megacolon
C) Chronic diarrhea
D) Malabsorption of fat-soluble vitamins

375. All of the following are classified as FDA category X drugs except:

A) Misoprostol (Cytotec)
B) Ciprofloxacin (Cipro)
C) Finasteride (Proscar)
D) Isotretinoin (Accutane)

376. You note during a physical examination pitting on the fingernails. This finding is best correlated with:

A) Iron-deficiency anemia
B) Psoriasis
C) Onychomycosis
D) Vitamin C deficiency

377. Which of the following is correct regarding the best site to listen for mitral regurgitation?

A) The apical area during S2
B) It is best heard at the base at S1
C) It is best heard at the apex at S1
D) It is best heard at the base at S2

378. Extreme tenderness and involuntary guarding at McBurney's point is a significant finding for possible:

A) Acute cholecystitis
B) Acute appendicitis
C) Acute gastroenteritis
D) Acute diverticulitis

379. All of the following can help relieve the symptom(s) of GERD except:

A) Losing weight
B) Stopping caffeine intake
C) Chewing breath mints
D) Stopping alcohol intake

380. A 34-year-old female is diagnosed with pelvic inflammatory disease (PID). The cervical Gen-Probe result is positive for *Neisseria gonorrhoeae* and negative for *Chlamydia trachomatis*. All of the following statements are true regarding the management of this patient except:

A) This patient should be treated for chlamydia even though the Gen-Probe for chlamydia is negative
B) Ceftriaxone (Rocephin) 250 mg IM and doxycycline 100 mg PO BID × 14 days are appropriate treatment for this patient

C) Advise the patient to return to the clinic for a repeat pelvic examination in 48 hours

D) Repeat the Gen-Probe test for *Chlamydia trachomatis* to ensure that the previous test was not a false-negative result

381. What Tanner stage is a girl at when her breasts have a secondary mound?

A) Tanner Stage II
B) Tanner Stage III
C) Tanner Stage IV
D) Tanner Stage V

382. A 36-year-old smoker is being evaluated for birth control choices. The patient has a history of chlamydial cervicitis. She has two small children. The best contraceptive method for this patient is:

A) Depo-Provera injections
B) Oral contraceptives
C) Intrauterine device (IUD)
D) Estrogen patches

383. Which of the following antibiotics can interact with theophylline?

A) Clarithromycin (Biaxin)
B) Metronidazole (Flagyl)
C) Amoxicillin (Amoxil)
D) Trimethoprim sulfamethoxzole (Bactrim DS)

384. You would recommend the pneumococcal vaccine (Pneumovax) to patients with all of the following conditions except:

A) Sickle cell anemia
B) Splenectomy
C) Patients infected with HIV
D) G6PD-deficiency anemia

385. A 40-year-old cashier complains of random episodes of dizziness and palpitations that have a sudden onset. The EKG shows P waves before each QRS complex and a heart rate of 170 beats per minute. A carotid massage decreases the heart rate to 80 beats per minute. This best describes:

A) Ventricular tachycardia
B) Paroxysmal atrial tachycardia
C) Atrial fibrillation
D) Ventricular fibrillation

386. A 25-year-old woman complains of dysuria, pruritis, and purulent vaginal discharge. Pelvic examination reveals a cervix with punctate superficial petechiae ("strawberry cervix"), an irritated and reddened vulvar area, and frothy discharge. Microscopic examination of the discharge reveals unicellular organisms. The correct pharmacologic therapy for the condition is:

A) Oral metronidazole (Flagyl)
B) Ceftriaxone sodium (Rocephin) injection

C) Doxycycline hyclate (Vibramycin)

D) Clotrimazole (Gyne-Lotrimin) cream or suppositories

387. All of the following conditions can cause secondary hypertension except:

A) Adrenal tumors

B) Renal artery stenosis

C) Mitral regurgitation

D) Sleep apnea

388. Metronidazole (Flagyl) produces the disulfuram (Antabuse) effect when combined with alcoholic drinks or medicine. You would educate the patient that:

A) She should avoid alcoholic drinks during the time she takes the medicine

B) She should avoid alcoholic drinks 1 day before, during therapy, and a few days after therapy

C) She should avoid alcoholic drinks after she takes the medicine

D) There is no need to avoid any food or drink

389. The treatment plan for patients with AIDS (acquired immunodeficiency syndrome) who have CD4 counts of <200/mm should emphasize:

A) Administering an MMR vaccine

B) Preventive therapy for toxoplasmosis

C) Preventive therapy for *Pneumocystis carinii* pneumonia (PCP)

D) Evaluation of the home environment

390. A positive obturator sign might signify which of the following conditions?

A) Acute appendicitis

B) Acute pancreatitis

C) Acute cholecystitis

D) Acute hepatitis

391. Where does spermatogenesis occur?

A) Epididymis

B) Vas deferens

C) Seminal vesicles

D) Testes

392. Prophylaxis for *Pneumocystis carinii* pneumonia includes all of the following drugs except:

A) Trimethoprim-sulfamethoxazole (Bactrim)

B) Dapsone

C) Aerosolized pentamidine

D) Nedocromil sodium (Tilade)

393. All of the following findings are associated with acute labyrinthitis or acute vestibular neuritis except:

    A) Acoustic nerve damage
    B) Symptoms are provoked by changes in head position
    C) Vertigo with nausea
    D) Nystagmus

394. While performing a routine physical examination on a 60-year-old hypertensive male, the nurse practitioner notices a bruit over the carotid area on the left side of the neck. There is no induration on the skin. This patient is at higher risk for:

    A) Temporal arteritis and brain aneurysms
    B) Dizziness and headaches
    C) Abdominal aneurysm and congestive heart failure
    D) Stroke and coronary heart disease

395. A 46-year-old kindergarten teacher was recently treated for an episode of acute otitis media (AOM) of the right ear. During her follow-up visit, she reports that she is on the fifth day of her menstrual cycle. During the physical examination, the patient's throat is a bright red color with no purulent discharge. The Quick Strep test is negative. The result of her urine dipstick shows a large amount of blood, 3+ leukocytes, and is positive for nitrites. On further questioning, the patient denies flank pain and fever, but is positive for dysuria and urinary frequency. The patient reports that she has a sulfa allergy and may also be allergic to penicillins. Which of the following is the best initial intervention?

    A) Send a urine specimen for culture and sensitivity to the laboratory and treat the patient for a urinary tract infection (UTI)
    B) Recheck the urine by sending another specimen to the laboratory and evaluate the patient further for strep throat
    C) Treat the patient for acute otitis media (AOM) and an acute urinary tract infection (UTI)
    D) Advise the patient that she needs further evaluation

396. Which of the following is the most common skin cancer in the country?

    A) Basal skin cancer
    B) Squamous skin cancer
    C) Melanoma
    D) None of the above

397. When starting an elderly patient on a new prescription of levothyroxine (Synthroid), the nurse practitioner should keep in mind that the rationale for starting an elderly patient on a lower dose is because of:

    A) Central nervous system (CNS) effects
    B) Cardiac effects
    C) Renal effects
    D) Hepatic effects

398. All of the following are useful in treating patients with chronic obstructive lung disease (COPD) except:

A) Anticholinergics
B) Short-acting B2 agonist
C) Oral steroids
D) Antihistamines

399. All of the following drugs interfere with the metabolism of oral contraceptives except:

A) Tetracycline
B) Rifampin
C) Phenytoin (Dilantin)
D) Corticosteroids

400. Which of the following is a recommended treatment by the Centers for Disease Control and Prevention (CDC) for a case of uncomplicated gonorrheal and chlamydial infection?

A) Metronidazole (Flagyl) 250 mg PO three times a day for 7 days
B) Valacyclovir (Valtrex) 500 mg PO twice daily for 10 days
C) Azithromycin 1 g orally OR Doxycycline 100 mg orally twice a day for 7 days
D) One dose of oral fluconazole (Diflucan) 150 mg

401. Which of the following is not a relative contraindication for oral contraceptive pills?

A) Active hepatitis A infection
B) Thrombosis related to an IV needle
C) Undiagnosed vaginal bleeding
D) Migraine headache without focal aura

402. A nurse practitioner is taking part in a community outreach program for a local hospital. Most of her audience has a diagnosis of hypertension. They are all interested in learning more about a proper diet. When discussing potential sources of potassium and magnesium, which of the following is the best advice?

A) Fruits, vegetables, and whole grains
B) Fruits, whole grains, and sausages
C) Bananas, beef, and yogurt
D) Mushrooms, fermented foods, and vegetables

403. A 35-year-old sexually active male presents with a 1-week history of fever and pain on his left scrotum along with frequency and dysuria. On examination of the genitals, the nurse practitioner notices that the scrotum is reddened, swollen, and tender to touch. The costovertebral (CVA) examination is negative and the patient denies nausea and vomiting. When the affected testicle is elevated toward the patient's body or when the patient uses his old football support brief, the pain is lessened. The urinalysis shows 2+ blood and a large amount of leukocytes. What is the most likely diagnosis?

A) Acute urinary tract infection
B) Acute pyelonephritis
C) Acute orchitis
D) Acute epididymitis

404. Julia M., a 16-year-old patient, is being treated for her first urinary tract infection. Julia had an allergic reaction with hives after taking sulfa as a child. Which of the following antibiotics would be contraindicated?

A) Cephalexin (Keflex)
B) Ampicillin (amoxil)
C) Trimethoprim-sulfamethoxazole (Bactrim)
D) Nitrofurantoin crystals (Macrobid)

405. All of the following are considered risk factors for breast cancer except:

A) Nulliparity
B) Early menarche
C) Polycystic ovaries
D) Premature menopause

406. The following statements about benign prostatic hypertrophy (BPH) are correct except:

A) It is seen in up to 50% of males older than 50 years old
B) Dribbling and nocturia are common patient complaints
C) Saw palmetto is always effective in reducing symptoms
D) The PSA value is usually slightly elevated

407. The hemoglobin A1c level that indicates prediabetes is:

A) 3.0% to 4.0%
B) 4% to 5.9%
C) 5.7% to 6.4%
D) 6.5% to 8.0%

408. At what Tanner stage does puberty start?

A) Tanner Stage I
B) Tanner Stage II
C) Tanner Stage III
D) Tanner Stage IV

409. All of the following conditions are recommended screening for a 40-year-old Black male except:

A) Obesity
B) Heart disease
C) Prostate cancer
D) Lung cancer

410. Acute prostatitis can present with all of the following signs and symptoms except:

A) Fever and chills
B) Tenderness of the scrotum on the affected side
C) Perineal pain
D) Slow onset of symptoms

411. Which of the following is the most common etiology of nongonococcal urethritis (NGU)?

A) *Escherichia coli*
B) *Chlamydia trachomatis*
C) *Neisseria gonorrhoeae*
D) Mycoplasma

412. Which of the following factors is considered a relative contraindication for combined oral contraceptive pills?

A) Undiagnosed vaginal bleeding
B) A hepatoma of the liver
C) Suspected history of transient ischemic attacks (TIAs)
D) Smoking

413. A 20-year-old Hispanic male complains of right knee pain after twisting it while playing soccer. The patient anxiously tells the nurse practitioner that the injured knee sometimes locks up when he walks or attempts to straighten the leg. This best describes:

A) Injury to the meniscus of the right knee
B) Injury to the patella of the right knee
C) Injury to the ligaments of the right knee
D) Rupture of the quadriceps tendon

414. Which of the following is the best course of treatment for this patient?

A) Refer him to an orthopedic specialist
B) Refer him to a chiropractor
C) Advise him that the clicking noise will resolve within 2 to 4 weeks
D) Advise him to use an Ace bandage wrap during the first 2 weeks for knee support and to see you again for reevaluation

415. All of the following are correct statements regarding oral contraceptives except:

A) The actual failure rate of oral contraceptives is 3%
B) Desogestrel belongs to the progesterone family of drugs
C) The newer low-dose birth control pills do not require backup during the first 2 weeks of use
D) Oral contraceptives are contraindicated for women 35 years of age or older who smoke

416. Which of the following hormones induces ovulation?

A) Follicle-stimulating hormone (FSH)
B) Luteinizing hormone (LH)
C) Estradiol
D) Progesterone

417. A cauliflower-like growth with foul-smelling discharge is seen during an otoscopic examination inside the middle ear of a new patient with a history of chronic otitis media infection. No tympanic membrane is visible and the patient reports hearing loss in the affected ear. Which of the following conditions is most likely?

    A) Chronic perforation of the tympanic member with secondary bacterial infection
    B) Chronic mastoiditis
    C) Cholesteatoma
    D) Cancer of the middle ear

418. All of the following are considered ethical concepts except:

    A) Beneficence
    B) Nonmalfeasance
    C) Honesty
    D) Advocacy

419. The best form of aerobic exercise for a patient with severe rheumatoid arthritis is:

    A) Yoga
    B) Swimming
    C) Riding a bicycle
    D) Passive range of motion

420. Benzodiazepines are useful in treating all of the following conditions except:

    A) Acute alcohol withdrawal/delirium tremens
    B) Status epilepticus
    C) Insomnia
    D) Mood disorders

421. All of the following patients are at higher risk of active tuberculosis disease except:

    A) Diabetic patients
    B) A healthy nurse whose PPD test becomes positive after a history of negative tests and denies tuberculosis signs and symptoms
    C) Patients with acute renal failure
    D) Patients who are alcoholics

422. All of the following are considered emancipated minors except:

    A) 15-year-old male who is married
    B) 14-year-old female who is a single parent
    C) 17-year-old male who is enlisted in the U.S. Army
    D) 13-year-old being treated for a sexually transmitted disease

423. All of the following factors are not associated with an increased risk of osteopenia in teenage girls except:

    A) Drinking one glass of low-fat milk daily
    B) Anorexia nervosa
    C) Exercise
    D) Normal BMI

424. A 36-year-old hospital janitor is being treated for an acute urinary tract infection (UTI) by the employee health nurse practitioner. The patient thinks that he had the same symptoms 4 months ago. Which of the following is the best intervention?

    A) Refer the patient to a urologist after treatment
    B) Prescribe the patient ofloxacin (Floxin) for 2 weeks instead of 1 week
    C) Advise the patient that he needs to void every 2 hours and drink more fluids
    D) Refer the patient to the local emergency department because he has a high risk of sepsis

425. Which of the following is a true statement regarding the beliefs of the majority of Jehovah's Witnesses patients?

    A) Transfusion of blood is prohibited even in cases of emergency
    B) Consumption of pork products is strictly prohibited
    C) Transfusion of blood is allowed in certain medical conditions
    D) Consumption of alcohol products is strictly prohibited

426. Which of the following is not a true statement?

    A) A protocol agreement with a physician is a requirement for nurse practitioners to practice in this country
    B) If a nurse practitioner is sued, the physician with whom he or she has a protocol agreement is not held liable
    C) Protocol agreements should be reviewed annually by both the nurse practitioner and the physician
    D) Protocol agreements help protect nurse practitioners from certain types of lawsuits

427. A postmenopausal female complains of intermittent vaginal bleeding for the past 6 months. Which of the following is recommended management for this condition?

    A) Cervical biopsy
    B) Pap smear
    C) Colposcopy
    D) Endometrial biopsy

428. Which of the following findings is not a characteristic of delirium?

    A) Sudden onset
    B) Patient is coherent
    C) Worse in the evenings
    D) It has a brief duration

429. The signs and symptoms of dementia include all of the following except:

    A) Personality changes
    B) Difficulty in verbalizing
    C) Difficulty in recognizing familiar objects
    D) Abstract thinking ability is increased

430. All of the following drugs are known to interact with theophylline either by decreasing the therapeutic blood level or by elevating it to toxic levels except:

   A) Clarithromycin (Biaxin)
   B) Carbamazepine (Tegretol)
   C) Captopril (Capoten)
   D) Ciprofloxacin (Cipro)

431. A women's health nurse practitioner is performing a pelvic examination on a middle-aged woman who recently became sexually active. On examination of the external vagina, a tender and warm cystic mass is found on the lower edge of the left labia majora. According to the patient, she does not use condoms because she is now on birth control pills. Which of the following is most likely?

   A) Skene's gland cyst
   B) Cystocele
   C) Lymphogranuloma venereum
   D) Bartholin's gland abscess

432. A 17-year-old high school student visits the local Planned Parenthood clinic. She tells the nurse practitioner who is evaluating her that she wants to be on birth control pills because she recently became sexually active with her boyfriend. Which of the following is a true statement?

   A) The nurse practitioner can examine and prescribe birth control pills to minors because there is no legal requirement for parental consent in cases concerning sexual activity and pregnancy
   B) Patients who are minors must obtain a signed consent from a parent before being examined or treated for possible pregnancy
   C) Some visits to a health care provider are allowed without parental consent as long as the patient is informed fully about the treatment options
   D) Planned Parenthood clinics are exempted from the consent rule as a result of a ruling from the landmark case of *Roe v. Wade*

433. A patient diagnosed with bacterial vaginosis should be advised that her sexual partner be treated with:

   A) Ceftriaxone (Rocephin) 250 mg IM with doxycycline 100 mg BID for 14 days
   B) Metronidazole (Flagyl) 500 mg PO twice a day for 7 days and 1 dose of azithromycin (Zithromax)
   C) Her partner does not need treatment
   D) Clotrimazole cream (Lotrimin) on his penis BID for 1 to 2 weeks

434. All of the following are correct statements regarding physiologic changes found in the elderly except:

   A) There is an increase of the fat-to-lean body ratio
   B) The metabolism of drugs by the liver decreases
   C) There is an increase in the production of cholesterol by the liver
   D) There is a loss of low-frequency hearing secondary to presbycusis

435. The following clinical signs are seen in patients with advanced Parkinson's disease except:

A) Pill-rolling tremor
B) Difficulty initiating involuntary movement
C) Shuffling gait
D) Increased facial movements

436. When a patient is instructed to smell a small amount of coffee grounds or a lemon, which of the following cranial nerves is being evaluated?

A) CN I
B) CN II
C) CN III
D) CN IV

437. A possible complication from Bell's palsy is:

A) Corneal ulceration
B) Acute glaucoma
C) Inability to swallow
D) Loss of sensation in the affected side

438. Which of the following is least likely to cause delirium?

A) Severe dehydration
B) Multiple brain infarcts
C) Metabolic derangements
D) Adverse drug reactions

439. A 38-year-old sexually active Asian woman with a history of infertility treatment and severe endometriosis complains to the nurse practitioner in the emergency department that she has right-sided pelvic pain that is steadily getting worse. She has also noticed small amounts of yellow vaginal discharge on her underwear for at least 1 week. The patient reports that she is expecting her period, which has not appeared for the last 2 months. Which of the following evaluations is best performed initially?

A) Follicle-stimulating hormone (FSH) and a culture with sensitivity testing of the vaginal discharge
B) Serum quantitative pregnancy test and cervical Gen-Probe testing
C) Pelvic ultrasound and serum quantitative pregnancy test
D) Microscopy of the vaginal discharge and complete blood count (CBC) with white cell differential

440. Which of the following conditions is the most important differential diagnosis to consider in a 38-year-old sexually active Asian woman with a history of infertility treatment and severe endometriosis with right-sided pelvic pain that is steadily getting worse and small amounts of yellow-colored vaginal discharge?

A) Tubal ectopic pregnancy and pelvic inflammatory disease (PID)
B) Mucopurulent cervicitis and tubal ectopic pregnancy
C) Human papilloma virus infection of the cervix and pelvic inflammatory disease (PID)
D) Ovarian cysts and severe endometriosis

441. Which of the following effects are seen in every woman using Depo-Provera (medroxyprogesterone injection) for more than 4 years?

A) Melasma
B) Amenorrhea
C) Weight loss
D) Headaches

442. The following are useful for treating migraine headache. Which one of the following is not considered to be effective therapy?

A) Propranolol (Inderal) prophylaxis
B) Cold packs to the forehead
C) Trimethobenzamide (Tigan) suppositories for nausea
D) Sodium restriction to decrease water retention

443. Which of the following groups of patients should avoid handling crushed or broken tablets of finasteride (Proscar) tablets directly?

A) Adult males
B) Elderly males
C) Elderly females
D) Reproductive-age females

444. The gag reflex is a function of which cranial nerve?

A) CN IX
B) CN X
C) CN XI
D) CN XII

445. A 75-year-old hypertensive male reports a history of an upper respiratory viral infection 4 weeks ago. He is currently complaining of a gradual onset of shortness of breath accompanied by very sharp midchest pain that increases in intensity when he lies down in a supine position. During the physical examination, a precordial rub is auscultated along with a soft S4. The most likely diagnosis would be:

A) Pulmonary embolism
B) A dissecting aneurysm
C) Acute pericarditis
D) Esophageal reflex

446. Which is recommended for a 65-year-old arthritic patient who complains of new onset of a painful and swollen left knee due to overworking in his garden for 3 days?

A) Quadriceps-strengthening exercises of the left knee followed by cold packs for 30 minutes on the swollen knee three times a day
B) Rest and elevation of the knee with intermittent application of cold packs × 15 minutes four times a day for the next 48 hours
C) Passive range-of-motion exercises after a warm tub bath
D) Warm showers to relax the quadriceps muscle followed by cold packs for the swelling

447. Irritable bowel syndrome (IBS) is most commonly seen in young women. These patients usually report a recent history of a stressful event in their lives as a precipitating factor for an acute exacerbation. Most complain of the following symptoms except:

A) Abdominal pain
B) Diarrhea or constipation
C) Relief of abdominal cramping after defecation
D) Severe vomiting

448. Peak expiratory flow (PEF) meters are useful for monitoring the progress or worsening of patients with asthma. The patients are instructed to try blowing as hard as they can at least three times. The personal best or highest volumes are recorded in a diary. All of the following factors are used to determine the PEF except:

A) Age
B) Gender
C) Height
D) Weight

449. A high school student presents to the nurse practitioner complaining of an acute onset of an itchy rash on the back of her neck. During the physical examination, the nurse practitioner notes a bright red maculopapular rash in a linear pattern on the back of the patient's neck. The student is wearing several pieces of jewelry. Which of the following is most likely?

A) Contact dermatitis
B) Erythema migrans
C) Atopic dermatitis
D) Scabies

450. All of the following are considered risk factors for urinary tract infections in women except:

A) Diabetes mellitus
B) Diaphragms and spermicide use
C) Pregnancy
D) Intrauterine device (IUD)

451. A serious sign to look for while performing a physical examination is enlarged sentinel nodes (Virchow's nodes). The sentinel nodes are located in which area of the body?

A) Right axillary area
B) Left supraclavicular area
C) Posterior cervical chain
D) Submandibular chain

452. Pete, a 30-year-old White male, is being seen for a physical examination by the nurse practitioner. He complains of pruritic macerated areas on his groin that are slowly getting larger. Which of the following is the most likely?

A) Tinea cruris
B) Tinea corporis
C) Tinea capitis
D) Tinea pedis

453. Cluster headaches are most often seen in:

A) Adolescent females
B) Middle-aged men
C) Elderly men
D) Postmenopausal women

454. A middle-aged female with a history of hypertension and osteoarthritis reports to the nurse practitioner that she is taking vitamin C for her common cold. She is currently taking a dose of 500 mg twice a day. Which of the following is a true statement?

A) The patient should continue taking the Vitamin C at the same doses
B) The patient should increase the dose of the Vitamin C to 1,000 mg twice a day
C) It does not matter, since there is no solid evidence regarding the efficacy of vitamin C in ameliorating the symptoms of the common cold
D) The patient should continue taking the Vitamin C and combine it with a multivitamin once a day to increase its effectiveness

455. Robert, a homeless man with an extensive history of alcohol abuse, is found in the local park, confused and combative. Family members report that Robert has not consumed any alcoholic drinks for at least 2 days because of a severe case of gastroenteritis. His behavior has progressively worsened and he is getting more uncontrollable. The most likely cause for Robert's behavior is which of the following?

A) Subdural hematoma
B) Delirium tremens secondary to acute withdrawal of alcohol
C) Thiamine intoxication
D) Gastrointestinal hemorrhage

456. A middle-aged woman is complaining of feeling anxious and irritable for several months. She reports weight loss and a fine tremor in her hands that bothers her even when she is at rest. She has lost weight without changing her usual diet or activity. The patient reports that her appetite has increased. Her menstrual cycles have become very irregular. Which of the following conditions is best described?

A) Hyperthyroidism
B) Obsessive-compulsive disorder (OCD)
C) Mood disorder
D) Maturity-onset diabetes of the young (MODY)

457. A middle-aged Hispanic patient with type 2 diabetes mellitus, chronic bronchitis, and hypertension is currently on hydrochlorothiazide 12.5 mg daily. The patient has gained 6 pounds since the last visit. The blood pressure is currently at 140/90, the pulse is 82 beats per minute, and the respiration is at 12 breaths per minute. Which of the following agents is the best choice for this patient?

A) Calcium channel blockers
B) Angiotensin reuptake blockers (ARBs)
C) Beta-blockers
D) Alpha-blockers

458. The cremasteric reflex is elicited by:

A) Asking the patient to open his mouth and touch the back of his pharynx with a tongue blade
B) Hitting the biceps tendon briskly with a reflex hammer and watching the lower arm for movement
C) Hitting the patellar tendon briskly with a reflex hammer and watching the lower leg for movement
D) Stroking the inner thigh of a male and watching the testicle on the ipsilateral side rise up toward the body

459. The nurse practitioner has diagnosed Tom, a 30-year-old farmer, with contact dermatitis on the left side of his face secondary to exposure to poison ivy. Which of the following is the best treatment plan for this patient?

A) Wash the rash with antibacterial soap twice a day to reduce risk of secondary bacterial infection
B) Apply hydrocortisone cream 1% BID to the rash until it is healed
C) Apply clotrimazole (Lotrimin) cream BID for 2 weeks on the rash
D) Use halcinonide (Halog) 1% ointment BID for 2 to 4 weeks

460. Pulsus paradoxus is best described as:

A) An increase in systolic blood pressure of >5 mm Hg on inspiration
B) A decrease in the diastolic blood pressure on exhalation
C) A decrease in the systolic blood pressure of >10 mm Hg on inspiration
D) An increase in diastolic blood pressure of >15 mm Hg on expiration

461. An 18-year-old sexually active male complains of the sudden onset of an extremely painful and swollen left scrotum on awakening that morning. On questioning, the patient denies any trauma, dysuria, and penile discharge, but says that he feels nauseated from the pain. The urine dipstick is negative for blood, leukocytes, and nitrites. On palpation, the nurse practitioner finds an extremely tender, swollen, and red left scrotum. There is no penile discharge. Which of the following conditions is most likely?

A) Epididymitis
B) Acute gastroenteritis
C) Testicular torsion
D) Orchitis

462. What type of follow-up should this patient receive?

    A) Refer him within 48 hours to a urologist
    B) Refer him to the emergency department as soon as possible
    C) Prescribe ibuprofen (Advil) 600 mg QID for pain
    D) Order a testicular ultrasound for further evaluation

463. A female teenager complains to the gym instructor that she recently noticed that one of her hips is higher than the other. She denies pain or any difficulty with ambulation and physical activity. The instructor instructs the girl to bend down forward with her spine in a straight line. On closer inspection, the instructor notices that the thoracic spine has a lateral curvature of about 10 degrees and suspects scoliosis. Which of the following is a true statement?

    A) The curvature is considered mild and will correct spontaneously over time as the patient continues to grow
    B) The girl needs to be referred for surgical correction as soon as possible before further damage to the spine results
    C) The usual clinical strategy is watchful waiting for curves of 10 degrees or less
    D) The patient always needs to wear a special brace for her back during the daytime

464. Which of the following cholesterol levels is classified as borderline?

    A) 180 to 199 mg/dL
    B) 200 to 239 mg/dL
    C) Over 240 mg/dL
    D) Over 300 mg/dL

465. The school health nurse practitioner is performing a sports physical on a teen who belongs to the school's swim team. She documents the girl as Tanner Stage II. The mother is advised that her daughter will probably start menarche within:

    A) 1 to 2 years
    B) 2½ to 3 years
    C) 3 to 4 years
    D) It is dependent on the girl's genetic makeup

466. All of the following do not require parental consent be obtained by the nurse practitioner except:

    A) A 17-year-old who wants to be treated for a sexually transmitted infection
    B) A 14-year-old who wants a serum pregnancy test
    C) A 15-year-old who wants birth control pills
    D) A 16-year-old who wants to be treated for dysmenorrhea

467. All of the following conditions fulfill the criteria for metabolic syndrome except:

    A) Glucose intolerance
    B) Microalbuminuria
    C) Hypertension
    D) Obesity

468. Transillumination is useful in helping diagnose which of the following conditions?

A) Sinusitis and hydrocele
B) Testicular tumor and acute otitis media
C) Nasal masses and other tumors in the facial region
D) Hydrocephalus and epididymitis

469. Which of the following is less likely to be found in a patient with emphysema-dominant chronic obstructive pulmonary disease (COPD)?

A) Exertional dyspnea
B) Weight loss
C) Prolonged expiration
D) A cough that is productive of large amounts of sputum

470. A split S2 is best heard at which of the following auscultatory areas?

A) The aortic area
B) The pulmonic area
C) The tricuspid area
D) The mitral area

471. Balanitis is caused by:

A) *Staphylococcus aureus*
B) *Streptococcus pyogenes*
C) *Candida albicans*
D) Diabetes

472. Which of the following is the most common type of anemia in the United States?

A) Iron-deficiency anemia
B) Thalassemia trait
C) Folate-deficiency anemia
D) Normocytic anemia

473. A newly diagnosed diabetic patient reports to the nurse practitioner that she had severe hives and swollen lips 1 year ago after taking trimethoprim/sulfamethoxazole (Bactrim) for a bladder infection. Which of the following statements is correct?

A) She cannot take any pills in the sulfonylurea class
B) She can take some of the pills in the sulfonylurea class
C) She can take any of the pills in the sulfonylurea class
D) None of the above

474. Which of the following is responsible for the symptoms of dysmenorrhea?

A) Estrogen
B) Human chorionic gonadotropin
C) Prostaglandins
D) Progesterone

475. Which of the following laboratory tests is the next step in working up a 55-year-old diabetic male with the following CBC results: Hgb 11 g/dL, Hct 38%, and an MCV of 102 fL?

A) Serum ferritin and peripheral smear
B) Hemoglobin electrophoresis
C) Serum folate and B12 level
D) Schilling test

476. Auscultation of normal breath sounds of the chest will reveal:

A) Bronchial breath sounds heard at the lower bases
B) High-pitched vesicular breath sounds heard over the upper lobes
C) Vesicular breath sounds heard over the trachea
D) Vesicular breath sounds in the lower lobe

477. The bell of the stethoscope is best used to auscultate which of the following heart sounds?

A) S3 and S4 and low-pitched tones
B) S3 and S4 only
C) S1 and S2 and high-pitched tones
D) S1 and S2 only

478. Vaginal candidiasis is best diagnosed in the primary care arena by the following method:

A) Microscopy
B) Tzanck smear
C) KOH (potassium hydroxide) smear whiff test
D) Clinical findings only

479. When an adolescent male's penis starts to grow in length along with the continued growth of the testicles and the scrotal sac, at which Tanner stage would this male be classified?

A) Tanner Stage I
B) Tanner Stage II
C) Tanner Stage III
D) Tanner Stage IV

480. A teenage male wants to be treated for acne. He has a large number of black and white comedones, especially on the cheeks and chin. The patient has treated himself in the past few months with several types of over-the-counter benzoyl peroxide and salicylic acid products with minimal results. Which of the following agents is the best choice for this patient?

A) Isotretinoin (Accutane) pulse therapy
B) Tetracycline
C) Retin-A 0.25% cream
D) Use a combination of benzoyl peroxide cream and topical vitamin C cream BID

481. The Romberg test is done to check which area of the central nervous system?

A) Frontal lobe
B) Temporal lobe
C) The midbrain
D) The cerebellum

482. All of the following vaccines are contraindicated in pregnant women except:

A) Influenza vaccine injections
B) Mumps
C) Varicella
D) Rubella

483. Females with polycystic ovary syndrome (PCOS) are at higher risk for the following:

A) Heart disease, infertility, uterine cancer, diabetes, and endometrial cancer
B) Fibroids and ovarian cancer
C) Premature menopause and anovulation
D) Oligomenorrhea, ovarian cancer, and cervical cancer

484. Which of the following is the best measure of the size of red blood cells in a sample?

A) Mean corpuscular hemoglobin concentration (MCHC)
B) Mean corpuscular volume (MCV)
C) Red cell distribution width (RDW)
D) Hematocrit

485. A college student who is on oral contraceptives calls the nurse practitioner's office asking for advice. She has forgotten to take her pills 2 days in a row during the second week of the pill cycle. Which of the following is the best advice?

A) Start a new pack of pills and dispose of the old one.
B) Take two pills today, then two pills the next day, and use condoms for the rest of the pill cycle.
C) Stop taking the pills right away and start a new pill cycle and use condoms.
D) Take one pill now and two pills the next day.

486. All of the following patients should be screened for diabetes mellitus except:

A) An obese male of Asian descent
B) An overweight middle-aged African American woman whose mother has type 2 diabetes
C) A woman who delivered an infant weighing 9½ pounds
D) A 30-year-old White female who smokes

487. A middle-aged medical assistant who is overweight complains to the nursing supervisor of a new onset of low back pain in the past 24 hours. She reports lifting some obese patients while working the previous night shift. She is advised to seek follow-up with the hospital's employee health nurse practitioner. Which of the following statements is correct?

A) Medical treatment for any work-related injury is covered under an employer's workers' comp insurance.

B) The injury is not covered by workers' comp because she has health insurance from the hospital.

C) The patient is not allowed to sue her employer for more benefits.

D) Workers' comp insurance premiums are paid by the employees of the hospital.

488. A sexually active 22-year-old man is asking to be screened for hepatitis B (HBV) because his new girlfriend has recently been diagnosed with hepatitis B infection. His laboratory results are the following: anti-HBV is negative, HBsAg is positive, HBeAg is negative. Which of the following is indicated?

A) The patient is immune to the hepatitis B virus

B) The patient is not infected with hepatitis B virus

C) The patient needs hepatitis B vaccine and hepatitis B immune globulin

D) The patient needs only hepatitis B immune globulin

489. A severe case of mitral regurgitation will radiate to which of the following areas?

A) Axilla

B) Neck

C) The middle of the back

D) The throat

490. You would advise a patient who is on a monoamine oxidase inhibitor (MAOI) prescription to avoid the following class of drugs because of an increased potential for neuroleptic syndrome. Which of the following class of drugs can cause this serious condition?

A) Benzodiazepines

B) Selective serotonin reuptake inhibitors (SSRIs)

C) Amphetamines

D) Lithium salts

491. An elderly patient complains of pain in the middle portion of her right buttock that radiates to the thigh. She denies trauma but reports that she has recently moved to a new apartment. The patient has noticed that the pain is worse after she sits for long periods. Which of the following is best described?

A) Sciatica

B) Acute muscle spasm

C) Cauda equina syndrome

D) Acute muscle strain

492. Which bacterium is commonly found to colonize the lungs of patient diagnosed with cystic fibrosis?

A) *Streptococcus pneumoniae*

B) *Chlamydia pneumoniae*

C) *Pseudomonas aeruginosa*

D) *Staphylococcus aureus*

493. Which of the following statements is false regarding physiologic changes in the body as people age?

A) The half-life of drugs is prolonged
B) There is an increase of cholesterol production by the liver
C) There is a mild increase in renal function
D) There is a slight decrease in the activity of the immune system

494. Which of the following cephalosporins is classified as a Category C drug?

A) Ceftriaxone (Rocephin)
B) Clarithromycin (Biaxin)
C) Azithromycin (Zithromax)
D) Cefuroxime axetil (Ceftin)

495. Which of the following is secondary to chronic gastroesophageal reflux disease (GERD) and is considered a precursor to esophageal cancer?

A) Barrett's esophagus
B) Esophageal varices
C) Basal cell metaplasia
D) Wilson's disease

496. Which of the following is recommended as prophylactic treatment for post-herpetic neuralgia?

A) Amitriptyline (Elavil)
B) Sertraline (Zoloft)
C) Naproxen sodium (Naprosyn)
D) Alprazolam (Xanax)

497. Which of the following findings on a thyroid scan may be indicative of a possible malignancy?

A) Simple cyst
B) Complex cyst
C) Cold nodule
D) Hot nodule

498. Carpal tunnel syndrome is inflammation of the:

A) Ulnar nerve
B) Radial nerve
C) Brachial nerve
D) Median nerve

499. Which of the following is found to be a helpful adjunct in the treatment of arthritis?

A) Glucosamine
B) B-complex vitamins
C) Vitamin C
D) Cod liver oil

500. An obese male presents in a primary care clinic complaining of sharp pain in his foot. He reports that he has had this pain for 3 weeks, and that it is worsened by prolonged standing and walking. In the morning, the pain is also worse when getting out of bed. It is located in the medial aspect on the sole of the right foot. Which of the following conditions is most likely?

A) Posterior tibial nerve compression
B) Plantar fasciitis
C) Morton's neuroma
D) Atrophic heel pad

501. Which of the following is recommended as first-line treatment for essential tremor?

A) Propranolol (Inderal)
B) Phenytoin (Dilantin)
C) Amitriptyline (Elavil)
D) Fluoxetine (Prozac)

502. The major difference between quasi-experimental design and experimental design is which of the following?

A) The quasi-experimental design is a type of observational study
B) The quasi-experimental design uses convenience sampling instead of random sampling to recruit subjects
C) The quasi-experimental design is also known as a survey
D) The quasi-experimental design does not have an intervention group

503. A mother brings in her 6-year-old daughter to see the nurse practitioner (NP). She complains that the school nurse found a few nits in her daughter's hair. The mother states that the school has a "no nits" policy regarding head lice and the child cannot go back to school until all the nits have been removed. The child was treated with permethrin shampoo (Nix) twice about 3 months ago. During the physical examination, the NP sees a few nits that are about 2 inches away from the scalp. The child denies itchiness on her scalp. Which of the following is the best action for the NP to take?

A) Prescribe lindane (Kwell) for the child because she may have head lice that are resistant to permethrin
B) Advise the mother to use a nit comb after spraying the child's hair with white distilled vinegar, waiting for 15 minutes, and then rinsing the child's hair
C) Advise the mother to re-treat the girl with permethrin cream instead of shampoo
D) Reassure the mother that the nits will probably drop off after a few weeks

504. What is the pedigree symbol for a diseased male?

A) An empty square
B) An empty circle
C) A filled-in square
D) A filled-in circle

505. A 25-year-old male who was involved in a car accident is brought into the local emergency department. He reports wearing a seatbelt and was the driver of the vehicle. The patient is complaining of pain on his right leg. The skin is intact, but the right foot is abducted slightly. The right knee is tender and swollen. Which of the following tests is/are the best choice for evaluating fractures and joint damage?

A) Plain radiographs of the right hip and knee
B) Ultrasound with a CT scan of the right leg
C) Plain radiograph of the right hip and leg with a magnetic resonance image (MRI) of the knee joint
D) Radiograph of the right hip and knee with special view of the hip

506. Systemic lupus erythematosus (SLE) is more common among the following racial backgrounds except:

A) African Americans
B) Asians
C) Hispanics
D) Mediterraneans

507. Which of the following physical examination findings is most specific for systemic lupus erythematosus (SLE)?

A) Swollen and painful joint involvement
B) Fatigue and myalgia
C) Stiffness and swelling of multiple joints
D) Malar rash

508. An older male is diagnosed with conductive hearing loss in the left ear by the nurse practitioner. Which of the following is the expected result on this patient when performing a Rinne test?

A) AC (air conduction) > BC (bone conduction)
B) Lateralization to the bad ear
C) BC > AC
D) Lateralization to the good ear

509. A physician is referring one of his patients to a nurse practitioner. What type of relationship will exist between the physician and nurse practitioner?

A) Consultative
B) Collaborative
C) Professional
D) Advocate

510. A homeless 47-year-old male with a history of injection drug use (IDU) and alcohol abuse presents to the public health clinic with a recent history of fever, night sweats, fatigue, and weakness. The patient has recently noticed some thin red streaks on his nailbed and red bumps on some of his fingers that hurt. During the cardiac examination, the nurse practitioner hears a Grade 3/6 murmur over the mitral area. The subcutaneous red-purple nodules are tender to palpation. The thin red lines on the nailbeds resemble subungual splinter hemorrhages. Which of the following conditions is most likely?

A) Pericarditis
B) Acute bacterial endocarditis
C) Rheumatic fever
D) Viral cardiomyopathy

511. Which of the following anatomic areas is involved with sensorineural hearing loss?

A) Outer ear
B) Middle ear
C) Inner ear
D) Cranial nerve VII

512. A 13-year-old adolescent female is brought in by her mother for a sports physical. The mother reports that the teen's last vaccines were given at the age of 6 years. Which of the following vaccines is recommended by the CDC for this patient?

A) Td and HPV vaccines
B) Tdap, MCV4, and the HPV vaccines
C) Tdap and the flu vaccine
D) DT and MCV4 vaccines

513. An 87-year-old male reports to the nurse practitioner that his grandson locks him in the bedroom when the grandson goes out of the house and sometimes withholds food from him if he does not give the grandson spending money. The patient appears frail, with poor grooming, and has a strong odor of urine on his clothing. Which of the following is the best action for the nurse practitioner to take?

A) Report the patient's grandson for elder abuse to protective health services of the state
B) Call the grandson from the waiting room and educate him about the importance of proper grooming for his grandfather
C) Advise the grandson that if the patient reports the same complaints the next time he is seen by the nurse practitioner, he will be reported for elder abuse to the state authorities
D) Advise the patient that he should call his son as soon as possible

514. A patient with chronic obstructive pulmonary disease (COPD) is referred for pulmonary function testing. Which of the following pulmonary function tests are abnormal in patients with COPD?

A) Reduction of the total lung capacity (TLC) and the residual volume (RV)
B) Complaints of mild to severe dyspnea with hypoxemia
C) Normal forced vital capacity (FVC) with no changes in the FEV1 (forced expiratory volume in 1 second)
D) Reduction of the FEV1 (forced expiratory volume in 1 second) with increase in the TLC (total lung capacity) and RV (residual volume)

515. The nurse practitioner is evaluating a middle-aged female who is complaining of gradual weight gain, lack of energy, dry hair, and an irregular period during an 8-month period. The routine annual laboratory testing showed the TSH result to be 10 mU/L. The nurse practitioner decides to order a thyroid profile. The TSH is 8.50 mU/L and the serum free T4 is decreased. During physical examination, the patient's BMI is 28. The heart and lung exams are both normal. Which of the following is the best treatment plan to use?

A) Advise the patient that since the TSH level has decreased, she does not have a thyroid problem anymore
B) Start the patient on levothyroxine (Synthroid) 0.25 mcg PO daily
C) Start the patient on Armour thyroid
D) Refer the patient to an endocrinologist

516. A 75-year-old patient has a history of benign prostatic hypertrophy (BPH). During physical examination, which of the following clinical findings during the prostatic exam is correct?

A) Prostate feels firm and uniformly enlarged
B) Prostate feels boggy and enlarged
C) Prostate feels harder than normal
D) Presence of tender nodules

517. A 55-year-old nurse brings her mother, who is 82 years of age, to the emergency department of a local hospital. She reports that she found her mother on the floor when she checked on her mother that morning. Her mother was awake and oriented, but needed help getting up. Her mother states that she thinks that she passed out. She is being evaluated by a physician who orders an electrocardiogram (EKG) and x-rays of both hips. Regarding laboratory testing, which of the following is important to perform initially?

A) Urinalysis
B) Serum electrolytes
C) Blood glucose
D) Hemoglobin and hematocrit

518. All of the following are clinical signs and symptoms seen early in testicular torsion except:

A) Nausea and vomiting
B) Absence of the cremasteric reflex
C) Affected testicle is elevated compared with the normal testicle
D) Affected testicle is swollen and feels cold to touch

519. The research term/symbol that is used to indicate the "total population" in a research study is:

A) The symbol called "n = "
B) The symbol called "N = "
C) The symbol called "p = "
D) The symbol called "P = "

520. A 22-year-old male presents to the urgent care clinic with burns caused by a hot oil spill while frying food. He denies facial involvement, dyspnea, or weakness. During physical examination, the nurse practitioner notices bright red skin with numerous bullae on the right arm and hand and bright red skin on the right thigh and the right lower leg. On a pain scale of 1 to 10, he reports the pain as "8." Based on the Rule of Nines, what is the TBSA of this patient's burns?

A) 36%
B) 27%
C) 18%
D) 9%

521. The atypical antipsychotic drugs have many adverse effects. Which of the following side effects is most likely to be seen in this drug class?

A) Orthostatic hypotension and sedation
B) Malignant hypertension and headache
C) Skin hyperpigmentation and alopecia
D) Severe anxiety and increased appetite

522. A 55-year-old woman who is on a prescription of clindamycin for a dental infection presents to the nurse practitioner with complaints of watery diarrhea for the past 4 days. She complains of abdominal cramping and bloating with diarrheal stools up to 10 times a day. She denies seeing blood or pus in her stool. There is no history of recent travel. The patient has been taking over-the-counter medicine with no relief. The nurse practitioner suspects that the patient has a mild case of *Clostridium difficile* colitis. Which of the following antibiotics is indicated for this infection?

A) Ciprofloxacin (Cipro) 400 mg PO BID × 7 days
B) Metronidazole (Flagyl) 500 mg PO TID × 10 days
C) Levofloxacin (Levaquin) 750 mg PO daily × 7 days
D) Trimethoprim–sulfamethoxazole (Bactrim DS) one tablet PO BID × 10 days

523. A 13-year-old patient has a throat culture that is positive for strep throat. She reports that her younger brother was recently diagnosed with strep throat and treated. The patient has a severe allergy to penicillin and reports that erythromycin makes her very nauseated. Which of the following antibiotics is the best choice?

A) Azithromycin (Zithromax)
B) Cephalexin (Keflex)
C) Cefuroxime axetil (Ceftin)
D) Levofloxacin (Levaquin)

524. All of the following groups are classified as "vulnerable populations" and have additional protections as human subjects except:

A) Prisoners
B) Pregnant women, fetuses, and children
C) Frail elderly
D) Mentally incompetent individuals

525. A 60-year-old female truck driver presents to the outpatient urgent care clinic of a hospital complaining of the worsening of her low-back pain the past few days. She describes the pain as "sharp and burning" and points to the left buttock. She reports that the pain started on the mid-buttock of the left leg and recently started to go down the lateral aspect of the leg toward the top of the foot. During physical examination, the ankle jerk and the knee jerk reflex are 1+ on the affected leg and 2+ on the other leg. The pedal, posterior tibialis, and popliteal pulses are the same on both legs. Which of the following tests should the nurse practitioner consider for this patient?

A) Order both a plain radiograph and computed tomography (CT) scan of the spine as soon as possible
B) Write a prescription for ibuprofen 800 mg PO QID with a muscle relaxant and advise the patient to follow up with her primary care provider within 3 days
C) Refer the patient to an orthopedic surgeon
D) Ordering an imaging study of the spine is premature because the majority of low back pain resolves within 10 to 12 weeks

526. A 70-year-old woman complains of left lower quadrant abdominal pain and fever for 2 days. Her blood pressure is 130/80, pulse 90 per minute, respirations 14 per minute, and temperature 100.5°F. During the abdominal exam, the left lower quadrant of the abdomen is tender to palpation. The NP does not palpate a mass, guarding, or rigidity. Rovsing's sign is negative. Bowel sounds are present in all quadrants. The nurse practitioner is familiar with the patient, who is alert and is asking appropriate questions about her condition. The nurse practitioner suspects that the patient has acute diverticulitis. Which of the following treatment plans is appropriate for this patient?

A) The patient should be referred to the physician as soon as possible
B) The patient has a mild case of acute diverticulitis and can be treated with antibiotics in the outpatient setting with close follow-up
C) This patient has a moderate to severe case of acute diverticulitis and needs to be admitted to the hospital for IV antibiotics
D) Refer the patient to the emergency department as soon as possible

527. What is the name of the physiologically active compound that is derived from soybeans?

A) Isoflavones
B) Estrogen
C) Progesterone
D) Resveratrol

528. All of the following conditions are contraindications for bupropion (Wellbutrin, Zyban) except:

A) Anorexia nervosa and bulimia
B) Seizure disorders
C) Peripheral neuropathy
D) Within 14 days after discontinuation of a monoamine oxidase inhibitor (MAOI)

529. The nurse practitioner is educating a new patient with Raynaud's phenomenon about lifestyle changes that have been found helpful in decreasing exacerbations of the disorder. Which of the lifestyle recommendations is false?

A) Caffeine-containing drinks and foods such as chocolate have been found to be helpful with decreasing the incidence of exacerbations

B) Wear gloves or mittens during cold weather and be careful when handling frozen foods

C) Stop smoking and exercise at least 3 times a week

D) Decrease emotional stress and lifestyle stressors

530. The Health Insurance Portability and Accountability Act (HIPAA) was passed by Congress in 2003. All of the following statements about HIPAA are correct except:

A) It provides federal protections for personal health information

B) It is applicable to all health care providers and payers who bill electronically and transmit health information over the Internet

C) Patients have the right to view their mental health and psychotherapy-related health information

D) It gives patients the right to view and to correct errors in their medical records

531. During the physical examination of a 60-year-old adult, the nurse practitioner performs an abdominal examination. The nurse practitioner is checking the left upper quadrant of the abdomen. During percussion, an area of dullness is noted beneath the lower left ribcage. Which of the following is a true statement regarding the spleen?

A) The spleen is not palpable in the majority of healthy adults

B) The spleen is 8 cm to 10 cm in the left midaxillary line at its longest axis

C) The spleen is 2 cm to 6 cm between the 9th to 11th ribs on the left midaxillary line

D) The splenic size varies depending on the patient's gender

532. All of the following drug classes are approved for treating hypertension. Which of the following antihypertensive drug classes is associated with the largest number of research studies?

A) ACE (angiotensin-converting enzyme) inhibitors

B) Angiotensin receptor blockers (ARBs)

C) Thiazide diuretics

D) Calcium channel blockers (CCBs)

533. When a domestic dog is suspected to be infected with the rabies virus, it can either be killed for a brain biopsy or it can be quarantined. What is the minimum number of days that a dog suspected of rabies must be quarantined?

A) 4 weeks

B) 21 days

C) 14 days

D) 10 days

534. Thiazide diuretics have been shown to have a beneficial effect on the bones. Hypertensive women with osteopenia or osteoporosis benefit from thiazide diuretics. What is the mechanism of action for its effect on the bones?

A) Thiazide diuretics decrease calcium excretion by the kidneys and stimulate osteoclast production

B) Thiazide diuretics increase both calcium and magnesium retention by the kidneys

C) Thiazide diuretics increase bone mineral density (BMD)

D) Thiazide diuretics influence electrolyte excretion by the kidneys

535. What is the best description of a variable?

A) It is an important part of every research study

B) It is the probability that a factor is important for the research data

C) It is the value or number that occurs the most frequently

D) It is a condition, characteristic, or factor that is being measured

536. A 30-year-old male with a history of gout is walking to the examination room and the nurse practitioner notices that he is limping. When the patient sits down, the nurse practitioner notes that the metatarsophalangeal joint of the great toe is very swollen and is bright red. The patient reports that he was attending a party the night before and drank. The patient is requesting a prescription to treat his painful toe. The nurse practitioner prescribes the patient indomethacin (Indocin) 50 mg TID PRN and colchicine. Regarding colchicine, which of the following instructions is correct?

A) Take one pill every 1 hour to every 2 hours until relief is obtained or adverse gastrointestinal effects occur, such as abdominal pain, nausea, or diarrhea

B) Take one pill every hour until relief is obtained up to 24 hours

C) Take one pill every 4 to 6 hours until the pain is relieved

D) Take two to three pills QID until relief is obtained or adverse GI effects occur, such as abdominal pain, nausea, or diarrhea

537. What type of testing is recommended before starting a patient on a prescription of hydroxychloroquine (Plaquenil)?

A) CBC

B) Serum creatinine and urine for microalbumin

C) Liver function tests

D) Comprehensive eye examination

538. A postmenopausal woman's dual-energy x-ray absorption (DXA or DEXA) result shows osteopenia. Which of the following *t*-scores is indicative of osteopenia?

A) *t*-score of −1.0 or higher

B) *t*-score between −1.0 and −2.5

C) *t*-score of less than −2.5

D) *t*-score of −2.50 to −3.50

539. An adult patient who was recently discharged from the hospital was prescribed clindamycin. The patient reports that he took his last dose yesterday. He presents in the primary care clinic with complaints of the recent onset of watery diarrhea from 10 to 15 times a day with abdominal cramping. He denies fever and chills. Which of the following conditions is most likely in this patient?

A) *Clostridium difficile*-associated diarrhea (CDAD)
B) Giardiasis
C) Pseudomembranous colitis
D) Irritable bowel syndrome

540. Which of the following individuals is more likely to be affected by alpha thalassemia anemia?

A) 53-year-old Greek patient
B) 25-year-old Chinese patient
C) 62-year-old Russian patient
D) 38-year-old African American patient

541. What is the significance of a positive Lachman's sign?

A) Instability of the affected knee caused by damage (i.e., rupture) to the anterior cruciate ligament (ACL) of the knee
B) Posterior cruciate ligament laxity that may cause locking of the affected knee
C) Achilles tendon rupture
D) Patellar tendon rupture

542. A positive Chvostek's sign is associated with:

A) Hypocalcemia
B) Hypernatremia
C) Hypokalemia
D) Hyperkalemia

543. The nurse practitioner calls a patient to discuss the results of routine laboratory tests that are all normal. She calls the patient twice and each time, the answering machine is on. Which of the following is the most appropriate action for the nurse practitioner to take?

A) Since they are all normal, leave the laboratory results on the answering machine
B) When the nurse practitioner is unable to speak with the patient directly, she should leave a message with her name and telephone number and instruct the patient to call back
C) Some clinics have a policy of not calling patients back if their laboratory results are normal
D) It is up to the physician to determine whether a laboratory result can be discussed with a patient on the telephone

544. Which of the following drugs that are used to treat attention deficit hyperactivity disorder (ADHD) is not classified as an amphetamine/stimulant?

A) Dexmethylphenidate (Focalin XR)
B) Mixed salts of amphetamine (Adderall)
C) Methylphenidate (Ritalin)
D) Atomoxetine (Strattera)

545. A 25-year-old male with schizophrenia comes in for a routine annual physical. He is a heavy smoker and has a BMI of 28. The patient has been on olanzapine (Zyprexa) for 10 years. Regarding the patient's prescription, which of the following laboratory tests is recommended for monitoring for adverse effects of atypical antipsychotics?

A) Fasting blood glucose, fasting lipid profile, and weight
B) Urinalysis, serum creatinine, 24-hour urine test for protein and creatinine clearance
C) Liver function tests only
D) Complete blood count (CBC) with differential, liver function tests, weight

546. Native Americans view illness or disease as being caused by which of the following?

A) Poor blood circulation in the body
B) A punishment by the "spirits" for wrongful actions against others or for failure to follow spiritual rules
C) An imbalance of the flow of energy in the body
D) An imbalance of the hot and cold energy forces in the body

547. A 74-year-old man presents with recurrent abdominal cramping associated with diarrhea that occurs from four to five times per day. He reports that currently he is having an exacerbation. The stools are bloody with mucus and pus. The patient reports that he has lost a little weight and is always fatigued. The patient denies recent travel or outdoor camping. Which of the following conditions is most likely?

A) Giardiasis
B) Irritable bowel syndrome (IBS)
C) Diverticulitis
D) Ulcerative colitis

548. A middle-aged male who is homeless reports to the local public health clinic complaining of a painless and shallow ulcer on the penile shaft for the past 2 weeks. He is sexually active and had unprotected intercourse with two male partners over the past few months. The patient is tested for HIV, syphilis, gonorrhea, hepatitis B, and herpes types 1 and 2. The syphilis and HIV tests are both positive. The gonorrhea, hepatitis B, and herpes test are negative. The nurse practitioner is aware of the Nationally Notifiable Infectious Conditions. Which of the following must be done regarding reporting of sexually transmitted infections?

A) Obtain the patient's permission before reporting the positive HIV and syphilis test results to the local public health department
B) Obtain the patient's and sexual partner's permission before reporting the positive test results to the local health department

C) Health care providers are mandated by law to report certain types of diseases to the local health department even if the patient does not give permission

D) The nurse practitioner should consult with the supervising physician about this issue

549. A medical assistant is calling out the names of patients who are in the waiting room. The medical assistant is following the HIPAA Privacy Rule if she performs which of the following actions?

A) Calls patients by their full names to show respect
B) Calls patients by their last names or surnames
C) If the patient prefers to be called by a nickname, uses that name to call him/her inside
D) Calls patients by using their first names only

550. A 14-year-old female with amenorrhea is tested for pregnancy and has a positive result. The patient tells the NP that she is seriously considering terminating the pregnancy. She tells the NP that she wants to be referred to a Planned Parenthood clinic. The NP's personal beliefs and religious beliefs are pro-life. Which of the following is the best plan for the NP to follow?

A) The nurse practitioner should tell the patient about her personal beliefs and advise the patient against getting an abortion
B) The NP advises the patient that an NP peer who is working with her can help answer her questions more thoroughly
C) The NP should excuse herself from the case
D) The nurse practitioner should refer the patient to an obstetrician

551. A 22-year-old female is going on a 5-day cruise for her honeymoon. She reports a history of severe motion sickness. Which of the following medicines can be prescribed for motion sickness?

A) Dimenhydrinate (Dramamine)
B) Metoclopramide (Reglan)
C) Odansetron (Zofran)
D) Scopolamine patch (Transderm Scop)

552. Which of the following is considered a spiritual illness by Latinos/Hispanics that can cause symptoms such as loss of appetite, crying, diarrhea, and weakness or death among infants and small children?

A) Mal ojo or mal de ojo
B) Chronic nightmares
C) Trabajo
D) Malo

553. A 45-year-old man fell asleep while smoking in his bedroom and started a fire. According to the patient, he refused to go to the emergency department because he had only minor burns. About 12 hours later, he presents to a walk-in urgent care center complaining of a new cough that is productive of saliva

with clear mucus with small carbonaceous black particles. The brows appear singed. Which of the following is the priority when evaluating this patient?

A) Perform a medical history, including prescription, OTC, and herbal medicines
B) Assess the patient for respiratory distress
C) Evaluate the patient for asthma and atopy
D) Use the Rule of Nines to evaluate the total body surface area (TBSA)

554. Which of the following benzodiazepines has the shortest half-life?

A) Lorazepam (Ativan)
B) Alprazolam (Xanax)
C) Triazolam (Halcion)
D) Clonazepam (Klonopin)

555. Multiple myeloma is a malignancy of the:

A) White blood cells (WBCs)
B) Red blood cells (RBCs)
C) Plasma cells
D) Platelets

556. In addition to surgical repair of a compound fracture that has broken through the skin, which of the following treatment plans is important to consider in this patient?

A) Application of a topical antibiotic BID until the wound is healed
B) Wound irrigation
C) Tdap vaccine
D) Tetanus vaccine and systemic antibiotics

557. A 62-year-old male with chronic obstructive pulmonary disease (COPD) complains to the nurse practitioner that his prescription of ipratropium bromide (Atrovent) is not working. He reports that he still feels short of breath even after using it four times a day for 3 months. Which of the following actions is the next step for the nurse practitioner to take?

A) Increase the patient's dose of ipratropium bromide (Atrovent) to 3 inhalations QID (four times a day)
B) Continue the ipratropium bromide and start the patient on oxygen by nasal cannula
C) Continue ipratropium bromide (Atrovent) and add an albuterol (Ventolin) inhaler two inhalations QID
D) Start the patient on oxygen by nasal cannula at bedtime and PRN (as needed) in the daytime

558. A coworker calls you, the nurse practitioner, and wants to know about a patient's progress. She tells you that they are neighbors and she is worried about the patient's health status. The coworker works in the same facility, but is not directly involved with this patient's care. Which of the following actions is the most appropriate?

A) Share with the coworker the patient's health status
B) Advise the coworker to call the patient right away and ask her for verbal permission

C) Inform the coworker that you cannot release any information about this patient because she is not directly involved in the patient's care

D) Reassure the coworker that the patient is doing fine and is getting better quickly

559. What is the name of the immune process that is responsible for anaphylactic reactions?

A) IgE-mediated reaction
B) Serious allergic reaction
C) Antibody reaction
D) Atopic reaction

560. A 76-year-old woman reports that for the previous 4 months she has noticed severe stiffness and aching in her neck and both shoulders and hips that is worsened by movement. She reports having a difficult time getting out of bed because of the severe stiffness and pain. It is difficult for her to put on a jacket or blouse or to fasten her bra. Along with these symptoms, she also has a low-grade fever, fatigue, loss of appetite, and weight loss. Starting yesterday, the vision in her right eye has progressively worsened. She has annual eye examinations and denies that she has glaucoma. Which of the following conditions is most likely?

A) Rheumatoid arthritis (RA)
B) Degenerative joint disease
C) Polymyalgia rheumatica (PMR)
D) Fibromyalgia

561. The most important job of an institutional review board (IRB) is:

A) Protecting the interests of the hospital or the research institution
B) Protecting the rights of the human subjects who participate in research done at their institution
C) Protecting the researcher and research team from lawsuits
D) Evaluating research protocols and methodology for appropriateness and safety

562. What is the most common cause of infertility among women in the United States?

A) Scarring of the fallopian tubes due to a history of pelvic inflammatory disease (PID)
B) Ovulation disorders
C) Age older than 35 years
D) Endometriosis

563. A 35-year-old male presents complaining of the acute onset of episodes of dizziness with nausea that started a few days after he got over a cold. The patient describes it as the sensation of the room moving or of the room spinning. It is worsened by sudden head movement. During the episodes, he gets very nauseated. He also has tinnitus with hearing loss on his right ear. The patient is a type 2 diabetic and is on a prescription of metformin 500 mg PO BID and an ACE inhibitor. The

blood glucose during the visit is 80 mg/dL. Which of the following conditions is most likely?

A) Vasovagal presyncopal episode
B) Meniere's disease
C) Atypical migraine
D) Hypoglycemia

564. All of the following physiologic changes are present in the lungs of the elderly except:

A) Decrease in the forced expiratory volume (FEV1)
B) Slight increase in the residual volume (RV)
C) Increase in lung compliance
D) Airways tend to collapse earlier (than young patients) with shallow breathing

565. A 50-year-old woman of Irish descent presents with history of lethargy, feeling weak, nausea, anorexia with diarrhea, and abdominal pain. The woman's skin appears tanned, but she denies prolonged sun exposure. During physical examination, the skin appears tanned with hyperpigmentation of the nipple area, on the gums, and on the lips. The electrolyte panel reveals hyperkalemia and hyponatremia. She reports craving salty foods. Which of the following is most likely?

A) Addison's disease
B) Cushing's disease
C) Metabolic syndrome
D) Cutaneous drug reaction

566. An adult female presents with complaints of "bad burns" that are very painful. A large pot of hot boiling water tipped over and spilled on her arms and her anterior chest and abdomen. During physical examination, the nurse practitioner notices bright red skin with numerous bullae on the left arm and hand and large patches of bright red skin on the anterior chest and abdominal area. On a pain scale of 1 to 10, she reports the pain as "9." Her vital signs are stable with tachycardia (pulse is 100 per minute). She does not appear to be in shock. Using the Rule of Nines, what is the total body surface area (TBSA) and the depth of the burns in this patient?

A) The patient has a TBSA of 15% with full-thickness burns of the left arm and left hand, and partial-thickness burns of the anterior chest and abdominal area
B) The patient has a TBSA of 20% with partial-thickness burns on the left arm, left hand, and mild burns on the anterior chest and abdominal area
C) The patient has a TBSA of 27% with partial-thickness burns on the left arm and left hand with superficial burns on the anterior chest and abdominal area
D) The patient has a TBSA of 18% with full-thickness burns of the left arm and left hand, and superficial burns on the anterior chest

567. Some nurse practitioners bill directly for their services. Regarding reimbursement, who is considered the third-party payer?

A) The patient
B) The health care provider
C) The health insurance companies, health plans, Medicare and Medicaid
D) The federal government

568. A 14-year-old is brought in by his mother, who reports that her child has been complaining for several months of recurrent bloating, stomach upset, and occasional loose stools. She reports that her son has difficulty gaining weight and is short for his age. She has noticed that his symptoms are worse after eating large amounts of crackers, cookies, and breads. She denies seeing blood in the child's stool. Which of the following conditions is most likely?

A) Amebiasis
B) Malabsorption
C) Crohn's colitis
D) Celiac disease

569. Which of the following pharmacologic agents is the best choice for an elderly patient with insomnia?

A) Diazepam (Valium)
B) Zolpidem (Ambien)
C) Temazepam (Restoril)
D) Diphenhydramine (Benadryl)

570. An elderly Hispanic male has been taking finasteride (Proscar) for several months. The nurse practitioner decides to check the prostate-specific antigen (PSA). The PSA result is 10 ng/mL. The patient's baseline PSA was 30 ng/mL. Which of the following is the next step?

A) Add the baseline PSA value to the treatment PSA value
B) The treatment PSA value is the correct value
C) Multiply the treatment PSA value by 2
D) Divide the baseline PSA value by the treatment PSA value

571. An adult patient is being evaluated for tuberculosis infection with a Mantoux test. The PPD (purified protein derivative) result is 10.5 mm. The patient denies weight loss, cough, and night sweats and has a negative chest x-ray. The patient reports that he is in the United States illegally and is fearful about discovery. What is the most appropriate action for the nurse practitioner to take?

A) The patient is an illegal alien/migrant and the nurse practitioner has the legal duty to report the patient to the local State Department responsible for illegal immigrants
B) Health care workers are legally mandated to report illegal immigrants to the state authorities
C) The nurse practitioner should call the state health department and report that the patient has a TB (tuberculosis) infection
D) Nurse practitioners have the ethical duty to provide quality health care to patients

572. Candidal intertrigo is the name for an infection that is caused by the yeast *Candida albicans*. What is the location of this type of *Candida* infection?

A) The scalp
B) The flexor areas of the elbows and the knees
C) The areas of the body where skin rubs together, such as under the breast or in the groin area
D) The hands

573. A nurse practitioner is teaching a 54-year-old woman with stress urinary incontinence about Kegel exercises. The patient is instructed to tighten her pelvic floor muscles for a count of 10 and then to relax them for a count of 10. The nurse practitioner instructs the patient that Kegel exercises should be done consistently every day at what frequency?

   A) Perform 30 exercises each time in the morning and the evening
   B) Perform 20 exercises each time two times a day
   C) Perform 15 exercises each time three to four times a day
   D) Perform 10 exercises each time three times a day

574. A 19-year-old student who is on a prescription of Triphasil is being seen for an annual gynecologic examination in the college health center. The nurse practitioner has obtained the Pap smear and is about to perform the bimanual examination. She gently removes the plastic speculum from the vagina. While performing the bimanual vaginal examination, the patient complains of slight discomfort during deep palpation of the ovaries. Which of the following is a true statement?

   A) The uterus and the ovaries are both very sensitive to any type of palpation
   B) The fallopian tubes and ovaries are not sensitive to light or deep palpation
   C) The ovaries are sensitive to deep palpation but they should not be painful
   D) The uterus and the ovaries are important organs of reproduction

575. All of the following statements about common health beliefs of many traditional Asian cultures are true except:

   A) An imbalance of the hot and cold (yin/yang) vital forces can cause illness, and treating a hot disease with a "cold" treatment (certain foods/herbs) can help to restore balance and cure the illness
   B) If the patient is very ill or dying, immediate family and extended family members will visit the patient daily in "shifts" to provide emotional support
   C) Babies and small children may wear an amulet such as a red string on the wrist or a piece of cloth on the neck or the wrist
   D) Surgical procedures are regarded as important treatment for many illnesses

576. A 45-year-old gardener is seen as a walk-in patient in a private clinic. He reports stepping on a nail that morning. His last tetanus vaccine was 7 years ago. Which of the following vaccines is recommended?

   A) DTaP
   B) DT
   C) Td
   D) Tdap

577. Acanthosis nigricans is associated with all of the following disorders except:

   A) Obesity
   B) Diabetes
   C) Colon cancer
   D) Tinea versicolor

578. The NP suspects that a middle-aged woman may have systemic lupus erythematosus (SLE). Which of the following laboratory tests is strongly associated with this disease?

    A) Sedimentation rate
    B) C-reactive protein
    C) Antinuclear antibody (ANA)
    D) SLE

579. An elderly Hmong, who is from Thailand, is seen by the nurse practitioner for a follow-up visit. He is accompanied by his eldest daughter. The patient presented 6 weeks ago with complaints of the recent onset of morning headaches. The patient was diagnosed with stage 2 hypertension and prescribed hydrochlorothiazide 25-mg tablet once a day. On this visit, Mr. Nguyen tells the nurse practitioner that the new medicine cured the headache and he stopped taking the medicine. What is the best plan to follow during this visit?

    A) Educate the patient about hypertension, how the medicine works on his body, and the importance of taking his pill daily
    B) Reassure the patient that he can resume his prescription medicine again the next morning
    C) Tell the patient that you will lower the dose of the hydrochlorothiazide to 12.5 mg daily
    D) Speak to the patient in a loud voice and confront him about his behavior

580. A 68-year-old woman has recently been diagnosed with polymyalgia rheumatica. The nurse practitioner is discussing the treatment options with the patient. Which of the following medications is the first-line treatment for this condition?

    A) Etanercept (Enbrel)
    B) Oral prednisone
    C) Indomethacin
    D) Methotrexate

581. Which of the following is a true statement regarding the first-pass metabolism process?

    A) Drugs that are administered by intramuscular injection all go through the process of first-pass metabolism
    B) After being swallowed, oral drugs are absorbed by the GI tract and metabolized by the bacteria in the small intestines before being released into the general circulation
    C) Drugs administered through the skin (patches) are metabolized by the dermis of the skin
    D) After a drug is taken by the oral route, it is absorbed in the small intestine and enters the liver through the portal circulation, where it is metabolized before being released into the general circulation

582. The nurse practitioner orders an ankle–brachial index (ABI) test for a patient. Which of the following disorders is the ABI test used for?

   A) Venous insufficiency
   B) Osteoarthritis of the arm or the ankle
   C) Peripheral arterial disease (PAD)
   D) Rheumatoid arthritis

583. A college student is seen as a walk-in appointment in a college health clinic. She complains of the abrupt onset of sore throat, nasal congestion, runny nose, and malaise. Vital signs are a temperature of 99.8°F, pulse 84, and respiratory rate 14 breaths per minute. The physical examination reveals an erythematous throat, swollen nasal turbinates, and rhinitis. The NP suspects viral upper respiratory infection (URI). All of the following treatments are appropriate except:

   A) Saline nasal spray (Ocean nasal spray)
   B) Pseudoephedrine (Sudafed)
   C) Ibuprofen (Advil)
   D) Oral prednisone (Medrol Dose Pack)

584. All of the following foods are best avoided by individuals with celiac sprue except:

   A) Rice cereal
   B) Blueberry muffins
   C) Organic wheat bread
   D) Rye bread

585. Medicare Part A will pay for all of the following services except:

   A) Minor surgery in a walk-in surgical center
   B) Plastic surgery to repair facial damage from a burn
   C) Kidney transplantation
   D) Medical supplies and drugs that are used while the patient is in the hospital

586. A 16-year-old male with a recent history of a cat bite is brought in by his father. The bite occurred about 2 hours before the visit. The nurse practitioner evaluates the wound and notes two small puncture wounds. There is no redness or purulent discharge. The father reports that the teenager received a tetanus booster when he was 12 years old. Which of the following is the correct action to take?

   A) Clean the wound with soap and water and apply topical antibiotic and a Band-Aid
   B) Since the wound is clean and does not appear infected, there is no need for antibiotics
   C) Give the patient a tetanus booster using the Tdap form of the vaccine
   D) Clean the wound with soap and water and prescribe Augmentin 500 mg PO BID × 10 days

587. A 15-year-old White male is brought in by his father for a physical examination. He is concerned that his son is "too short" for his age. The father reports that when he was the same age, he was much taller. His son wants to try out for the football team but the father is concerned because his son might be "too short" to join. Which of the following physical exam findings is worrisome?

    A) Small smooth testicles with no pubic or facial hair
    B) Smooth testicles with rugated scrotum that is a darker color than his normal skin color
    C) Smooth testicles with coarse and curly pubic hair
    D) Straight pubic and axillary hair with a long thin penis

588. Research nomenclature assigns which of the following symbols to indicate a subpopulation or a subgroup within the total population?

    A) The symbol called "n = "
    B) The symbol called "N = "
    C) The symbol called "p = "
    D) The symbol called "P = "

589. An elderly female patient who is a retired nurse has recently been discharged from the hospital. A few days later, she started having random and recurrent episodes of dizziness, but denies passing out. The patient describes the sensation of the room spinning or moving, which is worsened by sudden head movement. During the episodes, she gets very nauseated and sometimes vomits. The patient reports that she was given IV antibiotics and one of them was tobramycin. Which of the following medications would be helpful in treating her symptom of dizziness?

    A) Scopolamine patch (Transderm Scop)
    B) Meclizine (Antivert)
    C) Dimenhydrinate (Dramamine)
    D) Duloxetine (Cymbalta)

590. A 17-year-old high school student is considering her birth control options. She wants to know more about Seasonale. Which of the following statements is false?

    A) Taking Seasonale results in only four periods per year
    B) Her period will occur within the 7 days when she is on the inert pills
    C) It is a progesterone-only method of birth control and does not contain estrogen
    D) Take one tablet daily for 84 consecutive days followed by 7 days of inert pills

591. Which of the following diseases is associated with a high risk of giant cell arteritis?

    A) History of transient ischemic attacks (TIAs)
    B) Frequent migraine headaches with focal neurologic findings
    C) Polymyalgia rheumatica (PMR)
    D) Systemic lupus erythematosus (SLE)

592. Which of the following is a good example of how the "utilitarian" principle is applied?

   A) Helping a patient decide the type of treatment that he/she wants
   B) Using limited societal financial resources on programs that will positively affect the largest number of people possible with the lowest possible negative outcomes
   C) Minimize the bad outcome when choosing treatment choices for a patient
   D) Health caregivers should be more careful when using health care financial resources

593. All of the following clinical findings are classified as major criteria that are necessary to diagnose pelvic inflammatory disease (PID). Which of the following is classified as minor criteria?

   A) Cervical motion tenderness
   B) Adnexal tenderness
   C) Uterine tenderness
   D) Oral temperature of more than 101°F (more than 38°C)

594. What structure of the eye is responsible for 20/20 vision (sharpest vision)?

   A) Rods
   B) Cones
   C) Optic disc
   D) Fovea of the macula

595. A nurse practitioner, who is a recent graduate, is asking an experienced nurse practitioner's opinion about managing one of her patients who has multiple health problems. What type of relationship exists between the nurse practitioners?

   A) Collaborative relationship
   B) Consultative relationship
   C) Referral relationship
   D) Formal relationship

596. A 15-year-old female who attends a public school is referred to the nurse practitioner by one of her teachers. The teen has been missing school and is falling behind in her schoolwork. After closing the exam room door, the nurse practitioner starts to interview the teen. She is asking about her moods, her appetite, her sleep, about whether she has any plan of hurting herself or others, and other questions. What is the level of health prevention that the nurse practitioner is performing?

   A) Primary prevention
   B) Secondary prevention
   C) Tertiary prevention
   D) Dropout prevention program

597. All of the following signs and symptoms are present with an anticholinergic drug overdose except:

    A) Dilated pupils
    B) Flushing and tachycardia
    C) Hypertension
    D) Confusion

598. A woman who is in the third trimester of pregnancy presents to the nurse practitioner for a physical examination. During the physical examination, the nurse practitioner finds all of the following cardiac changes associated with pregnancy except:

    A) Systolic ejection murmur
    B) Diastolic murmur
    C) Displaced apical impulse
    D) Louder S1 and S2

599. An 80-year-old male with hypertension and hyperlipidemia presents with complaints of the quick onset of severe low-back pain that is accompanied by abdominal pain that is gradually worsening. The patient appears pale and complains that he does not feel well. During abdominal examination, the nurse practitioner detects a soft pulsatile mass just above the umbilicus as she palpates this area with her hand. Which of the following conditions is most likely?

    A) Abdominal aortic aneurysm
    B) Cauda equina syndrome
    C) Acute diverticulitis
    D) Adenocarcinoma of the colon

600. What is the pedigree symbol for a diseased or affected female?

    A) An empty square
    B) An empty circle
    C) A filled-in square
    D) A filled-in circle

601. The gold standard test for visualizing a torn meniscus or joint abnormalities is the:

    A) Computed tomography (CT) scan
    B) Magnetic resonance imaging (MRI) scan
    C) X-ray with special views of the affected knee
    D) Lachman's maneuver

602. What is the best description of Cullen's sign?

    A) The onset of hyperactive bowel sound before the onset of ileus
    B) A reddish-purple discoloration that is located on the flank area
    C) A bluish discoloration or bruising that is located on the umbilical area
    D) The acute onset subcutaneous bleeding seen during acute pancreatitis

603. Glucosamine sulfate is a natural supplement that is used for which of the following conditions?

A) Rheumatoid arthritis
B) Osteoarthritis
C) Osteoporosis
D) Metabolic syndrome

604. A charitable foundation plans to build a community youth center in a large urban area with a history of gang violence. What type of health prevention activity is being done in this area?

A) Primary prevention
B) Secondary prevention
C) Tertiary prevention
D) Health prevention

605. The Bacille-Calmette-Guérin (BCG) vaccine is used to immunize a person against which of the following?

A) Enterobiasis
B) Tuberculosis
C) Anthrax
D) Smallpox

606. A 13-year-old girl is brought in by the mother because her daughter is complaining of vaginal discharge and pain. The mother tells the nurse practitioner that her daughter is not sexually active yet. The mother is divorced and lives with her boyfriend and works full time. During the examination, the nurse practitioner notes that the vaginal introitus is red, with tears and a torn hymen. The cervix is covered with green discharge. The nurse practitioner suspects that the child has been sexually abused by the mother's boyfriend. What is the best action for the nurse practitioner to take?

A) Ask the mother questions about her boyfriend's behaviors
B) Advise the mother to watch how her boyfriend interacts with her daughter and to call within 1 week to discuss his behavior with her
C) Advise the mother that you suspect that her daughter has been sexually abused and that you are legally required to report the case to the child protection program
D) Report the child abuse to the local police department

607. A 75-year-old woman presents complaining of a soft lump on her abdomen that is located on the periumbilical area. She tells the nurse practitioner that she does not know how long she has had the lump or whether it has changed in size or shape. She denies abdominal pain, problems with defecation, loss of appetite, weight loss, or trauma. When performing an abdominal exam, what is the best method to differentiate between an abdominal wall mass from an intra-abdominal mass?

A) Palpate the abdominal wall while the patient is relaxed
B) Instruct the patient to lift her head off the table while tensing her abdominal muscles to visualize any masses and then palpate the abdominal wall

C) Instruct the patient to lie still for few seconds while palpating the abdominal wall

D) Palpate the abdomen deeply, then release the palpating hand quickly

608. Which of the following structures of the eyes is responsible for color vision?

A) Rods
B) Macula
C) Cones
D) Pupils

609. A new patient is being interviewed by the nurse practitioner. The patient reports that she had a gastrectomy procedure 5 years ago to treat severe obesity. Currently, her BMI is 25 and the patient denies complications from the procedure. The nurse practitioner is aware that the patient is at higher risk for which of the following disorders?

A) Folate-deficiency anemia
B) B12-deficiency anemia
C) Iron-deficiency anemia
D) Normocytic anemia

610. What is the most common type of skin cancer?

A) Basal cell skin cancer
B) Squamous skin cancer
C) Melanoma
D) Actinic keratoses

611. What is the median?

A) It is the number that occurs the most frequently
B) It is the middle number in a group of numbers
C) It is the average number in a group of numbers
D) It a measure of central tendency

612. Grey–Turner's sign is highly suggestive for which of the following conditions?

A) Acute pancreatitis
B) Acute appendicitis
C) Acute diverticulitis
D) Gastric cancer

613. A nurse practitioner is writing a referral for a middle-aged diabetic who has an A1c of 8.5% despite being on three antidiabetic medications. She is referring the patient to an endocrinologist. What type of relationship exists between the nurse practitioner and the endocrinologist?

A) Consultative relationship
B) Collaborative relationship
C) Referral relationship
D) Formal relationship

614. Which bacterium is the most common pathogen seen in otitis externa infections?

A) *Pseudomonas aeruginosa*
B) *Streptococcus pyogenes*
C) *Haemophilus influenza*
D) *Moraxella catarrhalis*

615. The Patient Protection and Affordable Care Act is President Obama's plan for national insurance coverage. All of the following are true statements about this law except:

A) Preexisting health conditions will be covered immediately
B) The health plan will start to be effective in the year 2013
C) Young adults up to the age of 26 years who live with their parents will be covered under their parents' health insurance plan
D) The health insurance plan mandates will fine employers who choose not to participate in the national health insurance plan

616. The following are considered instrumental activities of daily living (IADLs) except:

A) Grocery shopping
B) Managing one's finances
C) Grooming and hygiene
D) Using a telephone and a computer

617. The Rinne and the Weber tests are used to assess which of the following cranial nerve(s)?

A) CN III, IV, and VI
B) CN II
C) CN VIII
D) CN IX and X

618. A 68-year-old woman complains of leaking a small amount of urine whenever she sneezes, laughs, and/or strains. The problem has been present for many months. The patient denies dysuria, frequency, and nocturia. The urine dipstick test is negative for white blood cells, red blood cells, ketones, and urobilinogen. What is the name of this condition?

A) Urge incontinence
B) Overflow incontinence
C) Urinary incontinence
D) Stress incontinence

619. Medicare Part D will reimburse for which of the following services?

A) Preventive health care such as routine Pap smears and physical examinations
B) Prescription drugs
C) Alcohol misuse/abuse counseling
D) Over-the-counter drugs and vitamins

620. A 35-year-old woman is complaining of gradual weight gain, lack of energy, and amenorrhea. The urine pregnancy test is negative. The CBC shows a hemoglobin of 13.5 g and MCV 84. The nurse practitioner suspects that the patient may have hypothyroidism. The TSH is 10 mU/L. Which of the following is the next step in the evaluation?

A) Check the thyroid profile
B) Check the total T3 and T4 levels
C) Check for anti-thyroid peroxidase antibodies
D) Recheck the TSH in 4 to 6 months.

621. During a routine physical examination on an 82-year-old, the nurse practitioner palpates an irregular mass on midabdomen that is not tender and is about 2 cm in size. Which of the following is the best initial imaging test to further evaluate the abdominal mass?

A) CT scan of the abdomen
B) KUB study
C) Abdominal ultrasound
D) MRI of the abdomen

622. A research participant tells the nurse practitioner that he wants to withdraw from the study. Regarding this case, the nurse practitioner is aware that all research study consent forms should contain which of the following information?

A) The patient's demographic information
B) The possible risks from the study
C) Information that a research subject can voluntarily withdraw from the study at any time without any penalties or adverse consequences
D) The benefits from the study

623. All of the following factors are associated with a higher risk of osteopenia and osteoporosis except:

A) Excessive alcohol intake and cigarette smoking
B) Asian or Caucasian ancestry
C) Estrogen and progesterone deficiency
D) Older age

624. A skilled nursing facility (SNF) can provide all of the following except:

A) Physical therapy and other types of rehabilitation
B) Skilled nursing care and medical care
C) Reimbursement by Medicare
D) Provision of custodial care

625. All of the following are classified as activities of daily living (ADLs) except:

A) Ability to feed self (self-feeding)
B) Ability to manage bladder and bowel elimination
C) Personal hygiene and grooming
D) Grocery shopping

626. Positive psoas and obturator signs are highly suggestive of which of the following conditions?

A) Ectopic pregnancy
B) Acute appendicitis
C) Peritonitis
D) Abdominal aortic aneurysm

627. All of the following are true statements about sexuality in the older adult except:

A) Erectile dysfunction is very common
B) It may take longer to become aroused
C) Frail elderly are not interested in sexuality anymore
D) Dyspareunia is a common symptom of atrophic vaginitis

628. Which of the following drugs is most likely to cause sexual dysfunction in males?

A) SSRIs
B) ACE inhibitors
C) Amphetamines
D) Atypical antidepressants

629. Which of the following drugs is classified as a 5-alpha reductase inhibitor?

A) Terazosin (Hytrin)
B) Tamsulosin (Flomax)
C) Finasteride (Proscar)
D) Sildenafil (Viagra)

30

Answers With Rationale

1. **B) DeQuervain's tenosynovitis** De Quervain's tenosynotivits is a painful inflammation of the tendons on the thumb side of the wrist. There is usually discomfort every time the wrist is turned, grasping, or making a fist. The cause is unknown but occurs with repetitive hand or wrist movement.

2. **C) Even though the nurse practitioner is no longer insured by the same insurance company, any claims made against her on the dates that her malpractice insurance was active are still eligible for coverage** If a professional desires to change insurance companies, often the new insurer will take over the predecessor insurance company's responsibilities by writing its policy retroactively over the previous insurer. It picks up the retroactive date, the first date of coverage offered by the previous insurer, and charges a premium based on the number of previous years of coverage needed.

3. **A) It is the average blood glucose level during the previous 3 months** Glucose reacts with hemoglobin to form glycosylated hemoglobin. The lifespan of the red blood cell is 120 days. The HbA1c level is proportional to the average blood glucose concentration over the previous 4 weeks to 3 months.

4. **B) No endocarditis prophylaxis is indicated for any procedures** The current American Heart Association guidelines (2007) do not recommend endocarditis prophylaxis for most patients with aortic or mitral valve disease, including those with mitral valve prolapse or for patients with hypertrophic cardiomyopathy.

5. **C) Nursing home care** Medicare.gov website: Medicare Part A covers: inpatient care in hospitals, inpatient rehabilitation facilities, and long-term care hospitals. Hospice care services, home health care services and inpatient care in a religious nonmedical health care institution. It also covers inpatient care in a skilled nursing facility (not a custodial or long-term care facility).

6. **B) Acute appendicitis** Suspected ruptured appendix or a pelvic abscess irritates the lateral iliopsoas and obturator muscles. The patient should be in the supine position for testing. The iliopsoas muscle test is performed by the patient raising the leg from the hip while the examiner pushes downward against it. The obturator muscle test is performed with the right leg flexed at the hip and the knee at 90 degrees; the examiner rotates the leg laterally and medially. These muscle tests are positive if the patient experiences pain.

7. **B) It is an increase in the blood glucose level early in the morning due to the physiologic spike of growth hormone** The Dawn phenomenon is the end result of a combination of natural body changes that occur during the sleep cycle. Between 3 a.m. and 8 a.m., the body starts to increase the amounts of counter-regulatory hormones. Including growth hormone, cortisol, and catecholamines. These hormones work against insulin's action to drop blood sugars.

8. **B) Meningococcemia** Children and adolescents aged 5 to 19 years are at highest risk. The average incubation period for meningococcemia is 3 to 7 days (range of 1 to 10 days). Initial signs and symptoms include fatigue, fever, headache, and body aches. A rash appears as petechiae associated with low platelets and skin purpura associated with vasculitis. The rash may appear anywhere on the body, including the palms, soles, or inside the mouth. Symptoms of shock (low BP, tachycardia) are noted on physicial exam. A stiff neck (nuchal rigidity) is a sign associated with meningitis.

9. **B) *Mycoplasma* pneumonia** Pneumonia is suspected when abnormal sounds are auscultated in the lungs. The diagnosis is confirmed by x-ray. Cough, sputum production, fever, and pain on inspiration are also classic with pneumonia. A culture of the sputum is used to differentiate bacteria or fungi. *Mycoplasma pneumoniae* causes a slowly developing infection (vs. streptococcal pneumonia's abrupt onset with shaking chills/fever and rust-colored sputum).

10. **C) Beta-blockers** Beta-blockers can narrow bronchial airways and constrict blood vessels. Patients with asthma, emphysema, and chronic bronchitis should avoid beta-blockers if possible. Beta-blockers are the "-lol" drugs (propranolol, acebutolol, atenolol, metoprolol, nadolol, penbutolol, carvedilol, timolol, betaxolol, carteolol, pindolol).

11. **C) Administer an injection of epinephrine 1:1,000 intramuscularly immediately** Anaphylaxis is a medical emergency that requires immediate intervention. Prompt IM injection of epinephrine is the first-line medication. Anaphylaxis typically occurs through an IgE-dependent immunologic mechanism triggered by foods, stinging insects, or medications such as beta-blockers and ACE inhibitors. People with a history of allergies, asthma, or eczema are at greater risk than other people.

12. **B) Testicular torsion** The cremasteric reflex is tested by stroking the inner thigh (proximal to distal) with a blunt instrument such as a handle of the reflex hammer. The testicle and scrotum should rise on the stroked side. Testicular torsion is the twisting of the spermatic cord, which cuts off the blood supply to the testicle and surrounding structures within the scrotum.

13. **A) Spoon-shaped nails and pica** Symptoms of *iron-deficiency anemia* include tiredness, lethargy, shortness of breath, palpitations; less common symptoms include a smooth tongue (atrophic glosssitis), altered sense of taste, pica (desire to eat non-food items), and spoon-shaped nails (koilonychia).

14. **B) Check the patient's blood glucose** 4+ ketones in the urine indicates severe hyperglycemia, so the nurse should further assess the patient's status.

15. **D) Supplementing with fiber such as psyllium (Metamucil) is never recommended**   Diverticular disease increases with age (over 60 years). The dominant theory is that a low-fiber diet causes diverticular disease. The ingestion of psyllium (soluble fiber) helps prevent constipation. The American Dietetic Association recommends an intake of 20–35 grams of fiber per day. During a flare-up of diverticulitis, a low-fiber diet is recommended and fiber supplementation is not recommended.

16. **B) *Chlamydia trachomatis***   Physiologic factors related to cervical ectopy and columnar epithelium increases susceptibility to STIs. Coinfection with gonorrhea and chlamydia is extremely common; in fact, the CDC reports gonorrhea and chlamydia as the two most commonly reported infectious diseases in the United States.

17. **A) Educate the patient about Kegel exercises**   Stress and urge incontinence are caused by the relaxation/ loss of tone and ligaments of the pelvic floor that support the bladder, uterus, urethra, lower bowel, and vagina. Pelvic floor muscle-strengthening exercises are known as Kegel exercises. Kegels are performed by repeated contracting, holding, and relaxing of the pubococcygeus muscle (the muscle band of the perineal area).

18. **B) Higher than normal**   Alkaline phosphatase is a group of related enzymes. The bone form of the enzyme creates the alkaline conditions it requires to be most active with a chemical reaction involving the osteoblasts. Because of the rapid bone growth and increased depositing of calcium, there is a higher level.

19. **A) Calcium channel blockers**   Calcium metabolism has been reported in hypertension. The effect of hypertension is a modification of bone mass and bone quality. One factor is increased parathyroid hormone (PTH) serum levels. Calcium channel blockers decrease PTH and increase calcitonin levels; both are beneficial in stopping bone loss in osteoporosis.

20. **A) Instability of the knee due to anterior cruciate ligament damage**   The Lachman test is used to evaluate the motion of anterior translation (laxity) of the ACL. The maneuver should be tested on BOTH knees to compare the injured and the opposite knee to evaluate normal translation. Perform by bending the knee 30 degrees. Stabilize the femur with one hand and the other under the proximal tibia at the level of the joint line and then pull forward. The laxity is graded on a 0 (normal) to 3 scale (1.0–1.5 cm of translation).

21. **B) Tanner Stage III**   Tanner Stage III: The testicular volume increases, the scrotum enlarges, and the penis begins to lengthen. *Tanner stages*: Tanner I: Prepubertal small penis. Tanner II: The penis length remains unchanged. Tanner III: Penis begins to lengthen. Tanner IV: Penis increases in length *and* circumference. Tanner V: Adult scrotum and penis.

22. **C) Continue your anticoagulants as prescribed and report any bleeding in the gums and excessive bruising**   To be effective, anticoagulants must be taken exactly as prescribed. Teaching to report signs of bleeding is warranted.

23. **A) Laryngeal cancer** HPV exposure is a risk factor in laryngeal cancer. The human papilloma virus (HPV) DNA transforms the moist membranes of epithelial cells (cervix, anus, mouth, and throat). Juvenile type is r/t vertical transmission and the adult type is r/t orogenital contact. Subtype 16 HPV accounts for the majority of oral tumors, oropharynx cancers, and laryngeal cases.

24. **C) Osteoarthritis** Signs of osteoarthritis (OA) include stiffness of joints, especially in the morning and after sitting for long periods. Visible signs of OA are an element in the diagnosis. (RA and gout often rely more heavily on lab tests.) Heberden nodes (bony overgrowths) are classic signs of OA. They are located at the distal interphalangeal joints. They are felt as hard, nontender nodules usually 2–3 cm in diameter but sometimes encompassing the entire joint. Enlargement of the middle joint of a finger is called a Bouchard's node.

25. **B) Instability of the knee** The drawer test is used to identify mediolateral or anteroposterior plane instability of the knee. The test is performed on the unaffected and affected knee for comparison. The anterior drawer test evaluates the ACL. To perform the test, the patient lies supine and the knee is placed at 90-degree flexion. Grasp the posterior aspect of the tibia over the upper calf muscle; then, with a steady force, try to push the lower leg forward and backward. Anterior or posterior movement of the knee is positive. With the leg extended, stabilize the femur with one hand and the ankle with the other. Try to abduct and adduct the knee. There should be no medial or lateral movement.

26. **B) The force is being directed away from the body** Valgus stress test is to evaluate ligament damage. For the valgus stress test at 30 degrees, the examiner places the hands over the medial joint line while the other hand holds the foot/ankle. Valgus stress force is then applied laterally (away from the patient's body) to the joint through the foot, while the fingers palpate for an increase in joint line opening.

27. **D) Sexual abstinence** Healthy People 2020 has 4 overarching goals: 1) attain high-quality longer lives free of preventable disease, disability, injury, and premature death; 2) achieve health equity and eliminate disparities; 3) create social and physical environments that promote good health for all; and 4) promote quality of life, healthy development and healthy behaviors across life spans. Sexual abstinence is only 1 specific area for sexual health promotion.

28. **B) Creatinine** Diabetes is associated with cardiovascular and renal disease. A high serum creatinine (CR) level is one indication of kidney damage. Creatinine clearance is used to estimate filtering capacity. The glomerular filtration rate (GFR) is used to evaluate chronic kidney disease (CKD). GFR can be estimated from serum creatinine. The eGFR calculation uses creatinine measurement along with age and values assigned for sex and race. The National Kidney Foundation has determined different stages of CKD based on the value of eGFR.

29. **A) Chronic intake of nonsteroidal analgesics (NSAIDs) can cause the disorder** Inflammatory changes and gastric mucosal erosion are referred to as gastritis. Nonsteroidal anti-inflammatory drugs (NSAIDs) such as aspirin, ibuprofen, and naproxen are the most common agents associated with acute erosive gastritis.

NSAIDs are cycloxygenase-1 (COX-1) inhibitors (which increases the possibility of peptic ulcer formation) and reduce prostaglandin that protects the stomach. Regular use can lead to gastritis.

30. **D) Apraxia**   Apraxia is characterized by loss of the ability to execute or carry out learned purposeful movements despite the desire and the physical ability to perform the movements. Apraxia is not a sign or symptom of depression; it is a disorder of motor planning caused by damage to specific areas of the cerebrum.

31. **A) On deep inspiration by the patient, palpate firmly in the right upper quadrant of the abdomen below the costovertebral angle**   Murphy's sign is tested during an abdominal examination for biliary disorders. As the patient breathes in, the abdominal contents are pushed downward as the diaphragm moves down and the lungs expand. As the patient stops/hold the breath, the gallbladder comes in contact with the examiner's fingers and may elicit pain. To be considered positive, the same maneuver must not elicit pain when performed on the left side. A negative Murphy's test in the elderly is not useful for ruling out cholecystitis if history and other tests suggest the diagnosis.

32. **B) Acetaminophen (Tylenol)**   Acetaminophen is a analgesic that would treat the mother's pain. The other response choices—ibuprofen, naproxen, and aspirin— are all nonsteroidal anti-inflammatory drugs (NSAIDs). During the first trimester, NSAIDs have been associated with a risk of miscarriage. NSAIDs are contraindicated in the third trimester of pregnancy. They may cause premature closure of the fetal ductus arteriosus. Indomethacin (Indocin) is used in pregnancy to treat polyhydramnios by reducing fetal renal urine production via the inhibition of fetal renal blood flow. Indomethacin is also given to neonates whose ductus arteriosus has not closed within 24 hours of birth.

33. **A) Middle-aged to older women**   Hashimoto's thyroiditis or chronic lymphocytic thyroiditis is an autoimmune disease. An enlarged thyroid is most often the first sign of the disease. Hashimoto's disease is about seven times more common in women than in men. It can occur in teens and young women, but is more common in middle age.

34. **C) Severe vaginal atrophic changes**   Vaginal atrophy (atrophic vaginitis) is the thinning and inflammation of the vaginal walls due to a decline in estrogen. Vaginal atrophy occurs most often after menopause (may also decline during breastfeeding). The North American Menopause Society (NAMS) issued a position statement in 2007 about the treatment of vaginal atrophy with local vaginal estrogen.

35. **B) Hepatomegaly, arteriovenous (AV) nicking, bibasilar crackles**   Chronic, poorly managed hypertension damages both arteries and veins. Portal hypertension is abnormally high BP in the branches of the portal vein that brings blood from the intestines to the liver. Hepatomegaly is noted on palpation. Arteriovenous nicking is noted during an ophthalmologic examination when an arteriole is seen crossing the venule, resulting in impaction of the vein with bulging on either side of the crossing. This is most commonly seen with hypertensive retinopathy. Unrelieved pulmonary hypertension can lead to right-sided heart failure. As the heart failure progresses, bibasilar crackles in the lungs may be auscultated.

36. **C) Tinea cruris**   Tinea cruris is an infection of the groin with a dermatophyte fungus. The appearance is similar to ringworm (tinea corporis). Tinea cruris is most often seen in men.

37. **B) Bacterial vaginosis**   Bacterial vaginosis (BV) is characterized by the replacement of the normal hydrogen peroxide-producing *lactobacillus* with an overgrowth of anaerobic bacteria. BV is a vaginosis rather than a vaginitis. No symptoms may be present or the patient's history includes vaginal odor (fishy), increased vaginal discharge (milky white, thin adherent discharge or dark or dull gray discharge), and possible vaginal burning after intercourse. pH > 4.5, positive whiff test, clue cells on wet mount, epithelial cells dotted with large numbers of bacteria that obscure borders and should be more than 20% of clue cells.

38. **A) The NP needs to do cervical cultures to verify the presence of gonorrhea.**   Cultures should be taken at the time of the Pap smear, as the patient may not return for later diagnostic testing.

39. **B) Lichen sclerosus**   Lichen sclerosus often appears after menopause. It is a long-term problem of the skin that mostly affects the vulva and anal areas in women. They appear as small white spots early in the disease and grow into bigger patches. Itching is very common; however, other symptoms include discomfort, bleeding from skin tears, and blisters. A skin biopsy allows for differentiation from other dermatologic conditions.

40. **B) Closure of the semilunar valves**   A heart valve normally allows blood to flow in only one direction. A heart valve opens or closes incumbent upon differential blood pressure on each side. A form of heart disease occurs when a valve malfunctions and allows some blood to flow in the wrong direction. The S2 sound results from reverberation within the blood associated with the sudden block of flow reversal.

41. **A) Lower limb amputations**   Data from the 2011 National Diabetes Fact Sheet notes that more than 60% of nontraumatic lower limb amputation was performed in people with diabetes.

42. **D) Anesthesiologists' services**   Medicare.gov website: Medicare Part A covers anesthesia that is received while in an inpatient hospital. Medicare Part B covers outpatient care, durable medical equipment, home health services, and other medical services, including some preventive services such as mammograms, one every 12 months, for all women with Medicare age 40 and older.

43. **D) A grandmother who has recently been diagnosed with both hypertension and hypothyroidism**   Suicide statistics: Males take their own lives at nearly four times the rate of females. Suicide rates for females are highest between ages 45 and 54. American Indians/Alaska Natives and Hispanic and Blacks have a higher percentage of suicide attempts than their White, non-Hispanic counterparts. Risk factors include environmental risk factors, social/cultural risk factors, and biophysical risk factors, including mental disorders, alcohol and other substance use disorders, and family history of suicide.

44. **D) Subconjunctival hemorrhage** Bright red blood in a sharply defined area surrounded by normal-appearing conjunctiva indicates subconjunctival hemorrhage. The blood stays red because of direct diffusion of oxygen through the conjunctiva. Risk factors include diabetes, hypertension, illnesses that cause severe coughing or sneezing, blood-thinning medications and aspirin, and herbal supplements such as ginkgo.

45. **C) Advise the patient that it is a benign condition and will resolve spontaneously** Subconjunctival hemorrhages do not require any treatment. The blood in the eye will be absorbed within 10–14 days.

46. **A) Urine for culture and sensitivity** The urine for culture and sensitivity would be the first test to order. All presenting symptoms are consistent with a urinary tract infection. Trace amounts of protein are not unusual for a UTI. The patient's type 1 diabetes is negative for ketones, a syptom of dehydration. An IVP may be necessary to rule out a kidney stone.

47. **B) They affect the kidneys and can elevate blood pressure** All nonsteroidal anti-inflammatory drugs (NSAIDs) in doses that are adequate to reduce inflammation and pain can increase blood pressure in both normotensive and hypertensive patients. NSAIDs may also reduce the effect of all antihypertensive drugs except calcium channel blockers. The prohypertensive effect is dose dependent and probably involves the cyclooxygenase-2 (COX-2) in the kidneys, which reduces sodium excretion and increases intravascular volume.

48. **B) Bupropion (Zyban)** Bupropion (Zyban) is utilized to reduce craving for tobacco and to decrease withdrawal symptoms. The mechanism is not entirely known. Bupropion's ability to help stop smoking is not related to its antidepressant action.

49. **B) Tick** Rocky Mountain spotted fever is caused by *Rickettsia rickettsii*, which is carried by ticks. Risk factors include recent hiking or exposure to ticks in areas known to be infested. Bacteria can also infect people who crush ticks they have removed from pets. Symptoms develop around 2–14 days after tick bite: chills, confusion, fever, headache, muscle pain, and rash.

50. **B) It does not have a linear distribution** Atopic dermatitis is a long-term chronic skin disorder that involves scaly and itchy rashes. Skin changes may include: blisters with oozing and crusting, dry skin all over the body or bumpy skin on the back of the arms and front of the thighs, raw areas of the skin from scratching. Thickened or leather-like areas, called lichenification, can occur after long-term irritation and scratching. A skin biopsy can be done to confirm the diagnosis and rule out other causes.

51. **A) Varicella zoster virus infection of the cornea** A reactivation of latent varicella-zoster virus (VZV) results in a localized cutaneous rash erupting in a single dermatome, called herpes zoster (HZ) or shingles. HZ involving the first division of the trigeminal nerve causes herpes zoster ophthalmicus (HZO). HZO accounts for 10% to 25% of all cases of shingles. Sequelae include chronic ocular inflammation, visual loss, and debilitating pain.

52. **C) Pregnancy test**   Her positive physical findings of left adnexal tenderness and cervical motion tenderness and spotting suggest an ectopic pregnancy rather than pelvic inflammatory disease (PID). Amenorrhea should be treated as a pregnancy until proven otherwise.

53. **A) S3**   The S3 sound occurs at the beginning of diastole after S2; it is a lower pitch than S1 and S2 and is not of valvular origin. The third sound begins in youth, sometimes in pregnancy, and re-emerges later and may be a signal of cardiac problems such as heart failure. An S3 heart sound indicates increased volume of blood within the ventricles. An S3 heart sound is best heard with the bell of the stethoscope (used for lower-frequency sounds). The way to distinguish between a left- and right-sided S3 is to observe whether it increases in intensity with inspiration or expiration. A right-sided S3 will increase on inspiration, a left-sided S3 will increase on expiration.

54. **B) Elevation of the affected limb with episodic applications of cold packs for the next 48 hours**   RICE treatment is a cornerstone for musculoskeletal injury: REST: reduce activity, the injury should be splinted and no weight bearing. ICE: ice packs to reduce pain and swelling. Ice should be applied for 20-minute periods and should be removed for intervals of 40–60 minutes before reapplying. COMPRESSION: apply lightly in the form of an elastic wrap so that it accommodates swelling. ELEVATION: elevating the injured part above the level of the heart is standard to reduce swelling.

55. **A) G6PD-deficiency anemia**   Glucose-6-phosphate dehydrogenase deficiency (X-linked inherited disorder) is the most common enzyme deficiency worldwide; it causes a spectrum of disease, including neonatal hyperbilirubinemia, acute hemolysis, and chronic hemolysis. Normal amounts of G6PD protect red blood cells from certain drugs. The drugs that most often trigger reactions include sulfa drugs (including Bactrim and Septra), certain diuretics, and drugs for the prevention/treatment of malaria.

56. **D) Recommend immediate referral to the emergency department**   Priapism is considered a medical emergency. The cause is complex neurological and vascular factors. Priapism is associated with hematological disorders, especially sickle cell disease.

57. **A) St. John's wort**   St. John's wort may increase bleeding and interact with other drugs. The use of anesthesia in people who have used St. John's wort for 6 months or more may lead to heart complications during surgery. St. John's wort should be stopped at least 2 weeks prior to a scheduled surgery.

58. **B) Prevent anencephaly**   Folic acid (B vitamin) supplementation is used to prevent neural tube defects (NTDs), including spina bifida and anencephaly. Folic acid supplementation should begin preconception and continue during pregnancy. Folic acid prevents some NTDs by correcting abnormal homocysteine metabolism. Women need to take 0.4 mg/day during their childbearing years. There is an increased incidence of NTDs in diabetics, who require a higher dose to be therapeutic.

59. **A) Acute pyelonephritis**   Acute pyelonephritis does not involve any vascular change; however, *chronic* pyelonephritis (reflux nephropathy) is a factor for secondary hypertension. Pheochromocytoma is a rare tumor of the adrenal glands that results in a release of too much epinephrine and norepinephrine hormones that control heart rate, metabolism, and blood pressure (BP).

60. **B) *Chlamydia trachomatis***   Fitz-Hugh–Curtis syndrome consists of persistent right upper quadrant abdominal pain, perihepatitis, and genital tract infection. *Neisseria gonorrhoeae* and *Chlamydia trachomatis* have been identified as the causative agents.

61. **B) 5 mm**   Tuberculin skin tests are tests of delayed hypersensitivity. Purified protein derivative (PPD) tuberculin antigen is administered intradermally and injected to form a 6-mm to 10-mm wheal. TB skin test is read within 48 to 72 hours when the induration is most evident. Erythema without induration is generally considered to be of no significance. Induration of 5 mm or more in diameter indicates positive reaction and need for treatment of latent TB infection in high-risk groups.

62. **C) Varicella and nasal flu vaccine (FluMist)**   HIV/AIDS patients are immunocompromised and should not receive live virus vaccinations. Varicella vaccine is a live attenuated vaccine for chickenpox. FluMist is a live attenuated influenza vaccine. Persons with HIV/AIDS are not recommended to receive LAIV (FluMist). FluMist is approved only for use among healthy people ages 2–49 and who are not pregnant.

63. **A) Irritable bowel syndrome (IBS)**   The Rome Criteria defines IBS as 3 months of continuous or recurring symptoms of abdominal pain or irritation that may be relieved with a BM and two or more of the following symptoms (at least 25% of time): change in stool frequency (more than 3 BMs per day or fewer than 3 BMs a week), and may be related to change in consistency of stool (hard, loose and watery stools, or poorly formed stools), passage of mucus, bloating/abdominal distension, and altered stool passage (incomplete evacuation, straining, or urgency).

64. **D) HIV test**   This 13-year-old does not have any risk factors for HIV. She is not sexually active and is not an IV drug user.

65. **D) During the postpartum period**   The measles, mumps, and rubella (MMR) vaccine is contraindicated in pregnancy. The Advisory Committee on Immunization Practices recommends that pregnancy be avoided for 4 weeks after vaccination, that women who become pregnant within that period be advised of the theoretical risk to the fetus (congenital rubella syndrome), and that vaccination during pregnancy is generally not a reason to terminate the pregnancy.

66. **D) Eyeglasses and routine dental care**   Medicare Part B covers medically necessary services (i.e., service or supplies that are needed to diagnose or treat a medical condition that meets acceptable standards of medical practice) and preventive services such as flu shots. Part B does not cover eyeglasses or routine dental care.

67. **B) Normocytic anemia** In normocytic anemia, the mean corpuscular volume (MCV) is within defined normal limits, but the hemoglobin and hematocrit are decreased.

68. **B) Left heart failure** Heart failure signs and symptoms arise from congested organ and hypoperfused tissues. Left-sided heart failure (systolic heart failure) is the most common cause of HF. The ventricle loses some ability to contract and to pump the oxygenated blood out. Side effects include dyspnea, fatigue, chronic cough or wheezing, rapid or irregular heart rate, lack of appetite/nausea, mental confusion, edema, and rapid weight gain.

69. **C) Furosemide (Lasix)** Furosemide (Lasix) is a loop diuretic that provides rapid natriuresis and diuresis in heart failure, hypertension, liver disease, or renal problems such as nephrotic syndrome.

70. **B) Avoid foods with high potassium content** Foods that are high in potassium are not associated with migraines. Each of the other question responses—foods high in tyramine content, change in sleep patterns, and fermented foods—are all associated with migraine triggers. Other triggers include skipping meals/fasting, hormonal fluctuation, environmental factors, bright lights, odors/pollution, stress, stress letdown, overexertion, visual triggers such as eyestrain/bright glaring lights, etc.

71. **D) Prophylaxis is not recommended for this patient** Current American Heart Association guidelines (2007) do not recommend endocarditis prophylaxis for most patients with aortic or mitral valve disease, including those with mitral valve prolapse or for patients with hypertrophic cardiomyopathy.

72. **B) Koplik's spots** Koplik's spots are characterized as clustered, white lesions with a red base located on the buccal mucosa opposite the first and second molars. Koplik's spots appear in the prodromal stage of measles (rubeola).

73. **A) Hashimoto's disease** Hashimoto's thyroiditis or chronic lymphocytic thyroiditis is an autoimmune disease. An enlarged thyroid is most often the first sign of the disease. Other symptoms include: fatigue, depression, weight gain, cold intolerance, dry coarse hair, constipation, dry skin, muscle cramps, increased cholesterol, decreased concentration, and edema.

74. **C)** *Treponema pallidum* *Treponema pallidum* is a spirochete that is the cause of syphilis and is not associated with community-acquired pneumonia.

75. **D) Torsion of a testicular appendage** All prepubertal and young adult males with acute scrotal pain should be considered to have testicular torsion until proven otherwise. The finding of an ipsilateral absent cremasteric reflex is the most accurate sign of testicular torsion. It may also be diagnosed by the "blue dot" sign (i.e., tender nodule with blue discoloration on the upper pole of the testis). Treatment involves rapid restoration of blood flow to the affected testis. The optimal time frame is less than 6 hours after the onset of symptoms.

76. **C) Acute pancreatitis** The most common cause of acute pancreatitis (AP) is gallstones and excessive ETOH (ethanol) consumption. In addition, significantly elevated triglyceride levels can precipitate episodes of AP. Treatment of hyper-triglyceridemia-induced AP consists of immediate reduction of serum triglyceride levels and long-term medications and lifestyle modifications.

77. **B) Western blot test** A positive ELISA screening does not mean the person has HIV infection. A positive ELISA test is always followed by a Western blot test. A positive Western blot confirms an HIV infection. A negative Western blot means the ELISA test was a false-positive test.

78. **B) Order a serum TSH, a digoxin level, and an electrolyte panel** Hyperthyroidism is an established cause of atrial fibrillation (Afib). Digoxin slows the heart rate. Elderly patients may not be compliant with taking their medications as pre-scribed. The electrolyte panel must be completed because the imbalance of potas-sium (hypokalemia), calcium, and magnesium may lead to atrial fibrillation.

79. **B) Kernig's sign** The Kernig's sign is performed by flexing the leg at the knee and hip when the patient is supine. Then attempt to straighten the leg. Pain in the lower back and resistance to straightening the leg is a positive Kernig's sign, indi-cating meningeal irritation.

80. **B) Claims against the nurse practitioner are covered as long as she had an active malpractice policy at the time of the incident** Occurrence-based policies are written for a 1-year term and cover any claims that arise from services rendered during that 1-year term even, if at the time the claim was made, the insured was no longer with that company.

81. **B) *Chlamydia trachomatis*** Epididymitis is usually caused by the spread of bac-teria from the urethra or bladder. The most common infections include chlamydia and gonorrhea. Physical examination shows a red, tender, and sometimes swollen lump on the affected side of the scrotum. Tenderness is usually in a small area of the testicle where the epididymis (connects the testicle with the vas deferens) is attached.

82. **D) Initiate CPR (cardiopulmonary resuscitation) immediately** Although the patient is in respiratory distress, CPR is not warranted.

83. **A) Cluster headache** Cluster headaches' cardinal symptoms are an excruciat-ing unilateral, orbital, supraorbital, and/or temporal pain. The attack ranges from 15 minutes to 3 hours or more. Autonomic symptoms include ptosis (drooping eyelid), miosis (pupil constriction), lacrimation (tearing), and rhinorrhea in the nostril on the affected side of the face.

84. **C) Apply acetic acid to the penile shaft and look for acetowhite changes and confirm by biopsy** This method of testing is recommended by the Centers for Disease Control and Prevention's 2010 Sexually Transmitted Disease Treatment Guidelines.

85. **D) All of the above**   Obsessive-compulsive disorder is an anxiety disorder in which people have unwanted and repeated thoughts, feelings, ideas, sensations (obsessions), or behaviors that make them feel driven to do something (compulsions). Often the person carries out the behaviors to get rid of the obsessive thoughts, but this only provides temporary relief. Not performing the obsessive rituals can cause great anxiety.

86. **A) Paroxetine (Paxil CR)**   The first medication usually considered is a type of antidepressant called a selective serotonin reuptake inhibitor (SSRI). Paroxetine (Paxil) is in the SSRI drug class.

87. **B) She should not get pregnant within the next 4 weeks**   MMR should not be administered to women known to be pregnant. In addition, counsel women to avoid becoming pregnant for 28 days following vaccination.

88. **B) Mini-Mental Exam**   Begin with administering the MMSE for a baseline assessment, followed by taking a history from the patient and others.

89. **A) Recheck the patient's urine during the visit and then refer her to the nephrologist**   Although the patient is currently asymptomatic, her history of 3 UTIs in 8 months warrants testing while she is in the office. A nephrology consult is prudent. Diabetes is associated with microvascular disease, including renal failure. Consult with a nephrologist for chronic or recurrent UTIs, hematuria, kidney stones, hypertension, etc.

90. **D) Spinach, liver, and whole wheat bread**   Folic acid deficiency is associated with excessive alcohol intake and malnutrition. Folate occurs naturally in the following foods: beans and legumes, citrus fruits and juices, dark leafy vegetables (spinach), liver, poultry, pork, shellfish, wheat bran, and whole grains.

91. **B) A positive ELISA screening does not mean the person has HIV infection**   The ELISA test is always followed by a Western blot test to confirm the diagnosis.

92. **B) Gross obesity**   Metformin reduces weight, central adipose obesity, insulin, and LDL. Metformin is used in diabetes and metabolic syndrome

93. **A) Alpha-blockers**   Terazosin (Hytrin) is a long-acting selective alpha 1-receptor antagonist (alpha-blocker). Terazosin is used in the treatment of benign prostatic hyperplasia and hypertension.

94. **B) Chronic obstructive pulmonary disease**   80%–90% of COPD patients are long-time smokers. The lungs are hyperinflated, which changes the shape of the chest and diaphragm, making the mechanics of breathing more difficult. With the hyperinflated lungs, breathing can be exhausting. Excess mucus and obstructed airflow from a progressive thickening and stiffening of the airways diminish breath sounds. COPD creates a high hematocrit percentage because of the lack of a sufficient amount of oxygen/hypoxia due to damaged lungs.

95. **B) It is a precancerous lesion and should be followed up with her dermatologist**   Actinic keratosis is usually found on the face, scalp, back of hands, chest, or

other sun-exposed areas. They begin as flat and scaly, their color varies, and they develop into a hard wart-line or gritty rough surface. Some actinic keratoses may develop into squamous cell skin cancer. Risk factors include fair skin, severe sunburns early in life, older age.

96. **C) 9 provisions**   The nine provisions of the Nursing Code of Ethics are: rovision 1: Professional relationships with compassion and respect for every individual. Provision 2: Commitment to the patient. Provision 3: Promote and advocate for the patient. Provision 4: Individual responsibility and accountability. Provision 5: Preserve integrity and maintain competence. Provision 6: Maintain and improve healthly environments. Provision 7: Participate in the advancement of the profession. Provision 8: Collaborate with other professionals to meet health needs. Provision 9: Maintain integrity for practice and for shaping social policy.

97. **C) MCV (mean corpuscular volume)**   MCV is average red blood cell size. Anemia is defined based on the cell size. MCV less than the lower limit = microcytic anemia, MCV within normal range = normocytic anemia, and MCV greater than the lower limit of normal = macrocytic anemia.

98. **A) Angina pectoris**   Stable angina is chest pain or discomfort that often occurs with activity or stress. The most common cause of angina is coronary heart disease (CHD). With stable angina the pain does not occur more often or get worse over time. Unstable angina pain is sudden and gets worse over time.

99. **B) Consult with a cardiologist for further evaluation**   Blood tests that indicate tissue damage to the heart include troponin and creatine phosphokinase (CPK). Testing ordered should include ECG, nuclear stress test/stress echocardiogram, and coronary angiography. The patient would need a cardiology consultation for abnormal and/or invasive tests.

100. **D) Transient ischemic attack (TIA)**   TIA occurs when the blood flow to part of the brain stops for a brief period. Hypertension is the number 1 risk factor for TIAs and stroke. Symptoms of a TIA are the same as a stroke but last only a short time: vertigo, change in alertness, changes in feeling, confusion or memory loss, difficulty swallowing, difficulty writing, inability to recognize objects/people, incontinence, muscle weakness of face, arm, or leg (usually unilateral), trouble speaking or understanding others.

101. **A) Drinking organic juice**   Commercial orange juice is fortified with calcium and vitamin D. In general, organic products do not have any additives.

102. **B) Dextromethorphan and guaifenesin (Robitussin DM) 1 to 2 teaspoons every 4 hours**   After a physical examination, the over-the-counter dextromethorphan and guaifenesin (Robitussin DM) can be used for the patient's dry cough. Pseudoephedrine and diphenhydramine both can increase blood pressure. The patient does not need antibiotics; therefore, clarithromycin is not indicated.

103. **B) Mumps** Orchitis is inflammation of one or both of the testicles. Mumps is the most common virus that causes orchitis. Other causes of orchitis are sexually transmitted infections such as gonorrhea or chlamydia.

104. **A) An immune-mediated reaction precipitated by the destruction of a large number of spirochetes due to an antibiotic injection** Herxheimer reaction or Jarisch-Herxheimer reaction resembles bacterial sepsis and can occur after the initiation of antibiotics such as penicillin or tetracycline for treatment of tick-borne relapsing fever. An association has been found between the release of heat-stable proteins from spirochetes and the reaction. The death of these bacteria and their release of endotoxins manifest as fever, chills, rigor, hypotension, headache, tachycardia, vasodilation, myalgia, and exacerbation of skin lesions.

105. **B) Tell her to return 1 week after her period so her breasts can be rechecked** A breast mass may be palpated as normal premenstrual breast tissue; symptoms include tenderness and prominent breast tissue secondary to hormone levels (progesterone). After further assessment of the patient's history of last menstrual period, the patient has noticed a relationship to menses and breast symptoms. This patient also is having the breast masses in both breasts without skin changes and there is no nipple discharge.

106. **C) Abdominal aortic aneurysm** Pulsus paradoxus is an abnormally large decrease in systolic pressure and pulse-wave amplitude during inspiration. All of the other items can be associated.

107. **C) A large number of squamous epithelial cells whose surfaces and edges are coated with large numbers of bacteria along with a few leukocytes** Diagnosis of BV includes 3 of 4 Amsel criteria: 1) white, thick adherent discharge; 2) pH more than 4.5; 3) positive whiff test (amine odor mixed with 10% KOH); 4) clue cells greater than 20% on a wet mount (epithelial cells dotted with large numbers of bacteria that obscure cell borders); plus 5) Gram stain.

108. **D) Mitral valve prolapse (MVP)** Following a normal S1 and briefly quiet systole, the valve suddenly prolapses, resulting in a mid-systolic click. The click is so characteristic of MVP that even without a subsequent murmur, its presence alone is enough for the diagnosis. Immediately after the click, a brief crescendo-decrescendo murmur is heard, usually best at the apex.

109. **D) Renal artery stenosis** Renal artery stenosis is the narrowing of the kidney arteries. It is commonly noted in individuals more than 50 years of age and related to atherosclerosis and hypertension. Hematuria is not associated with renal artery stenosis.

110. **B) Pterygium** A pterygium is a noncancerous growth of clear, thin tissue that lies over the sclera. One or both eyes may be involved. Risk factors are exposure to sunlight and wind. The main symptom is a painless area of white tissue with blood vessels on the inner or outer edge of the cornea. No specific tests are usually needed; physical exam confirms the diagnosis. No treatment is needed unless it begins to block vision or cause symptoms.

111. **A) Discontinue his pravastatin and order a liver-function profile**   Pravastatin (Pravachol) is in the "statin" drug class. Pravastatin is prescribed to help lower LDL and triglycerides, and raise HDL. Statin side effects are associated with muscle pain/tenderness/weakness. They may lead to a more serious condition, rhabdomyolysis. It may also cause liver problems with possible side effects noted such as jaundice seen in the sclera or skin, dark urine, abdominal pain, and persistent nausea/vomiting. Statins must be discontinued and ordering the liver-function profile is indicated.

112. **A) Severe congestive heart failure**   Pioglitazone (Actos) is in the drug classification of thiazolidinediones (TZD) used in type 2 diabetes. TZD's side effects include edema and it has a Black Box Warning for causing or exacerbating congestive heart failure.

113. **A) Breast buds and some straight pubic hair**   Tanner Stage II is noted for breast and papilla elevated as a small mound and areola diameter increased (breast buds). Tanner II pubic hair for females is sparse, lightly pigmented straight hair along the medial border of the labia.

114. **A) Inflammation of the median nerve**   The Phalen maneuver is a diagnostic test for carpal tunnel syndrome. The Phalen's test is done by pushing the back of the hands together for 1 minute. By compressing the median nerve within the carpal tunnel, characteristic symptoms (burning, tingling, numbness over the thumb, index, middle and ring fingers) convey a positive test result.

115. **D) Clarithromycin (Biaxin) BID, amoxicillin BID, and omeprazole (Prilosec) QD daily**   First-line treatment for peptic ulcers caused by the bacterium *Helicobacter pylori* remains a combination of clarithromycin 500 mg and amoxicillin 1 g, or metronidazole (Flagyl) 400–500 mg and a proton pump inhibitor (PPI).

116. **C) Acute viral upper respiratory infection (URI)**   The cough associated with a viral URI is a mild to moderate, hacking cough. The cough is usually dry (no sputum). With post nasal drip, the cough may bring up some nasal secretions. The cough abates with the viral illness.

117. **D) Its effects only last 2 weeks and are reversible**   Aspirin use irreversibly blocks the formation of thromboxane A2 in platelets, producing an inhibitory effect on platelet aggregation.

118. **A) Albuterol inhaler (Proventil)**   Albuterol (Proventil) is a bronchodilator. It works by opening the air passages but does not have any steroidal/anti-inflammatory effect such as Azmacort or have any effect such as a leukotriene blocker (Singulair).

119. **C) Ceftriaxone (Rocephin)**   Ceftriaxone (Rocephin) is a cephalosporin. Rocephin is used in neonates and children for bacterial infections, meningitis, acute otitis media, gonoccal infection, and ophthalmia neonatorum; it is used in adolescents for pelvic inflammatory disease (PID), epididymitis, and for endocarditis prophylaxis.

120. **C) Systemic steroids**   Topical steroids such as Nasonex, Flonase, and Beconase are used in allergic rhinitis for their anti-inflammatory effect, thereby relieving nasal symptoms. Systemic steroids are not indicated.

121. **C) Group A beta-hemolytic *Streptococcus***   Erysipelas is cellulitis caused by group A *Streptococcus* bacteria in the upper dermis and superficial lymphatics. Diagnosis is general based on assessment; a skin biopsy is usually not indicated. Symptoms include vesicles, blisters, petechiae, pain, fever, chills, headache. The erythematous skin lesion enlarges rapidly and has a sharply demarcated raised edge. It is also known as "St. Anthony's fire." The rash is due to an exotoxin.

122. **C) Cauda equina syndrome**   Cauda equina is a serious condition caused by compression of the nerves in the lower portion of the spinal cord. It is considered a surgical emergency; if left untreated it can lead to permanent loss of bowel and bladder control and paralysis of the legs.

123. **B) Rovsing's sign**   The Rovsing sign is right lower quadrant pain intensified by left lower quadrant abdominal pressure. It is associated with peritoneal irritation and appendicitis.

124. **B) EBV (Epstein-Barr virus)**   EBV is a member of the herpes virus family and one of the most common viruses. During adolescence, the EBV causes infectious mononucleosis. In most cases of infectious mono, the clinical diagnosis can be made from the triad of fever, pharyngitis, and lymphadenopathy lasting 1–4 weeks. Serology tests include normal limits to moderately elevated WBC and increased number of lymphocytes, greater than 10% atypical lymphocytes, and a positive reaction to a mono spot test. The antibody response in primary EBV infection appears to be quite rapid.

125. **B) Adam's forward bend test**   The forward bend test is used often in schools to screen for scoliosis. During the test, the child should have just underwear on. The child bends forward with the feet together and knees straight while dangling the arms. Any imbalance in the rib cage or other deformities along the back could be a sign of scoliosis. The forward bend test is not sensitive to abnormalities in the lower back, missing about 15% of scoliosis. This is not recommended as the sole method for screening for scoliosis.

126. **A) Treat the patient with a 7-day course of antibiotics and order a urine test for culture and sensitivity (C&S) before and after treatment**   Prompt diagnosis and early therapy are warranted with a UTI/diabetic. A urine C&S prior to initiation of treatment, treatment, and post C&S to evaluate full treatment due to the susceptibility for UTIs increases with long duration and the greater severity of diabetes. Glycosuria and defective host immune factors predispose to infection. Treatment of asymptomatic bacteriuria in diabetic patients is not indicated.

127. **D) *Chlamydia trachomatis***   *Chlamydia trachomatis* initially infects the cervix and urethra. Signs of infection include abnormal vaginal discharge or a burning sensation with urination.

128. **C) The intracranial pressure (ICP) of the brain is increased**   The funduscopic examination is to visualize vessels and assess intracranial tension and is recommended in new-onset headaches. Papilledema is optic disc swelling cause by increased intracranial pressure. The swelling is usually bilateral. Signs include venous engorgement, loss of venous pulsation, hemorrhages over and/or adjacent to the optic disc, blurring of optic margins, elevation of the optic disc. On visual field exam there may be an enlarged blind spot.

129. **B) Gastroesophageal reflux disease (GERD)**   Classic signs of GERD include acid reflux (regurgitation) into the esophagus, heartburn, and nausea. Complications include ulcers, esophageal strictures, Barrett's esophagus, cough, asthma, throat and laryngeal inflammation. Risk factors include obesity, pregnancy, smoking, and alcohol use.

130. **A) Cataracts**   The red reflex is the light illuminating the retina. To test, have the patient look at a distant fixed point; direct the light of the ophthalmoscope at the pupil from about 30 cm/12 inches away. The retina appears as an orange-red color. Absence of the red reflex is often a result of an improperly positioned ophthalmoscope, but it may also indicate total opacity of the pupil due to a cataract or a hemorrhage into the vitreous humor.

131. **C) Alzheimer's disease**   Ten signs of Alzheimer's: 1) memory loss that disrupts daily life, 2) challenges in planning or problem solving, 3) difficulty completing familiar tasks, 4) confusion with time or place, 5) trouble understanding visual images and spatial relationships, 6) new problems with words or speaking/writing, 7) misplacing things and losing the ability to retrace steps, 8) decreased or poor judgment, 9) withdrawal from work/social activities, 10) changes in mood and personality.

132. **D) Leukoplakia of the tongue**   Leukoplakia mainly affects the mucus membranes of the mouth. It is thought to be caused by irritation. Leukoplakia are patches on the tongue, in the mouth, or on the inside of the cheek that occur in response to long-term irritation, including smoking, holding chewing tobacco or snuff in the mouth for a long period, or other tobacco use, especially pipes (smoker's keratosis).

133. **A) Doxycycline (Vibramycin) 100 mg PO BID × 21 days**   Erythema migrans is the rash characteristic of Lyme disease and appears usually 7–10 days after a tick bite. Lyme disease is caused by *Borrelia burgdorferi*, a spirochete. The rash appears either as a single expanding red patch or a central spot surrounded by clear skin that is in turn ringed by an expanded red rash (bull's eye). The choice of antibiotic depends on bacterial sensitivity. Doxycycline 100 mg BID for 14–21 days is the recommended treatment of adults.

134. **A) The Nurse Practice Act of the state where they practice**   The Nurse Practice Act is a statute enacted by the legislature of each state. The Act delineates the legal scope of the practice of nursing within the geographic boundaries of the jurisdiction. The purpose of the Act is to protect the public.

135. **B) Order a mammogram and refer the patient to a breast surgeon**   This patient needs a mammogram and a surgical consult. Paget's disease of the breast is a rare type of cancer involving the skin of the nipple and, usually, the areola. Paget's disease of the breast may be misdiagnosed at first because its early symptoms are similar to those caused by some benign skin conditions. Most people with Paget's disease of the breast also have one or more tumors inside the same breast, either ductal carcinoma in situ or invasive breast cancer.

136. **D) A 22-year-old female recently diagnosed with asthma**   The young person with asthma is not considered at high risk for TB. Risk factors for TB include a weakened immune system (e.g., diabetes, chronic kidney disease [CKD], cancer [CA], advanced age, malnutrition, biologic agents). Health care workers who come in contact with people with illness are at increased risk, as are those living/working in a residential care facility (e.g., prison, nursing home) or any site with overcrowding or poor ventilation such as a refugee camp/shelters, etc.

137. **C) This is a normal finding in some young athletes**   S2 is physiologically split in about 90% of people. The second heart sound is produced by the closure of the aortic and pulmonic valves. The sound produced by the closure of the aortic valve is termed "A2" and the sound produced by the closure of the pulmonic valve is termed "P2." The A2 sound is normally much louder than the P2 due to higher pressures in the left side of the heart, thus A2 radiates to all cardiac listening posts (loudest at the right upper sternal border) and P2 is usually only heard at the left upper sternal border.

138. **D) 4 risk factors**   The 4 risk factors for this patient are: 1) female, 2) overweight (BMI of 30), 3) hypertension, and 4) total cholesterol 230 g/dL (greater than 200 g/dL).

139. **D) Gastrointestinal upset**   Common side effects of metformin (Glucophage) include indigestion, nausea, vomiting, diarrhea, gas, headache, and a temporary metallic taste.

140. **A) Atrial fibrillation**   There are three pathological irregular rhythms: 1) ectopic beats (may be atrial, junctional, or ventricular), 2) atrial fibrillation, and 3) second-degree heart block. All are confirmed by EKG.

141. **C) A 21-year-old woman who is under treatment for a sexually transmitted infection**   Diabetic, pregnant, and rheumatoid patients are considered to be in immunocompromised states. This 21-year-old woman is being treated with antibiotics for her STI, which may also be the correct antibiotic for a concurrent urinary tract infection.

142. **B) Congestive heart failure**   In CHF the heart's ventricular function is inadequate. Symptoms include fatigue, diminished exercise capacity, shortness of breath, and edema. The kidneys begin to lose their normal ability to excrete sodium and water, leading to fluid retention. Lung congestion/pulmonary edema cause shortness of breath and decrease ability to tolerate exercise.

143. **A) Advise the patient that she had a normal exam**   The disc of a normal examination indicates sharp margins, a yellowish orange to a creamy pink, round or oval shape, and a cup-to-disc ratio less than 1/2. To test, have the patient look at a distant fixed point, direct the light of the ophthalmoscope at the fundus. The ophthalmoscope (set at +8 to +10) should be close to your eyes; your head and scope move together. Check for the red reflex/opacities, then adjust the diopter setting; approach more closely to inspect the disc, noting the color, shape, margins, and cup-to-disc ratio. Then inspect the vessels/pigmentation, then try to identify the macula as the patient looks at the light.

144. **A) The patient can see at 20 feet what a person with normal vision can see at 30 feet**   The Snellen fractions, 20/20, 20/30, etc., are measures of sharpness of sight. They relate to the ability to identify small letters with high contrast at a specified distance. When checking visual acuity, one eye is covered at a time and the vision of each eye is recorded separately, as well as both eyes together. In the Snellen fraction 20/20, the first number represents the test distance, 20 feet. The second number represents the distance that the average eye can see the letters on a certain line of the eye chart. So, 20/20 means that the eye being tested can read a certain size letter when it is 20 feet away. If a person sees 20/30, at 20 feet from the chart that person can read letters that a person with 20/20 vision could read from 30 feet away.

145. **B) Dawn phenomenon**   The Dawn phenomenon is the end result of a combination of natural body changes that occur during the sleep cycle. Between 3 a.m. and 8 a.m. the body starts to increase the amounts of counter-regulatory hormones, including growth hormone, cortisol, and catecholamines. These hormones work against insulin's action to drop blood sugars.

146. **A) HCV RNA**   The anti-HCV test detects the presence of antibodies to the hepatitis C virus, indicating exposure to HCV. The anti-HCV test cannot distinguish between someone with active or previous HCV infection (reported as positive or negative). The HCV RNA test is qualitative and used to distinguish between a current or past infection. It is reported as "negative" or "not detected." It may also be ordered after treatment is complete to see if the virus has been eliminated.

147. **D) Check the pedal and posterior tibial pulses**   Smoking is a risk factor for PVD. The physical examination for PVD includes inspection, palpation for temperature (cool suggests a poor circulation), pitting edema tested in dependent locations, capillary refill—should be less than 3 seconds. Check the arterial pulses: dorsalis pedis artery pulse (on dorsal surface of the foot, running lateral to the tendon of the first toe), posterior tibial artery pulse (posterior and inferior to the medial malleolus), popliteal artery pulse (behind the knees, usually done with both hands), and femoral artery pulse (in the femoral triangle).

148. **B) Montelukast (Singulair)**   Montelukast (Singulair) is in the drug class leukotriene modifiers and is used to treat asthma, asthma maintenance, bronchospasm prophylaxis, and COPD. It is an asthma controller functioning as a chemical mediator in inflammation. Theophylline is a member of the drug class methylxanthines.

It is also used to treat asthma, acute asthma, and maintenance as a bronchodilator. There is no contraindication/drug interaction of these two drugs/classes.

149. **C) Mitral regurgitation** Mitral regurgitation (MR) occurs when the mitral valve does not close properly. It is the abnormal leaking of blood from the left ventricle, through the mitral valve, and into the left atrium. When the ventricle contracts, there is regurge/back flow of blood back into the left atrium. MR is the most common form of valvular heart disease. Murmurs are graded/classified depending on how loud the murmur sounds with a stethoscope. The scale is 1–6 on loudness. A grade II/VI is a grade 2 on the 6-point scale.

150. **B) Ciprofloxacin (Cipro)** Anthrax is an infectious disease caused by a type of bacteria called *Bacillus anthracis*. Infection in humans most often involves the skin, gastrointestinal tract, or lungs. Cutaneous anthrax occurs when anthrax spores touch a cut or scrape on the skin. It is the most common type of anthrax infection. The main risk is contact with animal hides or hair, bone products, and wool, or with infected animals. Symptoms of cutaneous anthrax start 1 to 7 days after exposure: An itchy sore develops that is similar to an insect bite. This sore may blister and form a black ulcer (sore). The sore is usually painless, but it is often surrounded by swelling. A scab often forms, and then dries and falls off within 2 weeks. Complete healing can take longer. Most people with anthrax are treated with antibiotics. Several antibiotics are effective, including penicillin, doxycycline, and ciprofloxacin.

151. **B) Raynaud's disease** A feeling of cold in the hands and/or feet—or sensitivity to the cold—is a common complaint in people with hypothyroidism. Raynaud's disease involves an interruption in the blood flow to fingers and toes (sometimes nose and ears), due to spasms in the blood vessels. During a Raynaud's attack, the affected area typically turns white, and as oxygen fails to reach the extremities, they can turn blue, tingle, or painfully throb, and the affected area may swell. Symptoms can resolve quickly or may last for hours. Treatment includes proper thyroid treatment.

152. **B) Small red spots with bluish centers located by the posterior molaris** Koplik's spots are characterized as clustered, white lesions with a red base located on the buccal mucosa opposite the first and second molars. Koplik's spots appear in the prodromal stage of measles (rubeola).

153. **C) Squamous epithelial cells and endocervical cells** An optimal Pap smear sample contains sufficient mature and metaplastic squamous cells to indicate adequate sampling from the transformation zone and sufficient endocervical cells to indicate that the upper limit of the transformation zone was sampled, and to provide a sample for screening for adenocarcinoma and its precursors.

154. **A) T score of less than −2.50.** Several methods are available to measure bone density, but currently the most widely used technique is DEXA (dual energy x-ray absorptiometry). The *T-score* is the number of standard deviations below the average for a young adult at peak bone density. There are different T-scores depending on which group of young adults was used

as the reference. The *Z-score* is the number of standard deviations below an average person of the same age. Normal bone: T-score better than –1; osteopenia: T-score between –1 and –2.5; osteoporosis: T-score less than –2.5; and established (severe) osteoporosis *includes the presence of a nontraumatic fracture.*

155. **A) Trigeminal neuralgia** Trigeminal neuralgia is a nerve disorder that causes a stabbing or electric-shock-like pain in parts of the face. Symptoms are very painful, sharp electric-like spasms that usually last a few seconds or minutes, but can become constant. Pain is usually only on one side of the face, often around the eye, cheek, and lower part of the face. Pain may be triggered by touch or sounds. Painful attacks of trigeminal neuralgia can be triggered by common, everyday activities.

156. **D) Atypical bacterial infections** A potassium hydroxide (KOH) test is done to determine whether a fungus is causing a skin infection. Samples from an infected area are treated with KOH, which dissolves skin cells and leaves behind fungus cells (if any are present) that can been seen with a microscope. The KOH test may be used to diagnose fungal infections, such as thrush, tinea versicolor, ringworm, and bacterial vaginosis (positive whiff test).

157. **D) Bupropion hydrochloride (Wellbutrin)** Bupropion is used to treat major depressive disorder and seasonal affective disorder. The Zyban brand of bupropion is used to help people stop smoking by reducing cravings and other withdrawal effects.

158. **D) Auscultation** Auscultation is used to evaluate lung sounds, while tactile uses the hands. Fremitus is using the vibration of the chest wall when a person speaks and is heard through a stethoscope. Tactile fremitus is a type of vocal fremitus found over the area of secretions. Tactile fremitus is evaluated using the palmar surface of both hands over the back/lungs. In bronchophony (the ability to hear increased loudness of the spoken sounds), even a whisper can be heard through the stethoscope.

159. **B) Have the woman continue oral contraceptives** DVT is a contraindication for continuing oral contraceptives.

160. **C) Nongonococcal urethritis** A number of communicable diseases are required to be reported to the Public Health Department. A subset of those communicable diseases are then reportable to the Centers for Disease Control and Prevention (CDC). The most common bacterial cause of nongonococcal urethritis is *Chlamydia trachomatis*, but it may also be caused by *Ureaplasma urealyticum, Haemophilus vaginalis*, and *Mycoplasma genitalium*. Viral causes include herpes simplex and adenovirus; rarely a trichomonas vaginalis (parasite) may cause nongonococcal urethritis (NGU). It can also be caused by a mechanical injury such as a catheter or cystoscopy.

161. **A) Yogurt and sardines** Good sources of calcium include low-fat dairy products (yogurt), dark leafy vegetables, canned salmon or sardines with bones, soy products, and calcium-fortified cereals and orange juice. Just 3 ounces of canned sardines, including bones, drained of oil, provides 324 mg of calcium.

162. **A) Green leafy vegetables have high levels of vitamin K that can bind with the blood-clotting cascade and increase bleeding time**   Patients taking Coumadin to prevent blood clots should avoid certain foods rich in Vitamin K, according to the Agency for Healthcare and Research Quality. Vitamin K causes blood clotting and, therefore, interferes with Coumadin's therapeutic effect of thinning blood. Examples of foods high in vitamin K include liver, green leafy vegetables such as kale, spinach, cabbage, broccoli, asparagus, brussel sprouts, green onions, lettuce, mustard greens, collard greens, endive lettuce, and vegetable oils such as soybean oil and canola oil.

163. **B) Order a liver function profile**   Fluvastatin (Lescol) is in the "statin" drug class. Lescol is prescribed to help lower LDL and triglycerides, and raise HDL. Statin side effects are associated with muscle pain/tenderness/weakness. Statins may lead to a more serious condition called rhabdomyolysis. They may also cause liver problems with possible side effects noted, such as jaundice seen in the sclera or skin, dark urine, abdominal pain, and persistent nausea/vomiting. In such cases, statins must be discontinued; ordering of the liver function profile is indicated.

164. **D) Stop taking the medicine until the laboratory results are available**   This patient's symptoms suggest liver involvement; have the patient stop the statin until the lab results are back, then the patient and the clinician can make informed decisions.

165. **D) Ankylosing spondylitis**   Ankylosing spondylitis (AS) is a lifelong autoimmune disease and form of arthritis that causes inflammation, pain, and stiffness mainly in the spinal joints. In the early stages of AS, the pain and stiffness often start in the lower back, but over time it may move up the spine and into the neck. Most people with AS experience episodes of acute pain—known as flares—followed by periods when symptoms temporarily subside. There are no specific lab tests to identify ankylosing spondylitis. ESR is increased by the inflammation.

166. **B) Schedule the patient for a uterine ultrasound and uterine biopsy**   Postmenopausal bleeding should always be investigated because it could be a sign of endometrial carcinoma. Although endometrial carcinoma is the most serious cause of postmenopausal bleeding, an atrophic endometrium with dyssynchronous shedding is the most common cause. A less common cause is cervical or endometrial polyps. A uterine ultrasound is ordered to evaluate the lining of the endometrium and rule out polyps. A uterine biopsy is ordered to sample for pathology.

167. **A) Anticholinergics**   Anticholinergic drugs are another group of bronchodilators that are different from the beta-agonists. While the beta-agonists affect the bronchioles (small airways), anticholinergics affect the muscles around the bronchi (large airways). When the lungs are irritated, these bands of muscle can tighten, making the bronchi narrower. Anticholinergics work by stopping the muscles from tightening.

168. **A) Fever occurs in up to 80% of the patients**   The Td vaccine is adult tetanus and diphtheria. A mild fever may occur as a side effect of the vaccine; it occurs in up to about 1 in 15.

169. **A) Angiotensin-converting enzyme (ACE) inhibitors** Regimens based on ACE inhibitors or angiotensin receptor blockers (ARBs) slow the progression of diabetic nephropathy and reduce albuminuria. Microalbuminuria has an independent value to predict cardiovascular disease in patients with not only diabetes mellitus but also with essential hypertension and even in the general population. The Seventh Report of the Joint National Committee on Prevention, Detection, Evaluation and Treatment of High Blood Pressure has adopted microalbuminuria or estimated glomerular filtration rate less than 60 mL/min as one of the major cardiovascular risk factors.

170. **B) Bacterial vaginosis** Diagnosis of BV includes 3 of 4 Amsel criteria: 1) white, thick adherent discharge; 2) pH more than 4.5; 3) positive whiff test (amine odor mixed with 10% KOH); 4) clue cells greater than 20% on a wet mount (epithelial cells dotted with large numbers of bacteria that obscure cell borders); plus 5) Gram stain.

171. **A) Peripheral vision** A visual field test is an eye examination that can detect dysfunction in central and peripheral vision that may be caused by various medical conditions such as glaucoma, stroke, brain tumors, or other neurological deficits.

172. **C) Acne** Macules are small, flat, discolored areas on the skin that are level with the skin surface. Examples are freckles and some rashes. Acne is not level with the skin surface.

173. **A) Administer a booster dose of the Td vaccine** Those who have dirty wounds need a tetanus booster if they have not received a booster in the past 5 years. Dirty wounds include wounds that occur outdoors, wounds that contain dirt or foreign material, and wounds caused by bites. A booster of the tetanus vaccine is typically given in combination with a booster of diphtheria vaccine (Tdap).

174. **D) The left side of the sternum at the fifth ICS by the midclavicular line** The apex of the heart is the lowest superficial part of the heart. It is directed downward, forward, and to the left. The apex is overlapped by the left lung and pleura. The apex lies behind the fifth left intercostal space, slightly medial to the midclavicular line.

175. **B) Rosacea** The symptoms of rosacea affect primarily those of Caucasian or other ethnic groups with lighter-toned skin. Facial skin redness (erythema) is caused by hundreds of tiny dilated blood vessels near the surface of the facial skin that become inflamed or dilated due to many rosacea triggers. The symptoms of rosacea begin with facial skin redness and develop to more frequent flushing of the face, particularly the nose and cheeks.

176. **D) Iron-deficiency anemia** Koilonychia is a symptom of iron-deficiency anemia. Other symptoms of iron deficiency anemia include tiredness, lethargy, shortness of breath, palpitations; less common symptoms include a smooth tongue (atrophic glossitis), altered sense of taste, pica (desire to eat nonfood items), and spoon-shaped nails (koilonychia).

177. **B) Lung cancer**   The highest mortality is associated with lung cancer.

178. **C) It can be a normal variant if heard in a person aged 40 or older**   The S3 heart sound occurs at the beginning of diastole after S2 and is lower in pitch than S1 or S2, as it is not of valvular origin. The third heart sound is benign in youth, some trained athletes, and sometimes in pregnancy, but if it re-emerges later in life, it may signal cardiac problems like a failing left ventricle, as in dilated congestive heart failure (CHF).

179. **B) Inflammation of the sciatic nerve/herniated disc**   To perform the straight-leg test, have the patient lie supine on an exam table, and lift the patient's leg toward his/her head while the knee is straight. If the patient experiences sciatic pain when the straight leg is at an angle of between 30 and 70 degrees, then the test is positive and a herniated disc is likely to be the cause of the pain. The straight-leg test should be done on the pain-free side first to find out which range of movement is normal and to enable the patient to distinguish between "normal" stretching of muscles and a different sort of pain.

180. **A) An eye exam with an ophthalmologist**   Patients with type 2 diabetes should have an initial dilated and comprehensive eye examination by an ophthalmologist or optometrist shortly after the diagnosis of diabetes. Subsequent examinations for type 1 and type 2 diabetic patients should be repeated annually by an ophthalmologist or optometrist. Examinations will be required more frequently if retinopathy is progressing.

181. **D) She needs to be evaluated by a dermatologist**   This patient needs to be referred to a dermatologist. Any nonhealing ulcers require further evaluation. For example, squamous cell cancer (primarily found on sun-exposed areas such as the rim of the ear, face, scalp, lips, and mouth) often begins as a small, sandpaper-like growth called actinic keratoses. It then develops into a crusted or scaly patch with a red, inflamed base. It can also present as a growing tumor, a nonhealing ulcer, or just a crust. Any nonhealing ulcers warrant further evaluation.

182. **B) Albuterol (Ventolin) inhalers**   Albuterol (Ventolin) is a short-acting beta agonist. Short-acting bronchodilators are used only as needed as asthma "quick relief" or "rescue" medications, whereas long-acting bronchodilators are used every day to control asthma in conjunction with an inhaled steroid. Bronchodilators open up the airways so that it is easier for air to move through. Formoterol (Foradil) is a long-acting bronchodilator. Montelukast (Singular) is a leukotriene receptor antagonist (LTRA), and triamcinolone (AeroBid) is a corticosteroid.

183. **B) Degenerative joint disease**   Enlargement of the middle joint of a finger is called a Bouchard's node. Signs of osteoarthritis (OA) include stiffness of joints, especially in the morning and after sitting for long periods. Visible signs of OA are an element in the diagnosis. (RA and gout often rely more heavily on lab tests.) Heberden nodes (bony overgrowths) are classic signs of OA. They are located at the distal interphalangeal joints. They are felt as hard, nontender nodules usually 2–3 cm in diameter but sometimes encompass the entire joint.

184. **C) Macrocytic and normochromic cells** Anemias resulting from Vitamin B12 or folate deficiency are sometimes referred to as "macrocytic" or "megaloblastic" anemia because red blood cells are larger than normal. A diagnosis of pernicious anemia first requires demonstration of megaloblastic anemia with a complete blood count (CBC) with differential that evaluates the mean corpuscular volume (MCV), as well the mean corpuscular hemoglobin concentration (MCHC). Pernicious anemia is identified with a high MCV (macrocytic) and a normal MCHC (normochromic) anemia.

185. **B) Aortic stenosis** One of the most frequent pathologic systolic murmurs is due to aortic stenosis. The murmur of aortic stenosis is typically a mid-systolic ejection murmur, heard best over the "aortic area" or right second intercostal space, with radiation into the right neck. It has a harsh quality and may be associated with a palpably slow rise of the carotid upstroke. Additional heart sounds, such as an S4, may be heard secondary to hypertrophy of the left ventricle, which is caused by the greatly increased work required to pump blood through the stenotic valve.

186. **A) Hordeolum** A hordeolum is a common disorder of the eyelid. It is an acute focal infection (usually staphylococcal) involving either the glands of Zeis (external hordeola or styes) or, less frequently, the meibomian glands (internal hordeola). Histologically, hordeola represent focal collections of polymorphonuclear leukocytes and necrotic debris (i.e., abscesses).

187. **C) Propranolol (Inderal)** Propranolol (Inderal) is a beta-blocker. Sufficient evidence and consensus exist to recommend propranolol, timolol, amitriptyline, divalproex, sodium valproate, and topiramate as first-line agents for migraine prevention. The goal of preventive therapy is to improve patients' quality of life by reducing migraine frequency, severity, and duration, and by increasing the responsiveness of acute migraines to treatment. A full therapeutic trial may take 2 to 6 months.

188. **B) Cluster headache** Cluster headaches' cardinal symptoms are an excruciating, unilateral, orbital, supraorbital, and/or temporal pain. The attack ranges from 15 minutes to 3 hours or more. Autonomic symptoms include ptosis (drooping eyelid), miosis (pupil constriction), lacrimation (tearing), and rhinorrhea in the nostril on the affected side of the face.

189. **C) Clarithromycin (Biaxin)** Clarithromycin is a macrolide antibiotic chemically related to erythromycin and azithromycin. It is effective against a wide variety of bacteria, such as *Haemophilus influenzae, Streptococcus pneumoniae, Mycoplasma pneumoniae,* and *Staphylococcus aureus.* Clarithromycin has been used in combination with omeprazole (Prilosec) in treating *H. pylori* bacteria that cause stomach ulcers. Side effects (SE) are usually mild and transient. Common SE include nausea, diarrhea, abnormal taste, dyspepsia, abdominal pain, and headache.

190. **A) There is no delay in seeking medical treatment** Due to shame and secrecy of domestic violence, treatment is usually not sought or is delayed. The violent partner may refuse to let the partner out of his or her "control."

191. **A) A 50-year-old construction worker who drinks 1 beer nightly while watching sports programs on television**   The 50-year-old worker drinking one beer nightly is the least likely to become an abuser. The CAGE assessment is: C: Have you ever tried to Cut back on your use? A: Have you ever been Annoyed/Angered when questioned about your use? (30-year nurse has family that starts to annoy her). G: Have you ever felt Guilt about your use? E: Have you ever had an Eye-opener to get started in the morning? (70-year-old drinks rum in the morning). Binging may lead to more serious alcohol/drug consumption (19-year-old who binges).

192. **B) Hemoglobin electrophoresis**   Alpha thalassemia has MCV < 80 (microcytic) and decreased MCHC (hypochromic) confirmed by hemoglobin electrophoresis.

193. **D) Mitral stenosis**   The most common complication of mitral valve prolapse is mitral valve regurgitation (mitral insufficiency). An abnormal mitral valve increases the chance of getting endocarditis from bacteria, which can further damage the mitral valve. Doctors used to recommend that people with mitral valve prolapse take antibiotics before certain dental or medical procedures to prevent endocarditis (not a current practice). Stroke is a very rare complication of mitral valve prolapse.

194. **D) Scabies**   Scabies is a parasitic disease (infestation) of the skin caused by the human itch mite *Sarcoptes scabiei*. In typical scabies, the rash is generally characterized as red, raised bumps (papules). The scabies mite is generally transmitted from one person to another by direct contact with the skin of the infested person and can also be acquired by wearing an infested person's clothing (fomites), such as sweaters, coats, or scarves. Following the incubation period, the infested person will complain of pruritus (itching), which intensifies at bedtime under the warmth of the blankets. Common sites of infection are the webs of fingers, wrists, flexors of the arms, the axillae, lower abdomen, genitalia, buttocks, and feet.

195. **D) Renal system**   The two main adverse drug reactions associated with NSAIDs relate to gastrointestinal (GI) effects and renal effects of the agents. The main adverse drug reactions associated with use of NSAIDs relate to direct and indirect irritation of the GI tract. Ulceration risk increases with therapy duration, and with higher doses. NSAIDs can induce 2 different forms of acute kidney injury: hemodynamically-mediated, and acute interstitial nephritis, which is often accompanied by the nephrotic syndrome.

196. **D) All of the above**   The measles, mumps, and rubella (MMR) is recommended as one of the "catch-up" immunizations for that age group. The tetanus immunization that is recommended as a "catch-up" for that age group is the Tdap instead of just the Td.

197. **C) CN XI.**   Cranial nerve XI tests for spinal accessory. The procedure to test trapezius muscle strength is to have the patient shrug the shoulders against resistance. To test sternocleidomastoid muscle strength, have the patient turn the head to each side with resistance.

198. **B) A chest radiograph and sputum culture are indicated** Larger reactions (>10 mm) are considered positive in people with a known negative test in the past 2 years.

199. **C) Tertiary prevention** Primary prevention refers to methods to avoid occurrence of disease, including health promotion. Secondary prevention is used to diagnose and treat existing disease in its early stages before it causes significant morbidity. Tertiary prevention refers to methods to reduce negative impact of an existing disease by restoring function and reducing disease-related complications.

200. **B) 42-year-old obese woman taking prednisone 10 mg daily for severe asthma for 2 years** A few of the risk factors for osteoporosis are female gender, increasing age, Caucasian or Asian ethnicity, sedentary lifestyle, and long-term use of corticosteroids such as prednisone and cortisone (interferes with bone-building). The 42-year-old is at higher risk related to her gender and long-term use of steroids. If her obesity is related to a sedentary lifestyle instead of participation in weight-bearing exercise, she would have another risk factor.

201. **D) Gluten** Celiac disease, known as sprue, is an autoimmune disease that damages the small intestine and interferes with the absorption of nutrients. People with celiac disease cannot tolerate a protein called gluten, which is found in wheat, rye, and barley. If they eat foods or use products containing gluten, their immune system responds by damaging the lining of the small intestine. This damage to the small intestine decreases the absorption of all nutrients—resulting in an overall poor nutritional status. If not treated, a person with celiac disease can develop more severe nutritional deficiencies, such as osteoporosis (because of poor calcium absorption), iron-deficiency anemia, or multiple other vitamin and mineral deficiencies.

202. **D) Microaneurysms** Patients with diabetes often develop ophthalmic complications, such as corneal abnormalities, glaucoma, iris neovascularization, cataracts, and neuropathies. The most common and potentially most blinding of these is diabetic retinopathy. In the initial stages of diabetic retinopathy, patients are generally asymptomatic, but in more advanced stages of the disease patients may experience floaters, distorting, and/or blurred vision. Microaneurysms are the earliest clinical sign of diabetic retinopathy.

203. **C) A family history of migraines with aura** All of the items are contraindications; a family history does not substantiate avoiding oral contraceptives.

204. **A) Lung cancer** The report "Ten Leading Cancer Types for Estimated New Cancer Cases and Deaths by Sex, United States," from 2011, estimated that 28% of deaths for men and 26% of deaths for women are related to lung and bronchus cancer.

205. **D) Macrocytic and normocytic red blood cells** Anemia resulting from Vitamin B12 or folate deficiency is sometimes referred to as "macrocytic" or "megaloblastic" anemia because red blood cells are larger than normal. A diagnosis of pernicious anemia first requires demonstration of megaloblastic anemia with a

complete blood count (CBC) with differential that evaluates the mean corpuscular volume (MCV), as well the mean corpuscular hemoglobin concentration (MCHC). Pernicious anemia is identified with a high MCV (macrocytic) and a normal MCHC (normochromic).

206. **C) Elevated**   Headache is the most common chief complaint and presents in more than 2/3 of patients with temporal arteritis. The headache tends to be new or different in character than previous headaches and is typically sudden in onset, localizing to the temporal region. Any new headache in patients older than 50 years warrants a consideration of temporal arteritis. Erythrocyte sedimentation rate (ESR) greater than 50 mm/h is suspect. The normal sedimentation rate for males is 0 to 15 mm/h, and for females is 0 to 20 mm/h. The sedimentation rate can be slightly more elevated in the elderly.

207. **B) Rheumatoid arthritis**   When RA is active, symptoms can include fatigue, loss of energy, lack of appetite, low-grade fever, muscle and joint aches, and stiffness. Muscle and joint stiffness are usually most notable in the morning and after periods of inactivity. Arthritis is common during disease flares. Also during flares, joints frequently become red, swollen, painful, and tender. This occurs because the lining of the tissue of the joint (synovium) becomes inflamed, resulting in the production of excessive joint fluid (synovial fluid).

208. **D) Creutzfeldt-Jakob disease**   CJD is characterized by rapidly progressive dementia. Initially, individuals experience problems with muscular coordination; personality changes, including impaired memory, judgment, and thinking; and impaired vision. People with the disease also may experience insomnia, depression, or unusual sensations. CJD does not cause a fever or other flu-like symptoms. As the illness progresses, mental impairment becomes severe. Individuals often develop involuntary muscle jerks called myoclonus, and they may go blind. They eventually lose the ability to move and speak and enter a coma. Pneumonia and other infections often occur in these individuals and can lead to death.

209. **C) Indomethacin (Indocin)**   Nonsteroidal anti-inflammatory drugs (NSAIDs) such as indomethacin (Indocin) have been used for the treatment of *acute gout*. Allopurinol is used to prevent gout attacks, not to treat them once they occur. It may take several months or longer before the full benefit of allopurinol is felt. Allopurinol may increase the number of gout attacks during the first few months that it is taken, although it will eventually prevent attacks.

210. **A) Loss of joint mobility and renal failure**   Left untreated, gout can develop into a painful and disabling chronic disorder. Persistent gout can destroy cartilage and bone, causing irreversible joint deformities and loss of motion.

211. **D) International health promotion programs**   Healthy People has four overarching goals: 1) Attain high-quality, longer lives free of preventable disease, disability, injury, and premature death. 2) Achieve health equity and eliminate disparities. 3) Create social and physical environments that promote good health for all. 4) Promote quality of life and development of healthy behaviors across life spans.

212. **A) Bouchard's node** Enlargement of the middle joint of a finger is called a Bouchard's node. Signs of osteoarthritis (OA) include stiffness of joints, especially in the morning and after sitting for long periods. Visible signs of OA are an element in the diagnosis.

213. **A) Diabetes mellitus** Disease mortality rates are lower overall for Hispanics than for non-Hispanics, and considerably lower for the two major killers, cardiovascular disease and cancer. Diabetes, however, claims more lives among the Hispanic population. Diabetes is a primary health concern for Hispanics. This has been particularly documented among studies involving Mexican Americans where the risk of type 2 diabetes is 2 to 3 times higher than for non-Hispanic Whites.

214. **D) Initiate a prescription of nicotinic acid (niacin, Niaspan)** Niacin can raise HDL cholesterol by 15% to 35%. This makes niacin the most effective drug available for raising HDL cholesterol. Niacin also decreases LDL and triglyceride levels.

215. **D) The meniscus of the knee** The McMurray test is used to detect a torn meniscus. With the patient supine, flex one knee completely with the foot flat on the table near the buttocks. Maintain that flexion with your thumb and index finger stabilizing the knee on either side of the joint space. Hold the heel with your other hand, and rotate the foot and lower the leg to a lateral position. Extend the patient's knee to a 90-degree angle; notice any palpable or audible click or limited extension of the knee. Return the knee to full flexion and repeat the procedure, rotating the foot and lower leg to the medial position. A palpable or audible click in the knee or lack of extension is a positive sign.

216. **B) An endoscopy with tissue biopsy** The most accurate test for *H. pylori* involves microscope analysis of tissues sampled in an endoscopic biopsy of the stomach to detect the bacterium directly.

217. **C) June 2001** In June of 2001, the ANA House of Delegates voted to accept the 9 major provisions of a revised *Code of Ethics*. In July 2001, the Congress of Nursing Practice and Economics voted to accept the new language of the interpretive statements, resulting in a fully approved revised *Code of Ethics for Nurses with Interpretive Statements.*

218. **D) All of the above** The American Diabetic Association endorses all of these tests for diagnosis.

219. **B) A superficial vesicle filled with serous fluid greater than 1 cm in size** This is a blister—a circumscribed, fluid-containing, elevated lesion of the skin, usually more than 5 mm in diameter.

220. **B) Isoniazid (INH) prophylaxis is not recommended for persons aged 30 years or older because of higher risk of hepatic injury** The Centers for Disease Control and Prevention (CDC) and the American Thoracic Society joint guidelines for the treatment of latent TB infection state that baseline laboratory testing is not routinely indicated, even for persons aged more than 35 years, but may be considered

for patients who are taking other hepatotoxic medications or have chronic medical conditions. Baseline measurements of bilirubin and aspartate transaminase (AST) or alanine transaminase (ALT), along with monthly liver function test monitoring, are recommended for patients with preexisting liver disease, patients at risk for chronic liver disease, patients with HIV infection, pregnant or postpartum women, and regular users of alcohol.

221. **B) Western blot**   A positive ELISA screening does not mean the person has HIV infection. A positive ELISA test is always followed by a Western blot test. A positive Western blot confirms an HIV infection. A negative Western blot means the ELISA test was a false-positive test.

222. **B) Condyloma acuminata**   Condyloma acuminatum refers to an epidermal manifestation attributed to the epidermotropic human papilloma virus (HPV).

223. **D) Depo-Provera injections**   Depo-Provera is the brand name for a 150-mg aqueous injection of DMPA (depot medroxyprogesterone acetate). It is given as an intramuscular injection. Depo is given for contraception and for the management of endometriosis-related pain. Depo-subQ Provera is a variation of the original Depo shot given subcutaneously.

224. **D) Ovarian cysts**   There are a number of complications associated with pelvic inflammatory disease (PID), including repeated episodes of PID, abscess formation, and an increased risk of an ectopic pregnancy or infertility.

225. **D) Molluscum contagiosum**   Molluscum contagiosum is a viral skin infection. In adults, molluscum contagiosum appears on the face, neck, armpits, arms, and hands. Other common places include the genitals, abdomen, and inner thigh. They often begin as small, firm, dome-shaped growths; have a surface that feels smooth, waxy, or pearly; are flesh-colored or pink; have a dimple in the center (may be filled with a thick, white substance that is cheesy or waxy); and are painless but itch. Scratching or picking can spread the virus.

226. **C) Microcytic anemia**   Anemias can be classified according to the mean corpuscular volume (MCV) into microcytic, normocytic, and macrocytic anemias. A microcytic anemia is defined by an MCV of less than 80 fL. The differential diagnosis of a microcytic anemia includes iron-deficiency anemia (IDA), thalassemias, anemia of chronic disease (ACD), and sideroblastic anemias, including lead poisoning.

227. **B) Pelvis**   Hemorrhagic (hypovolemic) shock is due to acute blood or body fluid loss. The amount of blood loss after trauma is often difficult to determine. The hemorrhage after a blunt trauma is often underestimated. A femoral closed fracture, for example, may lose 1 to 2 liters of blood; a pelvic fracture can lose more than 2 liters of blood; whereas a simple rib fracture can lose up to 125 mL. The abdominal cavity may contain large amounts of blood without distension occurring; initially the blood does not irritate the peritoneum, making the diagnosis of haemoperitoneum difficult to establish.

228. **B) Gout**   Gout (also known as podagra when it involves the big toe) is character-ized by recurrent attacks of acute inflammatory arthritis—red, tender, hot, swollen joint. The metatarsal-phalangeal joint at the base of the big toe is the most com-monly affected (approximately 50% of cases).

229. **C) Grade IV**   A fine vibration, felt by an examiner's hand on a patient's body over the site of an aneurysm or on the precordium, results from turmoil in the flow of blood and indicates the presence of an organic murmur of grade IV or greater intensity. A thrill can also be felt over the carotids if a bruit is present and over an arteriovenous fistula in the patient undergoing hemodialysis.

230. **A) Aortic stenosis**   The murmur associated with aortic stenosis can be auscul-tated as harsh and high pitched in the right second intercostal space; it typically radiates to the carotid arteries and apex.

231. **D) Both hepatitis B and hepatitis C**   Of the primary hepatitis viruses, only B and C are associated with hepatocellular cancer.

232. **C) CNVII**   Bell's palsy is a form of facial paralysis resulting from a dysfunction of cranial nerve VII (the facial nerve) that results in the inability to control facial muscles on the affected side.

233. **C) Hepatitis B vaccination and hepatitis B immune globulin**   Hepatitis B sur-face antigen (HBsAg) is a marker of infectivity. If positive, it indicates either an acute or chronic hepatitis B infection. Antibody to hepatitis B surface antigen (anti-HBs) is a marker of immunity. Antibody to hepatitis B core antigen (anti-HBc) is a marker of acute, chronic, or resolved HBV infection; it may be used in prevaccina-tion testing to determine previous exposure to HBV. Interpretation of the hepatitis B panel for test results: A negative HBsAg and a negative anti-HBc and a negative anti-HBs indicates the patient is *susceptible*—not immune, has not been infected and is still at risk of future infection—*need vaccine*. Interpretation of the hepatitis C anti-HCV screening test that is negative indicates that the patient is not infected.

234. **D) Pregnancy**   Several types of anemia can develop during pregnancy: iron-defi-ciency anemia (microcytic anemia), folate-deficiency anemia (macrocytic anemia), and Vitamin B12 deficiency (also a macrocytic anemia).

235. **A) Apical and radial pulses at the same time, then subtracting the difference between the two**   The pulse deficit is the difference between the apical pulse and the radial pulse. These should be taken at the same time, which will require that 2 people take the pulse: one with a stethoscope and one at the wrist. Count for 1 full minute. The subtract the radial from the apical.

236. **D) Metronidazole (Flagyl)**   Treatment for bacterial vaginosis (BV) is metronida-zole (Flagyl) either orally or vaginally or treatment with clindamycin (Cleocin) either orally or vaginally. Treatment for the partner is not recommended by the CDC, since there is no decrease in recurrences with partner treatment and no effect on cure rates.

237. **A) Apply Candida or mumps antigen to the right forearm and the PPD (purified protein derivative) on the left forearm and read results in 48 to 72 hours**   Anergy testing is the practice of making intradermal injections of common antigens (e.g., mumps, Candida, or tetanus toxoid) along with PPD as a "positive control" for PPD. Commonly done in HIV-positive patients who are presumed to be more likely to be "anergic," that is, incapable of mounting a reaction to an intradermal antigen. Both arms are used—the PPD on one arm and the control on the opposite arm. Use of 2-step testing is recommended for initial skin testing of adults. This ensures that any future positive tests can be interpreted as being caused by a new infection, rather than simply a reaction to an old infection. The first test is read 48–72 hours after injection. If the first test is positive, consider the person infected. If the first test is negative, give a second test 1 to 3 weeks after the first injection.

238. **B) Mini-Mental Status Exam**   The Mini-Mental State Examination (MMSE) is used to screen for cognitive impairment/dementia. It is also used to estimate the severity of cognitive impairment at a specific time and to follow the course of cognitive changes in an individual over time, thus making it an effective way to document an individual's response to treatment. In about 10 minutes, the MMSE samples functions, including arithmetic, memory, and orientation.

239. **B) Treatment for mild acne**   That minors have the capacity and, indeed, the right to make important decisions about their own health care has been well established in federal and state policy. Many states specifically authorize minors to consent to contraceptive services, testing and treatment for HIV and other sexually transmitted diseases, prenatal care and delivery services, treatment for alcohol and drug abuse, and outpatient mental health care. With the exception of abortion, lawmakers have generally resisted attempts to impose a parental consent or notification requirement on minors' access to reproductive health care and other sensitive services. Because of its poor side-effect profile and teratogenicity, isotretinoin (Accutane) must be prescribed by a physician who is a registered member of the manufacturer's System to Manage Accutane-Related Teratogenicity program and have parental/guardian consent if the patient is under age 18.

240. **B) Serum creatinine and potassium level**   The K/DOQI (Kidney Disease Outcomes Quality Initiative) clinical practice guideline on hypertension-use of ACE inhibitors and ARB in CKD notes: After initiation or change in dose of ACE inhibitor or ARB therapy, follow-up measurements should be made in approximately *4–12 weeks* if SBP ≥120 mmHg, GFR ≥60 mL/min/1.73 m², change in GFR is <15% (GFR is measured by serum creatinine), and serum potassium ≤4.5 mEq/L. If SBP <120 mmHg, GFR <60 mL/min/1.73 m², change in GFR is ≥15%, or serum potassium >4.5 mEq/L, follow-up measurements should be at shorter intervals, and other interventions may be required.

241. **D) The patient's spouse has a right to override the attorney's decisions**   A power of attorney is a legal document that allows the appointment of another person to act as an agent to manage health, property, financial, and other affairs. The person granting the power to act is called the principal. The person who receives authorization to act on another's behalf is called the attorney-in-fact or agent. There

are different types of powers of attorney. A "durable" power of attorney stays valid even if the grantor becomes unable to handle his/her own affairs (incapacitated). If the grantor does not specify that the power of attorney is durable, it will automatically end if the grantor later becomes incapacitated. A general power of attorney gives the person chosen the power to manage the grantor's assets and financial affairs while the grantor is alive. A limited power of attorney allows the principal to give only specific powers to the agent.

242. **B) Chronic hypertension** Left ventricular hypertrophy develops in response to some factor, such as high blood pressure, that requires the left ventricle to work harder. As the workload increases, the walls of the chamber grow thicker, lose elasticity, and eventually may fail to pump with as much force as a healthy heart. High blood pressure, a blood pressure reading greater than 140/90 mmHg, is the greatest risk factor.

243. **C) Chronic coughing** Asthma is among the most common causes of chronic cough in adult nonsmokers. Although cough usually accompanies dyspnea and wheezing, it may present in isolation as a precursor of typical asthmatic symptoms, or it may remain the predominant or sole symptom of asthma. Cough-variant asthma is a type of asthma in which the main symptom is a dry, nonproductive cough. (A nonproductive cough does not expel any mucus from the respiratory tract.) People with cough-variant asthma often have no other "classic" asthma symptoms, such as wheezing or shortness of breath.

244. **D) The Board of Nursing** APRN practice is typically defined by the Nurse Practice Act and governed by the Board of Nursing, but other laws and regulations may affect practice, and other boards may play a role. For instance, in some states nurse-midwives are regulated by a Board of Midwifery or public health.

245. **A) Premedicate himself 20 to 30 minutes before starting exercise** One to 2 puffs of an inhaled short-acting beta agonist 10 to 15 minutes before exercise is enough to prevent symptoms for up to 4 hours. These inhaled bronchodilator medications can rapidly ease symptoms during an asthma attack.

246. **A) It is a slow or sudden painless loss of central vision** Atrophic macular degeneration (AMD) occurs when the macula—the central portion of the retina that is important for reading and color vision—becomes damaged. AMD is a single disease, but it can take two different forms: dry and wet. The atrophic or dry form of macular degeneration is the most common. There is a gradual withering of the visual cells and the blood vessels of the choroid (the vascular layer of tissue behind the retina). Usually the atrophic form results in only moderate loss of central vision. Although there is no medical or surgical treatment for the dry form of macular degeneration, eyesight may be helped somewhat by low-vision aids. These devices include magnifying lenses, brighter light for reading, or an electronic magnifier using a TV screen.

247. **C) Acute sinusitis** The classic symptoms of acute sinusitis in adults usually follow a cold that does not improve, or one that worsens after 5 to 7 days of symptoms. Symptoms include: bad breath or loss of smell; cough, often worse at night; fatigue and generally not feeling well; fever; headache (pressure-like

pain, pain behind the eyes, toothache, or facial tenderness); nasal congestion and discharge; and sore throat and postnasal drip. Symptoms of chronic sinusitis are the same as those of acute sinusitis, but tend to be milder and last longer than 12 weeks.

248. **C) A thyroid storm**   Thyroid storm is a life-threatening condition that develops in cases of untreated thyrotoxicosis (hyperthyroidism). This is an emergency condition. Call 911 or another emergency number. A thyroid storm is usually brought on by a stress such as trauma or infection. Symptoms are severe and include agitation, change in alertness (consciousness), confusion, diarrhea, fever, tachycardia, restlessness, shaking, sweating.

249. **B) Fluorescein stain**   Corneal abrasions result from cutting, scratching, or abrading the thin, protective, clear coat of the exposed anterior portion of the ocular epithelium. These injuries cause pain, tearing, photophobia, foreign-body sensation, and a gritty feeling. Symptoms can be worsened by exposure to light, blinking, and rubbing the injured surface against the inside of the eyelid. The diagnosis of corneal abrasion can be confirmed by visualizing the cornea under cobalt-blue filtered light after the application of fluorescein, which will cause the abrasion to appear green. If examination is limited by pain, instillation of a topical anesthetic (e.g., proparacaine [Ophthetic], tetracaine [Pontocaine]) may be needed. During the examination, it is important to assess for and remove any foreign bodies, some of which may leave a rust residue.

250. **B) Inability to swallow**   Signs and symptoms of Bell's palsy come on suddenly and may include rapid onset of mild weakness to total paralysis on one side of the face occurring within hours to days, making it difficult to smile or close the eye on the affected side. Other symptoms are facial droop and difficulty making facial expressions, pain around the jaw or in or behind the ear on the affected side, increased sensitivity to sound on the affected side, headache, a decrease in ability to taste, and changes in the amount of tears and saliva produced. In rare cases, Bell's palsy can affect the nerves on both sides of the face.

251. **A) Angiotensin-converting enzyme (ACE) inhibitor**   Hypertension is an important risk factor for the development and worsening of many complications of diabetes, including diabetic eye disease and kidney disease. Most people with diabetes develop high blood pressure during their lives. ACE inhibitors have been shown not only to be useful drugs to treat high blood pressure, but also to prevent or delay the progression of kidney disease in people with diabetes.

252. **C) Moderate persistent asthma**   The Global Initiative for Asthma has four clinical classifications of severity: intermittent, mild persistent, moderate persistent, and severe persistent. Daily symptoms, with more than 1 nighttime episode of symptoms per week, 60%–80% FEV1, and greater than 30% FEV1 variability and need for short-acting beta-2 agonist for symptom control, is classed as moderate persistent severity in patients greater than 12 years of age.

253. **D) Psoriasis**   The Auspitz sign is simply bleeding that occurs after psoriasis scales have been removed. It occurs because the capillaries run very close to the surface of the skin under a psoriasis lesion, and removing the scale essentially

pulls the tops off the capillaries, causing bleeding. Auspitz's sign is also found in other scaling disorders such as actinic keratoses.

254. **D) Any of the above**   In addition to conducting a physical examination and taking a thorough history and symptoms into account, one or more laboratory tests are used to diagnose Hashimoto's thyroiditis. The 3 most common diagnostic tests that detect this common thyroid disorder are: serum thyroid-stimulating hormone test (TSH), antithyroid antibodies tests, and the free T4 hormone test.

255. **C) Acute glaucoma**   The optic disc is the anatomical location of the eye's "blind spot," the area where the optic nerve and blood vessels enter the retina. The optic disc can be flat or it can have a certain amount of normal cupping. But glaucoma, which is due to an increase in intraocular pressure, produces additional pathological cupping of the optic disc. The pink rim of the disc contains nerve fibers. The white cup is a pit with no nerve fibers. As glaucoma advances, the cup enlarges until it occupies most of the disc area.

256. **B) The nurse practitioner may be exempted from the lawsuit if documentation is thorough and can be verified**   Medical malpractice extends to every health care profession, including nurse practitioners. As NPs assume an expanded role in the health care industry, related legal issues increase.

257. **B) Thyroid-stimulating hormone (TSH)**   A TSH level is the best screening test for detecting hypothyroidism. A normal TSH rules out primary hypothyroidism in asymptomatic patients. Abnormal TSH should be followed by determination of thyroid hormone levels. Overt hypothyroidism is defined as a clinical syndrome of hypothyroidism associated with elevated TSH and decreased serum levels of T4 or T3. Subclinical hypothyroidism is defined as a condition without typical symptoms of hypothyroidism, elevated TSH (>5 µU/mL), and normal circulating thyroid hormone. Overt thyrotoxicosis is defined as the syndrome of hyperthyroidism associated with suppressed TSH and elevated serum levels T4 or T3. Subclinical thyrotoxicosis is devoid of symptoms, but TSH is suppressed although there are normal circulating levels of thyroid hormone.

258. **B) Brudzinski's maneuver**   A stiff neck or nuchal rigidity is a sign of meningitis and intracranial hemorrhage. The Brudzinski sign may also be present when neck stiffness is assessed. Flexion of the hips and knees when flexing the neck is a positive Brudzinski sign for meningeal irritation.

259. **A) Women aged 50 years or older**   Women have a greater risk of developing thyroid disease than men. Being age 50 and above increases the risk of thyroid disease for both men and women. Pregnancy/postpartum period increases the risk of developing autoimmune thyroid disease; the risk of temporary thyroiditis increases slightly with pregnancy and during the first year postpartum.

260. **B) Order a 24-hour urine for microalbumin**   In the occurrence of proteinuria of diabetic nephropathy, damage to the three main renal functional cells—glomerular endothelial cells, epithelial cells, and renal tubular cells—plays a key role. A

microalbumin urine test is done to check for protein (albumin) in the urine. Early detection may change treatment in an effort to preserve as much kidney function as possible.

261. **A) The destruction of Rh-positive fetal red blood cells that are present in the mother's circulatory system**   Rh$_o$(D) immune globulin (RhoGAM) is used to prevent the immunological condition known as rhesus disease or hemolytic disease of the newborn. RhoGAM is a solution of IgG anti-D (anti-RhD) antibodies that suppresses the mother's immune system from attacking Rh-positive blood cells that have entered the maternal blood stream from fetal circulation. In a Rh-negative mother, RhoGAM can prevent temporary sensitization of the maternal immune system to RhD antigens, which can cause Rh disease in the current or subsequent pregnancies.

262. **A) Bacterial pneumonia**   Pneumonia is an inflammatory condition of the lung especially affecting the alveoli. Pneumonia is associated with fever, chest symptoms, and consolidation on a chest x-ray. Infectious agents include bacteria, viruses, fungi, and parasites.

263. **B) Vesicular breath sounds**   There are two normal breath sounds. Breath sounds heard over the tracheobronchial tree are called bronchial breathing and breath sounds heard over the lung tissue are called vesicular breathing.

264. **C) Less than 130/80**   The JNC 7 report delineates specific high-risk conditions that are compelling indications for the use of other antihypertensive drug classes (angiotensin-converting enzyme inhibitors, angiotensin-receptor blockers, beta-blockers, calcium channel blockers); 2 or more antihypertensive medications will be required to achieve goal BP (less than 140/90 mm Hg, or less than 130/80 mm Hg) for patients with diabetes and chronic kidney disease. For patients whose BP is more than 20 mm Hg above the systolic BP goal or more than 10 mm Hg above the diastolic BP goal, initiation of therapy using two agents, one of which usually will be a thiazide diuretic, should be considered; regardless of therapy or care, hypertension will be controlled only if patients are motivated to stay on their treatment plan.

265. **A) Nedocromil sodium (Tilade)**   Nedocromil sodium (Tilade) is a mast cell stabilizer. Mast cell stabilizers can be used to treat mild to moderate inflammation in the bronchial tubes and other allergy symptoms. These medications can also be used to prevent asthma symptoms during exercise and can be given before exposure to an allergen when it cannot be avoided. It may take several weeks before the full effects are felt.

266. **A) A patch of leukoplakia**   Leukoplakia mainly affects the mucous membranes of the mouth. It is thought to be caused by irritation. Leukoplakia are patches on the tongue, in the mouth, or on the inside of the cheek that occur in response to long-term irritation, including smoking, holding chewing tobacco or snuff in the mouth for a long period, or other tobacco use, especially pipes (smoker's keratosis).

267. **A) Document the nurse coworker's behavior and file an incident report**   Since the coworker is only suspected of narcotics addiction, the documentation of the date/behaviors observed will be needed for further evaluation, which may include reporting to the Board of Nursing and placement in the impaired nurse program.

268. **B) Mitral stenosis**   The low-frequency rumbling murmur of mitral stenosis is mid-diastolic and progresses with the severity from a short decrescendo murmur to a longer crescendo murmur. The murmur is best heard at the apical region and is not radiated. The apex is behind the fifth left intercostal space, 8 to 9 cm from the midsternal line, slightly medial to the midclavicular line. Since it is low pitched, it is heard best with the bell of the stethoscope.

269. **D) A 37-year-old male biker with a concussion due to a fall who appears agitated and does not appear to understand instructions given by the medical assistant checking his vital signs**   A concussion is a traumatic brain injury (TBI) that may result in a bad headache, altered levels of alertness, or unconsciousness. The following are emergency symptoms for which immediate medical care should be sought: changes in alertness and consciousness, seizures, muscle weakness on one or both sides, persistent confusion, repeated vomiting, unequal pupils, unusual eye movements, problems with walking, or coma.

270. **B) Decreased mobility of the tympanic membrane as measured by tympanogram**   Acute suppurative otitis media is an acute infection affecting the mucosal lining of the middle ear and the mastoid air system. Suppurative stage: The tympanic membrane bulges and ruptures spontaneously through a small perforation in the pars tensa. Ear discharge is usually present. Diagnosis is usually made simply by looking at the eardrum through an otoscope. The eardrum will appear red and swollen, and may appear either abnormally drawn inward or bulging outward. Using the tympanogram with the otoscope allows a puff of air to be blown lightly into the ear. Normally, this should cause movement of the eardrum. In an infection, or when there is fluid behind the eardrum, this movement may be decreased or absent.

271. **C) Status asthmaticus**   Status asthmaticus is a medical emergency in which asthma symptoms are refractory to initial bronchodilator therapy in the emergency department. Typically, patients present a few days after the onset of a viral respiratory illness, following exposure to a potent allergen or irritant, or after exercise in a cold environment. Frequently, patients have underused or have been under-prescribed anti-inflammatory therapy. Normally, the pulsus paradoxus (i.e., the difference in systolic blood pressure between inspiration and expiration) does not exceed 15 mm Hg. In patients with severe asthma, a pulsus paradoxus of greater than 25 mm Hg usually indicates severe airway obstruction.

272. **D) Varicocele**   An abnormal tortuosity and dilation of the veins of the pampiniform plexus within the spermatic cord is termed *varicocele*. It is most common on the left side and may be associated with pain. It occurs in boys and young men and is associated with reduced fertility. The condition, often visible only when the patient is standing, is classically described as "bag of worms."

273. **D) Decreased anxiety and depression are common symptoms of abuse in the elderly** In an abusive situation, the patient may experience increased anxiety, may not want the NP to see his or her unclothed body, may not speak in front of the abuser, and may exhibit depression and despair.

274. **A) Closure of the atrioventricular valves** A heart valve normally allows blood to flow in only one direction. A heart valve opens or closes incumbent upon differential blood pressure on each side. A form of heart disease occurs when a valve malfunctions and allows some blood to flow in the wrong direction. The S1 heart sound is caused by turbulence caused by the closure of mitral and tricuspid valves at the start of systole.

275. **D) Melanoma** People with Down syndrome (trisomy 21) develop a syndrome of dementia that has the same characteristics of Alzheimer's disease that occurs in individuals without Down syndrome. The only difference is that Alzheimer's disease occurs much earlier in people with Down syndrome; patients with Down syndrome begin to have symptoms in their late 40s or early 50s. In the United States, atlantoaxial instability (AAI) with or without subluxation has been reported in as many as 10%–30% of individuals with Down syndrome. Children with Down syndrome are at a much higher risk for congenital heart disease. Types of defects include atrioventricular septal defects (most common), ventricular septal defects, atrial septal defects, patent ductus arteriosus, and tetralogy of Fallot.

276. **D) Families change over time because of the influence of environmental factors** The family developmental framework provides a guide to examine and analyze the basic changes and developmental tasks common to most families during their life cycle. Although each family has unique characteristics, normative patterns of sequential development are common to all families. These stages and developmental tasks illustrate common family behaviors that may be expected at specific times in the family life cycle. The stages go from beginning families, families with children (multiple age categories), to aging families.

277. **D) Elevated creatinine and BUN (blood–urea–nitrogen)** Acute infectious mononucleosis symptoms consist of lymphadenopathy, fever, hepatosplenomegaly, malaise, and abdominal discomfort in adolescents and young adults. Host immune response to the viral infection includes CD8+ T lymphocytes with suppressor and cytotoxic functions, the characteristic atypical lymphocytes found in the peripheral blood. Epstein-Barr virus (EBV) antibodies may be ordered when symptoms suggest mono, but there is a negative mono test. A positive test for IgM antibodies is most likely a current, or a very recent, EBV infection. With a positive IgG concentration, it is highly likely that the patient recently had an EBV infection.

278. **A) Lateralization to one ear** The Weber test is a quick screening test for hearing. It can detect unilateral conductive hearing loss (middle ear hearing loss) and unilateral sensorineural hearing loss (inner ear hearing loss). In the Weber test, a vibrating tuning fork is placed in the middle of the forehead, above the upper lip under the nose over the teeth, or on top of the head equidistant from the patient's ears on top of thin skin in contact with the bone. In a normal patient, the Weber

tuning fork sound is heard equally loud in both ears, with no one ear hearing the sound louder than the other (lateralization). In a patient with hearing loss, the Weber tuning fork sound is heard louder in one ear (lateralization) versus the other.

279. **D) Cheilosis**   Cheilosis is the fissuring and dry scaling of the vermilion surface of the lips and angles of the mouth, a characteristic of riboflavin deficiency.

280. **C) Medroxyprogesterone (Depo-Provera)**   Depo-Provera is the brand name for a 150-mg aqueous injection of DMPA (depot medroxyprogesterone acetate). It is given as an intramuscular injection. Depo is given for contraception and for the management of endometriosis-related pain; however, one side effect of Depo is decreased bone mineral density.

281. **D) These fractures always require surgical intervention to stabilize the joint**   Typically, a scaphoid fracture occurs when the scaphoid is compressed against a bone of the forearm (the radius). This often occurs with direct contact to the palm of the hand, such as a fall on the hand with the arm outstretched. The most common signs and symptoms of a scaphoid fracture include pain, swelling, and tenderness over the thumb side of the wrist. Crunchiness and pain with gripping motions are also common symptoms that may be found with such an injury. A scaphoid fracture may mistakenly be diagnosed as a sprain and not found on an x-ray on initial examination. This fracture may be more accurately diagnosed with a bone scan if it does not appear on an x-ray. The treatment for scaphoid fractures depends largely on the severity and shape of the fracture line. Fractures that are not displaced (those where the break line is small) are immobilized (casting). Nondisplaced fractures that do not heal after 3 to 4 months often require surgical intervention, and the use of other modalities, such as electrical stimulation.

282. **B) Increase only the NPH insulin in the morning**   Regular insulin is rapid/short-acting insulin. Depending on the type of regular insulin, the onset is 10 to 15 minutes and peaks within an average of 1.5 hours with a duration of 3 to 5 hours. NPH insulin is an intermediate-acting insulin. Depending on the type of NPH insulin, the onset is 1.5 to 3 hours. NPH peaks in 4 to 12 hours and the duration is from 18 to 24 hours. By increasing the morning NPH, the peak will occur in the afternoon, bringing down the blood glucose (BG).

283. **C) Her son can participate in some sports after he has been checked for cervical instability**   Atlantoaxial instability (AAI) denotes increased mobility at the articulation of the first and second cervical vertebrae (atlantoaxial joint). The American Academy of Pediatrics issued a position statement in 1984 on AAI and Down syndrome (DS): All children with DS who wish to participate in sports should have cervical spine x-rays. Repeated x-rays are not indicated for children with DS who have had previously normal neck x-ray. Persons with DS who have no evidence of AAI may participate in all sports.

284. **A) Erythema migrans**   Erythema migrans is the rash characteristic of Lyme disease, which appears usually 7 to 10 days after a tick bite. Lyme disease is caused

by *Borrelia burgdorferi,* a spirochete. The rash appears either as a single expanding red patch or a central spot surrounded by clear skin that is in turn ringed by an expanded red rash (bull's eye). The choice of antibiotic depends on bacterial sensitivity. Doxycycline 100 mg BID for 14 to 21 days is the recommended treatment for adults.

285. **A) Cimetidine (Tagamet), digoxin (Lanoxin), diphenhydramine (Benadryl)** Drugs to avoid in the elderly population are listed on the Beer's Criteria Medication list. The American Geriatrics Society updates the Beer's Criteria list based on evidence-based recommendations. Elderly patients taking cimetidine are at risk for neuropsychiatric changes, which may be temporarily reversed by physostigmine. Older patients are also more likely to develop toxicity and diagnosis of digoxin toxicity can be difficult in this group. Benadryl can worsen glaucoma, a consideration for elderly individuals. Thick oral secretions are also a side effect, making the medication unsafe for the elderly with lung disease. It can also cause high blood pressure, a common ailment associated with aging.

286. **A) ARBs (angiotensin receptor blockers)** Beta-blockers are often used as migraine prophylaxis; however, second-degree block at the level of the atrioventriocular node (AVN) may be due to digoxin, beta-blockers, or calcium channel blockers. No beta-/alpha-blockers would be used.

287. **D) CN V** Cranial nerve V is the trigeminal nerve and is used to test corneal reflex. The procedure to test cranial nerve V is inspection for muscle atrophy and tremors. Palpate the jaw muscles for tone and strength when the patient clenches teeth. Test superficial pain and touch sensation in each branch. Test temperature sensation if there are unexpected findings to pain or touch. Use a whisp of cotton to test the corneal reflex.

288. **D) Gamma glutamyl transpeptidase (GGT)** The GGT is used to evaluate liver damage. Lipases are involved in biological processes ranging from routine metabolism of dietary triglycerides to inflammation. The main lipase includes human pancreatic lipase (HPL). The pancreas makes amylase to hydrolyze dietary starch into disaccharides and trisaccharides, which are converted by other enzymes to glucose to supply the body with energy.

289. **A) Dry cough** A dry, persistent cough is a well-described class effect of the angiotensin-converting enzyme (ACE) inhibitor medications. The mechanism of ACE inhibitor-induced cough remains unresolved, but likely involves the protussive mediators bradykinin and substance P, agents that are degraded by ACE and therefore accumulate in the upper respiratory tract or lung when the enzyme is inhibited; and prostaglandins, the production of which may be stimulated by bradykinin.

290. **A) Al-Anon is designed for family members of alcoholics** Al-Anon/Alateen, known as Al-Anon Family Groups, is an international "fellowship of relatives and friends of alcoholics who share their experience, strength, and hope in order to solve their common problems."

291. **D) McMurray's test**   The McMurray test is used to detect a torn meniscus. With the patient supine, flex one knee completely with the foot flat on the table near the buttocks. Maintain that flexion with your thumb and index finger stabilizing the knee on either side in the joint space. Hold the heel with your other hand, and rotate the foot and lower leg to a lateral position. Extend the patient's knee to a 90-degree angle; notice any palpable or audible click or limited extension of the knee. Return the knee to full flexion and repeat the procedure, rotating the foot and lower leg to the medial position. A palpable or audible click in the knee or lack of extension is a positive sign.

292. **C) The document's objectives are applicable only to people of the United States of America**   Healthy People has 4 overarching goals: 1) Attain high-quality longer lives free of preventable disease, disability, injury, and premature death. 2) Achieve health equity and eliminate disparities. 3) Create social and physical environments that promote good health for all. 4) Promote quality of life, healthy development, and healthy behaviors across life spans.

293. **A) The NP needs to do cervical cultures to verify gonorrhea**   Cultures should be taken at the time of the Pap smear, as the patient may not return for later diagnostic testing.

294. **A) Advocacy for civil rights**   There are nine provisions to the ANA's Code of Ethics. Provision 1: Professional relationships with compassion and respect for every individual. Provision 2: Commitment to the patient. Provision 3: Promote and advocate for the patient. Provision 4: Individual responsibility and accountability. Provision 5: Preserve integrity and maintain competence. Provision 6: Maintain and improve healthy environments. Provision 7: Participate in the advancement of the profession. Provision 8: Collaborate with other professionals to meet health needs. Provision 9: Maintain integrity for practice and for shaping social policy.

295. **B) A family history of migraines with aura**   A family history versus a personal history is not considered an absolute contraindication.

296. **B) Lung cancer**   "Ten Leading Cancer Types for the Estimated New Cancer Cases and Deaths by Sex, United States," 2011, estimates 28% of deaths for men and 26% for women related to lung and bronchus cancer.

297. **C) Cervical cancer**   There are more than 30 types of human papilloma virus (HPV). HPV types in the anogenital region have been strongly associated with low-grade and high-grade cervical change, cervical neoplasia, anogenital, and other cancers.

298. **A) Reactivation of EBV (Epstein–Barr virus) infection**   Reactivation of an EBV is not a criterion for the diagnosis of AIDS. EBV is a member of the herpes virus family and one of the most common viruses. When the EBV occurs during adolescence, it causes infectious mononucleosis.

299. **B) Hypertrophic cardiomyopathy**   Congenital cardiovascular disease is the leading cause of nontraumatic sudden athletic death, with hypertrophic cardiomyopathy being the most common cause. Despite public perception to the contrary,

sudden death in young athletes is exceedingly rare. It most commonly occurs in male athletes, who have estimated death rates nearly fivefold greater than the rates of female athletes.

300. **A) 15 to 18 cm in the midclavicular line** This range is considered the normal span for adults.

301. **A) Cerebellum** The main clinical features of cerebellar disorders include incoordination, imbalance, and troubles with stabilizing eye movements. Tandem gait is where the toes of the back foot touch the heel of the front foot at each step. Neurologists sometimes ask patients to walk in a straight line using tandem gait as a test to help diagnose ataxia, especially truncal ataxia, because sufferers of these disorders will have an unsteady gait.

302. **C) Osgood–Schlatter disease** Osgood–Schlatter disease is a painful swelling of the bump on the upper part of the shinbone, just below the knee. This bump is called the anterior tibial tubercle. Osgood–Schlatter disease is thought to be caused by small injuries due to repeated overuse before the area has finished growing.

303. **A) Scarlatina** Scarlatina (scarlet fever) is a rash that usually first appears on the neck and chest, then spreads over the body. It is described as "sandpapery" in feel. The texture of the rash is more important than the appearance in confirming the diagnosis. The rash can last for more than a week. As the rash fades, peeling (desquamation) may occur around the fingertips, toes, and groin area. Another sign is a bright red tongue with a "strawberry" appearance.

304. **B) This is a normal finding** Full movement of the eyes is controlled by the integrated function of cranial nerves III (oculomotor), IV (trochlear), and VI (abducens). Holding the patient's chin to prevent movement of the head, ask the patient to watch your finger as it moves through the 6 cardinal fields of gaze. Then ask the patient to look to the extreme lateral (temporal) positions. A few horizontal nystagmic beats are within normal limits (WNL).

305. **A) Acute cholecystitis** Murphy's sign is tested during an abdominal examination for biliary disorders. As the patient breathes in, the abdominal contents are pushed downward as the diaphragm moves down and the lungs expand. As the patient stops/holds the breath, the gallbladder comes in contact with the examiner's fingers and may elicit pain. To be considered positive, the same maneuver must not elicit pain when performed on the left side.

306. **D) Ciprofloxacin (Cipro)** Ciprofloxacin, doxycycline, and penicillin G procaine have been approved by the Food and Drug Administration (FDA) for prophylaxis of inhalational *Bacillus anthracis* infection. The CDC recommendations for anthrax prophylaxis include ciprofloxacin or doxycycline; amoxicillin (in three daily doses).

307. **B) Acute pancreatitis** Periumbilical ecchymosis (bluish periumbilical discoloration), Cullen's sign, is most often considered a sign of hemorrhagic pancreatitis.

308. **B) Dancing** Aerobics, weight-bearing, and resistance exercises are all effective in increasing the bone mineral density (BMD) of the spine in postmenopausal women. Walking is also effective for the hip. Dancing is a weight-bearing exercise.

309. **C) Pneumococcal (Pneumovax) and influenza vaccines** The tetanus (Td) immunization is good for about 10 years. October/November is the beginning window of the flu season and the pneumococcal (pneumonia) vaccine is indicated for patients older than 65 years.

310. **C) Paroxysms of coughing that are dry or productive of mucoid sputum** A cough is the main symptom of acute bronchitis. It may be dry at first (does not produce mucus) and after a few days may bring up mucus from the lungs (productive cough). The mucus may be clear, yellow, or green. Sometimes small streaks of blood may be present.

311. **A) Arcus senilis (senile arcus)** Arcus senilis (*arcus senilis corneae*) is a white, gray, or blue opaque ring in the corneal margin (peripheral corneal opacity), or white ring in front of the periphery of the iris. It is present at birth, but then fades; however, it is quite commonly present in the elderly. It can also appear earlier in life as a result of hypercholesterolemia. Unilateral arcus is a sign of decreased blood flow to the unaffected eye due to carotid artery disease or ocular hypotony.

312. **D) Gold salt injections** Gold is used to reduce inflammation and slow disease progression in people with rheumatoid arthritis. Gold is not usually the first treatment given to people with rheumatoid arthritis, since methotrexate and other disease-modifying, anti-rheumatic drugs (DMARDs) are available.

313. **C) Night vision** There are two types of photoreceptors in the human retina: rods and cones. Cones are active at higher light levels (photopic vision), and are capable of color vision and night vision. Cones are responsible for high spatial acuity. The central fovea is populated exclusively by cones. There are three types of cones that we will refer to as the short-wavelength sensitive cones, the middle-wavelength sensitive cones, and the long-wavelength sensitive cones or S-cones, M-cones, and L-cones for short. Rods are responsible for vision at low light levels (scotopic vision). They do not mediate color vision, and have a low spatial acuity.

314. **D) Second-degree burns on the lower arm** Burns are described according to the depth of injury to the dermis and are loosely classified into first, second, third, and fourth degrees. A second-degree (superficial partial-thickness) burn extends into the superficial (papillary) dermis. Appearance is red with clear blisters, blanches with pressure, moist texture, painful sensation. It takes 2 to 3 weeks to heal.

315. **B) Second intercostal space, left sternal border** S2 is physiologically split in about 90% of people. The second heart sound is produced by the closure of the aortic and pulmonic valves. The sound produced by the closure of the aortic valve is termed A2 and the sound produced by the closure of the pulmonic valve is

termed P2. The A2 sound is normally much louder than the P2 due to higher pressures in the left side of the heart; thus, A2 radiates to all cardiac listening posts (loudest at the right upper sternal border) and P2 is usually only heard at the left upper sternal border.

316. **C) <120/80** JNC VII Guidelines recommend that BP readings be less than 120/80.

317. **A) A severe sunburn with blistering** Burns are described according to the depth of injury to the dermis and are loosely classified into first, second, third, and fourth degrees. A second-degree (superficial partial-thickness) burn extends into the superficial (papillary) dermis. Appearance is red with clear blisters, blanches with pressure, has moist texture, painful sensation. It takes 2 to 3 weeks to heal.

318. **B) Her son's physical development is delayed and should be evaluated by a pediatric endocrinologist** Puberty may be delayed for several years and still occur normally, in which case it is considered constitutional delay, a variation of healthy physical development. Delay of puberty may also occur due to malnutrition, many forms of systemic disease, or to defects of the reproductive system (hypogonadism) or the body's responsiveness to sex hormones. Hypogonadism is when the sex glands produce little or no hormones. In men, these glands (gonads) are the testes. An endocrinology consult is warranted.

319. **A) Temporal arteritis (giant cell arteritis)** Temporal arteritis (TA) is inflammation and damage to blood vessels that supply the head area, particularly the large or medium arteries that branch from the neck and supply the temporal area. Headache is the most common chief complaint and presents in over two thirds of patients with temporal arteritis. The headache tends to be new or different in character than previous headaches and is typically sudden in onset, localizing to the temporal region. Vision difficulties that occur with TA include blurred, double, or reduced vision. Blindness may occur in one or both eyes. Any new headache in patients older than 50 years warrants a consideration of temporal arteritis. The patient should be instructed to stop smoking.

320. **D)** *Chlamydia trachomatis* Although chlamydia may seem like an obvious candidate to cause systemic infections since it can ascend to the uterus and affect a variety of sites including the eyes and the rectum, the specific type of chlamydia that causes genital infections is not generally thought to cause systemic infections. The predominant infections are urethritis, cervicitis, and proctitis, but chlamydial infection can spread locally to the Bartholin glands, endosalpinges, or epididymis. Up to 40% of untreated chlamydial cervicitis cases will ascend into the upper genital tract, where considerable tubal damage can occur with very few symptoms.

321. **B) CN VIII** The CN VIII cranial nerve is the acoustic nerve. The Rinne test is performed by placing the base of a vibrating tuning fork against the patient's mastoid bone to evaluate bone conduction. Ask the patient to tell you when the sound is no longer heard. Then place the tuning fork in the front of the ear to evaluate air conduction. Air conduction should be twice as long as bone-conduction sound.

322. **C) Thiamine intoxication** This patient would not have thiamine intoxication on presentation. Thiamine is administered to prevent Wernicke-Korsakoff syndrome, usually found in chronic alcoholics. Wernicke-Korsakoff syndrome (alcoholic encephalopathy) can cause a seizure, vision changes, ataxia, and impaired memory.

323. **B) Oral tetracycline** One antibiotic often prescribed for the treatment of moderate to severe acne is tetracycline. The medication is not recommended for acne that is not moderate or severe. It helps control acne by curbing the growth of bacteria and reducing inflammation, which results in fewer pimples and less redness. Because of its poor side effect profile and teratogenicity, isotretinoin (Accutane) must by prescribed by a physician who is a registered member of the manufacturer's System to Manage Accutane-Related Teratogenicity program and have parental/guardian consent if the patient is under age 18.

324. **B) The typical lesions are bullae** Shingles rash starts as small blisters on a red base, with new blisters continuing to form for 3 to 5 days. The blisters follow the path of individual nerves—dermatome pattern—and appear in a bandlike pattern on an area of skin. The entire path of the affected nerve may be involved, or there may be areas in the distribution of the nerve with blisters and areas without blisters. Shingles is a skin rash caused by a nerve and skin inflammation from the varicella zoster virus (VZV) and belongs to the herpes family of viruses.

325. **A) Hidradenitis suppurativa** Considered a severe form of acne (acne inversa), hidradenitis suppurativa occurs deep in the skin around the sebaceous glands and hair follicles. The parts of the body affected—the groin and armpits—are the main locations of apocrine sweat glands. Hidradenitis suppurativa tends to start after puberty, persist for years and worsen over time. Excess weight, stress, hormonal changes, heat, or excessive perspiration can worsen symptoms. Sometimes hidradenitis suppurativa occurs with other diseases, such as Crohn's disease or Graves' disease.

326. **C) Edema of the ankles and headaches** Cardiovascular side effects can be significant with nifedipine (Procardia XL) and have included peripheral edema (7% to 29%), hypotension (less than 1% to 5%), palpitations (less than 1% to 7%), myocardial infarction (4%), congestive heart failure (2%), and noncardiogenic edema (0.6% to 8%).

327. **A) Vigorous massage of the prostate** A prostate massage should never be done in a patient with suspected acute prostatitis, since it may induce sepsis. Acute prostatitis is associated with chills, fever, pain in the lower back and genital area, urinary frequency and urgency (often at night), burning or painful urination, body aches, and a demonstrable infection of the urinary tract, as evidenced by white blood cells and bacteria in the urine. Acute prostatitis is considered a medical emergency. It should be distinguished from other forms of prostatitis such as chronic bacterial prostatitis and chronic pelvic pain syndrome (CPPS).

328. **A) Prostate-specific antigen (PSA)** Prostate cancer is the most common malignancy in men and the second leading cause of cancer-specific deaths in U.S. males. The United States Preventative Services Task Force recommended that the PSA

blood test no longer be offered to men for early detection of prostate cancer. This federal agency concluded that the benefits of early detection of prostate cancer are outweighed by the risks of both diagnosis and treatment. However, the American Urological Association recommends regular PSA screening for all men over 40.

329. **C) Macrolides** The Infectious Diseases Society of the American/American Thoracic Society consensus guidelines for the management of community-acquired pneumonia (CAP) in adults notes that if the patient is previously healthy with no risk factors for drug-resistant *Staphylococcus pneumoniae* (DRSP) infection treatment, the use of a macrolide antibiotic (azithromycin, clarithromycin, or erythromycin) for CAP is preferred.

330. **D) Neovascularization and microaneurysms** The severity of nonproliferative diabetic retinopathy (NPDR) can be graded as mild, moderate, severe, or very severe. In mild disease, microaneurysms are present with hemorrhage or hard exudates (lipid transudates). In moderate NPDR, these findings are associated with cotton-wool spots (focal infarcts of the retinal nerve fiber layer or areas of axoplasmic stasis) or intraretinal microvascular abnormalities (vessels that may be either abnormally dilated and tortuous retinal vessels or intraretinal neovascularization).

331. **B) This is a normal finding due to the skeletal growth spurt in this age group** Alkaline phosphatase is a group of related enzymes. The bone form of the enzyme creates the alkaline conditions it requires to be most active with a chemical reaction involving the osteoblasts. Because of the rapid bone growth and increased deposit of calcium, there is a higher alkaline phosphatase level.

332. **B) Irrigate with normal saline and apply Silvadene cream BID** Silvadene (silver sulfadiazine): Initial cream for suspected partial and full-thickness burns (2nd and 3rd degree). Action: Contains silver sulfadiazine in micronized form, which has broad microbial activity. It is bactericidal against many gram-negative and gram-positive bacteria as well as being effective against yeasts. Silvadene is a sulfa drug and should not be used on someone who has a sulfa allergy. It should also be used on external areas only.

333. **A) Advise the patient that he is immune to hepatitis C and no further testing is indicated** The anti-HCV test detects the presence of antibodies to the hepatitis C virus, indicating exposure to HCV. The anti-HCV test cannot distinguish between someone with active or previous HCV infection (reported as positive or negative).

334. **C) Atrophy of the sebaceous glands** Sebaceous glands produce less oil as one ages. Men experience a minimal decrease, usually after the age of 80. Women gradually produce less oil beginning after menopause. This can make it harder to keep the skin moist, resulting in dryness and itchiness.

335. **D) It reviews information via a nongovernmental agency** The state board of nursing is a regulatory agency created by the state government and is devoted to monitor nurses' personal and professional behaviors. State boards of nursing have

"the legislative power to initiate, regulate, and enforce the provisions of the Nurse Practice Act."

336. **A) The veins are larger than the arterioles**   The fundus of the eye is opposite the lens, and includes the retina, optic disc, macula and fovea, and the posterior pole. The eye's fundus is the only part of the human body where the microcirculation can be observed directly. The retinal arteries and veins emerge from the nasal side (left) of the optic disc. Vessels directed temporally have an arching course; those directed nasally have a radial course. Arteries are brighter red and narrower than veins.

337. **D) Ovarian hormonal imbalance**   Ovarian hormonal imbalance is not a risk factor for Afib. Risk factors include older age, heart disease, hypertension, chronic conditions such as sleep apnea, alcohol use (especially binge drinking), and family history.

338. **A) Gonorrhea**   Gonorrhea is caused by the bacteria *Neisseria gonorrhoeae*. Health care providers in every state in the United States are required by law to tell their state board of health about anyone diagnosed with gonorrhea. Symptoms of gonorrhea usually appear 2–5 days after infection; however, in men, symptoms may take up to a month to appear. Early symptoms include dysuria, increased urinary frequency/urgency, white/yellow/green penile discharge, red or edematous penile urethra, tender/swollen testicles. If the infection spreads systemically, fever, rash, and arthritis-like symptoms may occur.

339. **D) Acute abdomen**   Suspected ruptured appendix or a pelvic abscess irritates the lateral iliopsoas muscle. The patient should be in the supine position; place your hand over the lower thigh for testing. The iliopsoas muscle test is performed by asking the patient to raise the leg, flexing at the hip, while you push downward against the leg. An alternate technique is to have the patient lie on the left side and ask the patient to raise the right leg from the hip while you press downward against it. The iliopsoas muscle test is positive if the patient experiences lower quadrant pain.

340. **B) CN III, CN IV, and CN VI**   Cranial nerves III (oculomotor), IV (trochlear), and VI (abducens) innervate the extrocular muscles. Inspect the eyelids for drooping. Inspect pupil size for equality and their direct and consensual response to light and accommodation.

341. **A) Hemoglobin electrophoresis**   Review the complete blood count and reticulocyte count for clues to the diagnosis or complicating diseases. Hemoglobin electrophoresis and isoelectric focusing are the most commonly used tests for the diagnosis of sickle hemoglobinopathies. Although the definitive diagnosis of thalassemia syndromes requires direct DNA-based techniques, hemoglobin electrophoresis is a useful ancillary test to differentiate thalassemias from the sickle hemoglobinopathies and to help differentiate among the thalassemias.

342. **C) Overweight patients**   Metformin (glucophage) often causes weight loss. Metformin may rarely cause a serious, life-threatening condition called lactic

acidosis. Patients with dehydration, renal disease, and alcoholism (especially binge drinking) increase their risk for developing lactic acidosis.

343. **C) Bacterial pneumonia**   The most common cause of bacterial pneumonia is a type of bacteria known as *Streptococcus pneumoniae*. *Haemophilus influenzae, Chlamydia pneumoniae, Mycoplasma pneumoniae,* and *Legionella pneumophila* are some other major bacteria that cause pneumonia. Typical pneumonia comes on very quickly; the patient has high fever/chills, productive cough with yellow or brown sputum, shortness of breath, and may have chest pain with breathing/coughing. Older people can have confusion or a change in their mental abilities. With bacterial pneumonia it is important to determine whether bacteria are present in the urine to identify appropriate antibiotics to treat the bacteria.

344. **B) Azithromycin ER (Zmax)**   This is the first antipneumonia antibiotic approved for single-dose delivery.

345. **B) Beta-blockers**   Beta-blockers require a gradual reduction in dose. Suddenly stopping taking a beta-blocker can sometimes cause problems such as palpitations, a rise in blood pressure, or a recurrence of angina pains.

346. **D) Migraine headaches**   Migraines are not a contraindication to Betimol (timolol). Contraindications include bronchial asthma, asthma history, severe COPD, uncompensated heart failure, second- or third-degree AV block, sinus bradycardia, and cardiogenic shock. Caution should be used if the following conditions are present: closed-angle glaucoma, peripheral vascular disease, bronchospastic disease, diabetes, hyperthyroidism, and myasthenia gravis.

347. **A) Anticholinergic effects**   Antihistamines' anticholinergic side effects include dry mouth and throat, increased heart rate, pupil dilation, urinary retention, constipation, and, at high doses, hallucinations or delirium.

348. **A) The patient becomes very agitated, confused, and aggressive after sunset and throughout the night with resolution of symptoms in the morning**   Sundowning is a psychological phenomenon associated with increased confusion and restlessness in patients with some forms of dementia. Most commonly associated with Alzheimer's disease, but also found in those with mixed dementia, the term "sundowning" was coined due to the timing of the patient's confusion. Sundowning seems to occur more frequently during the middle stages of Alzheimer's disease and mixed dementia. Symptoms include increased general confusion as natural light begins to fade/shadows increase. Agitation and mood swings—yelling and becoming upset with the caregiver—are not uncommon, plus fatigue, tremors, increase in restlessness. Restlessness can lead to pacing or wandering.

349. **A) Document in the patient's record his behaviors and the action taken by the nurse**   Patients have the right to refuse their medications. Bipolar disorder tends to get worse if it is not treated. Explain that there is a good chance that manic and depressive episodes will become more frequent and severe over time.

350. **B) Educate the mother that it is a benign finding**   S2 is physiologically split in about 90% of people. The second heart sound is produced by the closure of the

aortic and pulmonic valves. The sound produced by the closure of the aortic valve is termed A2, and the sound produced by the closure of the pulmonic valve is termed P2. The A2 sound is normally much louder than the P2 due to higher pressures in the left side of the heart; thus, A2 radiates to all cardiac listening posts (loudest at the right upper sternal border) and P2 is usually only heard at the left upper sternal border.

351. **A) Informed consent**   The most important goal of informed consent is that the patient has an opportunity to be an informed participant in his/her own health care decisions. It is generally accepted that complete informed consent includes a discussion of the following elements: the nature of the decision/procedure; reasonable alternatives to the proposed intervention; the relevant risks, benefits, and uncertainties related to each alternative; assessment of patient understanding; and the acceptance of the intervention by the patient.

352. **A) Reduce intake of potassium because of its cardiac effects**   Lifestyle modifications for HTN include losing weight (especially waistline), regular exercise, DASH diet—lots of whole grains, fruits, vegetables, and low-fat dairy, limited saturated fat. Potassium can lessen the effects of Na on HTN. Calcium helps to produce the heartbeat, and magnesium regulates it. Reduce sodium; limit to 2,300 mg/day. Limit ethanol (ETOH).

353. **C) Tertiary prevention**   Art therapy is an example of tertiary prevention. Primary prevention involves methods to avoid occurrence of disease, including health promotion. Secondary prevention is used to diagnose and treat existent disease in early stages before it causes significant morbidity. Tertiary prevention involves methods to reduce the negative impact of an existing disease by restoring function and reducing disease-related complications.

354. **C) Osteoporosis**   Kyphosis is a curving of the spine that causes a bowing or rounding of the back, which leads to a hunchback (dowager hump) or slouching posture. Adult kyphosis can be caused by degenerative diseases of the spine such as disc disease or arthritis, fractures caused by osteoporosis/osteoporotic compression fracture, injury/trauma, and slipping of one vertebra forward on another (spondylolisthesis).

355. **C) Thayer-Martin culture**   Thayer-Martin Selective Agar is an enriched medium for the selective isolation of *Neisseria* species.

356. **D) Loretta Ford, PhD**   Loretta Ford, NP, EdD, FAAN, is considered the founder of the nurse practitioner movement, and has received many awards for her work. Ford has graduate degrees in nursing and a Doctorate in Education from the University of Colorado and was certified as a Public Health Nurse. In the early 1960s, she and pediatrician Henry K. Silver were colleagues at the University of Colorado. With a regional shortage of family care physicians and pediatricians hampering health care delivery to rural and underserved areas, they saw that innovation was needed to solve the problem. They got a small grant from the university in 1965 and created a demonstration project, focusing on extending the role of the nurse in the community. They published their findings and developed an educational curriculum for nurse practitioners.

357. **A) Benign prostatic hypertrophy (BPH) and hypertension**   Terazosin is used in men to treat the symptoms of an enlarged prostate (benign prostatic hyperplasia or BPH), which include difficulty urinating (hesitation, dribbling, weak stream, and incomplete bladder emptying), painful urination, and urinary frequency and urgency. It also is used alone or in combination with other medications to treat high blood pressure. Terazosin is in a class of medications called alpha-blockers. It relieves the symptoms of BPH by relaxing the muscles of the bladder and prostate. It lowers blood pressure by relaxing the blood vessels so that blood can flow more easily through the body.

358. **C) Basilar migraine headaches**   Symptoms related to papilledema when caused by increased pressure include headache (but not a basilar migraine headache) and nausea with vomiting and a machinery-like sound. Papilledema is an optic disc swelling that is secondary to elevated intracranial pressure. Some important causes of increased pressure from cerebral spinal fluid and papilledema are brain tumors and brain infections, such as a brain abscess, meningitis, or encephalitis. A pressure increase resulting from bleeding or from very high blood pressure can also cause papilledema.

359. **A) The blue dot sign**   All prepubertal and young adult males with acute scrotal pain should be considered to have testicular torsion until proven otherwise. The finding of an ipsilateral absent cremasteric reflex is the most accurate sign of testicular torsion. It may also be diagnosed by the "blue dot sign" (i.e., tender nodule with blue discoloration on the upper pole of the testis). Treatment involves rapid restoration of blood flow to the affected testis. The optimal time frame for treatment is less than 6 hours after the onset of symptoms.

360. **A) Left heart failure**   Heart failure (HF) signs and symptoms arise from congested organs and hypoperfused tissues. Left-sided heart failure (systolic heart failure) is the most common cause of HF. The ventricle loses some ability to contract and lacks the power to pump the oxygenated blood out. Side effects include dyspnea, fatigue, chronic cough or wheezing, rapid or irregular heart rate, lack of appetite/nausea, mental confusion, edema, and rapid weight gain.

361. **D) Hypertension**   Hypertension is not associated with an increase in mortality with pneumonia. More complications occur in very young or very old individuals who have multiple areas of the lung infected simultaneously. Individuals with other chronic illnesses (including cirrhosis of the liver, congestive heart failure), individuals without a functioning spleen, and individuals who have other diseases that result in a weakened immune system experience complications. Patients with immune disorders, various types of cancer, transplant patients, and AIDS patients also experience complications. An alcohol-impaired pulmonary immune system is no defense against pneumonia-producing bacteria.

362. **A) *Streptococcus pneumoniae***   Community-acquired pneumonia (CAP) is the sixth most common cause of death in the United States and the leading cause of death from infectious diseases. It is associated with significant morbidity and mortality, and poses a major economic burden to the healthcare system. *Streptococcus pneumoniae* is the leading cause of CAP.

363. **B) Initiate a prescription of hydrochlorothiazide 12.5 mg PO daily** HDTZ is a thiazide diuretic. Thiazide diuretics are recommended as initial therapy for uncomplicated hypertension, either alone or in combination with other agents, by the JNC-7 guidelines. The Cochrane collaboration, WHO, and the U.S. guidelines also support low-dose thiazide-based diuretics as first-line treatment for hypertension.

364. **B) Antibiotics** Experts recommend that antibiotics not be used for acute bronchitis. Antibiotics reduce coughing slightly, but most people who have bronchitis improve without antibiotics. In people who also have symptoms of a common cold but have no signs of pneumonia, antibiotics generally are not effective.

365. **A) Microalbuminuria and diabetes** Cardiovascular (CV) risk prevention requires a multifaceted strategy to reach guideline committee (JNC 7 and ATP III) goals to reduce CV disease. Cardiovascular risk factors include HTN, smoking, obesity, physical inactivity, dyslipidemia, diabetes, microalbuminuria or estimated GFR less than 60 m/min, age (over 55 for men/65 for women), family history of premature CV death (men under age 55/women under age 65).

366. **D) CAGE test** The CAGE assessment is: C: Have you ever tried to Cut back on your use? A: Have you ever been Annoyed/Angered when questioned about your use? G: Have you ever felt Guilty about your use? E: Have you ever had an Eye-opener to get started in the morning? Binging may lead to more serious alcohol/drug consumption.

367. **B) Initiate a prescription of metformin (Glucophage) 500 mg PO BID** Standards of Medical Care in Diabetes 2012 notes that in a patient with classic symptoms of hyperglycemia or hyperglycemic crisis, a random plasma glucose greater than 200 mg/dL is diagnostic. At the time of type 2 diabetes diagnosis, initiate metformin therapy along with lifestyle interventions, unless metformin is contraindicated.

368. **B) Strenuous exercise is contraindicated for most type 1 diabetics because of a higher risk of hypoglycemic episodes** With increasing emphasis on fitness and competitive sports, more diabetic individuals are engaging in intense physical activity with greater frequency. The therapeutic approaches that derive from the latter observations, that is, to increase consumption of rapidly assimilated carbohydrate in the period around which exercise is performed and/or to adjust insulin doses downward in anticipation of exercise could actually exacerbate the hyperglycemia that follows intense exercise. Though not quantified, many diabetic athletes report hyperglycemia following intense exercise.

369. **C) *Pseudomonas aeruginosa*** *Pseudomonas aeruginosa* is an uncommon cause of CAP but is a particularly difficult bacteria to treat.

370. **C) Adrenal glands** Over time, the effects of hypertension can include a heart attack, kidney failure, and congestive heart failure. The body structures most vulnerable to high blood pressure include the blood vessels (including eyes), heart, brain, and kidneys. Catecholamines are a class of hormones secreted by the adrenal

glands. They include adrenaline and noradrenaline, which regulate heart rate, blood pressure, sweating, and other reactions that prepare the body for physical activity. Corticosteroids, like cortisol, and mineralocorticoids, such as aldosterone, are also secreted by the adrenal glands. Cortisol helps the body cope with stress, while aldosterone regulates blood pressure and blood levels of sodium and potassium.

371. **B) Dial 911**   This patient is exhibiting classic symptoms of a myocardial infarction and needs immediate treatment—call 911.

372. **D) Misoprostol (Cytotec)**   Misoprostol is recommended for short-term, uncomplicated PUD because it decreases gastric acid production and enhances mucosal resistance to injury.

373. **D) Furosemide (Lasix)**   There were no interactions found in our database between erythromycin and Lasix. The cytochrome P450 enzyme system plays a significant role in drug metabolism, particularly with regard to drug interactions. Erythromycin has been shown to potentiate the pharmacodynamic effects of warfarin. Erythromycins inhibit the metabolism of theophylline, increasing the risk for theophylline toxicity. Modification of the antibiotic erythromycin with the CYP450 system also detoxifies such diverse drugs as codeine, diazepam (Valium), paclitaxel (Taxol), and several anti-HIV drugs. This will slow down the detoxification of drugs, which may cause them to have stronger effects than expected.

374. **A) Severe ulcers in the stomach or duodenum**   Zollinger-Ellison syndrome is a condition in which there is increased production of the hormone gastrin. Complications from Zollinger-Ellison include intestinal bleeding or perforation from the stomach or duodenum. Proton pump inhibitors are the first choice for treating Zollinger-Ellison syndrome. PPIs reduce acid production by the stomach, and promote healing of ulcers in the stomach and small intestine.

375. **Ciprofloxacin (Cipro)**   Ciprofloxacin (Cipro) is a fluoroquinolone class antibiotic and is an FDA pregnancy category C. The *pregnancy category* of a pharmaceutical agent is an assessment of the risk of fetal injury due to the pharmaceutical if it is used as directed by the mother during pregnancy. Category A = adequate well-controlled studies failed to demonstrate a risk to the fetus in the first trimester and no evidence of risk in the later trimesters. Category B = animal studies have shown an adverse effect, but adequate and well-controlled studies in pregnant women have failed to demonstrate a risk to the fetus in any trimester. Category C = animal studies have shown an adverse effect on the fetus, but there are no adequate and well-controlled studies in humans, and potential benefits may warrant use of the drug in pregnant women despite potential risks. Category D = there is positive evidence of human fetal risk based on adverse reaction data from investigational or marketing experience, but potential benefits may warrant use of the drug in pregnant women despite potential risks. Category X = studies in animals for humans have demonstrated fetal abnormalities; the risks involved clearly outweigh the potential benefits.

376. **B) Psoriasis**   Nail abnormalities are problems with the color, shape, texture, or thickness of the fingernails or toenails. Psoriasis may cause pitting, splitting of the nail plate from the nailbed, and chronic destruction of the nail plate (nail dystrophy).

377. **C) It is best heard at the apex at S1** Following a normal S1 and briefly quiet systole, the valve suddenly prolapses, resulting in a midsystolic click. The click is so characteristic of MVP that even without a subsequent murmur, its presence alone is enough for the diagnosis. Immediately after the click, a brief crescendo–decrescendo murmur is heard, usually best at the apex.

378. **B) Acute appendicitis** McBurney's point is the name given to the point over the right side of the abdomen that is 1/3 of the distance (approximately 2 inches) from the anterior superior iliac spine to the umbilicus. This point roughly corresponds to the most common location of the base of the appendix where it is attached to the cecum. (During pregnancy the location of the appendix changes as the uterus grows.)

379. **C) Chewing breath mints** The mint flavoring in breath mints and chewing gum triggers acid reflux. Acid-reflux diets usually list peppermint, spearmint, and other mints as foods to avoid. Foods that also aggravate acid reflux include chocolate, fatty or fried foods, whole milk, oils, creamed foods or soup, and many fast foods. Citrus fruit and juices and coffee and other caffeinated drinks may also irritate an esophagus inflamed by acid reflux. Among obese patients in a weight-loss program, about 2/3 of those with gastroesophageal reflux disease (GERD) reported complete symptom resolution by the end of the intervention. Alcohol relaxes the lower esophageal sphincter, allowing the reflux of stomach contents into the esophagus. It also increases the production of stomach acid.

380. **D) Repeat the Gen-Probe test for *Chlamydia trachomatis* to ensure that the previous test was not a false-negative result** Repeating the Gen-Probe test for chlamydia is not recommended. The 2010 CDC STD treatment guidelines for pelvic inflammatory disease (PID) state: PID comprises a spectrum of inflammatory disorders of the upper female genital tract, including any combination of endometritis, salpingitis, tubo-ovarian abscess, and pelvic peritonitis. Delay in diagnosis and treatment probably contributes to inflammatory sequelae in the upper reproductive tract. Treatment should be initiated as soon as the presumptive diagnosis has been made, because prevention of long-term sequelae is dependent on early administration of appropriate antibiotics. All regimens used to treat PID should also be effective against *N. gonorrhoeae* and *C. trachomatis* because negative endocervical screening for these organisms does not rule out upper-reproductive-tract infection. Outpatient, oral therapy can be considered for women with mild to moderately severe acute PID, because the clinical outcomes among women treated with oral therapy are similar to those treated with parenteral therapy. **Recommended regimen**: Ceftriaxone (Rocephin) 250 mg IM in a single dose PLUS doxycycline 100 mg orally twice a day for 14 days WITH or WITHOUT metronidazole 500 mg orally twice a day for 14 days.

381. **C) Tanner Stage IV** The Stage of breast and pubic hair development in the female is related to her chronological age, age at menarche, and evidence of the height spurt. Breasts begin development before pubic hair. In Tanner Stage IV, the areola and papilla form a secondary mound.

382. **A) Depo-Provera injections** The synthetic hormonal substance in Depo-Provera (depot medroxyprogesterone acetate or DMPA) is the better choice of the 4. The patient is a smoker and should not be on oral contraceptives/estrogen. With her history of chlamydial cervicitis, she is not a candidate for an IUD (would increase risk for PID).

383. **A) Clarithromycin (Biaxin)** Clarithromycin may block the breakdown of theophylline by the liver. If this happens, blood levels of theophylline could be increased and this could cause an increase in side effects, including stomach irritation, loss of appetite, nervousness, and irritability. More serious or potentially dangerous side effects include seizures, a rapid heartbeat, a decrease in blood pressure, and an abnormal heart rhythm. However, theophylline may cause clarithromycin to be removed from the body at a faster rate than normal. If this happens, then potentially less clarithromycin would be available for the body to use and blood levels could become too low. This could make clarithromycin less effective at fighting an infection.

384. **D) G6PD-deficiency anemia** The pneumonia vaccine would be especially recommended for all of the patient's conditions listed with the exception of C6PD deficiency (hemolytic anemia). The pneumonia vaccination is a vaccine indicated for active immunization for the prevention of disease caused by *Streptococcus pneumoniae*. Immunocompromised individuals or individuals with impaired immune responsiveness due to the use of immunosuppressive therapy may have reduced antibody response. This would include patients with sickle cell anemia, post splenectomy, and patients with HIV.

385. **B) Paroxysmal atrial tachycardia** In paroxysmal supraventricular tachycardia (PSVT), abnormal conduction of electricity causes the atrium, and secondarily the ventricles, to beat very rapidly. It is paroxysmal, because the rapid rate can occur sporadically and without warning. It may last a few seconds or many hours. A person experiencing PSVT may feel his or her heart rate go from 60 to 200 beats per minute or more. It typically also has a sudden termination from the fast heart rate back to normal rhythm. PSVT often presents with the complaints of palpitations, described as a rapid heart rate often felt in the throat, and may be associated with lightheadedness, weakness, SOB, and chest pain. Most supraventricular tachycardias have a narrow QRS complex on EKG, but supraventricular tachycardia with aberrant (abnormal appearing) conduction (SVTAC) can produce a wide-complex tachycardia that may mimic ventricular tachycardia (VT). The Valsalva maneuver should be the first vagal maneuver tried. Carotid sinus massage, carried out by firmly pressing the bulb at the top of *one* of the carotid arteries in the neck, is effective but is often not recommended due to risks of stroke in those with plaque in the carotid arteries.

386. **A) Oral metronidazole (Flagyl)** A single dose of metronidazole is effective in the majority of cases of *Trichomonas* infections. The strawberry cervix is considered to be selectively associated with trichomonas. The etiology is the parasitic protozoan flagellate, *T. vaginalis*. Symptoms include a foul-smelling vaginal discharge (often fishy); burning and soreness of the vulva, perineum, and thighs; dyspareunia and dysuria. Wet prep microscopic examination should reveal highly motile cells, slightly larger than leukocytes, smaller than epithelial cells.

387. **C) Mitral regurgitation** Mitral regurgitation does not cause secondary hypertension. One of the principal causes of secondary hypertension is related to adrenal gland tumors or dysfunctions such as Cushing's syndrome, primary aldosteronism (Conn's syndrome), and pheochromocytoma. Renovascular hypertension is a type of secondary hypertension caused by narrowing (stenosis) of one or both arteries leading to the kidneys. Renovascular hypertension can cause severe hypertension and irreversible kidney damage. Sleep apnea causes part of the nervous system to be overactive and release certain chemicals that increase blood pressure.

388. **B) She should avoid alcoholic drinks 1 day before, during therapy, and a few days after therapy** The patient should avoid alcoholic drinks during and for at least 3 days after therapy with metronidazole (Flagyl). Flagyl and alcohol together cause severe nausea and vomiting, flushing, fast heartbeat (tachycardia), and shortness of breath. The reaction has been described as being similar to the effects of Antabuse.

389. **C) Preventive therapy for *Pneumocystis carinii* pneumonia (PCP)** Once a patient's CD4 count declines significantly, prophylaxis for opportunistic infections is initiated and continues indefinitely. Strongly recommended standard of care for *Pneumocystis carinii* pneumonia (PCP): Indication CD4+ count less than 200/µL or oropharyngeal candidiasis. First-choice preventive regimen: TMP-SMZ 1 DS or SS PO q day.

390. **A) Acute appendicitis** Suspected ruptured appendix or a pelvic abscess irritates the lateral iliopsoas and obturator muscles. The patient should be in the supine position for testing. The iliopsoas muscle test is performed by the patient raising the leg from the hip while the examiner pushes downward against it. The obturator muscle test is performed with the right leg flexed at the hip and the knee at 90 degrees; the examiner rotates the leg laterally and medially. These muscle tests are positive if the patient experiences pain.

391. **D) Testes** Spermatogenesis takes place within several structures of the male reproductive system. The initial stages occur within the testes and progress to the epididymis, where the developing gametes mature and are stored until ejaculation. When ejaculation occurs, sperm is forcefully expelled from the tail of the epididymis into the deferent duct. Sperm then travels through the deferent duct up the spermatic cord into the pelvic cavity, over the ureter to the prostate behind the bladder. Here, the vas deferens joins with the seminal vesicle to form the ejaculatory duct, which passes through the prostate and empties into the urethra.

392. **D) Nedocromil sodium (Tilade)** Nedocromil sodium (Tilade) is a mast cell stabilizer and is used to treat mild to moderate inflammation in the bronchial tubes and other allergy symptoms. *Pneumocystis* pneumonia (PCP) is the most common opportunistic infection in people with HIV. Drugs used to treat PCP include trimethroprim-sulfamethoxazole (TMP/SMX), dapsone, pentamidine, and atovaquone.

393. **A) Acoustic nerve damage** The other symptoms listed are common with labrynthitis; made worse with moving the head, sitting up, rolling over, or looking upward.

394. **D) Stroke and coronary heart disease** A bruit is a murmur heard over the carotid artery in the neck, suggesting arterial narrowing. It is usually secondary to atherosclerosis. Stroke is likely if the narrowing is severe and the condition is untreated. Bruits at the bifurcation of the common carotid artery are best heard high up under the angle of the jaw. At this level the common carotid artery bifurcates and gives rise to its internal branch. If one hears a bruit only in the base of the neck, or along the course of the common carotid artery, it is referred to as "diffuse." Diffuse bruits are not a very specific indicator of internal carotid artery disease. Bruits heard only at the bifurcation are more specific for internal carotid artery origin stenosis.

395. **A) Send a urine specimen for culture and sensitivity to the laboratory and treat the patient for a urinary tract infection (UTI)**   The evaluation of gross hematuria requires a complete history and physical exam. The urinalysis (U/A) is a critical component of the workup of gross hematuria and should be the initial test. A urine culture will also determine the need for switching of antibiotics. Recent pharyngitis or skin infection may also suggest postinfectious glomerulonephritis.

396. **A) Basal skin cancer**   An estimated 2.8 million cases of basal cell carcinoma (BCC) are diagnosed in the United States each year. In fact, it is the most frequently occurring form of all cancers. More than one out of every three new cancers are skin cancers, and the vast majority are BCCs. BCCs are abnormal, uncontrolled growths or lesions that arise in the skin's basal cells, which line the deepest layer of the epidermis. BCCs often look like open sores, red patches, pink growths, shiny bumps, or scars. Usually caused by a combination of cumulative UV exposure and intense, occasional UV exposure, BCC can be highly disfiguring if allowed to grow, but almost never metastasize beyond the original tumor site.

397. **B) Cardiac effects**   Because people have varying degrees of hypothyroidism and other thyroid problems, Synthroid is not a "one-size-fits-all" medication. Instead, the Synthroid dosage must be individualized. Exercise caution when administering levothyroxine (Synthroid) to patients with cardiovascular disorders and to the elderly in whom there is an increased risk of occult cardiac disease.

398. **D) Antihistamines**   Avoid use of antihistamines and decongestants with COPD because they can thicken mucus, making it even more difficult to cough up secretions.

399. **D) Corticosteroids**   Corticosteroids are not implicated in interference with the metabolism of oral contraceptives. The pharmacokinetics and clinical significance of the major drug interactions seen with oral contraceptives include drugs interfering with pill efficacy, and/or the oral contraceptive pills interfering with the action of other drugs. Drugs affecting contraceptive efficacy include anticonvulsants (Dilantin), antibiotics (tetracycline), rifampicin, griseofulvin, ascorbic acid, and acetaminophen.

400. **C) Azithromycin 1 g orally OR Doxycycline 100 mg orally twice a day for 7 days**   Drug therapy is based on the 2010 CDC STD guidelines for treatment.

401. **B) Thrombosis related to an IV needle**   Thrombosis related to either a known trauma or IV needle does not represent a contraindication for use of oral contraceptives.

402. **A) Fruits, vegetables, and whole grains**   Lifestyle modifications for HTN include losing weight (especially waistline), regular exercise, DASH diet—lots of whole grains, fruits, vegetables; low-fat dairy; and limited saturated fat. Potassium can lessen the effects of Na on HTN. Calcium helps to produce the heartbeat, and magnesium regulates it.

403. **D) Acute epididymitis**   Epididymitis is usually caused by the spread of bacteria from the urethra or bladder. The most common infections include chlamydia and gonorrhea. Physical examination shows a red, tender, and sometimes swollen lump on the affected side of the scrotum. Tenderness is usually in a small area of the testicle where the epididymis (connects the testicle with the vas deferens) is attached.

404. **C) Trimethoprim-sulfamethoxazole (Bactrim)**   With the allergic history to a sulfa drug, it would be safest to avoid Bactrim.

405. **D) Premature menopause**   Potential benefits of premature menopause include a 30% to 50% lower risk of breast cancer among women who undergo menopause before age 50 and a decreased risk of ovarian cancer for women who undergo bilateral oophorectomy.

406. **C) Saw palmetto is always effective in reducing symptoms**   Many herbs have been tried for treating an enlarged prostate. Saw palmetto has been used by millions of men to ease BPH symptoms and is often recommended as an alternative to medication. Some studies have shown that it helps with symptoms, but there is evidence that this popular herb is no better than a placebo in relieving the signs and symptoms of BPH. Further studies are needed.

407. **C) 5.7% to 6.4%**   The recommended range for a hemoglobin A1c is 4.0% to 5.9%. Prediabetes is 5.7% to 6.4% and higher indicates diabetes.

408. **B) Tanner Stage II**   Tanner Stage I is considered prepubescent. Tanner Stage II is considered the onset of puberty.

409. **D) Lung cancer**   The National Comprehensive Cancer Network (NCCN) guidelines note that lung cancer screening is appropriate to consider for those high-risk patients who are potential candidates for definite treatment. Category 1: High-risk factors include: age 55 to 74 years **and** more than 30 pack-year history of smoking **and** smoking cessation less than 15 years. Category 2B high-risk factors include: age greater than 50 years **and** more than 20 pack-year history of smoking **and** one additional risk factor (other than second-hand smoke).

410. **D) Slow onset of symptoms**   Acute prostatitis symptoms include fever, chills, tenderness of scrotum on affected side, and abrupt onset of symptoms.

411. **B)** *Chlamydia trachomatis*   The most common bacterial cause of NGU is *Chlamydia trachomatis*, but it can also be caused by *Ureaplasma urealyticum, Haemophilus vaginalis,* and *Mycoplasma genitalium.*

412. **D) Smoking**   Smoking (and being over the age of 35) is a relative contraindication for oral contraceptives. Undiagnosed uterine bleeding, hepatoma, and previous/present history of thromboembolism are all absolute contraindications.

413. **A) Injury to the meniscus of the right knee**   Individuals who experience a meniscus tear usually experience pain and swelling as their primary symptoms. Another common complaint is joint locking, or the inability to completely straighten the joint. This is due to a piece of the torn cartilage physically impinging the joint mechanism of the knee.

414. **A) Refer him to an orthopedic specialist**   Treatment of an injury to the meniscus varies depending on the extent and location of the meniscus tear. If the tear is minor and the pain and other symptoms resolve quickly, muscle-strengthening exercises may be all that is needed to recover fully. In this case, a patient is usually referred to physical therapy. A large meniscus tear that causes symptoms or mechanical problems with the function of the knee joint may require arthroscopic surgery for repair.

415. **C) The newer low-dose birth control pills do not require backup during the first 2 weeks of use**   New OCPs require a 7-day back-up method for birth control.

416. **B) Luteinizing hormone (LH)**   LH origin is the anterior pituitary gland. In females, an acute rise in LH triggers ovulation and development of the corpus luteum.

417. **C) Cholesteatoma**   An abnormal skin growth in the middle ear behind the eardrum is called cholesteatoma. Repeated infections and/or a tear or pulling inward of the eardrum can allow skin into the middle ear. Cholesteatomas often develop as cysts or pouches that shed layers of old skin, which build up inside the middle ear. Over time, the cholesteatoma can increase in size and destroy the surrounding delicate bones of the middle ear, leading to hearing loss that surgery can often improve. Permanent hearing loss, dizziness, and facial muscle paralysis are rare, but can result from continued cholesteatoma growth.

418. **D) Advocacy**   Patient advocacy may encompass, but is not limited to, patients' rights advocacy. Patient advocacy is not merely the defense of infringements of patient rights. Advocacy for nursing stems from a philosophy of nursing in which nursing practice is the support of an individual to promote his or her own well-being, as understood by that individual.

419. **A) Yoga**   The American College of Rheumatology states that exercise is beneficial for everyone, including those with RA, and currently recommends 150 minutes of moderate-intensity aerobic activity each week. Safe forms of aerobic exercise, such as walking, aerobic dance, and aquatic exercise, help arthritis patients to control weight, and improve sleep, mood, and overall health.

420. **D) Mood disorders**   Benzodiazepines are a class of drugs that work on the central nervous system, acting selectively on gamma-aminobutyric acid-A (GABA-A). Benzodiazepines are similar in pharmacological action but have different potencies,

and some benzodiazepines work better in treatment of particular conditions. Benzodiazepines are used as sedatives, hypnotics, anxiolytics, anticonvulsants, and muscle relaxants. They are not prescribed for mood disorders.

421. **C) Patients with acute renal failure** Of the patients at highest risk, the acute renal failure patient is the correct response. DM was associated with an increased risk of TB regardless of study design and population. People with DM may be important targets for interventions such as active case finding, and treatment of latent TB and efforts to diagnose, detect, and treat DM may have a beneficial impact on TB control. People who drink more than 40 g of alcohol per day and/or have an alcohol disorder are at greater risk for active tuberculosis, according to the results of a systematic review reported in *BMC Public Health*. As in the case of the nurse, a positive skin test does not necessarily mean that a person has active TB. More tests must be done to check whether there is active disease. However, she is at increased exposure and risk.

422. **D) 13-year-old being treated for a sexually transmitted disease** As soon as an individual turns 18, she/he legally becomes an adult and is automatically emancipated from parental custody and control. Likewise, when a minor marries or joins the armed forces (with parental consent and permission from the court), she/he becomes emancipated from his/her parents. In many states, a pregnant minor is considered an emancipated minor for the purposes of providing informed consent for her own treatment and the treatment of the fetus during the pregnancy and childbirth. For this principle to apply, however, the minor pregnant mother cannot have a cognitive disability that prevents her from giving informed consent for or refusing treatment.

423. **B) Anorexia nervosa** While many of the medical complications of anorexia nervosa are reversed by weight restoration, osteoporosis is a very serious one, which may persist even after successful treatment of the eating disorder.

424. **A) Refer the patient to a urologist after treatment** Because urinary tract infections are relatively rare in young men with normal urinary tracts, a referral to a urologist is warranted. Additional tests that should be conducted may include intravenous pyelography, renal ultrasound, CT, or cystoscopy.

425. **A) Transfusion of blood is prohibited even in cases of emergency** Just as the *Watchtower* revoked its ruling in the 1980s that organ transplants are wrong, over the last few years it has made significant changes regarding the acceptable use of blood. Every Jehovah's Witness should seriously consider the implications of the *Watchtower* making such life-and-death doctrinal changes before deciding to refuse blood when lives are at stake.

426. **D) Protocol agreements help protect nurse practitioners from certain types of lawsuits** Protocols should be developed because the nurse practitioner has the ability to examine, diagnose, and establish treatment plans for patients; friction may develop among the various health care professionals. Should these professionals become codefendants in professional liability litigation, an adversarial situation may result. In some jurisdictions, physicians may carry lower limits of professional

liability coverage than a nurse practitioner. In such cases, the nurse practitioner may become the focus of the defendant's claim in order to reach additional liability insurance coverage.

427. **D) Endometrial biopsy**   An endometrial biopsy is warranted for postmenopausal bleeding (PMB). PMB refers to any uterine bleeding in a menopausal woman (other than the expected cyclic bleeding that occurs in women taking sequential postmenopausal hormone therapy). The most common causes are atrophic endometrium, endometrial proliferation or hyperplasia, endometrial or cervical cancer. Other causes include atrophic vaginitis, trauma, endometrial polyps, friction ulcers of the cervix associated with prolapse of the uterus, and blood dyscrasias.

428. **B) Patient is coherent**   Most patients with delirium have associated cognitive deficits such as altered perception (including hallucinations, illusions, and delusions); memory loss (especially distorted memories, approximate answers, and misidentification of people or places); language deficits (especially writing); disorientation; difficulty with calculations, abstraction, insight, and judgment; and mood disorders, which can include fear, elation, anxiety, or depression. Some patients have relatively preserved orientation, language, and other cognitive functions, but they simply cannot maintain focus on a conversation.

429. **D) Abstract thinking ability is increased**   Most patients with delirium have associated cognitive deficits such as altered perception; memory loss; language deficits (especially writing); disorientation; difficulty with calculations, abstract thinking, insight, and judgment.

430. **C) Captopril (Capoten)**   Captopril (Capoten) is an ACE inhibitor. The interaction between ACE inhibitors and theophylline is related to an increase in potassium. They are not known to increase/decrease theophylline levels.

431. **D) Bartholin's gland abscess**   Bartholin's duct cysts and gland abscesses are common problems in women of reproductive age. Bartholin's glands are located bilaterally at the posterior introitus and drain through ducts that empty into the vestibule at approximately the 4 o'clock and 8 o'clock positions. These normally pea-sized glands are palpable only if the duct becomes cystic or a gland abscess develops. Obstruction of the distal Bartholin's duct may result in the retention of secretions, with resultant dilation of the duct and formation of a cyst. The cyst may become infected, and an abscess may develop in the gland. A Bartholin's duct cyst does not necessarily have to be present before a gland abscess can develop.

432. **A) The nurse practitioner can examine and prescribe birth control pills to minors because there is no legal requirement for parental consent in cases concerning sexual activity and pregnancy**   At the federal level, the focal point of debate over minors' access to confidential services has been the Title X family planning program. Since its inception in 1970, services supported by Title X have been available to anyone who needs them without regard to age. As a result, Title X-supported clinics provide contraceptive services and other reproductive health care to minors on a confidential basis, although they encourage minors to involve their parents in their decision to seek services.

433. C) Her partner does not need treatment The usual medical regimen for treatment is the antibiotic metronidazole (400 mg twice a day, once every 12 hours) for 7 days. A one-time 2-g dose is no longer recommended by the CDC because of low efficacy. Extended-release metronidazole is an alternative recommendation. In contrast to some other infectious diseases affecting the female genitals, according to some sources, treatment of the sexual partners is not necessarily recommended.

434. D) There is a loss of low-frequency hearing secondary to presbycusis Presbycusis may affect any older person, but is more likely to occur in persons who have been exposed to loud noise for long periods in their lives—often related to working in noisy environments. Other risk factors associated with presbycusis include cigarette smoking, heart disease, and high blood pressure (hypertension). A person may be unable to clearly identify the age-related hearing loss and therefore other features should be noted. These include listening to the TV or radio at a loud volume to be able to hear, difficulty understanding the speech of others and complaining that others are speaking in a garbled or mumbled manner, some sounds seeming extremely loud when they are not to others, and difficulty with hearing high-pitched sounds.

435. D) Increased facial movements Increased facial movements are not associated with advanced Parkinson's disease. The primary Parkinson's disease symptoms include tremors, muscle rigidity, bradykinesia (slowness of movement), and postural instability—may be mild at first, but will gradually become more intense and debilitating.

436. A) CN 1 CN 1 is the olfactory nerve. Test the ability to identify familiar aromatic odors; one naris is tested at a time with the patient's eyes closed. The patient should be able to perceive an odor on each side, usually identifying it. The sense of smell may diminish with age.

437. A) Corneal ulceration Due to the paralysis caused by the seventh cranial nerve damage, the eyelid on the affected side may not close voluntarily. This leads to dryness, which can further result in ulceration.

438. B) Multiple brain infarcts Multiple brain infarcts are the least likely cause for delirium. Delirium is most likely caused by a combination of factors that make the brain vulnerable and factors that trigger a malfunction in brain activity. It is often caused by a disease process outside the brain, such as poor nutrition or dehydration, aging, multiple medical problems, infection (UTI, pneumonia) or drug effects, particularly anticholinergic or other CNS depressants (benzodiazepines and opioids) and alcohol or drug use/withdrawal.

439. C) Pelvic ultrasound and serum quantitative pregnancy test The most critical step in beginning the workup is to have a high clinical suspicion for ectopic pregnancy (e.g., in any woman of childbearing age). Bedside pelvic sonography is the imaging test of choice to investigate early pregnancy. Patients with indeterminate ultrasonography findings (empty uterus, gestational sac less than 8 mm without a yolk sac) should have a beta-hCG level drawn and should be followed up closely with gynecology to monitor serial beta-hCG levels and ultrasonography.

440. **A) Tubal ectopic pregnancy and pelvic inflammatory disease (PID)**   Her positive physical findings of left adnexal tenderness and discharge suggest an ectopic pregnancy versus pelvic inflammatory disease (PID). Amenorrhea should be treated as a pregnancy until proven otherwise.

441. **B) Amenorrhea**   As women continue using Depo-Provera Contraceptive Injection, fewer experience irregular bleeding and more experience amenorrhea. By month 12, amenorrhea was reported by 55% of women, and by month 24, amenorrhea was reported by 68% of women using Depo-Provera Contraceptive Injection.

442. **D) Sodium restriction to decrease water retention**   Migraine is a type of headache characterized by constriction of vessels in the brain, followed by painful dilation and inflammation of the same blood vessels. Scientists do not cite any direct correlation between sodium levels and migraine headaches, but the amount of salt one consumes may be a factor in some types of headache pain. Salty foods can act as a migraine trigger in some people. Others might experience nonmigraine headaches when sodium levels get too high or too low.

443. **D) Reproductive-age females**   Finasteride (Proscar) can be absorbed through the skin, and women or children should not be permitted to handle Proscar tablets. Proscar prevents the conversion of testosterone to dihydrotestosterone (DHT) in the body. DHT is involved in the development of benign prostatic hyperplasia (BPH). Proscar has been given a pregnancy Category X classification based on its risks to an unborn fetus. Women should not handle crushed or broken Proscar tablets when they are pregnant or may potentially be pregnant. DHT is important for male genital development; if Proscar is taken during pregnancy, it may cause abnormalities to the external genitals of a male fetus.

444. **B) CNX**   Cranial nerve X (10) is the vagus nerve. To evaluate the nasopharyngeal sensation, tell the patient you will be testing the gag reflex. Touch the posterior wall of the patient's pharynx with an applicator as you observe for upward movement of the palate and contraction of the pharyngeal muscles. The uvula should remain in the midline, and no drooping or absence of an arch on either side of the soft palate should be noted.

445. **C) Acute pericarditis**   The patient most likely has acute pericarditis. A pericardial friction rub is the hallmark of acute pericarditis, which can result from an acute infection. Pericardial rub occurs when two inflamed layers of the pericardium slide over each other, causing a scratching, grating, or crunching sound that ranges from faint to loud. It is best heard between the apex and along the lower left sternal border during deep inspiration. This also causes sharp precordial or retrosternal pain that usually radiates to the left shoulder, neck, and back. The pain worsens when the patient breathes deeply, coughs, or lies flat. It abates when the patient sits up and leans forward.

446. **B) Rest and elevation of the knee with intermittent application of cold packs ×
15 minutes four times a day for the next 48 hours**   The patient should be prescribed the **RICE** treatment. **Rest** for the first 24 to 48 hours after the injury and
gradually increase activity. **Ice** for the first 48 hours: apply ice 20 minutes at a time
for 3 to 4 hours. (The ice pack can be a bag of frozen vegetables.) **Compression**—
use an Ace bandage as indicated. **Elevate**—try to get sprains higher than the heart
if possible and elevate at night by using pillows under the leg/arm.

447. **D) Severe vomiting**   Vomiting is not a symptom associated with irritable bowel
syndrome (IBS). IBS is a disorder that leads to abdominal pain and cramping,
changes in bowel movements, and other symptoms. The main symptoms of IBS
are abdominal pain, fullness, gas, and bloating that have been present for at least 3
days a month for the last 3 months. People with IBS may switch between constipation and diarrhea, or mostly have 1 or the other.

448. **D) Weight**   Weight is not used in the determination of the estimated/expected
peak expiratory flow (peak flow). Age, height, and gender are used to calculate
expected peak flow to help quantify asthma exacerbation severity.

449. **A) Contact dermatitis**   Contact dermatitis is a condition in which the skin
becomes red, sore, or inflamed after direct contact with a substance. There are two
kinds of contact dermatitis: irritant and allergic.

450. **D) Intrauterine device (IUD)**   An IUD is not a risk factor for UTIs. Besides
increased urine glucose, diabetes may increase the risk of UTIs through additional mechanisms, including impaired immune cell delivery, inefficient white
blood cells, and inhibition of bladder contractions that allow urine to remain
stagnant in the bladder. Diaphragms are associated with an increased risk of
UTIs. Urinating before inserting the diaphragm and also after intercourse
may reduce this risk. Hormonal and mechanical changes increase the risk of
urinary stasis and vesicoureteral reflux. These changes, along with an already
short urethra (approximately 3 to 4 cm in females) and difficulty with hygiene
due to a distended pregnant belly, increase the frequency of UTIs in pregnant
women. Indeed, UTIs are among the most common bacterial infections during
pregnancy.

451. **B) Left supraclavicular area**   Virchow's node (or signal node) is a lymph node in
the left supraclavicular fossa (the area above the left clavicle). It takes its supply
from lymph vessels in the abdominal cavity. The finding of an enlarged, hard node
(also referred to as Troisier's sign) has long been regarded as strongly indicative of
the presence of cancer in the abdomen, specifically gastric cancer, that has spread
through the lymph vessels.

452. **A) Tinea cruris**   Tinea cruris (jock itch) is a common skin infection that is caused
by a type of fungus called tinea. The fungus thrives in warm, moist areas of the
body and as a result, infection can affect the genitals, inner thighs, and buttocks.
Infections occur more frequently in the summer or in warm, wet climates. Tinea
cruris appears as a red, itchy rash that is often ring shaped.

453. **B) Middle-aged men**   Cluster headache is a condition that involves, as its most prominent feature, an immense degree of pain that is almost always on only one side of the head. Cluster headaches occur periodically; spontaneous remissions interrupt active periods of pain. The cause of the condition is currently unknown. It affects approximately 0.1% of the population, and men are more commonly affected than women. The headaches typically start before age 30.

454. **C) It does not matter, since there is no solid evidence regarding the efficacy of vitamin C in ameliorating the symptoms of the common cold**   This patient is taking 1,000 mg of vitamin C. Vitamin C was first touted for the common cold in the 1970s. But despite its widespread use, experts say there is very little proof that vitamin C actually has any effect on the common cold. Studies have suggested a possible link between people with higher intakes of vitamin C from food or supplements and lower blood pressure. But the evidence of this effect from clinical trials has been mixed. Previous short-term studies in humans and guinea pigs have shown that vitamin C might protect against osteoarthritis of the knees. In contrast, a new study shows that prolonged use of vitamin C supplements may aggravate osteoarthritis.

455. **B) Delirium tremens secondary to acute withdrawal of alcohol**   Delirium tremens is a severe form of alcohol withdrawal that involves sudden and severe mental or nervous system changes. Symptoms most often occur within 72 hours after the last drink. However, they may occur up to 7 to 10 days after the last drink. It is especially common in those who drink 4 to 5 pints of wine or 7 to 8 pints of beer (or 1 pint of "hard" alcohol) every day for several months. Delirium tremens also commonly affects people who have had alcoholism for more than 10 years.

456. **A) Hyperthyroidism**   Symptoms of hyperthyroidism are nervousness, irritability, increased perspiration, heart racing, hand tremors, anxiety, difficulty sleeping, thinning of the skin, fine brittle hair, and muscular weakness—especially in the upper arms and thighs. More frequent bowel movements may occur, but diarrhea is uncommon. Weight loss, sometimes significant, may occur despite a good appetite; vomiting may occur; and, for women, menstrual flow may lighten and menstrual periods may occur less often.

457. **B) Angiotensin reuptake blockers (ARBs)**   Hypertension is a comorbidity of type 2 diabetes, and blood pressure lowering has been shown to reduce cardiovascular (CV) and renal disease progression in this population. Angiotensin-converting enzyme (ACE) inhibitors have demonstrated reduction in CV mortality and myocardial infarction, stroke, and heart failure in patients with diabetes. Evidence suggests that angiotensin receptor blockers (ARBs) have similar CV protective effects, particularly in patients who are postmyocardial infarction and in those with heart failure, and ARBs' renoprotective effects have reduced proteinuria in patients with or without diabetes.

458. **D) Stroking the inner thigh of a male and watching the testicle on the ipsilateral side rise up toward the body**   The cremasteric reflex test is done by stroking the inner thigh (proximal to distal) with a blunt instrument such as a handle of the reflex hammer. The testicle and scrotum should rise on the stroked side.

459. **B) Apply hydrocortisone cream 1% BID to the rash until it is healed** Topical hydrocortisone cream is only indicated for the temporary relief of external anal and genital itching and itching associated with minor skin irritations; inflammation and rashes due to poison ivy, oak, sumac, insect bites, detergents, cosmetics, jewelry, soaps, seborrheic dermatitis, eczema, and psoriasis.

460. **C) A decrease in the systolic blood pressure of >10 mm Hg on inspiration** Pulsus paradoxus is a marked decrease in pulse amplitude during quiet inspiration or a decrease in the systolic pressure greater than 10 mm Hg, a typical finding in cardiac tamponade. Heart sounds may be heard over the precordium when the radial pulse is not felt.

461. **C) Testicular torsion** The cremasteric reflex test is done by stroking the inner thigh (proximal to distal) with a blunt instrument such as a handle of the reflex hammer. The testicle and scrotum should rise on the stroked side. Testicular torsion is a twisting on the spermatic cord, which cuts off the blood supply to the testicle and surrounding structures within the scrotum.

462. **B) Refer him to the emergency department as soon as possible** The diagnosis of testicular torsion is often made clinically, but if it is in doubt, an ultrasound is helpful in evaluating the condition. Irreversible ischemia begins at 6 hours after a torsion. Emergency diagnosis and treatment are usually required within 4 to 6 hours to prevent necrosis.

463. **C) The usual clinical strategy is watchful waiting for curves of 10 degrees or less** The treatment prescribed for scoliosis, kyphosis, or lordosis varies with the individual patient. Severity and location of the curve, age, potential for further growth, and general health of the patient must all be taken into account. A mild curvature (up to 20 degrees) generally warrants only periodic observation to evaluate for signs of further progression. Bracing is the usual treatment for children and adolescents with curves of 25–40 degrees, and in other special circumstances.

464. **B) 200 to 239 mg/dL** The Adult Treatment Panel (ATP) III guidelines define a cholesterol level of 200 to 239 as borderline.

465. **A) 1 to 2 years** Menarche typically occurs within 2 to 3 years after thelarche (breast budding; Tanner Stage II). The areola widens, darkens slightly, and elevates from the rest of the breast as a small mound. The mound (nipple) may be visible, and lying under the areola is a bud of breast tissue (breast bud) that is palpable (noticeable to the touch).

466. **D) A 16-year-old who wants to be treated for dysmenorrhea** Dysmenorrhea that requires more than OTC anti-inflammatory (NSAIDs) and nonprescription therapies may involve more invasive testing and would probably require parental consent, especially if the evaluation/treatments involve billing to insurance.

467. **B) Microalbuminuria** As of 2011, the Adult Treatment Panel III criteria (ATP III), the American Heart Association criteria, and the recent harmonized international criteria for the definition of the metabolic syndrome included blood pressure,

waist circumference, fasting plasma glucose, serum triglycerides, and high-density lipoprotein (HDL) cholesterol, but excluded microalbuminuria.

468. **A) Sinusitis and hydrocele** Transillumination is used for evaluation of the frontal and maxillary sinusitis as well as for a hydrocele. Since light is able to pass through the delicate skin covering the hollow sinus cavities, a light source held against the upper cheek will produce a red dot on the palate if the sinuses are normal (filled with air rather than obstructed). The transillumination test is used to differentiate a hydrocele from hernia—you see an illuminated scrotum with the testicle in the center surrounded by water in the hydrocele.

469. **D) A cough that is productive of large amounts of sputum** Patients with COPD have increased mucus production because of an over abundant amount of mucus-producing glands in their airways compared with healthy people. This results in a chronic cough. A cough is the body's defense mechanism developed in an attempt to clear the airways. A common problem for people with COPD is thick sputum, making sputum difficult to cough up and out.

470. **B) The pulmonic area** S2 is physiologically split in about 90% of people. The second heart sound is produced by the closure of the aortic and pulmonic valves. The sound produced by the closure of the aortic valve is termed A2, and the sound produced by the closure of the pulmonic valve is termed P2. The A2 sound is normally much louder than the P2 due to higher pressures in the left side of the heart; thus, A2 radiates to all cardiac listening posts (loudest at the right upper sternal border) and P2 is usually only heard at the left upper sternal border.

471. **C) *Candida albicans*** Balanitis is swelling (inflammation) of the foreskin and head of the penis. Balanitis is usually caused by poor hygiene in uncircumcised men. Other possible causes include *Candida* (fungal infection) and bacterial infection, harsh soaps, and uncontrolled diabetes. Symptoms include redness of the foreskin or penis, other rashes on the head of the penis, foul-smelling discharge, and pain.

472. **A) Iron-deficiency anemia** Iron-deficiency anemia is the most common form of anemia.

473. **C) She can take any of the pills in the sulfonylurea class** The patient can take sulfonylureas. The sulfonamide component in the typical sulfa antibiotics is of a slightly different molecular structure than that in sulfonylureas. Although cross-reactivity is technically possible, current literature does not consider this likely, and sulfonylureas are typically well tolerated in patients with a sulfa allergy.

474. **C) Prostaglandins** The etiology of primary dysmenorrhea is not precisely understood, but most symptoms can be explained by the action of uterine prostaglandins, particularly $PGF_{2\text{-alpha}}$. During endometrial sloughing, the disintegrating endometrial cells release $PGF_{2\text{-alpha}}$ as menstruation begins. $PGF_{2\text{-alpha}}$ stimulates myometrial contractions, ischemia, and sensitization of nerve endings. The clinical evidence for this theory is quite strong.

475. **A) Serum ferritin and peripheral smear** The assessment is for iron-deficiency anemia. The ferritin should be tested. Examination of the peripheral smear is an

important part of the workup of patients with anemia. Examination of the erythrocytes shows microcytic and hypochromic red blood cells in chronic iron-deficiency anemia.

476. **D) Vesicular breath sounds in the lower lobe** There are two normal breath sounds. Breath sounds heard over the tracheobronchial tree are called bronchial breathing and breath sounds heard over the lower lobes of lung tissue are called vesicular breathing.

477. **A) S3 and S4 and low-pitched tones** The bell is most useful for picking up low-pitched sounds; for example, S3, S4, mitral stenosis. The diaphragm is most useful for picking up high-pitched sounds; for example, S1, S2, aortic or mitral regurgitation, pericardial friction rubs.

478. **A) KOH (potassium hydroxide) smear whiff test** Generally, wet preps use 1 to 2 slides to evaluate *Candida*. Under the microscope, observe for presence and number of white blood cells (WBCs), trichomonads, candidal hyphae, or clue cells. Yeast or hyphae also may be seen on the wet prep. The KOH prep is made by adding a drop of KOH solution to a drop of saline suspension of the vaginal discharge. The KOH lyses epithelial cells in 5 to 15 minutes and allows easier visualization of candidal hyphae.

479. **C) Tanner Stage III** Tanner Stage III: The testicular volume increases, the scrotum enlarges, and the penis begins to lengthen. Tanner I: Prepubertal small penis. Tanner II: The penis length remains unchanged. Tanner III: Penis begins to lengthen. Tanner IV: Penis increases in length *and* circumference. Tanner V: Adult scrotum and penis.

480. **C) Retin-A 0.25% cream** Use Retin-A 0.25%. Guidelines for care of acne vulgaris management note: The effectiveness of topical retinoids in the treatment of acne is well documented. These agents act to reduce obstruction within the follicle and therefore are useful in the management of both comedonal and inflammatory acne. Systemic antibiotics are a standard of care in the management of moderate and severe acne.

481. **D) The cerebellum** The cerebrum is the largest part of the brain and is associated with conscious thought, movement, and sensation. Balance is initially evaluated by the Romberg test. Ask the patient (eyes open then closed) to stand, feet together and arms at the sides. Loss of balance, a positive Romberg sign, indicates cerebellar ataxia or vestibular dysfunction. If the patient staggers or loses balance with the Romberg test, postpone other tests of cerebellar function requiring balance.

482. **A) Influenza vaccine injections** Not all vaccinations are safe to get during pregnancy. However, the flu vaccine can be given before, during, and after pregnancy.

483. **A) Heart disease, infertility, uterine cancer, diabetes, and endometrial cancer** The risk of heart attack is four to seven times higher in women with PCOS than women of the same age without PCOS. Women with PCOS are at greater risk of having high blood pressure and have high levels of LDL and low levels of HDL cholesterol. Lack of ovulation is usually the reason for fertility problems in women

with PCOS. More than 50% of women with PCOS will have diabetes or prediabetes (impaired glucose tolerance) before the age of 40. Women with PCOS are also at risk for endometrial cancer. Irregular menstrual periods and the lack of ovulation cause women to produce the hormone estrogen, but not progesterone. Without progesterone, the endometrium becomes thick, which can cause heavy or irregular bleeding. Over time, this can lead to endometrial hyperplasia and cancer.

484. **B) Mean corpuscular volume (MCV)**   There are three red blood cell indices: mean corpuscular volume (MCV), mean corpuscular hemoglobin (MCH), and mean corpuscular hemoglobin concentration (MCHC). The MCV shows the size of the red blood cells. The MCH value is the amount of hemoglobin in an average red blood cell. The MCHC measures the concentration of hemoglobin in an average red blood cell. These numbers help in the diagnosis of different types of anemia. Red cell distribution width (RDW) can also be measured, which shows whether the cells are all the same or different sizes or shapes.

485. **B) Take two pills today, then two pills the next day, and use condoms for the rest of the pill cycle**   In the case of 2 missed pills in the first 2 weeks of the packet, take two pills at the regular time for 2 days. Use back-up contraception for the remainder of the cycle. If two or more pills are missed in the third week, take two pills daily until all OCPs are taken; restart the pill cycle with one pill daily within 7 days; use back-up contraceptive until OCs are restarted with a new pack and the first 7 days of that packet have been taken.

486. **D) A 30-year-old White female who smokes**   The 30-year-old White female who smokes has the lowest risk for diabetes among the four patients. Risk for diabetes mellitus includes: people with impaired glucose tolerance (IGT) and/or impaired fasting glucose (IFG), people over age 45, people with a family history of diabetes, people who are overweight, people who do not exercise regularly, people with low HDL cholesterol or high triglycerides or high blood pressure, certain racial and ethnic groups (e.g., non-Hispanic Blacks, Hispanic/Latino Americans, Asian Americans and Pacific Islanders, and American Indians and Alaska Natives), and women who had gestational diabetes or who have had a baby weighing 9 pounds or more at birth.

487. **A) Medical treatment for any work-related injury is covered under an employer's workers' comp insurance**   State law governs workers' compensation systems, and thus what injuries are covered by workers' compensation differ from state to state. Generally, though, an injury that arises "out of the course of employment" will be covered under your state's workers' compensation system. This means that injuries that happened while you were performing your job duties, or diseases/illnesses that arise from conditions at your job, will likely amount to a workers' compensation claim.

488. **C) The patient needs hepatitis B vaccine and hepatitis B immune globulin**   This patient is susceptible and needs the hepatitis B vaccine and the hepatitis B immune globulin.

489. **A) Axilla**   Mitral regurgitation is best heard at the apex with radiation into the axilla.

490. **B) Selective serotonin reuptake inhibitors (SSRIs)** Monoamine oxidase inhibitors (MAOIs) should not be combined with other psychoactive substances except under expert care. MAOIs are a class of antidepressants. They are particularly effective in treating atypical depression. Because of potentially lethal dietary and drug interactions, MAOIs have historically been reserved as a last line of treatment and are used only if other classes of antidepressants, such as SSRIs, have failed.

491. **A) Sciatica** Usually, sciatica only affects one side of the lower body, and the pain often radiates from the lower back all the way through the back of the thigh and down through the leg. Common sciatica symptoms: Lower back pain, if experienced at all, is not as severe as leg pain; constant pain in only one side of the buttock or leg, but rarely both the right and left sides; pain that originates in the low back or buttock and continues along the path of the sciatic nerve—down the back of the thigh and into the lower leg and foot; pain that feels better when patients lie down or are walking, but worsens when standing or sitting; sciatic pain that is typically described as sharp or searing, rather than dull; some experience a "pins-and-needles" sensation, numbness or weakness, or a prickling sensation down the leg.

492. **C) *Pseudomonas aeruginosa*** *Pseudomonas aeruginosa* is the major pathogen in the cystic fibrosis (CF) lung. Prevalence is high and, once acquired, chronic infection will almost always ensue. *P. aeruginosa* settles into the thick mucus trapped in the airways. Once it sets up house in the respiratory tract, *P. aeruginosa* is hard to get rid of. Respiratory failure caused by the infection is often the ultimate cause of death in many people with CF.

493. **D) There is a slight decrease in the activity of the immune system** Our immune system's ability to perform declines with age. These changes happen at all levels, from chemical changes in how our cells communicate with one another to changes in immune organs altogether.

494. **B) Clarithromycin (Biaxin)** Clarithromycin (Biaxin) is a macrolide antibiotic and is in FDA pregnancy category C. All of the other antibiotics listed are pregnancy class B. The *pregnancy category* of a pharmaceutical agent is an assessment of the risk of fetal injury due to the pharmaceutical, if it is used as directed by the mother during pregnancy. Category A = Adequate, well-controlled studies failed to demonstrate a risk to the fetus in the first trimester and no evidence of risk in the later trimesters. Category B = Animal studies have shown an adverse effect, but adequate and well-controlled studies in pregnant women have failed to demonstrate a risk to the fetus in any trimester. Category C = Animal studies have shown an adverse effect on the fetus, but there are no adequate and well-controlled studies in humans, and potential benefits may warrant use of the drug in pregnant women despite potential risks. Category D = There is positive evidence of human fetal risk based on adverse reaction data from investigational or marketing experience, but potential benefits may warrant use of the drug in pregnant women despite potential risks. Category X = Studies in animals or humans have demonstrated fetal abnormalities, so the risks involved clearly outweigh the potential benefits.

495. **A) Barrett's esophagus** Barrett's esophagus is most often diagnosed in people who have long-term gastroesophageal reflux disease (GERD) — a chronic

regurgitation of acid from the stomach into the lower esophagus. Only a small percentage of people with GERD will develop Barrett's esophagus.

496. **A) Amitriptyline (Elavil)** Amitriptyline (Elavil) is a tricyclic antidepressant. Post-herpetic neuralgia (PHN) is a chronic neuropathic pain syndrome that occurs after reactivation of varicella zoster virus infection with damage to sensory ganglia in nerve roots. Burning pain typically precedes the rash by several days and can persist for several months after the rash resolves. With post-herpetic neuralgia, a complication of herpes zoster, pain may persist well after resolution of the rash and can be highly debilitating. Tricyclic antidepressants or anticonvulsants, often given in low dosages, may help to control neuropathic pain.

497. **C) Cold nodule** Nodules that produce excess thyroid hormone—called hot nodules—show up on the thyroid scan because they take up more of the isotope than normal thyroid tissue does. Cold nodules are nonfunctioning and appear as defects or holes in the scan. Hot nodules are almost always noncancerous, but a few cold nodules are cancerous. The disadvantage of a thyroid scan is that it cannot distinguish between benign and malignant cold nodules.

498. **D) Median nerve** By compressing the median nerve within the carpal tunnel, characteristic symptoms—burning; tingling; numbness over the thumb, index, middle, and ring fingers—convey a positive test. The Phalen maneuver is a diagnostic test for carpal tunnel syndrome. The Phalen test is done by pushing the back of the hands together for 1 minute. Symptoms indicate a positive result for carpal tunnel.

499. **A) Glucosamine** Glucosamine is a sugar naturally produced by the body. It is one of the building blocks of cartilage. Cartilage covers and protects the ends of the bones, allowing bones to move smoothly against each other. Glucosamine comes in two forms—glucosamine sulfate and glucosamine hydrochloride.

500. **B) Plantar fasciitis** The plantar fascia is the flat ligament that connects the heel bone to the toes. It supports the arch of the foot. Most people with plantar fasciitis have pain when they take their first steps after they get out of bed or sit for a long time. Stiffness and pain occur after taking a few steps, but the feet may hurt more as the day goes on. It may hurt the most when climbing stairs or after standing for a long time.

501. **A) Propranolol (Inderal)** Propranolol (Inderal) is approved for "treatment" of essential tremor. It helps control the symptoms. Essential tremors are permanent and cannot be cured. Before prescribing, order an EKG. Do not use beta-blockers if a patient has second- or third-degree heart block or chronic lung disease.

502. **B) The quasi-experimental design uses convenience sampling instead of random sampling to recruit subjects** The quasi-experimental design uses an intervention (it is not an observational study or a survey). It has many similarities with an experimental study except that the human subjects are recruited by convenience and not at random (as in an experimental study).

503. **B) Advise the mother to use a nit comb after spraying the child's hair with white distilled vinegar, waiting for 15 minutes, and then rinsing the child's hair**   According to the CDC, nits that are more than ¼ inches from the child's scalp are usually not viable. The child also does not have an itchy scalp. One method of removal is to soak the child's head with distilled vinegar (and then rinse after), which will break down the protein of the nit casings, making it easy to comb them out of the hair.

504. **C) A filled-in square**   A filled-in square is a diseased or affected male and a filled-in circle is a diseased or affected female. An empty square is a healthy male and an empty circle is a healthy female.

505. **C) Plain radiograph of the right hip and leg with a magnetic resonance image (MRI) of the knee joint**   The stem is asking for two things "...when evaluating fractures and joint damage." Plain x-rays are the first exam ordered for suspected or obvious bony fractures. An MRI scan is the best test for any type of joint pathology (swollen right knee).

506. **D) Mediterranean**   Lupus is more common among women of African American, Asian, and Hispanic racial background compared with those of Mediterranean background (Italians, Greeks, etc.).

507. **D) Malar rash**   A malar rash is the butterfly-shaped rash on the middle of the face that is caused by a type of photosensitivity reaction. It is associated with SLE. The other answer options are also found with other diseases, such as rheumatoid arthritis, polymyalgia rheumatica, etc.

508. **C) BC > AC**   A normal result in the Rinne is AC greater than BC. When there is a conduction hearing loss (cerumenosis, otitis media), the result will be BC greater than AC. The reason is that the sound waves are blocked (e.g., cerumen, fluid in middle ear). Therefore, the patient cannot hear them as well as through bone conduction.

509. **B) Collaborative**   A collaborative relationship exists when a health caregiver refers a patient to others (physicians, specialists, physical therapy, etc.) to help with patient treatment and management. Consult reports and progress reports are sent to the primary caregiver to report the patient's progress. Consultative relationships are informal, such as talking to a colleague about a patient's treatment.

510. **B) Acute bacterial endocarditis**   Bacterial endocarditis is also known as infective endocarditis (IC). It is a serious bacterial infection of the heart valves and the endocardial surface. The most common bacteria are *Staphylococcus* and *Streptococcus* species. Subcutaneous red painful nodules on the finger pads are called "Osler's nodes." Subungual splinter hemorrhages on the nailbeds are caused by microemboli. "Janeway's lesions" are caused by bleeding under the skin (usually located on the palms and the soles) and are painless red papules and macules. Other findings are conjunctival hemorrhages, petechaie, cardiac friction rubs, arrhythmias, murmurs, and others. Three blood cultures obtained at separate sites 1 hour apart are used to identify the causative organism. Some

of the risk factors are damaged or prosthetic valves, history of rheumatic fever, injection drug use, etc.

511. **C) Inner ear**   Sensorineural hearing loss (i.e., presbycussis) involves damage to both the hair cells in the cochlea (sensory portion) and cranial nerve VIII (8) (neural).

512. **B) Tdap, MCV4, and the HPV vaccines**   Vaccine questions usually are not this complicated, but there are several lessons that can be learned with this question. The 2012 CDC recommendations for the ages 13 to 18 years are the Tdap catch-up (if not received at age 11 to 12 years), HPV or Gardisil catch-up (if not received at age 11 to 12 years), and the MCV4 or meningococcal conjugate vaccine (Menactra). Only one dose of Tdap is recommended (lifetime). Thereafter, the Td form of the vaccine is indicated every 10 years.

513. **A) Report the patient's grandson for elder abuse to protective health services of the state**   Speaking with the grandson and warning him about elder abuse and reporting may result in harm to the patient and/or refusal to return to the clinic in the future for follow-up of the patient. Option D is a vague answer (call his son as soon as possible for what?).

514. **D) Reduction of the FEV1 (forced expiratory volume in 1 second) with increase in the TLC (total lung capacity) and RV (residual volume)**   COPD findings during pulmonary function testing are the reduction of the FEV1 (forced expiratory volume in 1 second) and reduction of the FVC (forced vital capacity). There is an increase in the TLC (total lung capacity) and RV (residual volume). The lungs of patients with emphysema have lost their recoil (decreases FEV1). The lungs are always full of air that is hard to "squeeze out" of the lungs (increases residual volume and total lung capacity). To summarize (COPD): reduction in the FEV1 and FVC with increased in the RV and TLC.

515. **B) Start the patient on levothyroxine (Synthroid) 0.25 mcg PO daily**   The patient is symptomatic (weight gain, lack of energy, and irregular periods) with low free T4. Even though the TSH went down slightly, the free T4 remains low. An elevated TSH and low free T4 are indicative of hypothyroidism. The next step is to start her on levothyroxine (Synthroid) 0.25 mcg daily and recheck the TSH in 6 weeks. The goal is to normalize the TSH (between 1.0 to 3.5) and to ameliorate the patient's symptoms (increased energy, feels better, etc.). Armour thyroid (desiccated thyroid) is a natural supplement composed of dried (desiccated) pork thyroid glands. It is used in alternative medicine as an alternative to synthetic levothyroxine/T4 (Synthroid).

516. **A) Prostate feels firm and uniformly enlarged**   The prostate should feel firm and will be uniformly enlarged. A boggy and warm prostate is present with acute prostatitis.

517. **C) Blood glucose**   Checking the blood glucose is indicated for patients with syncopal and near-syncopal episodes. The NP performs a thorough history of the incident (diabetic, rapid onset or slow, position, provocation), medical history, health history, and the medications.

518. **D) Affected testicle is swollen and feels cold to touch** The affected testicle will be swollen, but it will feel very warm to the touch. A cold testicle is abnormal and is indicative of gangrene (after 24 hours).

519. **B) The symbol called "N ="** The correct symbol used to indicate total number of subjects in a study (total population) is "N." For example, a research study has a total number of subjects or total population of 100 (N = 100). The small letter n is used to indicate a subpopulation. For example, a study with a total population of N = 100 that is divided into 2 groups of 50 subjects (n = 50).

520. **B) 27%** This patient has a total body surface area (TBSA) of 27% and should be referred to the emergency department as soon as possible. Check the "ABCs" and monitor the patient for shock. Do not puncture bullae.

521. **A) Orthostatic hypotension and sedation** Orthostatic hypotension and sedation are common side effects of atypical antipsychotics such as olanzapine (Zyprexa), quetiapine (Seroquel), and risperidone (Risperdal). It is also a common side effect of the older antipsychotics like haloperidol (Haldol). Antipsychotics do not cause severe anxiety and hyperphagia (increased appetite). They lower anxiety and cause sedation, sleepiness, anorexia, and hypotension and increase the risk of sudden death in frail elders.

522. **B) Metronidazole (Flagyl) 500 mg PO TID x 10 days** First-line treatment for a mild case of *Clostridium difficile* colitis is metronidazole (Flagyl) 500 mg PO TID x 10 days. Discontinuation of the offending antibiotic (if possible) or switching to another antibiotic class is recommended. The role of probiotic supplementation is controversial. Complications are pseudomembranous colitis, toxic megacolon, and fulminant colitis.

523. **A) Azithromycin (Zithromax)** If the patient has a severe penicillin allergy, there is a 10% chance of cross-reactivity to cephalosporins (especially first generation). Since the patient is a child, the levofloxacin is contraindicated. Nausea is a common adverse reaction to erythromycin (it is not an allergic reaction). The best option is to use azithromycin because of its minimal GI adverse effects. Azithromycin has fewer drug interactions compared with other macrolides.

524. **C) Frail elderly** Frail elderly who are mentally competent are not considered a vulnerable population group.

525. **A) Order both a plain radiograph and computed tomography (CT) scan of the spine as soon as possible** The patient has a severe case of sciatica that is worsening quickly (may progress to cauda equina). In addition, older age and an abnormal neurological exam are red flags for potentially serious underlying pathology (osteoporosis fracture, cancer, infection, spondylolisthesis). Because the patient's symptoms are worsening, a CT (computed tomography) scan is the best choice. A plain radiograph can only detect bony pathology, but a CT scan can detect nerve root compression, herniated disc, cancer, and spinal stenosis (narrowing of the spinal canal). In addition, the patient needs to follow up with a neurologist as soon as possible.

526. **B) The patient has a mild case of acute diverticulitis and can be treated with antibiotics in the outpatient setting with close follow-up** The patient has a mild case of acute diverticulitis and can be treated as an outpatient with antibiotics and a clear fluid diet. If outpatient treatment is selected, careful patient selection and close follow-up (within 24 to 48 hours) are very important. Instruct patients to go to the hospital if symptoms get worse, if fever increases, if unable to tolerate PO treatment, and if pain worsens. Order CBC (leukocytosis, neutrophilia, and possible shift to the left), chemistry profile, and urinalysis (to rule out renal causes).

527. **A) Isoflavones** Soy isoflavones mimic the action of estrogen in the body. It is derived from soybeans and soybean products (soy milk, tofu). Resveratrol is found in red grapes and red wine. It is thought to help prolong life and is thought to be one of the reasons that the Mediterranean diet increases longevity.

528. **C) Peripheral neuropathy** Bupropion increases the risk of seizures. Contraindications are seizures, anorexia nervosa, and bulimia. Avoid with any condition that increases seizures such as after abrupt withdrawal of alcohol or sedatives and certain head avoiding injuries. For peripheral neuropathy, atypical antidepressants such as duloxetine (Cymbalta) and TCAs such as amitriptyline (Elavil) are used to treat this condition.

529. **A) Caffeine-containing drinks and foods such as chocolate have been found helpful with decreasing the incidence of exacerbations** Lifestyle changes associated with decreasing exacerbations are wearing gloves or mittens during cold weather, taking care with handling frozen foods (wear gloves), avoiding vasoconstricting agents (caffeine, smoking, cocaine, amphetamines), and avoiding emotional stress. Exercise and reducing emotional stress are recommended. Usually involves the fingers and/or toes due to severe arteriolar vasospasm causing ischemia. During an exacerbation, the fingers change color into white, blue, and red (think of the American flag as a reminder). Raynaud's is classified either as primary (Raynaud's disease) or secondary (Raynaud's phenomenon). Secondary Raynaud's individuals have a higher risk of autoimmune disorders such as scleroderma, Sjogren syndrome, and systemic lupus erythematosus. Affects mostly young women (ages 15 to 30 years).

530. **C) Patients have the right to view their mental health and psychotherapy-related health information** Mental health and psychotherapy/psychiatric records do not have to be released to patients even if they request them. Otherwise, any type of medical records can be released if requested by the health insurance or health plan for billing purposes and reimbursement. HIPAA applies to all health care providers, health plans, health insurance companies, medical clearinghouses, and others who bill electronically and transmit health information over the Internet.

531. **A) The spleen is not palpable in the majority of healthy adults** The spleen is located on the left upper quadrant of the abdomen under the diaphragm and is protected by the lower ribcage. In the majority of adults, it is not palpable. The spleen's longest axis is from 11 cm to 20 cm. Any spleen larger than 20 cm is enlarged. The best test for evaluating splenic (or hepatic) size is the abdominal ultrasound. Disorders that can cause splenomegaly include mononucleosis, sickle

cell disease, congestive heart failure, bone marrow cancers (myeloma, leukemia), and several other diseases.

532. **C) Thiazide diuretics**   Thiazide diuretics have been used to treat hypertension for many decades and numerous placebo-controlled studies have documented their effectiveness as an antihypertensive drug.

533. **D) 10 days**   The minimum number of days to quarantine an animal suspected of rabies is 10 days. If the animal is healthy and has no symptoms of rabies at 10 days, it is not infected with the rabies virus and can be returned to the owner.

534. **A) Thiazide diuretics decrease calcium excretion by the kidneys and stimulate osteoclast production**   This positive side effect of thiazides results in a decrease in calcium bone loss and an increase in the bone mineral density.

535. **D) It is a condition, characteristic, or factor that is being measured**   A variable is a condition, characteristic, or the factor that is being measured. An independent variable is the one being manipulated that is not affected by the others. A dependent variable is the result or the outcome from the manipulation of the independent variable.

536. **A) Take one pill every 1 to 2 hours until relief is obtained or adverse gastrointestinal effects occur, such as abdominal pain, nausea, or diarrhea**   Colchicine acts as an anti-inflammatory and helps to suppress gouty attacks. It is usually taken as one tablet (0.6 mg) every 1 to 2 hours until relief is obtained (or adverse gastrointestinal effects occur, such as abdominal pain, nausea, or diarrhea). Prescribe the patient only 10 tablets at a time (do not refill) during a flare-up. The maximum dose is 6 mg/day. Many patients will develop GI adverse effects even before the pain is relieved. Colchicine can also be taken daily in small amounts for prophylaxis.

537. **D) Comprehensive eye exam**   A comprehensive eye exam by an ophthalmologist is recommended because hydroxychloroquine can adversely affect the retina (scotomas or visual field defects, loss of central vision, loss of color vision). Higher doses and long-term use increase the risk of retinal toxicity.

538. **B) *t*-score between –1. 0 and –2.5**   Osteopenia is defined as a *t*-score between –1. 0 and –2.5. Osteoporosis is defined as a *t*-score of less than –2.5.

539. **A) *Clostridium difficile*-associated diarrhea (CDAD)**   Important risk factors for *Clostridium difficile*-associated diarrhea (CDAD) and *C. difficile* colitis are antibiotic therapy and hospitalization. Almost any antibiotic can cause the condition, but the most common are clindamycin, cephalosporins, and fluroquinolones. Diarrhea can occur during therapy as well as after therapy (5 to 10 days; up to 10 weeks). Pseudomembranous colitis is a complication of *C. difficle* colitis.

540. **B) 25-year-old Chinese patient**   Alpha thalassemia minor/trait or disease is more prevalent among Asians such as Chinese and Filipinos. Beta thalassemia minor/trait or disease is more common in persons from the countries in the Mediterranean area, such as Greeks and Italians.

541. **A) Instability of the affected knee caused by damage (i.e., rupture) to the anterior cruciate ligament (ACL) of the knee**   A positive Lachman's sign is highly suggestive of damage to the anterior cruciate ligament of the knee. The anterior drawer sign may also be positive. There is laxity of the abnormal knee joint (compared with the normal knee). The Lachman test or maneuver is considered more sensitive for ACL damage compared with the anterior drawer test.

542. **A) Hypocalcemia**   Chvostek's sign is contraction of the facial muscles when the facial nerve is tapped briskly in front of the ear (anterior to the auditory canal). Low calcium levels cause tetany and neuromuscular disturbances. Acute hypocalcemia with symptoms (tetany, weakness, arrythymias) should be referred to the emergency department. Conditions such as acute or chronic renal failure, vitamin D or magnesium deficiency, or acute pancreatitis, increase risk of hypocalcemia.

543. **B) When the nurse practitioner is unable to speak with the patient directly, she should leave a message with her name and telephone number and instruct the patient to call back**   It is against HIPAA regulations to leave laboratory results on an answering machine even if they are normal routine laboratory tests. HIPAA is also known as the "Privacy Rule."

544. **D) Atomoxetine (Strattera)**   Strattera is classified as a norepinephrine reuptake inhibitor. It is not a stimulant or an amphetamine. Strattera is contraindicated during/within 14 days of taking an MAOI, narrow-angle glaucoma, or heart disorder in which increases in BP or heart rate will worsen it, or with pheochromocytoma. Children and teenagers should be monitored for suicidal thoughts/plans.

545. **A) Fasting blood glucose, fasting lipid profile, and weight**   Patients on atypical antipsychotics commonly gain weight and are at risk for obesity, hyperglycemia, and type 2 diabetes. Zyprexa will increase lipids (cholesterol, low-density lipoprotein [LDL], and triglycerides). Atypical antipsychotics also increase the risk of death among frail elderly and elderly living in nursing homes.

546. **B) A punishment by the "spirits" for wrongful actions against others or for failure to follow spiritual rules**   Native Americans believe that illness is a punishment. Shamans "cure" the illness by performing rituals and using herbal medicines. Medicine pouches that are tied to the patient by a string are believed to help cure the illness. Do not remove without the patient's (or parent's) permission.

547. **D) Ulcerative colitis**   The most important clue for ulcerative colitis is bloody stools that are covered with mucus and pus, along with the systemic symptoms (fatigue, low-grade fever).

548. **C) Health care providers are mandated by law to report certain types of diseases to the local health department even if the patient does not give permission**   Physicians and laboratories are legally mandated to report certain types of diseases. STDs, HIV infection/AIDS, gonorrhea, and syphilis must be reported to the local health department even if the patient does not give permission. Partner tracing and notification are done by the local health department. The CDC website contains a list of nationally

reportable diseases. Other diseases that are on the CDC 2012 list of reportable diseases that must be reported are TB; diphtheria; hepatitis A, B, and C; measles; mumps; pertussis; Lyme disease; Rocky Mountain spotted fever; and many others.

549. **D) Calls patients by using their first names only**   Patients who are in waiting rooms or rooms with other people should be called by their first names only to protect their privacy.

550. **B) The NP advises the patient that an NP peer who is working with her can help answer her questions more thoroughly**   In general, discussing personal beliefs is considered unprofessional behavior. Respecting the patient's right to choose is an example of patient autonomy.

551. **D) Scopolamine patch (Transderm Scop)**   Scopolamine patch (Transderm Scop) is a prescription medicine that is used for motion/sea sickness. It is a small circular-shaped patch that is placed behind the ear and is effective for 3 days. Advise the patient to apply it 4 hours before the trip, so that it takes effect in a timely manner. Since the question is asking about a "prescribed" med, over-the-counter medicines (OTCs) such as Dramamine is an incorrect answer. Zofran is indicated for cancer-related nausea and vomiting (chemo, radiation, surgery).

552. **A) Mal ojo or mal de ojo**   *Mal ojo* or *mal de ojo* is a spiritual illness that can cause symptoms such as loss of appetite, crying, diarrhea, colic, fear, weakness, or death. A curandero or curandera is usually consulted and does spiritual cleansing of the patient. It may take several cleansings (*limpia*) to cure the patient. *Trabajo* means "work" and *malo* means "bad" and these options are being used as distractors.

553. **B) Assess the patient for respiratory distress**   Assess the patient for respiratory distress ASAP. Follow the "ABCs" and assess the patient for any life-threatening symptoms. Smoke inhalation lung injury is the main cause of death in thermal burn victims.

554. **C) Triazolam (Halcion)**   Triazolam (Halcion) has an average half-life of about 2 hours. Xanax has a half-life of 12 hours. Ativan has a half-life of 15 hours. Klonopin has a half-life of 34 hours.

555. **C) Plasma cells**   Myeloma is a cancer of the plasma cells (or mature B-cells/lymphocytes), which affects the bone marrow. Plasma cells produce antibodies and reside mainly in the bone marrow. Signs/symptoms are bone pain, fractures, hypercalcemia, depressed immunity, and anemia. The bone marrow produces WBCs (neutrophils, lymphocytes, eosinophils, basophils), RBCs, and platelets. The typical patient is an older adult who is aged 60 years or older.

556. **D) Tetanus vaccine and systemic antibiotics**   A break in the skin with a compound fracture is an indication for a tetanus vaccine (if last dose was more than 5 years ago) and systemic antibiotics.

557. **C) Continue ipratropium bromide (Atrovent) and add albuterol (Ventolin) inhaler 2 inhalations QID**   Continue the Atrovent and add an albuterol (Ventolin)

inhaler. Treatment of COPD starts with an anticholinergic (ipratropium bromide). The next step is to add a short-acting beta-2 agonist (albuterol).

558. **C) Inform the coworker that you cannot release any information about this patient because she is not directly involved in the patient's care** HIPAA regulations require that information not be released to anyone not directly involved in patient care unless the patient has given specific permission for release to that person.

559. **A) IgE-mediated reaction** Anaphylaxis is an IgE-mediated reaction (also known as IgE-mediated type 2). IgE immediate reactions such as anaphylaxis trigger mast cell degranulation and release of potent mediators such as histamines, leukotrienes, and prostaglandins, which immediately induce constriction of smooth muscle, swelling, vasodilation, and other pathologic changes in the body that may be fatal.

560. **C) Polymyalgia rheumatica (PMR)** PMR is associated with a high risk of giant cell arteritis (GCA) or temporal arteritis (15%–30%). The new onset of vision loss and the location of the pain (neck, both shoulders/hips) are the most important clues. PMR is a rheumatic condition that involves joints and the arteries. Temporal arteritis can cause permanent blindness. The sedimentation rate is very high (40 mm/hr to 100 mm/hr). Almost all will have elevated C-reactive protein levels (up to 99%). These patients are managed by rheumatologists via long-term steroids.

561. **B) Protecting the rights of the human subjects who participate in research done at their institution** Each research institution has an institutional review board (IRB) whose job is to review all the research that is conducted in that institution. Their most important role is to protect the rights of the human subjects who participate in research that is done at their institution (e.g., research hospitals, universities).

562. **B) Ovulation disorders** Ovulation disorders are the top cause of female infertility (25%). There is no ovulation (anovulation) or infrequent ovulation that results in oligomenorrhea (PCOS). The second cause is endometriosis (15%). About 10% of women in the United States (ages 15 to 44 years) have difficulty getting pregnant (CDC, 2009). PCOS is one of the most common causes of female infertility. Infertility in males is often caused by a varicocele (heats up the testes) and abnormal and/or low sperm count.

563. **B) Meniere's disease** The classic triad of symptoms of Meniere's disease are vertigo, tinnitus, and hearing loss. The condition can resolve spontaneously or may be chronic. BPV has similar symptoms except that it does not cause hearing loss. Vertigo is due to the dysfunction of the labyrinthine system. Differential diagnoses are many (Meneire's, acute labyrinthitis, acoustic neuroma, etc.). Vasovagal syncope does not cause hearing loss or tinnitus, nor is it episodic.

564. **C) Increase in lung compliance** There is a decrease in lung compliance as we get older, therefore the FEV1 also decreases. There is minimal change in the total

lung volume. Airways tend to collapse earlier (than in young patients) with shallow breathing, which increases the risk of pneumonia.

565. **A) Addison's disease** Addison's disease is also known as primary adrenal insufficiency. The most common cause of damage to the adrenal cortex (the outer layer of the gland) is autoimmune destruction. The adrenal cortex produces glucocorticoids (cortisol) and mineralocorticoids (aldosterone). Aldosterone regulates sodium retention and potassium excretion through the kidneys (affects blood pressure). Electrolyte abnormalities are high potassium and low sodium. In primary disease (Addison's), serum cortisol is low, ACTH is high, and serum aldosterone is low. If the patient is not treated, severe stress (illness, accident) may cause an adrenal crisis ("Addisonian" crisis), which can be fatal.

566. **D) The patient has a TBSA of 18% with full-thickness burns of the left arm and left hand, and superficial burns on the anterior chest** The TBSA is calculated according to the Rule of Nines; the depth of the burns is determined from the clinical presentation details.

567. **C) The health insurance companies, health plans, Medicare and Medicaid** Third-party payers are the entities that actually pay the bills: health insurance companies, health plans (HMO or PPO), Medicare and Medicaid. The first party is the patient. The second party is the health care provider.

568. **D) Celiac disease** Celiac disease is also known as celiac sprue. Patients should avoid foods containing gluten, which causes malabsorption (diarrhea, gas, bloating, abdominal pain, etc.). Foods to avoid are wheat, rye, and barley. Oats do not damage mucosa in celiac disease. Antigliadin IgA and IgG are elevated in almost all patients (90%).

569. **B) Zolpidem (Ambien)** Ambien has a quick onset of action (15 minutes) and a short half-life of 2 hours. Avoid diphenhydramine in the elderly because in this population there is higher incidence of adverse effects (confusion, prolonged sedation). Avoid long-acting benzodiazepines such as diazepam (half-life 12 hours) and temazepam (half-life of 10 hours). Hypnotics can be used PRN up to 2 weeks; benzodiazepines can cause addiction and withdrawal symptoms.

570. **C) Multiply the treatment PSA value by two** Before starting a prescription of Proscar, obtain the baseline PSA. Recheck the PSA again within 2 to 3 months during treatment to assess the patient's response (treatment PSA). For this example, the corrected treatment PSA is 20 (multiply 10 x 2 = 20). When comparing the corrected treatment PSA (20) with the baseline PSA (30), the value is lower (means the prostate shrunk in size). The patient's symptoms will also improve, including less nocturia, less dribbling, and stronger urinary stream.

571. **D) Nurse practitioners have the ethical duty to provide quality health care to patients** Currently, health care givers are not legally required to report illegal aliens to the state or local authorities. This patient does not have the signs and symptoms of active TB disease (cough, weight loss, night sweats) and has a negative chest x-ray. Therefore, he has latent TB infection and is not contagious. Only

active TB disease (has signs/symptoms) is required to be reported to the state public health department.

572. **C) The areas of the body where skin rubs together, such as under the breast or in the groin area** Candidal intertrigo infections are more common in the obese and in women with pendulous breasts. It is found in areas where skin rubs against skin (under breasts, groin area, and on stomach folds in the obese). It is more common in warm and humid weather (summer).

573. **D) Perform 10 exercises each time three times a day** Weak pelvic floor muscles increase the risk of urinary and fecal incontinence. Educate a female patient that the pelvic floor muscles are the ones that she uses when she consciously holds/ stops the flow of urine when she urinates. Warn her that the anal sphincter will also tighten with the vaginal muscles. Advise the patient to relax the abdomen and the thighs when doing the exercises. Kegel exercises are also recommended as conservative treatment for patients (male and female) with fecal incontinence.

574. **C) The ovaries are sensitive to deep palpation but they should not be painful** The ovaries are usually slightly sensitive to deep palpation, but they should not be painful. Unilateral adnexal pain accompanied by cervical motion tenderness and purulent endocervical discharge is suggestive of PID.

575. **D) Surgical procedures are regarded as important treatment for many illnesses** The Vietnamese regard surgery as the last resort and regard loss of blood as depleting the vital forces of the body and causing illness. Western medicine is considered as "hot" and patients may discontinue or reduce the doses of their medicine without asking. An imbalance of the hot and cold (yin/yang) causes illness. Treating a "yin" disease (common cold) means avoiding eating yin foods (melons, cucumbers) because they will worsen it. Instead, yin diseases are treated with yang foods (meat, spicy foods) so that the body becomes more balanced. If the patient is very ill or dying, immediate family and extended family members will visit the patient daily in "shifts" to provide emotional support. Babies and small children may wear an amulet such as a red string on the wrist or a piece of cloth that ties on the neck or the wrist.

576. **D) Tdap** The CDC recommends that one of the tetanus boosters be replaced with the Tdap (once in a lifetime). Thereafter, the Td form of the vaccine is indicated every 10 years. The DTaP (diphtheria-tetanus-acellular pertussis) and DT (diphtheria-tetanus) forms of the tetanus vaccine are not given after the age of 7 years. Puncture wounds are at higher risk for tetanus because *Clostridium tetani* bacteria are anaerobes (deep puncture wounds are not exposed to air compared with superficial wounds).

577. **D) Tinea versicolor** Acanthosis nigricans is a skin condition that is benign. It appears as hyperpigmented velvety areas of skin that are usually located on the neck and the axiallae. It is a sign of insulin resistance. It is rarely associated with some types of adenocarcinoma of the gastrointestinal tract. Tinea versicolor is a superficial infection of the skin (stratum corneum layer) that is caused by dermatophytes (fungi) of the tinea family. Another name for it is "sunspots."

578. **C) Antinuclear antibody (ANA)** The ANA is usually positive in lupus patients. Other types of autoantibody testing recommended for these patients in addition to antinuclear antibody (ANA) tests are antiphospholipid antibodies, antibodies to double-stranded DNA, and anti-Smith (Sm) antibodies. Patient with suspect lupus should be referred to a rheumatologist. The sedimentation rate and the C-reactive protein are nonspecific findings of inflammation and are present in autoimmune diseases, infections, and others.

579. **A) Educate the patient about hypertension, how the medicine works on his body, and the importance of taking his pill daily** When Hmong (Thailand, Burma, Vietnamese) see a medical doctor for a symptom, they expect to be treated and "cured" of their illness. When the symptoms disappear, many will stop taking the medicine. When medication is to be taken on a long-term basis, it is important to educate the patient (and the daughter/son) about the disease (in this case, hypertension), how the medicine works on the body, and the reason why he/she has to take his medicine daily. Vietnamese are very polite and consider speaking in a loud voice, staring, or confrontation to be rude behavior.

580. **B) Oral prednisone** Patients with PMR are treated with oral steroids (glucocorticoids). One of the hallmarks of the disorder is the dramatic improvement of symptoms after starting treatment with oral prednisone. Usually, the symptoms can be controlled with long-term (2–3 years) low-dose oral prednisone, which can be tapered when symptoms are under control. For most patients, PMR is a self-limited illness (from a few months to 3 years).

581. **D) After a drug is taken by the oral route, it is absorbed in the small intestine and enters the liver through the portal circulation, where it is metabolized before being released into the general circulation** First-pass metabolism (first-pass effect) determines how much of the active drug is available to the body (bioavailability). Depending on drug and other factors, a drug may be poorly metabolized or extensively metabolized by the liver.

582. **C) Peripheral arterial disease (PAD)** The ankle–brachial index (ABI) is a test that is used to stratify the severity of arterial blockage in the lower extremities for patients with peripheral arterial disease (PAD). An ABI score of 1.0 to 1.4 is normal. Any value less than 1.0 is abnormal. A score of 0.5 or less is indicative of severe PAD.

583. **D) Oral prednisone (Medrol Dose Pack)** Symptomatic treatments for viral URI are saline nasal sprays (Ocean spray), decongestants (pseudoephedrine), NSAIDs (Advil), increasing fluids, and alternative herbal remedies (echinachea, astralagus, elderberry syrup, high doses of Vitamin C).

584. **A) Rice cereal** Patients can eat any food except those that contain the protein gluten. Foods containing wheat, barley, and rye should be avoided.

585. **A) Minor surgery in a walk-in surgical center** Medicare Part A will pay for medically necessary inpatient care and supplies. Therefore, any type of surgery that is done in outpatient settings, such as a walk-in surgical center, will not be

reimbursed. If plastic surgery is medically necessary (e.g., plastic surgery to repair facial damage from a burn), then it will be reimbursed. Costs for organ transplantation such as kidney transplants are reimbursed.

586. **D) Clean the wound with soap and water and prescribe Augmentin 500 mg PO BID x 10 days**   Cat wounds are more likely to become infected compared with dog bites, plus the bite is located on an extremity.

587. **A) Small smooth testicles with no pubic or facial hair**   Small, smooth testicles with no pubic or facial hair (Tanner Stage I) is a worrisome finding at the age of 15 years since it signifies that the boy is not in the pubertal stage yet. The average age of onset of puberty among boys is 12 years (range 10 to 14 years). The maximum growth spurt in boys occurs about 2 years after the onset of puberty. Boys start about 1 year later than girls and continue to grow until their early 20s (college).

588. **A) The symbol called "n ="**   The correct symbol to indicate a subpopulation of a sample is the small letter "n." For example, if a research study has a total population of 100 (N = 100), but it is divided into 2 equal groups, then each group has 50 subjects (n = 50 for each group).

589. **B) Meclizine (Antivert)**   The case is describing vertigo. Meclizine (Antivert) 12.5 mg to 50 mg TID to QID is used to treat vertigo. Do not forget to also treat nausea, which can be severe. Antinausea medicines like dimenhydrinate (Dramamine) or prochlorperazine (Compazine) are effective. Advise the patient that these drugs can cause drowsiness.

590. **C) It is a progesterone-only method of birth control and does not contain estrogen**   Seasonale is an extended-cycle form of birth control. It contains both levonorgestrel and ethinyl estradiol. There are 84 pink tablets (active) and 7 white pills (inert). In general, more spotting (breakthrough bleeding) is experienced with extended-cycle pills during the first few months of use (compared with the monthly birth control pills).

591. **C) Polymyalgia rheumatica (PMR)**   Giant cell arteritis (also known as temporal arteritis) is more common among patients with PMR. It can cause permanent blindness if it is not treated. PMR patients are taught how to recognize it. The quick onset of vision loss on one eye accompanied by a tender indurated artery and scalp tenderness on the same side are classic symptoms. The screening test is the sedimentation rate and C-reactive protein test. Both will be markedly elevated.

592. **B) Using limited societal financial resources on programs that will positively affect the largest number of people possible with the lowest possible negative outcomes**   Generally, the utilitarian principle refers to societal programs that will affect or benefit the largest number of people in a positive manner. It is not used to refer to an individual or to one person.

593. **D) Oral temperature of more than 101°F (more than 38°C)**   PID is a clinical diagnosis. The presence of at least one of the major criteria (cervical motion

tenderness, adnexal tenderness, uterine tenderness) when combined with the history is highly suggestive of PID. Minor criteria are not necessary, but they help to support the diagnosis of PID (oral temperature of more than 101°F [more than 38°C], mucopurulent cervical or vaginal discharge, elevated sedimentation rate, elevated C-reactive protein, large amount of WBC on saline microscopy of the vaginal fluid, or laboratory documentation of cervical infection with *N. gonorrhoeae* or *C. trachomatis*).

594. **D) Fovea of the macula**   The fovea is located in the center of the macula and is responsible for the sharpest vision ("20/20 vision") in the eyes. In the fovea, the only receptors are the cones, which allow us to see things in color and in detail. The macula is responsible for central vision.

595. **B) Consultation relationship**   A consultative relationship is an informal process between two or more providers who exchange information about a patient occasionally.

596. **B) Secondary prevention**   The nurse practitioner is evaluating the teenager for major depression. Since the teenager already has the disease (depression), this is a screening test. All screening tests/labs (mammography, Pap smears, etc.) are secondary prevention activities.

597. **C) Hypertension**   Drugs with strong anticholinergic properties include diphenhydramine, scopolamine, TCAs, antipsychotics, etc. The mnemonic is "dry as a bone, red as a beet, mad as a hatter, blind as a bat." Look for low-grade temperature.

598. **B) Diastolic murmur**   Diastolic murmurs are more likely to be pathologic. The heart is displaced in a more transverse position that is lateral to the midclavicular line. The systolic ejection murmur is due to increased stroke volume caused by increased cardiac output and higher basal heart rate.

599. **A) Abdominal aortic aneurysm**   Elderly males who are ex-smokers are at higher risk for abdominal aortic aneurysm. It is usually asymptomatic and is discovered incidentally during a routine chest x-ray or abdominal ultrasound. Although small aneurysms are usually not detectable during abdominal exams, the larger aneurysms may be palpable during an abdominal exam, but abdominal obesity will obscure the findings. The symptoms point toward a rapidly dissecting aneurysm. The best action in this case is to call 911 stat.

600. **D) A filled-in circle**   A filled-in circle is a diseased/affected female and an empty circle is a healthy female. A tip to remember is that females make eggs (or follicles), which resemble a circle. By default, the square symbol is the male.

601. **B) Magnetic resonance imaging (MRI) scan**   MRIs provides good visualization of soft tissues of the body (most cancers, brain, cartilage, muscles, inflammation, etc.). It is best used in tissues with high water content. Patients with metal implants such as cochlear implants and cardiac pacemakers should be carefully screened. The MRI does not use radiation, but uses strong magnetic and radio waves to visualize body structures.

602. **C) A bluish discoloration or bruising that is located on the umbilical area**   Cullen's sign is the acute onset of bluish discoloration that is located on the umbilical/periumbilical area that is caused by bruising underneath the skin. The bluish discoloration that is located on the flank area is called the Grey-Turner sign. It is a sign of a severe case of pancreatitis.

603. **B) Osteoarthritis**   Glucosamine sulfate has been found to have a beneficial effect on cartilage growth and repair. It may also have an anti-inflammatory effect. Many patients with osteoarthritis who take it claim that it helps to relieve joint pain. It can take from 1 to 3 months of taking the medicine to feel its effects. Glucosamine is a compound made up of glucose and an amino acid.

604. **A) Primary prevention**   A community youth center with good staffing can be an effective method of drawing the children out of the streets into a safer environment. It can reduce the risk of children falling victim to gang violence. In addition, staff members can serve as role models or mentors for the older children.

605. **B) Tuberculosis**   The BCG vaccine is given routinely in some countries where tuberculosis is endemic (or epidemic). One of the few exceptions for the BCG vaccine in the United States is for health care workers who see a high percentage of patients who are infected with *M. tuberculosis* strains resistant to both isoniazid and rifampin. BCG is considered a biohazardous material (U.S. Black Box Warning) and proper handling and disposal must be followed.

606. **C) Advise the mother that you suspect that her daughter has been sexually abused and that you are legally required to report the case to the child protection program**   The NP is legally required to report the case to the child protection program. If the child is in danger, child protective services may ask for a court order to take the child away for protection until the investigation is completed. Talking about the boyfriend's behavior will not be effective and may put the child and/or mother in danger if the boyfriend suspects that he is being watched.

607. **B) Instruct the patient to lift her head off the table while tensing her abdominal muscles to visualize any masses and then palpate the abdominal wall**   An abdominal wall mass will become more prominent when the abdominal wall muscles are tense. If it is an intra-abdominal mass, it will be pressed down by the muscles and will become less obvious or disappear. Some of the most common abdominal wall masses are hernias (epigastric, umbilical, incisional). This patient had a periumbilical hernia (soft, painless lump on her abdomen that is located on the periumbilical area).

608. **C) Cones**   Rods and cones are photoreceptor cells of the retina. The cones of the eyes are responsible for color vision. Cones are very sensitive to colors (red, blue, or green) and work better in brighter light. Rods are good for night vision and for vision in low-light conditions because they are sensitive to light and dark. To remember them, note that both cone and color start with the letter "C."

609. **B) B12-deficiency anemia**   Intrinsic factor is made by the parietal cells, which are located on the fundus of the stomach. Intrinsic factor is needed to effectively

absorb vitamin B12 (dairy, meat). Since the gastric fundus is damaged in these patients, they are at higher risk of B12-deficiency anemia (MCV greater than 100).

610. **A) Basal cell skin cancer** Skin cancer is the most common type of cancer over-all, but the most common type of skin cancer is basal cell carcinoma of the skin. Regarding mortality, the skin cancer that causes the most deaths (from skin can-cer) is melanomas (65% of skin cancer deaths).

611. **B) It is the middle number in a group of numbers** The median is the middle score of a group of numbers. For example, for this group of numbers (2, 3, 6, **7**, 7, 8, 10), the number "7" is the median value.

612. **A) Acute pancreatitis** Grey–Turner's sign is the acute onset of bluish discolor-ation that is located on the flank area and is caused by bruising. It is usually asso-ciated with severe acute pancreatitis, but it can also be found in some cases of ruptured ectopic pregnancy.

613. **B) Collaborative relationship** A collaborative relationship is a formal process of sharing responsibility for treating a patient together (sharing progress report); for example, referring a patient to a specialist or for rehabilitation.

614. **A) *Pseudomonas aeroginosa*** The most common bacteria is *Pseudomonas*. The second most common bacteria is *Staphylococcus aurea*s. Polymyxin and neomycin combination ear drops (Cortisporin) are the first-line treatment for otitis externa. Other ear drops that are also effective are the quinolone ear drops (ofloxacin, cip-rofloxacin topical drops).

615. **B) The health plan will start to be effective in the year 2013** President Obama's national health insurance plan is known the "Patient Protection and Affordable Care Act." It covers preexisting health conditions immediately and prohibits an insurance company from rejecting people with preexisting health conditions. There is a penalty for employers (and individuals) who choose not to participate in the national health plan.

616. **C) Grooming and hygiene** Grooming and hygiene are classified as basic activi-ties of daily living (ADLs). Grocery shopping, paying bills, using telephones, or driving a car are all IADLs.

617. **C) CN VIII** The Rinne and Weber tests are used to assess cranial nerve 8 or the acoustic nerve. The patient's hearing is tested by air conduction (Rinne and Weber) and bone conduction (Rinne only).

618. **D) Stress incontinence** The signs and symptoms of stress incontinence occur when the stress caused by sneezing, laughing, and/or straining results in the leak-ing of a small amount of urine through a weakened sphincter.

619. **B) Prescription drugs** Medicare Part D is a voluntary program that charges a premium. Like all Medicare services, patients need to enroll during the "open enrollment" periods during the year (there is a penalty for late enrollment). There

is a drug formulary and not all drugs are available or reimbursed. Use of generic drugs is preferred since there is a spending limit. Medicare Part B will reimburse for alcohol misuse/abuse treatment.

620. **A) Check the thyroid profile** The upper limit of the serum TSH level is about 5.0 mU/L (range of 0.5 to 5.0). With an elevated TSH of 10, it is important to rule out hypothyroidism. The next step in this patient's evaluation is to order a thyroid profile test. Serum assays measure bound and unbound (free) forms of thyroxine (T4) and triiodothyronine (T3). Classic findings of hypothyroidism are a low total T4, low T3-resin uptake (THBI), and low free T4 index.

621. **C) Abdominal ultrasound** The ultrasound or sonogram is used as an initial imaging test for abdominal tumors. A CT scan can be ordered at a later time, but it is not considered an initial imaging test in the primary care area.

622. **C) Information that a research subject can voluntarily withdraw from the study at any time without any penalties or adverse consequences** It should be written on the consent forms that the research subject can voluntarily withdraw from the study at any time without any penalties or adverse consequences. In addition, the human subject should be verbally informed of this right.

623. **C) Estrogen and progesterone deficiency** Bone loss is not associated with progesterone deficiency (only estrogen deficiency). Risk factors include excessive alcohol intake, cigarette smoking, ancestry (Asian or Caucasian), older age, anorexia nervosa, small bone frame, etc.

624. **D) Provision of custodial care** Custodial care is done by nursing homes. Skilled nursing facilities (SNFs) are reimbursed by Medicare and can provide skilled nursing and medical care. If a patient is discharged from a hospital, but needs therapy and skilled care, he or she is usually transferred to an SNF. SNFs have transfer agreements with local hospitals. Nursing home patients are usually medically stable and need skilled or medical care. These patients are unable to perform from two to six ADLs. Patients with Alzheimer's and other types of dementia are usually cared for in nursing homes.

625. **D) Grocery shopping** Grocery shopping, housework, and managing one's finances are considered instrumental ADLs (IADLs).

626. **B) Acute appendicitis** Both the psoas and obturator signs are associated with acute appendicitis. When the appendix becomes inflamed or ruptured, the blood and pus irritate the psoas and/or obturator muscles, which are both located in the retroperitoneal area. Both muscles are hip flexors and assist with hip movement.

627. **C) Frail elderly are not interested in sexuality anymore** Some studies have shown that older adults in their 80s can remain sexually active. By the age of 70 years, about 80% of males have ED.

628. A) SSRIs   A common side effect of SSRIs (Prozac, Paxil, Zoloft, etc.) is sexual dysfunction in males. For depressed males, atypical antidepressants such as bupropion (Wellbutrin) cause less sexual dysfunction.

629. C) Finasteride (Proscar)   Finasteride (Proscar) belongs to the drug class called 5-alpha reductase inhibitors. It helps to lower serum testosterone, which helps to decrease the size of the prostate. It is also used for male-pattern baldness. A smaller prostate results in less obstructive voiding symptoms such as weak stream, frequency, and nocturia. Both terazosin (Hytrin) and tamsulosin (Flomax) are alpha-blockers and may start to control symptoms in as little as 3 days. They work by relaxing the smooth muscle tissue of the prostate gland, which enlarges the diameter of the urethra.

References

Administration on Aging (AOA). www.aoa.gov

Agency for Healthcare Research and Quality (AHRQ). U.S. Department of Health and Human Services. www.ahrq.gove

Aging and Cancer. Cancer.net. http://www.cancer.net/coping

American Academy of Family Physicians (AAFP). *Immunization schedules/preventive care recommendations.* http://www.aafp.org/online/en/home/clinical/immunizationres.html

American Academy of Nurse Practitioners (AANP). www.aanp.org

American Academy of Nurse Practitioners National Certification Program. www.aanpcertification.org

American Academy of Pediatrics (AAP). http://www.cispimmunize.org/

American Academy of Pediatrics (AAP). (2004). Management of hyperbilirubinemia in the newborn infant 35 or more weeks of gestations. *Pediatrics, 114*, 297-316.

American Academy of Pediatrics (AAP). www.aap.org

American Association of Colleges of Nursing. (2010, March). *Adult-gerontology primary care nurse practitioner competencies.* Developed in collaboration with the Hartford Institute for Geriatric Nursing at New York University and the National Organization of Nurse Practitioner Faculties. Washington, DC: Author.

American Association of Retired Persons. (AARP). *The 1987 nursing home reform act.* www.aarp.org

American Cancer Society. (2012). *Cancer facts and figures 2012.* Atlanta, GA: Author.

American Cancer Society. www.cancer.org

American College of Obstetricians and Gynecologists. (ACOG). http://www.acog.org

American Diabetes Association. (2012). *Clinical practice recommendations.* http://care.diabetesjournals.org/content/35/Supplement_1/S4.full.pdf+html

American Diabetes Association. (2012). Standards of medical care in diabetes. *Diabetes Care, 35* (Suppl. 1), S11-S63. doi:10.2337/dc12-s011

American Heart Association. http://www.heart.org

American Nurses Association. (ANA). www.nursingworld.org

American Nurses Association. (ANA). *Scope and standards of practice.* http://www.nursingworld.org/scopeandstandardsofpractice

American Nurses Credentialing Center. (ANCC). http://www.nursescredentialing.org/

American Pregnancy Association. *Promoting pregnancy wellness.* www.americanpregnancy.org

American Thoracic Society. http://www.thoracic.org/go/copd

Anaphylaxis Treatment Guideline. *The diagnosis and management of anaphylaxis: An updated practiced parameter.* http://www.guideline.gov/content.aspx?id=6887

Aronson, M. D., Fletcher, R. H., & Fletcher, S. W. (Eds.). (2012). *The Sanford guide to antimicrobial therapy* (40th ed.). UpToDate. Retrieved from http://www.uptodate.com/online/

ATP IV. *CVD risk assessment and dyslipidemia: Update 2012.*

Behrman, R. E., & Kliegman, R. M. (1998). *Nelson essentials of pediatrics* (3rd ed.). Philadelphia: W. B. Saunders.

Boynton, R. W., Dunn, E. S., Pulcini, J., St. Pierre, S., & Stephens, G. R. (2009). *Manual of ambulatory pediatrics* (6th ed.). Philadelphia: Lippincott Williams & Wilkins.

Bull, M. J., & Committee on Genetics. Health supervision for children with Down syndrome. *Pediatrics* [online article]. Accessed November 2012 at American Association for Pediatric Ophthalmology and Strabismus, www.aapos.org

Centers for Disease Control and Prevention. (CDC). *Birth defects: Diagnosis.* http://www.cdc.gov/ncbddd/birthdefects/diagnosis.html

Centers for Disease Control and Prevention. (CDC). *Breastfeeding recommendations.* http://www.cdc.gov/breastfeeding/recommendations/index.htm

Centers for Disease Control and Prevention. (CDC). http://www.cdc.gov/vaccines

Centers for Disease Control and Prevention. (CDC). *Management of occupational exposure to HIV and recommendations for postexposure prophylaxis.* http://www.cdc.gov/mmwr/

Centers for Disease Control and Prevention. (CDC). (2010). *Sexually transmitted disease treatment guidelines.* Atlanta, GA: Author.

Centers for Disease Control and Prevention (CDC). *Smoking and tobacco use.* www.cdc.gov

Complementary and alternative medicine. *MedlinePLUS.* http://www.nlm.nih.gov/medlineplus/complementaryandalternativemedicine.html

Domino, F. J., Baldor, R. A., Golding, J., Grimes, J. A., & Taylor, J. S. (Eds.). (2011). *The 5-minute clinical consult 2012.* Philadelphia: Lippincott Williams & Wilkins.

Drug-Nutrient Interaction Task Force, Warren Grant Magnuson Clinical Center, National Institutes of Health. Important information to know when you are taking: Coumadin and vitamin K. *Important drug and food information.* http://ods.od.nih.gov/pubs/factsheets/coumadin1.pdf

Enzenauer, R. W. (Roy Hampton, Sr., Ed.). Neonatal conjunctivitis. *Medscape Reference.* http://emedicine.medscape.com/article/1192190-overview

Family Practice Notebook. www.fpnotebook.com

Fay, V., Tardiff, K., Henderson, M. J., & Jansen, M. (2010). *Gerontological nurse practitioner review and resource manual.* Washington, DC: Institute for Research, Education and Consultation at The American Nurses Credentialing Center.

Ferguson, C. M. *Inspection, auscultation, palpation, and percussion of the abdomen,* ch. 93. http://www.ncbi.nlm.nih.gov/books/NBK420/

Ferri, F. (2011). *Ferri's clinical advisor.* Philadelphia: Elsevier Mosby.

Fletcher, S. W., & Elmore, J. G. (2003). Mammographic screening for breast cancer. *New England Journal of Medicine, 348*, 1672.

Gilbert, D. N., Meollering, R. C., & Eliopoulos, G. M. (Eds.). (2012). *The Sanford guide to antimicrobial therapy.* Sperryville, VA: Antimicrobial Therapy, Inc.

Hay, W. W., Jr., Hayward, A. R., Levin, M. J., & Sondheimer, J. M. (Eds.). (2001). *Current pediatric diagnosis & treatment* (15th ed.). New York: Lange Medical Books/McGraw-Hill.

Healthychildren.org. www.healthychildren.org

Joint National Committee on Prevention, Detection, Evaluation, and Treatment of High Blood Pressure. (JNC). *Seventh report.* Washington, DC: National Heart, Lung, and Blood Institute.

Joint National Committee on Prevention, Detection, Evaluation, and Treatment of High Blood Pressure. (JNC). *Seventh report—Express.* http://www.nhlbi.nih.gov/guidelines/index.htm

Joint Task Force on Practice Parameters; American Academy of Allergy, Asthma and Immunology; American College of Allergy, Asthma and Immunology; & Joint Council of Allergy, Asthma and Immunology. (2005, March). The diagnosis and management of anaphylaxis: An updated practice parameter. *Journal of Allergy and Clinical Immunology, 115* (Suppl. 3), S483-S523. http://www.aaaai.org/conditions-and-treatments/allergies/anaphylaxis.aspx

LeBlond, R. F., Brown, D. D., & DeGowin, R. L. (2008). *DeGowin's diagnostic examination* (9th ed.). [Paperback]. McGraw-Hill Professional.

Lenshin, L. *Down syndrome: Health issues.* http://www.ds-health.com/

Managing asthma long term in youth ≥ 12 years of age and adults. (2007). In National Asthma Education and Prevention Program (NAEPP), *Expert panel report 3: Guidelines for the diagnosis and management of asthma* (pp. 326-362). Bethesda, MD: National Heart, Lung, and Blood Institute.

McPhee, S. J., Papadakis, M. A., & Rabow, M. W. (Eds.). (2012). *Current medical diagnosis & treatment* (51st ed.). New York: Lange Medical Books/McGraw-Hill.

Medicaid.gov. www.medicaid.gov

Medicare.gov. The official U.S. government site for Medicare. www.medicare.gov

MedlinePLUS. http://www.nlm.nih.gov/medlineplus

MedlinePlus. Trusted health information for you. http://vsearch.nlm.nih.gov/

Morbidity and Mortality Weekly Report. http://www.cdc.gov/mmwr

Morris, P. B. http://www.acli.com/Events/Documents/Tue22812%20-%20Lipidology%20-%20Pamel%20Morris.pdf

National Aphasia Association. www.aphasia.org

National Cholesterol Education Panel. (2002). *Third report of the expert panel on detection, evaluation, and treatment of high cholesterol in adults (Adult Treatment Panel III).* Washington, DC: National Heart, Lung, and Blood Institute.

National Guidelines Clearinghouse. *Infectious Diseases Society of America and American Thoracic Society consensus guidelines on the management of community-acquired pneumonia in adults.* http://www.journals.uchicago.edu/doi/pdf/10.1086/511159

National Heart, Lung, and Blood Institute (NHLBI), National Institutes of Health. http://www.nhlbi.nih.gov/health/public/lung/copd

National Heart, Lung, and Blood Institute (NHLBI), National Institutes of Health. *National asthma education and prevention program expert panel report 3: Guidelines for the diagnosis and management of asthma.* http://www.nhlbi.nih.gov/guidelines/index.htm

National Heart, Lung, and Blood Institute (NHLBI), National Institutes of Health. *Third report of the expert panel on detection, evaluation, and treatment of high blood cholesterol in adults (Adult treatment panel III): Full report.* http://www.nhlbi.nih.gov/guidelines/cholesterol/index.htm

National Institutes of Health. *Bioethics resources on the web.* Retrieved from http://bioethics.od.nih.gov

National Institutes of Health. http://health.nih.gov/topic/ImmunizationVaccination

National Reye's Syndrome Foundation. http://www.reyessyndrome.org/

Ledford, H. (2013). Cholesterol limits lose their luster. *Nature, 494,* 410-411. doi:10.1038/494410a

NCPAD. *Disability/condition: Down syndrome and exercise.* http://www.ncpad.org/disability/fact_sheet.php?sheet=139&view=all

Nicoll, D., McPhee, S. J., & Pignone, M. (2004). *Pocket guide to diagnostic tests* (4th ed.). [Paperback]. New York: McGraw-Hill Medical.

Prescriber's Letter. https://prescribersletter.therapeuticresearch.com/home.aspx

Prescriber's Letter online. https://prescribersletter.therapeuticresearch.com/

Prescribing References, Inc. (2011-2012, Winter). *Nurse practitioners' prescribing reference (NPPR).* New York: Haymarket Media.

PubMed Central. CFP*MFC. http://www.ncbi.nlm.nih.gov/pmc/articles/PMC1783707/

PubMed Central. http://www.ncbi.nlm.nih.gov

Rice, S. G. (2008). Medical conditions affecting sports participation. *Pediatrics, 121*(4), 841-848. http://www.ncbi.nlm.nih.gov/pubmed?term=18381550

Schwartz, M. W. (Ed.), Bell, L. M., Jr., Bingham, P. M., Loomes, K. M., et al. (Assoc. Eds.). 2008). *5-minute pediatric consult* (6th ed.). Philadelphia: Lippincott Williams & Wilkins.

Stiles, S. *JNC 8, ATP 4 guidelines (still) soon to be released.* Retrieved from www.theheart.org

Stone, C. K., & Humphries, R. (2005). *Current essentials of emergency medicine (LANGE Essentials).* New York: Lange Medical Books/McGraw-Hill.

The March of Dimes. http://www.marchofdimes.com

The Merck Manuals Online Medical Library. *The Merck manual for health care professionals.* Retrieved from http://www.merckmanuals.com/professional/

The Joint Commission. http://www.jointcommission.org

Touhy, T. A., & Jett, K. F. (2009). *Ebersole and Hess' gerontological nursing & healthy aging* (3rd ed.). St. Louis, MO: Mosby.

UpToDate.com. http://www.uptodate.com/online/

U.S. Department of Health and Human Services. Health information privacy. www.hhs.gov

U.S. Department of Health and Human Services. http://www.womenshealth.gov

U.S. Department of Health and Human Services. *OCR privacy brief: Summary of the HIPAA privacy rule.* Washington, DC: U.S. Department of Health and Human Services, Office for Civil Rights.

U.S. Department of Health and Human Services. Office of Civil Rights. www.hhs.gov

U.S. Drug Enforcement Administration (DEA). www.justice.gov/dea

U.S. Food and Drug Administration. www.fda.gov

WebMD. www.webmd.com

Willms, J. L. (1996). *Pocket guide to physical diagnosis.* Philadelphia: Lippincott Williams & Wilkins.

Abbreviations

AAA	abdominal aortic aneurysm
AACN	American Association of Colleges of Nursing
AAHSA	American Association of Homes and Services for the Aging
AAI	atlantoaxial instability
AANPCP	American Academy of Nurse Practitioners Certificate Program
ABCs	airway–breathing–circulation
ABI	ankle–brachial index
AC	air conduction
ACA	Affordable Care Act of 2010
ACD	anemia of chronic disease
ACE	angiotensin-converting enzyme
ACEI	angiotensin-converting enzyme inhibitor
ACL	anterior cruciate ligament
ACNP	acute care nurse practitioner
ADD	attention deficit disorder
ADHD	attention deficit hyperactivity disorder
ADLs	activities of daily living
AF	atrial fibrillation
AFB	acid-fast bacillus
A–GNP	adult–gerontology nurse practitioner
AGPCNP	adult–gerontology primary care nurse practitioner
AGS	American Geriatrics Society
ALF	assisted-living facility
ALT	alanine aminotransferase
ALT	alanine transaminase
AMD	age-related macular degeneration
AMD	atrophic macular degeneration
ANA	American Nurses Association
ANA	antinuclear antibody/antinuclear antigen
ANC	absolute neutrophil count
ANCC	American Nurses Credentialing Center
ANP	adult nurse practitioner
Anti-HBc	antibody to hepatitis B core antigen
Anti-HBs	antibody to hepatitis B surface antigen
Anti-HCv	antibody to hepatitis C virus
Anti-TNF	antitumor necrosis factor
AoA	Administration on Aging
AOM	acute otitis media
AP	acute pancreatitis
A–P	anterior–posterior

APMHNP	adult psychiatric mental health nurse practitioner
APRN	advanced practice registered nurse
APS	Adult Protective Services
ARB	angiotensin receptor blocker/ angiotensin II converting blocker
AS	ankylosing spondylitis
ASA	acetylsalicylic acid
ASCUS	atypical squamous cells of undetermined significance
ASMP	arthritis self-management program
AST	alanine aminotransferase *or* aspartate aminotransferase
ATS	American Thoracic Society
AUC	area under the curve
AUDIT	alcohol use disorders identification
AV	arteriovenous *or* atrioventricular
AVD	atrioventricular node
AZT	azidothymidine
BC	bone conduction
BCC	basal cell carcinoma
BCV	Bacille–Calomette–Guerin
BDTC	black dot tiniacapitis
BG	blood glucose
BID	*bis in die* (twice a day)
BM	bowel movement
BMD	bone mineral density
BMI	body mass index
BMR	basal metabolic rate
BON	Board of Nursing
BP	blood pressure
BPH	benign prostatic hyperplasia
BPV	benign positional vertigo
BSE	breast self-examination
BTB	breakthrough bleeding
BUN	blood–urea–nitrogen
BV	bacterial vaginosis
CA	cancer
CABG	coronary artery bypass graft
CAD	coronary artery disease
CAM	complementary/alternative medicine
CAP	community-acquired pneumonia
CBC	complete blood count
CCB	calcium channel blocker
CCNE	Commission on Collegiate Nursing Education
CCRC	continuing-care retirement community
CDAD	*Clostridium difficile*-associated diarrhea
CDC	Centers for Disease Control and Prevention
CD4	helper T lymphocyte express cluster determinant 4
CE	continuing education
CF	cystic fibrosis
CFU	colony-forming units
CHADS2	congestive heart failure, hypertension, age, diabetes, stroke score
CHF	congestive heart failure
CK	creatinine kinase
CKD	chronic kidney disease
CMS	Centers for Medicare & Medicaid Services

CNS	central nervous system
CNS	clinical nurse specialist
CO	cardiac output
COBRA	Consolidated Omnibus Budget Reconciliation Act
COC	combined oral contraceptives
CON	certificate of need
COPD	chronic obstructive pulmonary disease
CPK	creatinine phosphokinase
CPPS	chronic pelvic pain syndrome
CPT	current procedural terminology
CRP	C-reactive protein
C&S	culture and sensitivity
CSF	cerebrospinal fluid
CT	computed tomography
cTnT	cardiac-specific isoforms of troponin
CTS	carpal tunnel syndrome
CVA	cerebrovascular accident
CVA	costovertebral angle
CXR	chest x-ray
DASH	dietary approaches to stop hypertension
D&C	dilation and currettage
DDS	doctor of dental surgery
DEA	Drug Enforcement Administration
DEET	N, N-diethyl-meta-toluamine
DES	diethylstilbestrol
DEXA	dual-energy x-ray absorptiometry
DFA-TP	direct fluorescent antibody testing
DGI	disseminated gonorrheal infection
DHEA	dehydroepiandrosterone
DHT	dihydrotestosterone
DIP	distal interphalangeal joints
DJD	degenerative joint disease
DM	diabetes mellitus
DMARDs	disease-modifying antirheumatic drugs
DMD	doctor of dental medicine
DME	durable medical equipment
DMPA	depot medroxyprogesterone acetate
DMV	department of motor vehicles
DO	doctor of osteopathy
DON	director of nursing
DOT	directly observed treatment
DRE	digital rectal examination
DS	Down's syndrome
DTaP	diphtheria–tetanus–acellular pertussis
DTR	deep tendon reflexes
DVT	deep vein thrombosis
DXA	dual x-ray absorptiometry
EBM	evidence-based medicine
EBV	Epstein–Barr virus
ECG/EKG	electrocardiogram
ED	emergency department *or* erectile dysfunction
EEG	electroencephalogram
EF	ejection fraction

eGFR	estimated glomerular filtration rate
ELISA	enzyme-linked immunosorbent assay
EOMs	extraocular muscles/extraorbital muscles
EPA	Environmental Protection Agency
EPO	erythropoietin
EPT	expedited partner treatment
ERT	estrogen-replacement therapy
ESR	erythrocyte sedimentation rate
ETOH	ethanol
FBG	fasting blood glucose
FDA	Food and Drug Administration
FEV1	forced expiratory volume in 1 second
fL	femtoliters
FNP	family nurse practitioner
FOBT	fecal occult blood test
FPMHNP	family psychiatric mental health nurse practitioner
FSH	follicle-stimulating hormone
FTA–ABS	fluorescent antibody–absorption antibody
FVC	forced vital capacity
GAD	generalized anxiety disorder
GCA	giant cell arteritis
GERD	gastroesophageal reflux disease
GFR	glomerular filtration rate
GGT	gamma-glutamyl transaminase *or* gamma-glutamyltranspeptidase
GH	growth hormone
GI	gastrointestinal
GITT	Geriatric Interdisciplinary Team Training
GLP-1	glucagonlike peptide 1
GNP	gerontologic nurse practitioner
GSE	genital self-examination
G6PD	glucose-6-phosphate dehydrogenase
gtts	drops/minute
GU	genitourinary
HA	headache
HAART	highly active antiretroviral therapy
HbeAg	hepatitis B "e" antigen
HbF	fetal hemoglobin
HBM	health belief model
HbS	sickle hemoglobin
HBsAG	hepatitis B surface antigen
hct	hematocrit
hCG	human chorionic gonadotropin
HCP	health care personnel
HCTZ	hydrochlorothiazide
HCV	RNA hepatitis C ribonucleic acid
HDL	high-density lipoprotein
HDTZ	hydrochlorothiazide
HEENT	head, ear, eye, nose, throat
HEPA	high-efficiency particulate air
HGH	human growth hormone
H&H	hemoglobin and hematocrit
HIPAA	Health Insurance Portability and Accountability Act
HMG-CoA	5-hydroxy-3-methylglutaryl-coenzyme A

HMO	health maintenance organization
HPA	hypothalamic–pituitary–adrenal
HPL	human pancreatic lipase
HRT	hormone-replacement therapy
HS	half strength
HSV	herpes simplex virus
HTN	hypertension
HUD	Department of Housing and Urban Development
Hz	hertz
HZ	herpes zoster
HZO	herpes zoster ophthalmicus
IADLs	instrumental activities of daily living
IBS	irritable bowel syndrome
IC	infective endocarditis
ICP	intracranial pressure
ICS	intercostal space
I&D	incision and drainage
IDA	iron-deficiency anemia
IDP	idiopathic thrombocytopenic purpura
IDSA	Infectious Disease Society of America
IDU	intravenous drug user
IF	intrinsic factor
IFG	impaired fasting glucose
IgE	immunoglobulin E
IgG	immunoglobulin G
IgGAnti-HAV	hepatitis A antibody IgG type
IgM	Anti-HAV hepatitis A antibody IgM type
IGRA	interferon-gamma release assays
IGT	impaired glucose tolerance
IM	intramuscular
INH	isoniazid
INH	isonicotinylhydrazine
INR	international normalized ratio
I&O	intake and output
IOP	intraocular pressure
IRB	institutional review board
ITP	idiopathic thrombocytopenia purpura
IU	international unit
IUD	intrauterine device
IV	intravascular *or* intravenous
IVP	intravenous pyelogram
JC	Joint Commission
JCAHO	Joint Commission on the Accreditation of Health Care Organizations
JVD	jugular venous distention
K/DOQI	Kidney Disease Outcomes Quality Initiative
KOH	potassium hydroxide
KUB	kidney, ureter, and bladder x-ray study
LABA	long-acting beta agonists
LAIV	live attenuated influenza virus
LCL	lateral collateral ligament
LDL	low-density lipoprotein
LFT	liver function test

LH	luteinizing hormone
LMP	last menstrual period
LOC	level of consciousness
LPN	licensed practical nurse
LTCF	long-term-care facility
LTRA	leukotriene receptor antagonist
LVH	left ventricular hypertrophy
MAOI	monoamine oxidase inhibitor
MCH	mean corpuscular hemoglobin
MCHC	mean corpuscular hemoglobin concentration
MCL	medial collateral ligament
MCV	mean cell volume/mean corpuscular volume
MCV4	meningococcal conjugate vaccine quadrivalent
MDI	metered-dose inhaler
MDMA	3, 4-methylenedioxy-N-methamphetamine
MDRD	modification of diet in renal disease
MDS	minimum data set
MDS–CHESS	Scale Minimum Data Set—Changes in Health, End-Stage Disease, Symptoms and Signs Scale
MEE	middle ear effusion
MHC	mean hemoglobin concentration
MI	myocardial infarction
MIC	minimum inhibitory concentration
MMA	methylmalonic acid
MMR	measles, mumps, rubella
MMSE	Mini-Mental State Examination
MODY	maturity-onset-diabetes of the young
MR	mitral regurgitation
MRSA	methicillin-resistant *Staphylococcus aureus*
MSM	men who have sex with men
MSW	master of social work
MVI	multivitamin
MVP	mitral valve prolapse
MVTR	moisture vapor transmission rate
NAAT	nucleic acid amplification tests
NAFLD	nonalcoholic fatty liver disease
NAMS	North American Menopause Society
NCOA	National Council on Aging
NG	nasogastric
NGU	nongonococcal urethritis
NL	normal limits
NLNAC	National League for Nurses Accrediting Commission
NONPF	National Organization of Nurse Practitioner Faculty
NPDR	nonproliferative diabetic retinopathy
NPH	neutral protamine Hagedorn
NRTIs	nucleoside reverse transcriptase inhibitors
NSAIDs	nonsteroidal anti-inflammatory drugs
NTD	neural tube defect
N/V	nausea/vomiting
NYHA	New York Heart Association
OA	osteoarthritis
OBRA	Omnibus Budget Reconciliation Act
OC	oral contraceptive

OCD	obsessive-compulsive disorder
OD	*oculus dexter* (right eye)
OGTT	oral glucose tolerance test
OHL	oral hairy leukoplakia
OS	*oculus sinister* (left eye)
OSHA	Occupational Safety and Health Administration
OT	occupational therapy
OTC	over-the-counter
OU	*oculus uterque* (both eyes)
PA	pernicious anemia
PA	physician assistant
PAT	paroxysmal atrial tachycardia
PCL	posterior cruciate ligament
PCOS	polycystic ovarian syndrome
PCP	phencyclidine
PCR	polymerase chain reaction
PE	pulmonary embolism
PEF	peak expiratory flow
PEFR	peak expiratory flow rate
PEP	postexposure prophylaxis
PFT	pulmonary function test
PHN	postherpetic neuralgia
PID	pelvic inflammatory disease
PIP	proximate interphalangeal joints
PMB	postmenopausal bleeding
PMR	polymyalgia rheumatic
PNP	pediatric nurse practitioner
PO	*per os* (by mouth)
PPD	purified protein derivative
PPI	proton pump inhibitor
PPO	preferred provider organization
PPSV	pneumococcal polysaccharide vaccine
PRN	*pro re nata* (as needed)
PSA	prostate-specific antigen
PSVT	paroxysmal supraventricular tachycardia
PT	physical therapy
PT	prothrombin time
PTH	parathyroid hormone
PTT	partial thromboplastin time
PUD	peptic ulcer disease
PVD	peripheral vascular disease
QID	*quarter in die* (four times a day)
RA	rheumatoid arthritis
RAI	resident assessment instrument
RAIV	radioactive iodine uptake
RCA	root cause analysis
RDW	red blood cell distribution width
RF	rheumatoid factor
RMSF	Rocky Mountain spotted fever
RNA	ribonucleic acid
ROM	range of motion
RPR	rapid plasma reagent
RUQ	right upper quadrant

RV	residual volume
SAH	subarachnoid hemorrhage
SC or SQ	subcutaneous
SCA	sickle cell anemia
SDH	subdural hematoma
SE	sentinel event
SERM	selective estrogen receptor modulator
SGOT	serum glutamic-oxaloacetic transaminase
SGPT	serumglutamic-pyruvic transaminase
SOB	shortness of breath
SoFAS	solid fats and added sugars
SLE	systemic lupus erythematosus
SMAST	Shortness Michigan Alcoholism Screening Test
SNF	skilled-nursing facility
SNRI	selective norepinephrine reuptake inhibitor
SOAPE	subjective, objective, assessment planning, and evaluation
SPF	sun protection factor
SQ or SC	subcutaneous
SSRI	selective serotonin reuptake inhibitor
STD	sexually transmitted disease
STI	sexually transmitted infection
SVTC	supraventricular tachycardia with aberrant conduction
TA	temporal arteritis
TB	tuberculosis
TBSA	total body surface area
TCA	tricyclic antidepressant
TCH	trichloroacetic acid
TCM	traditional Chinese medicine
TCO	test content outline
Td	tetanus–diphtheria
Tdap	tetanus–diphtheria–pertussis
TED	thromboembolitic deterrent
TIA	transient ischemic attack
TIBC	total iron binding capacity
TID	*ter in die* (three times a day)
TIG	tetanus immunoglobulin
TIV	trivalent inactivated vaccine
TLC	total lung capacity
TM	tympanic membrane
TMP/SMX	trimethoprim-sulfamethazole
TNF	tumor necrosis factor
TNM	tumor–nodes–metastasis
TnT	troponin
TSH	thyroid-stimulating hormone
TST	tuberculosis skin test
TTM	Transtheoretical Model
TZDs	thiazolidenediones
UA	urinalysis
URI	upper respiratory infection
USDHHS	U.S. Department of Health and Human Services
USPSTF	U.S. Preventive Services Task Force
UTI	urinary tract infection
UV	ultraviolet

VAERS   vaccine adverse event reporting system
VDRL   Venereal Disease Research Laboratory test
VT   ventricular tachycardia
VTE   venous thromboembolism
WBC   white blood bell
WHO   World Health Organization
WHR   waist-to-hip ratio
WIC   Special Supplemental Food Program for Women, Infants, and
Children
WNL   within normal limits
ZDV   zidovudine

Index

Note: Page numbers followed by "*f*" and "*t*" denote figures and tables, respectively.